MW01232869

The Genetics of Osteoporosis and Metabolic Bone Disease

The Genetics of Osteoporosis and Metabolic Bone Disease

Edited by

Michael J. Econs, MD

Indiana University School of Medicine, Indianapolis, IN

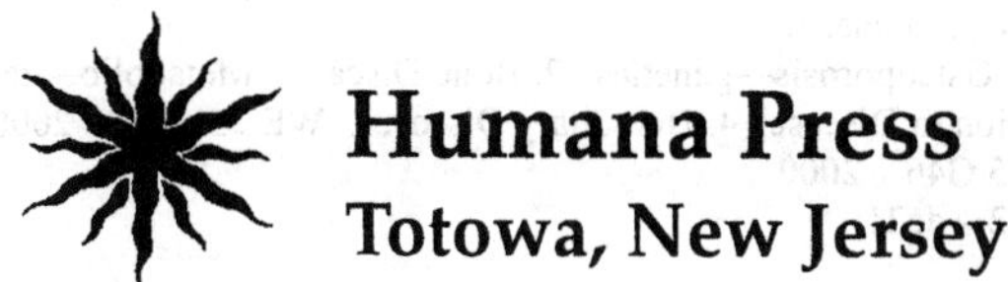

Humana Press

Totowa, New Jersey

999 Riverview Drive, Suite 208
Totowa, New Jersey 07512

This publication is printed on acid-free paper. ∞
ANSI Z39.48-1984 (American Standards Institute) Permanence of Paper for Printed Library Materials.

Cover designed by Patricia F. Cleary

For additional copies, pricing for bulk purchases, and/or information about other Humana titles, contact Humana at the above address or at any of the following numbers: Tel. 973-256-1699; Fax: 973-256-8341; E-mail: humana@humanapr.com or visit our website at http://www.humanapress.com

Printed in the United States of America. 10 9 8 7 6 5 4 3 2 1

Library of Congress Cataloging in Publication Data

Main entry under title:
The genetics of osteoporosis and metabolic bone disease / edited by Michael J. Econs.
p. cm.
Includes bibliographical references and index.
ISBN 0-89603-702-9 (alk. paper)
1. Bones—Metabolism—Disorders—Genetic aspects. 2. Osteoporosis—Genetic aspects.
I. Econs, Michael J.
[DNLM: 1. Osteoporosis—genetics. 2. Bone Diseases, Metabolic—genetics. 3. Genetic Predisposition to Disease. 4. Hereditary Diseases. WE 250 G328 2000]
RC931.M45 G46 2000
616.7'16042—dc21

99-058332

Preface

The explosive growth in the field of molecular biology over the last two decades has started to make a great impact on clinical medicine. Genes have been cloned for diseases that were poorly understood only a decade ago. Additionally, investigators are increasingly aware that there are strong genetic components to complex disorders, such as osteoporosis, that are not classically thought of as genetic disorders. New insights into the pathogenesis of metabolic bone diseases have been obtained from investigations into the molecular biology of these diseases and new therapies will become available based on these new insights.

In *The Genetics of Osteoporosis and Metabolic Bone Disease,* I have assembled an internationally renowned group of experts to write the various chapters. Each of the authors is an expert in his/her field who is currently performing research on the content of their chapter and have made important contributions to the understanding of the clinical features and pathophysiology of metabolic bone disease and genetics.

The first part of *The Genetics of Osteoporosis and Metabolic Bone Disease* addresses issues related to genetic contributions to the development of osteoporosis and the many factors that must be considered when searching for genes that predispose to osteoporosis. The second section addresses recent advances in the clinical and molecular biological aspects of inherited metabolic bone disorders. The last section reviews the latest techniques for finding genes that predispose to metabolic bone diseases.

Michael J. Econs, MD

Dedications

This book is dedicated to Lee Win Liu, MD, who has made many sacrifices as I have pursued genes that cause metabolic bone disease. She has worked with me on numerous reunions of families with metabolic bone disorders. These family reunions have almost always occurred during weekends or holidays.

The book is also dedicated to Robert and Steven Econs, who have enriched our lives beyond what we could ever have imagined.

Contents

Contributors

JEAN-PHILIPPE BONJOUR • *Division of Bone Diseases, WHO Collaborating Center for Osteoporosis and Bone Diseases, Department of Internal Medicine, University Hospital, Geneva, Switzerland*

EDWARD M. BROWN • *Endocrine-Hypertension Division, Department of Medicine, Brigham and Women's Hospital, Boston, MA*

GILBERT COTE • *Associate Professor of Medicine, Section of Endocrine Neoplasia and Hormonal Disorders, University of Texas M. D. Anderson Cancer Center, Houston, TX*

PAUL A. DAWSON • *Section on Connective Tissue Disorders, Heritable Disorders Branch, NICHD, NIH, Bethesda, MD*

MARTIN DELATYCKI • *Victorian Clinical Genetics Service, Murdoch Institute, Royal Children's Hospital, Flemington Road, Parkville, Victoria, Australia*

MICHAEL J. ECONS • *Departments of Medicine and Medical and Molecular Genetics, Indiana University School of Medicine, Indianapolis, IN*

FIONA FRANCIS • *Institut Cochin de Génétique Moléculaire, INSERM U. 129, CHU Cochin Port-Royal, Paris, France*

SERGE FERRARI • *Division of Bone Diseases, WHO Collaborating Center for Osteoporosis and Bone Diseases, Department of Internal Medicine, University Hospital, Geneva, Switzerland*

ROBERT F. GAGEL • *Section of Endocrine Neoplasia and Hormonal Disorders and Department of Internal Medicine Specialties, University of Texas M.D. Anderson Cancer Center, Houston, TX*

FRANCIS H. GANNON • *Department of Orthopaedic Surgery, Pathology and Laboratory Medicine, University of Pennsylvania School of Medicine, Philadelphia, PA*

JOHN L. HOPPER • *The University of Melbourne, Melbourne, Australia*

KANDASWAMY JAYARAJ • *GRECC, VAMC, Division of Geriatrics, Duke University Medical Center, Durham, NC*

HARALD JÜPPNER • *Endocrine Unit, Department of Medicine and Children's Service, Massachusetts General Hospital and Harvard Medical School, Boston, MA*

FREDERICK S. KAPLAN • *Department of Orthopaedic Surgery, University of Pennsylvania School of Medicine, Philadelphia, PA*
SHIGEAKI KATO • *Institute of Molecular and Cellular Biosciences, The University of Tokyo, Tokyo, Japan*
L. LYNDON KEY, JR. • *Department of Pediatrics, General Clinical Research Center, Medical University of South Carolina, Charleston, SC*
SACHIKO KITANAKA • *Institute of Molecular and Cellular Biosciences, The University of Tokyo, Tokyo, Japan*
ROBIN J. LEACH • *Department of Cellular and Structural Biology, University of Texas Health Science Center at San Antonio, San Antonio, TX*
SUZANNE M. LEAL • *Rockefeller University, New York, New York*
MARTINE LEMERRER • *Hospital Necker, Paris, France*
MICHAEL A. LEVINE • *Division of Pediatric Endocrinology, Department of Pediatrics, The Johns Hopkins University School of Medicine, Baltimore, MD*
KENNETH LYLES • *GRECC, VAMC, Division of Geriatrics, Duke University Medical Center, Durham, NC*
JOAN C. MARINI • *Section on Connective Tissue Disorders, Heritable Disorders Branch, NICHD, NIH, Bethesda, MD*
STUART H. RALSTON • *Bone Research Group, Department of Medicine and Therapeutics, University of Aberdeen, Scotland, UK*
RENÉ RIZZOLI • *Division of Bone Diseases, WHO Collaborating Center for Osteoporosis and Bone Diseases, Department of Internal Medicine, University Hospital, Geneva, Switzerland*
JOHN G. ROGERS • *Victorian Clinical Genetics Service, Murdoch Institute, Royal Children's Hospital, Victoria, Australia*
PETER S. N. ROWE • *Dept of Biochemistry and Molecular Biology, University of London, Royal Free Hospital Medical School, Hampstead, London, UK*
STEVEN J. SCHEINMAN • *Department of Medicine, SUNY Upstate Medical University, Syracuse, NY*
EGO SEEMAN • *Austin and Repatriation Medical Centre, University of Melbourne, Melbourne, Australia*
CAROLINE SILVE • *INSERM U. 426, Faculté de Médecine Xavier Bichat, Paris, France*
FREDERICK R. SINGER • *John Wayne Cancer Institute at St. John's Health Center, Santa Monica, CA*
EILEEN M. SHORE • *Department of Orthopaedic Surgery, Department of Genetics, University of Pennsylvania School of Medicine, Philadelphia, PA*

Roger Smith • *Medical Research Council Bone Research Laboratory, University of Osvord, Nuffield Orthopaedic Centre, Headington, Oxford, UK*

Marcy C. Speer • *Department of Medicine, Duke University Medical Center, Durham, North Carolina*

Tim M. Strom • *Abteilung Medizinische Genetik, Kinderklinik, Ludwig-Maximilians-Universität, Muenchen, Germany*

Rajesh V. Thakker • *MRC Molecular Endocrinology Group, MRC Clinical Sciences Centre, Imperial College School of Medicine, Hammersmith Hospital, London, UK*

James Triffitt • *Medical Research Council Bone Research Laboratory, University of Osvord, Nuffield Orthopaedic Centre, Headingdon, Oxford, UK*

J. Andoni Urtizberea • *Association Francaise Contre les Myopathies, Evry, France*

Lee S. Weinstein • *Metabolic Diseases Branch, National Institute of Diabetes, Digestive and Kidney Diseases, National Institutes of Health, Bethesda, MD*

Kenneth E. White • *Department of Medicine, Indiana University School of Medicine, Indianapolis, IN*

Michael P. Whyte • *Metabolic Research Unit, Shriners Hospital for Children and, Division of Bone and Mineral Diseases, Washington University School of Medicine, St. Louis, MO*

Contributors

[illegible] • Medical Research Council Bone Research Laboratory, University of Oxford, Nuffield Orthopaedic Centre, Headington, Oxford, UK

[illegible] • Department of Medicine, Duke University Medical Center, Durham, North Carolina

[illegible] • [illegible] Medizin [illegible] Kinderklinik, [illegible] Medizinische Hochschule Hannover, Germany

[illegible] • MRC [illegible] Endocrinology Group, MRC Clinical [illegible] School of Medicine [illegible] Hospital [illegible], UK

[illegible] • Medical Research Council Bone Research Laboratory, University of Oxford, Nuffield Orthopaedic Centre, Headington, Oxford, UK

[illegible]

[illegible] • [illegible] National Institutes of Health, Bethesda, MD

[illegible] • Department of Medicine, Indiana University School of Medicine, Indianapolis

[illegible] White • [illegible] Children and Division of [illegible] Washington University School of Medicine, St. Louis, MO

CHAPTER 1

Genetic and Environmental Determinants of Variance in Bone Size, Mass, and Volumetric Density of the Proximal Femur

Ego Seeman

1. Introduction

The genetic and environmental factors responsible for age, gender and race specific differences in bone fragility and fracture rates of the proximal femur are unknown. There are several possible reasons.

First, the phenotype is inadequately defined. Areal bone mineral density (BMD), the surrogate measure of bone fragility used as a predictor of fracture, is a summation of the modeling and remodeling that occurs during growth and aging on the periosteal and endosteal (endocortical, intracortical, trabecular) surfaces of bone. The differing and largely independent modeling and remodeling on these surfaces — during growth, aging, and disease, in men and women, and in different races, suggests the surfaces are regulated differently. Areal BMD is an ambiguous phenotype as it is the net result of the bone added and removed from these surfaces. Its use obscures the pathogenetic basis of bone fragility rather than revealing it. Insight into the regulators of the bone surface remodeling is unlikely to be obtained until the age, gender, and race specific means and variances of these specific phenotypes are described and quantified. Potential genetic and environmental factors hypothesized to explain the variances can then be investigated.

Second, there is no experimental evidence to support the notion that gender and racial differences in areal BMD are responsible for the corresponding gender and racial differences in fracture rates. Gender and racial differences in areal BMD are likely to be largely accounted for by corresponding differences in bone

The Genetics of Osteoporosis and Metabolic Bone Disease
Ed.: M. J. Econs © Humana Press Inc., Totowa, NJ

size. Little evidence exists for gender or racial differences in volumetric BMD. If volumetric BMD does differ, its structural basis (differences in cortical thickness, true cortical density, trabecular number, or thickness) is largely undefined, except for evidence to support greater trabecular thickness in blacks than whites.

Third, a causal relationship is assumed to exist between gender, racial, and secular differences in hip axis length (HAL) and corresponding differences in hip fracture rates. This association has not been tested in a prospective study. Gender, racial, and secular differences in HAL are likely to be due to corresponding differences in leg length. Adjustments by total height may over- or underestimate gender and racial differences in HAL depending on the comparisons made because leg length is greater in men than women, and greater in blacks than whites or Asians.

Fourth, the search for genetic factors has not been driven by specific testable hypotheses concerning any age-, gender-, or race-specific biological process such as periosteal apposition, endocortical remodeling. Lack of knowledge of the structural differences that are responsible for the differences in bone fragility between genders and races hampers attempts to find genes that are responsible for these differences.

What Is the Problem — Hip Fractures?

Hip fractures are the most serious consequence of bone fragility in terms of morbidity, mortality, and financial burden *(1,2)*. The incidence of hip fractures:

1. increases with advancing age in women and men,
2. is higher in women than men,
3. is higher in whites than blacks or Asians,
4. varies from country to country,
5. varies more between countries than between genders, and
6. secular trends in hip fracture incidence have been variously reported to increase, decrease, or remain unchanged during the past 50 yr *(1)*.

Assuming accurate case ascertainment, these gender-, race-, country-, and time-specific estimates of hip fracture incidence are likely to reflect differences in the incidence of falls, the severity of trauma, and underlying bone fragility. This chapter is confined to the discussion of the genetic and environmental factors that may account for differences in bone fragility that may, in turn, contribute to this perplexingly diverse epidemiology of hip fractures.

What Are the Questions?

What are the structural elements that contribute to bone strength of the proximal femur? Do they differ according to age, gender, and race? What are the age-,gender-, and race-specific genetic and environmental factors that account for the variance in these structures, i.e., between young and old, women and men, and between races? Do the differences in these structures, and the differences in genetic and environmental factors account for the age-,gender-, and racial-differences in hip fracture rates? What structural differences are found at the proximal femoral between individuals with and without hip fractures? Have there been secular changes in these structures that may explain secular trends in the age-, gender-, and race-specific incidence of hip fractures?

The majority of these questions have no answers because:

1. there are methodological problems in measuring the phenotypes — the specific structural elements responsible for bone strength,
2. there are methodological problems in identifying associations between candidate genes and these structural elements, and
3. measuring the "dose" of an environmental exposure is difficult.

A most challenging problem is to demonstrate, by experimental design, that the higher hip fracture rate in women than men, or in whites compared to other racial groups is attributable to any gender or racial difference in a phenotype such as bone mineral content (BMC), bone size, areal BMD, bone mineral apparent density (BMAD), or volumetric BMD. Causality is usually inferred when the observation is "consistent with" or "fits" the preconceived notion.

Defining Causality Using an Ambiguous Phenotype — Vagaries of "Areal BMD"

As fractures are uncommon annual events, fracture rates are exceedingly difficult endpoints to use in the study of the pathogenesis or treatment of bone fragility. As areal BMD predicts the breaking strength of bone in vitro, and fractures in vivo, this surrogate endpoint of bone strength has been most widely studied at this time. Although some insights have been obtained, areal BMD may not be the appropriate phenotype needed to answer questions regarding the genetic and environmental factors contributing to pathogenesis of bone fragility.

Areal BMD is a summation of the periosteal and endosteal (endocortical, intracortical, trabecular) surface modeling and remodeling during growth and aging. It is the summation or net result of the amounts of bone added to, and removed from, these surfaces. As each of these surfaces is regulated differently and responds differently to environmental factors, this integrated endpoint is likely to obscure the ability to detect true causal relationships between genetic and environmental factors and the modeling and remodeling behavior on these surfaces. Areal BMD is incorrectly perceived to be an unambiguous and tightly regulated phenotype. It is not. It is a "gemish," a mixture, and failure to recognize its limitations is likely to seriously mislead the thinking in the field.

The structural basis underlying the development of the macro-and microarchitecture of the skeleton during growth and the loss of mass and structural integrity during aging, are not conveyed by the areal BMD measurement. This phenotype has resulted in the following flawed notions *(3)*:

1. Areal BMD increases during growth; it does not, bone size increases;
2. Peak areal BMD is higher in men than women; it is not, bone size is greater;

3. Areal BMD is stable until menopause in women; it is not, bone loss at the proximal femur is well documented before menopause;
4. Women lose more trabecular bone from the axial skeleton than men; no, trabecular bone loss is similar in women and men *(3)*;
5. Cortical bone loss is greater in women than men; no, net loss is greater because endocortical resorption is greater and subperiosteal formation is less in women than men;
6. Blacks have higher areal BMD than whites, who in turn have higher areal BMD than Asians — this is largely (but not entirely) due to differences in bone size rather than due to differences in volumetric BMD *(3)*.

Growth in Femoral Width and Cortical Thickness and The Constancy of Volumetric Density

The increase in size and bone mass of the proximal femur produces the picture of increasing areal BMD during growth (Fig. 1, upper panels) *(4)*. As the femur increases in length and diameter, cortical thickness increases so that the amount of bone within the growing bone increases in absolute terms (i.e., compared with its value in grams in younger individuals) but the increase in external size is matched by a commensurate increase in cortical thickness so that the amount of bone in the bone, i.e., the volumetric BMD of the femur does not change (Fig. 1, lower panels).

The increase in cortical thickness is achieved by expansion of periosteal diameter with less expansion of the endocortical (medullary) diameter of long bones such as the metacarpals and femur *(5)*. (If the endocortical diameter and periosteal diameter expanded in parallel, cortical thickness would not increase despite the bone enlarging so that volumetric BMD would fall.) Endocortical contraction occurs in females and perhaps to a lesser extent in males, in early puberty with a sharp rise in cortical width so that by maturity, about 75% of metacarpal cortical width is due to periosteal expansion while 25% is due to endocortical contraction in females. Whether the pattern of development is similar at the femur is less certain. Provisional data suggests that the process is similar at the femoral midshaft but endocortical (medullary) contraction occurs later than at the metacarpal, consistant with the later growth and maturation of proximal than distal limb segments *(6)* (Fig. 2). The clinical relevance of this regional growth may emerge when exposure occurs to disease or risk factors; regions or surfaces further from their peak may be affected more greatly than regions nearer their peak. Medullary contraction may fail to occur at one or more sites depending on the timing of exposure.

If volumetric BMD of the growing bone is constant from birth to adulthood, i.e., independent of age, then the position of an individual's volumetric BMD in the population distribution at any age is likely to be determined prenatally. That is, the factors that determine whether an individual has a femoral volumetric BMD at the 5th or 95th percentile are likely to be deter-

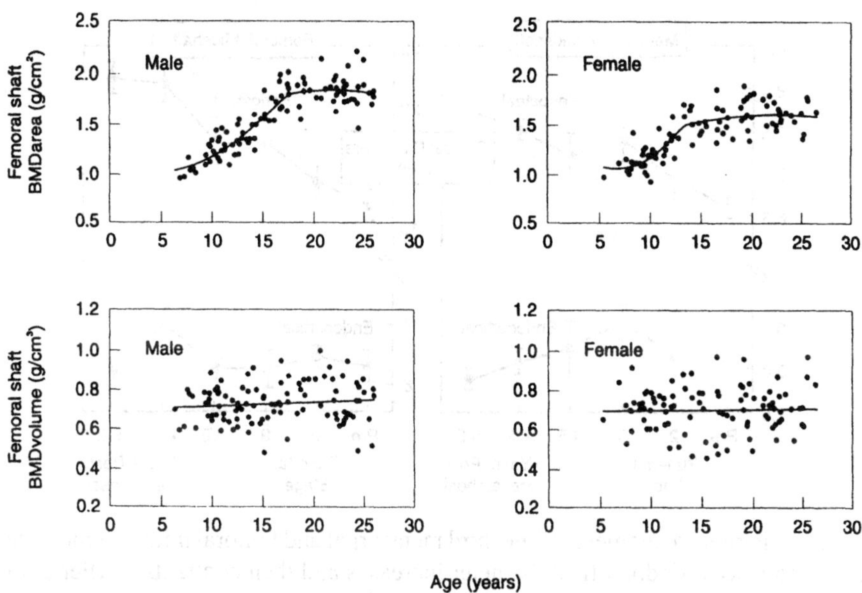

Fig. 1. Areal and volumetric bone mineral density (BMD) of the femoral shaft versus age in males and females. (Adapted with permission from ref. *4*.)

mined before birth — unless an individual's volumetric BMD can change percentiles. This does not occur for height unless there is illness or recovery from illness. The structural differences responsible for femoral volumetric BMD being in the 5th percentile compared to 95th percentile are not known. Until these morphological differences between individuals within a decade as well as across decades are defined, identifying the genetic and environmental causes for these differences will be difficult.

The evidence that genetic factors may determine the variance in areal BMD in old age is partly based on studies in mother-daughter pairs. Areal BMD z scores or standardized deviations (SD, mean ± SEM) in 74 women mean age 73 yr with hip fractures was about – 0.5 SD at the femoral neck, – 1.0 SD at the femoral shaft, and – 0.4 SD at the lumbar spine *(7)*. Respective z scores in 41 daughters mean age 44 yr, were – 0.4 SD, – 0.4 SD, and + 0.23 SD. The deficit at the femoral shaft in the daughters (relative to their peers) was about half the deficit of the mothers (relative to their peers) — consistent with the genetic hypothesis *(8)*. Daughters of women with spine fractures had deficits in areal BMD at the spine of about – 0.8 SD. The deficits at the proximal femur were similar to those reported in daughters of women with hip fractures *(9)*. The differing temporal patterns of growth of the axial and appendicular skeleton may be antecedents for deficits at the femur but not spine, or deficits at both sites *(3,6)*.

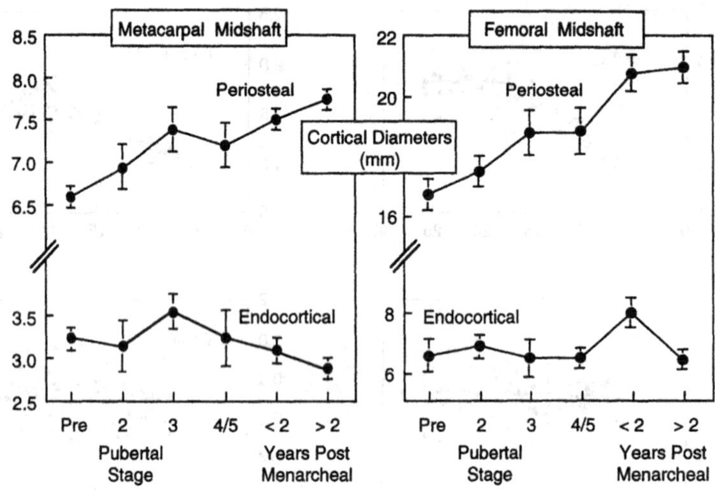

Fig. 2. Periosteal diameter of the third metacarpal and femoral midshaft increases as age advances. Endocortical diameter increases and then contracts; earlier at the metacarpal than femoral midshaft. (Adapted with permission from ref. *6*.)

Differences in Bone Mass, Size, and Volumetric Density

Patients with and without Fractures

As areal BMD measurement does not entirely adjust for bone size, it remains possible that the resemblance in the areal BMD in the mother-daughter pairs may be explained by resemblance in bone size, rather than resemblance in volumetric BMD (and therefore cortical thickness, trabecular number, and thickness). Women and men with spine fractures have smaller vertebral bone size than age- and gender-matched controls *(10,11)*. Men with hip fractures may have smaller femoral neck width than controls while women with hip fractures may have larger femoral neck width than controls *(12)*. Thus, the lower areal BMD in women with spine fractures and men with spine or hip fractures may be at least partly due to the smaller bone size rather than reduced volumetric BMD. The lower areal BMD in women with hip fractures (with larger bones) may be an underestimate — the deficit in volumetric BMD may be less than the deficit in areal BMD.

The smaller size may be due to attainment of a smaller bone size during growth, the failure of periosteal appositional growth during aging, or both. There is less bone in the bone because peak bone mass attained during growth may be reduced, and/or bone loss may have been excessive. The structural basis of less bone in bone may be thinner cortices, fewer or thinner trabeculae, or reduced true bone density of bony tissue. The observation that men with hip fractures have smaller femoral neck width, whereas women with hip fractures have larger femoral neck width, requires independent confirmation. The possible mechanisms responsible are uncertain. However, to speculate, hypogonadism during growth may contribute to the smaller bone size in men because testosterone regulates periosteal growth. The larger bone size in women may be the result of delayed epiphyseal fusion and continued growth in size due to estrogen deficiency.

Gender Differences

The failure of densitometry to entirely account for differences in bone size may also be responsible for the notion that proximal femoral areal BMD is higher in males than females. Gender comparisons of bone mass, size, and volumetric BMD in males and females are shown in Fig. 3 *(12)*. There are gender differences in bone mass and volume but not volumetric BMD. Peak spine and proximal femoral volumetric BMD is similar in men and women *(13)*. Iliac crest trabecular bone volume, trabecular number, and thickness do not differ in men and women *(14)*. Radial volumetric BMD is also no different in boys and girls *(15)*. However, Butz et al. reported higher trabecular and total radial volumetric BMD in men than women using peripheral quantitative computed tomomgraphy *(16)*. Zanchetta et al. found no differences in radial areal BMD in boys and girls, whereas gender differences in femoral areal BMD emerged at 16 yr of age *(17)*. Whether differences in pubertal stage were accounted for is unclear. As puberty occurs 2 yr later in boys than girls, matching boys and girls by pubertal stage means that there will be mismatch by age, matching by age means there will be mismatch by pubertal stage. Close examination of whether there are gender differences in proximal femoral volumetric BMD is needed. If so, the morphological basis of any gender differences — cortical thickness, trabecular number and thickness, or true density of these bony structures need to be defined.

Gender differences in bone size are probably present prenatally and have been described during the first years of life *(18,19)*. In addition, men have bigger bones than women because puberty occurs two years later, growth velocity is greater and continues longer. As puberty is associated with cessation of growth in leg length, this two additional years of growth results in men having greater leg length than women. Puberty is associated with accelerated trunk growth. Delayed puberty may result in longer legs and a shorter trunk, but final height may not be compromised. Of the 13 cm difference in height between women and men, 10 cm is due to prepubertal growth. Of the 13 cm difference, 8 cm is due to the greater leg length, and 5 cm is due to the greater trunk length in men *(20,21)*. The later puberty in the male than female results in differences in segment lengths. A male of the same height as a female is likely to have longer legs and greater areal BMD of the femur because of the size difference — volumetric BMD is similar *(12,13)*.

Testosterone results in increased periosteal width while estrogen is growth limiting in the female resulting in reduced femoral periosteal width. As shown in Fig. 4, gonadectomy in the growing male rat results in smaller femoral bone mass

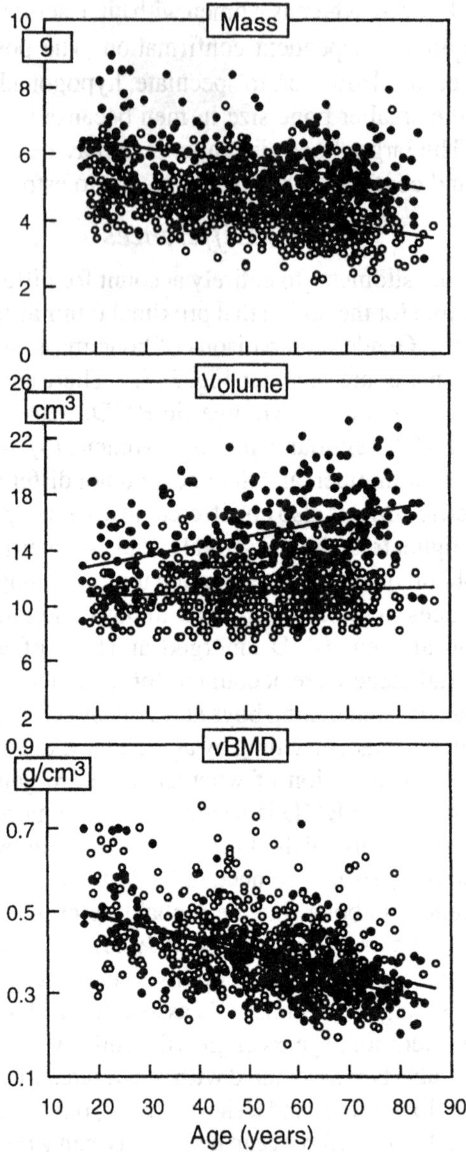

Fig. 3. Femoral neck bone mass, volume, and volumetric bone mineral density (VBMD) in men (closed circles) and women (open circles). From Duan and Seeman (adapted with permission from ref. *12*).

and volume with less bone in the (smaller) bone. Gonadectomy in the female rat results in a bigger femur (with little change in the growth rate of the spine). The larger femur produces in the seemingly anomalous finding of normal BMC or

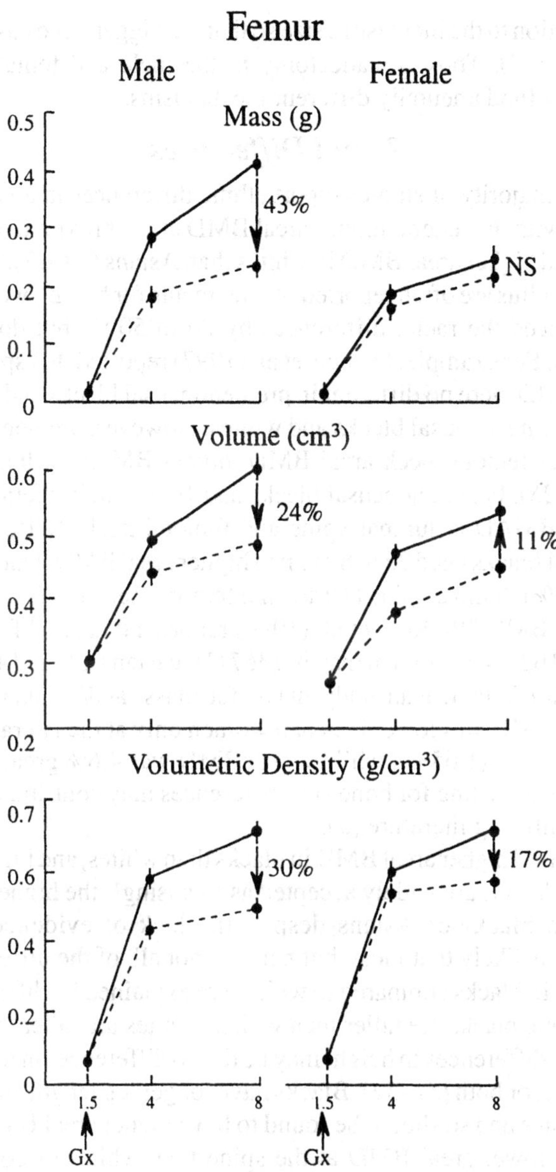

Fig. 4. Gonadectomy (Gx) results in reduced femoral mass, volume, and volumetric density in the growing male rat but no change in bone mass relative to controls, increased volume and reduced volumetric density in the growing female rat. Gx, dashed line; control, full line. (Adapted with permission from ref. 22.)

areal BMD following gonadectomy (a larger femur is compared with a smaller femur in the control) but volumetric BMD is reduced because the increase in mass is not in proportion to the increase in size so that the bigger bone has relatively less bone within it *(22)*. Thus, gonadectomy in the male and female rat result in osteoporosis by fundamentally different mechanisms.

Racial Differences

The vast majority of studies report ethnic differences in areal BMD at one or more sites, with, in general higher areal BMD at the proximal femur in blacks than whites, and higher areal BMD in whites than Asians *(23–27)*. No differences at the spine or radius are often reported. Adjustments for height, weight, projected bone area reduced the racial differences by 20 to 50 %, but do not generally eliminate them. For example, Daniels et al. (1997) reported that spinal (and distal radial) areal BMD were no different in premenopausal blacks and whites, and no different in postmenopausal blacks and whites. However, premenopausal blacks had 12% higher femoral neck areal BMD, higher BMAD at lumbar spine and femoral neck *(28)*. Postmenopausal blacks had 16.5% higher femoral neck areal BMD, higher BMAD at lumbar spine and femoral neck. Nelson et al. (1995) reported that 34 blacks aged 23 to 80 yr had higher areal BMD than 160 white men at the radius (5%), lumbar spine (10%), and femoral neck (20%) before and after adjustment for BMI *(29)*. Ross et al. (1996) reported that areal BMD was 3.7 to 6.6% lower in 162 Asian women than in 1367 Caucasian and aged 45 to 59 yr *(30)*. On adjusting for height, lean body mass, fat mass, and/or quadriceps muscle strength, areal BMD was lower in Asian women only at the lateral spine (4.4%), arm (2.2%), and leg (1.65%), while wrist aBMD was 4.6% greater. These inaccurate means of adjusting for bone size differences may contribute to the contradictory and confusing literature *(3)*.

The reported higher areal BMD in blacks than whites, and higher areal BMD in whites than Asians are widely accepted as ''causing'' the higher fracture rates in whites than blacks or Asians despite the lack of evidence for a causal relationship. It is likely that most, but perhaps not all, of the differences in areal BMD reported in blacks compared to whites are explained by differences in bone size. On average, blacks are taller than whites, whites are taller than Asians and Hispanics. The differences in height may be due to differences in upper body size, lower body size, or both *(31–34)*. Blacks have longer leg length and shorter trunk length that whites and so should be found to have higher areal BMD at the femur and similar or lower areal BMD at the spine than whites of comparable total height. Asians have shorter legs and longer trunks than whites so that if Asians and whites are matched for height, reduced proximal femoral areal BMD and higher lumbar spine areal BMD should be found given the average segment length differences.

Black children may have more advanced skeletal age than white children of comparable chronological age *(35)*. In a study of 1942 blacks and 3046 whites, skeletal age was about 0.5 SD more advanced in blacks than whites. Height was about 0.25 SD more advanced in blacks of both genders. Thus, comparisons of black and white children, males and females, must take skeletal maturation, chronological age, and pubertal staging into consideration. Until size differences are taken into account by measurement of the size of the bone itself, differences in 'density' should be viewed sceptically.

Secular increases have occurred in total height, sitting height, and leg length during the last 50 yr in whites, blacks, and Asians *(36–38)*. The epidemiology of the secular changes are as perplexingly varied as is the epidemiology of hip fractures; with gender-specific, race-specific- upper and/or lower body segment specific increases reported. Secular increases have been reported in upper and lower body segments in females and males. However, in some studies, secular changes were confined to one gender or one body segment. Within a community, secular trends may be found in the lower, but not higher, socioeconomic group. Secular changes in the frequency or severity of falls, in the magnitude of bone loss during aging, in factors regulating peak bone mass, size, shape, volumetric BMD, body proportions, or age at menarche may contribute to the trends in the epidemiology of hip fractures *(1,2)*.

The genetic, hormonal, and environmental factors that may contribute to racial differences in bone size are not unknown. The evidence that structural differences exist between races is fragmentary and contradictory. No histomorphometric data are available for the proximal femur. However, findings in the iliac crest suggest that premenopausal blacks have greater trabecular thickness but not numbers than white women *(39)*. By contrast, no racial differences were detected in other studies *(40–42)*. A difference in true bone density may result in a higher volumetric BMD in men than women or in blacks than whites. Blacks have been reported to have a lower mineralized matrix apposition rate, a longer bone formation period which may allow a greater deposition of bone mineral. In part, the increase in areal BMD following bisphosphonates may be due to the slower bone turnover, allowing more complete mineralization of bone *(43)*. Harris et al. reported that a thymidine–cytosine polymorphism exists in the first of the two potential translation initiation sites of the VDR gene detectable using the endonuclease, FokI *(44)*. The FokI genotype was determined in 72 black and 82 white premenopausal women. In the whole group, ff women had 7.4% lower femoral neck areal BMD than FF women. In whites, ff women had 12.1% lower femoral neck areal BMD than FF. Lumbar areal BMD did not differ by genotype. FokI genotype reduced the racial difference in femoral neck areal BMD by 35%. The authors concluded that the polymorphism influenced peak areal BMD and differences in its distribution may partly explain racial variations in areal BMD. Any association with bone size was not reported (*see* Chapter 3 for more detail on the VDR). Rosen et al. reported differences in femoral volumetric BMD of up to 50% in C3H compared to B6 mouse strains *(45)*. F1 progeny females had intermediate IGF-I and femoral BMD values between the parental strains. F2 progeny with highest BMD had highest IGF-I with about 35% of the variance in femoral BMD attributed to serum IGF-I. The IGF-I in calvariae, tibiae, and femora was 32% higher in C3H. The authors conclude that the difference in volumetric BMD between strains may be related to systemic and skeletal IGF-I synthesis. Whether this reflects a causal relationship is unclear. The morphological basis of the higher volumetric BMD at this cortical site was not clearly defined. It may be due to a thicker cortex or a cortex of higher true mineral density, or both.

If size is an important factor accounting for gender and racial differences in areal BMD, then what factors account for the differing fracture epidemiology? Is the difference in bone size the main morphological variable accounting for differences in bone fragility? What genetic and environmental factors account for gender and racial differences in bone size, for the variance in cortical thickness, trabecular number, and trabecular thickness; the structural components of volumetric BMD? If true density is higher then the determinants of variance in mineralization need to be studied.

Hip Axis Length

HAL, is the distance from greater trochanter to inner pelvic brim. HAL increases during growth to reach a peak length at 15 yr *(46)*. Height was the only independent predictor of HAL. Height adjusted correlations for HAL in 176 monozygotic (MZ) pairs vs 128 dizygotic (DZ) pairs were 0.79 (95% CI 0.73, 0.84) vs 0.54 (95% CI 0.39, 0.68). About 80% of variation in HAL was attributable to additive genetic factors. This fell to 51% on adjusting for shared environmental factors. The authors suggested that about 10% of the increased risk of hip fracture associated with maternal hip fracture history may be due to genes determining HAL. In a study of adult twins, MZ correlations for areal BMD and geometry ranging between 0.36 to 0.81 and were higher than the DZ trait correlations except femoral neck *(47)*. Heritability was between 0.72 and 0.78 for regional areal BMD, the center of mass of the femoral neck, and the resistance of the femoral neck to forces experienced in a fall, but not for femoral neck length. Arden et al. reported that heritability in 128 identical and 122 nonidentical pairs of female twins aged 50 to 70 years was 0.62 (CI 0.22, 1.02) for HAL and was unchanged after adjustment for areal BMD suggesting that variances for bone architecture as well as areal BMD are genetically determined *(48)*.

HAL is reported to be an independent predictor of hip fracture. Differences in HAL have been observed between genders, races, and between hip fracture cases and controls. Faulkner et al. reported that HAL was 3.4% greater in 64 hip fracture cases compared with 134 controls *(49)*. For each SD increase in HAL, fracture risk increased 1.8-fold (95% CI 1.3, 2.5), for each SD fall in BMD, fracture risk increased 2.7-fold (95% CI 1.7, 4.3). Boonen et al. compared 105 women with spine fractures (type I or postmenopausal osteoporosis, 30 with hip fractures (type II or senile osteoporosis) and 75 controls. Femoral neck areal BMD was no different in the two osteoporotic groups, but HAL was greater in the type II group relative to the others *(50)*. The women with spinal fractures were the same height as the hip fracture cases. If the hip fracture cases had been matched with women in the spinal fracture group who were shorter (but who would have been the same height had they not had spinal fracture), then the difference in HAL may have been even greater.

The 40% lower rate of hip fracture in Asian women and 50% lower hip fracture rates in black women relative to white women are inferred to be due to a greater HAL in whites. HAL was 6.7 ± 0.4 in 135 whites, 6.3 ± 0.3 in 74 Asians, and 6.4 ± 0.4 cm in 50 blacks ($P < 0.01$ for Asians and blacks compared with whites with differences persisted after height adjustments *(51)*. The shorter HAL conferred an odds ratio for hip fracture of 0.53 (95% CI, 0.37 to 0.76, Asian) and of 0.68 (95% CI, 0.55 to 0.85, blacks) compared to whites. Nelson et al. reported that 34 black and 160 white men aged 23 to 80 yr had no difference in HAL *(29)*. Mikhail et al. found greater HAL and femoral neck width in 50 black compared to white premenopausal women *(52)*.

In a study of 57 Japanese and 119 white women, whites had greater femoral neck BMC (3.91 vs 3.02 g), cross-sectional moment of inertia (0.99 vs 0.57 cm^4), femoral neck length (5.6 vs 4.4 cm), and femoral neck angle (130 vs 128 degrees). The lower risk of femoral neck fracture in Japanese women was attributed to a shorter femoral neck and a smaller femoral neck angle *(53)*. Daniels et al. reported that premenopausal whites had longer femoral neck axis length than blacks (6.5 ± 0.4 vs 6.1 ± 0.4 cm) *(28)*. Among postmenopausal subjects, femoral neck axis length was 6.5 ± 0.4 cm in whites and 6.0 ± 0.3 cm in blacks. Chin et al. reported that femoral neck length in premenopausal women was 61.5 mm in 52 Chinese, 61.5 mm in 50 Indians, 66.0 mm in 71 Europeans, and 68.2 mm in 52 Polynesians *(54)*. HAL in the respective groups was 98.0, 94.5, 102.3, and 106.4 mm. The Polynesians were heavier and taller than other groups, followed by the Europeans. The lower incidence of hip fracture in Asians was attributed to shorter femoral neck length. The very low incidence of hip fracture in Polynesians could not be reconciled with the larger HAL. Reid et al. (1994) reported a secular increase in HAL and femoral neck length between 1953 and 1990 and suggested that the increased HAL could account for much of the increase in fracture rates in the last 40 yr *(55)*.

The notion of a "longer" or "shorter" HAL may be a function of the size of the femur itself. Height adjustments are unlikely to be a satisfactory way of adjusting for differences in bone size because of racial differences in body segment lengths. Women have shorter legs than men so a shorter HAL is difficult to reconcile with the higher hip fracture rates in women than men. Asians have shorter legs than whites of comparable height. Thus, the shorter HAL may reflect this difference in bone size. Finding a shorter HAL in blacks may be a conservative bias as blacks have longer legs than whites. A secular increase in HAL may occur along with a secular increase in lower body size. Whether these differences in HAL "cause" the gender, racial and secular differences in hip fractures is speculative. There have been no randomized trials undertaken where a group of subjects were stratified by HAL matching by design so that important factors influencing hip fracture risk equally represented in both groups (e.g., bone mass, size, density, age, and illnesses).

Bone Loss — The Net Effect of Endosteal Resorption and Periosteal Apposition

Bone loss from the proximal femur is well documented before menopause in women and probably begins in men soon after attainment of peak areal BMD. Ravn et al. report proximal femoral areal BMD in 1238 healthy white women aged 21 to 75 yr *(56)*. Premenopausal women aged 21 to 54 yr showed bone loss in the femoral neck (0.3%/yr) and Ward's triangle (0.6%/yr). Postmenopausal areal BMD loss ranged from 9 to 13% in the first five years after menopause, rising to 17 to 30% after 20 yr. Tsai et al. measured bone mass and areas of the proximal femur in 202 Chinese men and 507 Chinese women aged 21 to 70 yr *(57)*. Areal BMD was 10 to 15% lower than published values in Caucasians. Femoral neck and trochanteric areal BMD were lower in women than men although premenopausal women had higher femoral neck areal BMD than men. At Ward's triangle, areal BMD in men was similar to that in premenopausal women. areal BMD decreased with age at a rate of –0.2 to –1.0% per year, with a smaller decrement in men than women.

The mechanisms responsible for bone loss in young adulthood are not well documented because they are difficult to detect in an individual. In part, the changes may be an artefact of a fall in marrow cellularity and increase in marrow adipose cells of the proximal femur, which will result in a lower areal BMD *(58)*. Moreover, it is possible that cortical mineral accrual and consolidation may still be occurring in adults between the ages of 20 to 30 yr while trabecular bone may reach its adult peak in earlier adulthood and start to decrease, whereas cortical accrual continues. Densitometric methods will integrate the subtle cortical accrual and trabecular bone loss to suggest no changes have occurred. Furthermore, the age of attainment of peak areal BMD and commencement of bone loss also varies by race *(59)*.

Both men and women lose bone with advancing age. Subperiosteal expansion occurs in men during aging and perhaps less so in women *(12,60)*. The reason women lose more bone than men is because endocortical resorption is greater, and, periosteal formation is less than in men (Fig. 5). Finding greater periosteal expansion at puberty in boys than girls *(5)*, and greater periosteal expansion during aging in men than women, suggests that this may be partly a testosterone dependent process. The smaller bone size in men with spine or hip fractures may be partly due to reduced subperiosteal expansion. Whether this in turn may be due to testosterone deficiency or growth hormone deficiency is also unknown. Heaney et al. reported 21 yr follow-up in 170 Caucasian women aged 35 to 45 yr. Femoral neck and shaft external diameters increased with age (0.135%/yr and 0.229%/yr). Women with bb genotype of the Bsm1 polymorphism of the vitamin D receptor had greater shaft expansion and a greater increase in cortical area *(61)*. Whether this association is causal is uncertain. If causal the physiological mechanisms mediating this greater expansion are undefined. This was not a randomized trial

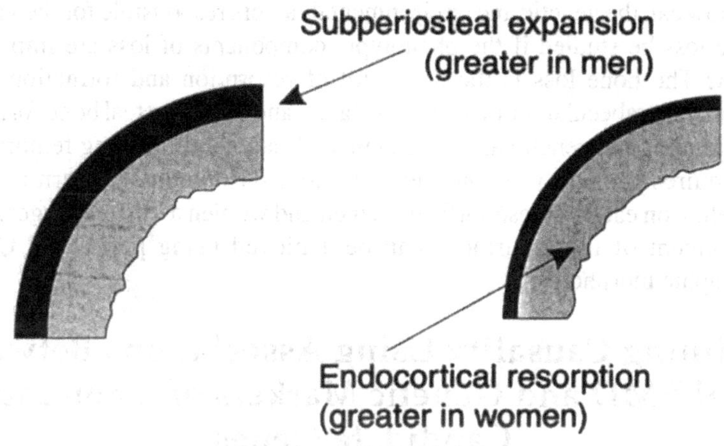

Fig. 5. Left, men. Right, women. Cortical bone loss is less in men than women because endocortical resorption is greater in women than men, and subperiosteal formation is greater in men than women. (Adapted with permission from ref. *60*.)

so that the greater expansion associated with the bb genotype may be due to unmeasured confounders.

The commonly held view that proximal femoral bone loss decelerates in old age is based on cross sectional data. Prospective studies suggest that bone loss accelerates in old age and that the bone loss is probably predominantly cortical in origin. Ensrud et al. showed that rates of decline in areal BMD at the proximal femur, measured in 5698 community-living white women aged >61 yr, increased with age from 2.5 mg/cm² per year in women aged 67–69 yr to 10.4 mg/cm² per year in women aged >85 yr *(62)*. Greenspan et al. report femoral areal BMD in 85 healthy, community living women aged 66 to 93 yr showed annual rates of bone loss at total hip (– 0.74%) and intertrochanter (–1.14%). Cross-sectional analysis indicated annual rates of bone loss were about – 0.8% at the femoral neck, total hip, trochanter, intertrochanteric region, and Ward's triangle *(63)*.

Continued bone loss may be due to secondary hyperparathyroidism, which increases cortical bone remodeling and activation frequency. Endosteal bone resorption and intracortical remodeling increase bone fragility in the proximal femur. Cortical bone surfaces increase as intracortical and endocortical resorption continues increasing the surface available for resorption to take place with a subsequent increase in bone turnover and bone loss. The increased numbers of sites undergoing remodeling are partly due to secondary hyperparathyroidism with imbalance at the BMU forming the morphological basis of the bone loss. The reduced bone formation results in a negative bone balance and bone loss and may be due to reduced osteoblastic progenitor cell availability *(64,65)*. Trabecular bone loss may contribute less to bone loss as trabeculae are lost.

How can the genetic and environmental factors responsible for the variance of bone loss be studied if the phenotypic components of loss are imprecisely defined? The bone loss is the net result of resorption and formation on the endocortical, trabecular, intracortical surfaces, and subperiosteal bone formation. Understanding the genetic and environmental factors influencing femoral bone loss requires the study of the genetic and environmental determinants of remodeling on each of these surfaces in men and women at different ages. Direct measurement of these surfaces can be achieved using peripheral QCT or radiographic morphometry.

Defining Causality Using Associations Between Areal BMD and Genetic Markers of Unmeasured Candidate Genes

Reports of possible associations between candidate genes and bone surface modeling and remodeling are nonexistent. Most of the studies that have been done have used areal BMD as the phenotype. A true association between genotypes and areal BMD may exist but methodological problems such as small study samples may have precluded the detection of this association in many studies, especially if the effect on areal BMD is small. (The small effect may nevertheless be important if the genotype is common.) Susceptibility gene-environment interactions have been proposed to account for the null or contradictory data. These gene-environment interactions may occur but are very difficult to identify because small study samples, low frequency of a susceptibility gene, and low exposure to an environmental factor may preclude the detection of this interaction. The difficulty in identifying an increased risk due to gene-environment interaction is even greater if the exposure results in an increased fracture risk through nongenomically mediated mechanisms. These methodological limitations may result in negative results interpreted as "no effect" rather than "no detectable effect."

The genes and gene products that regulate the gain in bone size or mass during growth, and the loss of bone mass during aging are not known. Associations between proximal femoral areal BMD and polymorphisms of the vitamin D receptor, estrogen receptor, and type 1 collagen genes are inconsistent, contradictory, or negative *(66,67)*. Associations between vitamin D receptor genotypes and areal BMD have been reported in some, but not all, studies. In many studies, one genotype was compared with the other one or two; the choice of genotype groupings were dictated by the data. Few, if any studies, explain more than 1–3% of the variance in areal BMD and it is now most unlikely that any single genetic marker can be used to predict an individual's hip fracture risk—either by association with higher or lower BMD, higher or lower bone turnover, or experimentally proven higher or lower hip fracture incidence.

Moreover, the search for genes associated with bone fragility has not been driven by a hypothesis regarding bone fragility. For example, periosteal diameter may be an important determinant of bone strength, and gender or racial differences in periosteal diameter may be related to differences in fracture rates. Do some individuals have a greater periosteal growth response to growth hormone/IGF-1? Are there growth hormone/IGF-1 or androgen receptor polymorphisms associated with greater periosteal bone growth? Cortical thickness is determined by periosteal expansion before, during, and after puberty and endocortical contraction during puberty in females. Are there IGF-1, estrogen receptor, or androgen receptor polymorphisms associated with differing degrees of accrual of cortical thickness? These surfaces are easily measured with accuracy and precision.

Although several studies have suggested that bone loss at the proximal femur occurs more rapidly in individuals with the vitamin D receptor BB genotype, these studies are based on post hoc analyses. Likewise, studies purporting an association between a genotype and areal BMD response to dietary calcium or vitamin D have not been designed with prior stratification by genotype and then randomization to placebo versus intervention. The lack of stratification and randomization means that measured or unmeasured confounders may explain any observed difference in rates of loss or treatment effects associated with, and falsely ascribed to, a genotype.

Genetic and Environmental Components of Variance

Quantifying total variance and estimating its genetic and environmental components can be achieved by studying correlations between twins. If the MZ correlation exceeds the DZ correlation, the excess is due to shared genes. If the only reason twins are correlated is shared genes, then $r_{mz} = 2\ r_{dz}$. If the DZ correlation is greater than one half the MZ correlation, then the amount by which it is greater must be attributed to the effects of environmental factors shared by twins: the common environmental variance. For a discussion of the pros and cons of twin studies *see* Chapter 2.

Hopper et al. reported that total variance in femoral neck areal BMD increased during and after pubertal growth (Fig. 6, gray bars) *(68)*. Most of the total variance was attributable to genetic factors (black bars). However, the genetic variance in twins aged 13–17 yr was less than in twins aged 10–13 yr, while the common environmental variance was higher in the 13–17 yr olds (white bars). The covariance increased in MZ twins as did the total variance, whereas the covariance of DZ twins increased during adolescence but then decreased in early adulthood. Identical twins may choose a similar lifestyle in adulthood so that they remain similar, whereas DZ twins may pursue independent lifestyles and become increasingly dissimilar. As shown in Fig. 7, total variance (black bars) differs in magnitude from site to site as do the genetic (whites bars), common and individual environmental components of the total variance (gray and hatched bars respectively). Genetic variance in elderly twins accounts for most of the total variance

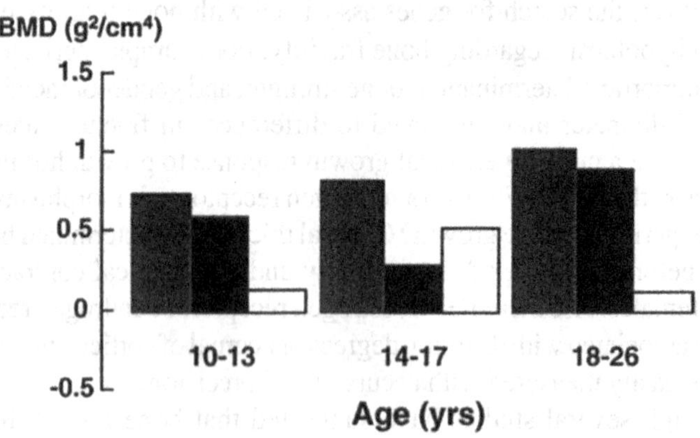

Fig. 6. Total variance (grey bars) in areal bone mineral density (BMD) at the femoral neck is largely accounted for by genetic variance (black bars). In twins aged 13–17 yr, there was a significant common environmental component of variance (white bars). (Adapted with permission from ref. *68*.)

in areal BMD, but a large common environmental component of variance was identified at the forearm *(69)*. The factors responsible for the differences in the size of the variance and the genetic and environmental components are unknown.

In a study in adult twins, total variance ($g^2/cm^4 \times 10^4$) was lower at the femoral neck than lumbar spine (Fig. 8) *(70)*. For femoral neck areal BMD, the genetic variance was 108 after adjusting for age alone (black bars) or 63% of the total variance (108 + 64 = 172). After adjusting for age and lean mass the genetic variance decreased by 16% from 108 to 92 (gray bars) but the common environmental variance remained unchanged. At the lumbar spine, the additive genetic variance was 200, about twice that observed at the femoral sites. Adjusting for lean mass reduced the additive genetic variance by only 2%. Thus, areal BMD is associated with lean mass, the more so at the femoral sites. A reduction in variance of proximal femoral areal BMD, but not spine areal BMD, after adjusting for lean mass suggests that exercise may be important at the former site. If this was the case, however, then the fall in variance on adjusting for lean mass should have been in the environmental component (although one cannot exclude the possibility that genetic factors also explain variation in exercise). The fall in the genetic component suggests that there are genetic determinants of both areal BMD and lean mass. That is, there are genes that influence variation in both areal BMD and lean mass.

To explore this possibility we studied 56 monozygotic (MZ) and 56 dizygotic (DZ) female twin pairs, mean age 45 yr (range 24–67), same-trait correlations in MZ pairs were double those in DZ pairs for femoral neck areal BMD (0.62 vs 0.33) and lean mass (0.87 vs 0.30; all $P < 0.001$). Areal BMD and lean mass correlate in the same individual, i.e., in self ($r = 0.43$). In MZ pairs the age-

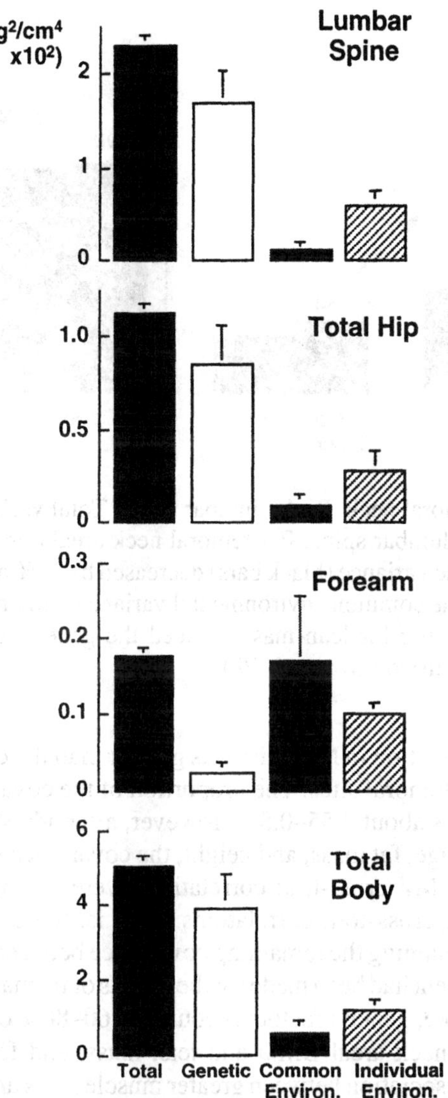

Fig. 7. Total variance (black bars) and its components; genetic (white bars), common environmental (gray bars) and individual environmental (hatched bars). Genetic variance in elderly twins accounts for most of the total variance in areal BMD, but a large common environmental component was identified at the forearm. (Adapted with permission from ref. *69*.)

adjusted areal BMD of one twin correlated with the age-adjusted lean mass of the other ($r = 0.31$ in MZ pairs, i.e., approx 75% of the cross-trait correlation in self, and almost double that in the DZ pairs ($r = 0.19$). When adjusting for age alone,

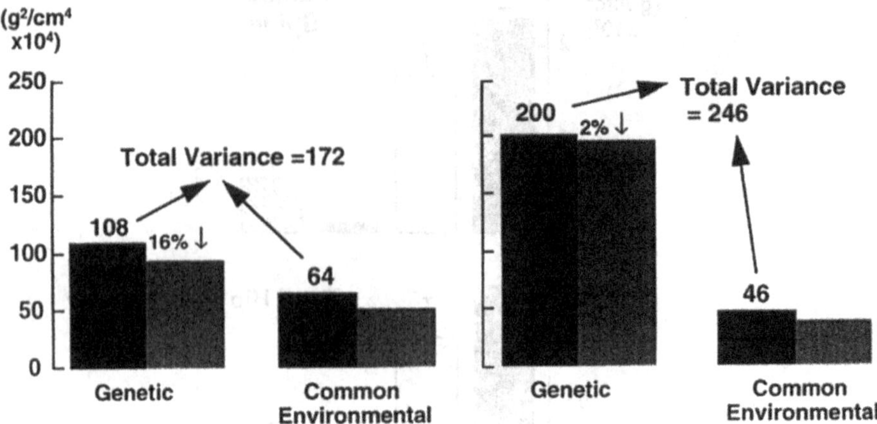

Fig. 8. Left, femoral neck. Right, lumbar spine. Total variance was lower at the femoral neck than lumbar spine. For femoral neck areal bone mineral density, the age-adjusted genetic variance (black bars) decreased by 16% after adjusting for lean mass (gray bars); the common environmental variance remained unchanged. At the lumbar spine adjusting for lean mass reduced the genetic variance by only 2%. (Adapted with permission from ref. *70*.)

the cross-trait correlation in MZ pairs was greater than the cross-trait correlation in DZ pairs at the femoral sites. The proportion of the covariance attributable to genetic factors, was about 0.55–0.85. However, after adjusting both areal BMD and lean mass for age, fat mass, and height, the covariance was reduced by more than half, and the MZ cross-trait correlations were no longer different to the corresponding DZ cross-trait correlations. That is, there was no evidence for genetic factors explaining the remaining covariance between areal BMD and lean mass once adjustment had been made for the effects of fat mass and height on these two traits. Therefore, genetic factors account for 60–80% of the individual variances of femoral neck areal BMD and lean mass, and for over 50% of their covariance. The association between greater muscle mass and greater areal BMD is likely to be determined by genes regulating size.

Using the Twin Model to Control for Genes and Measure Environmental Exposure

It may be difficult to detect the contribution of an environmental factor in explaining the variance in areal BMD or in a specific skeletal structure given that:

1. Genetic differences within the population result in a large amount of trait variation across the population,
2. The level of exposure (i.e., "dose") to an environmental factor is difficult to measure,

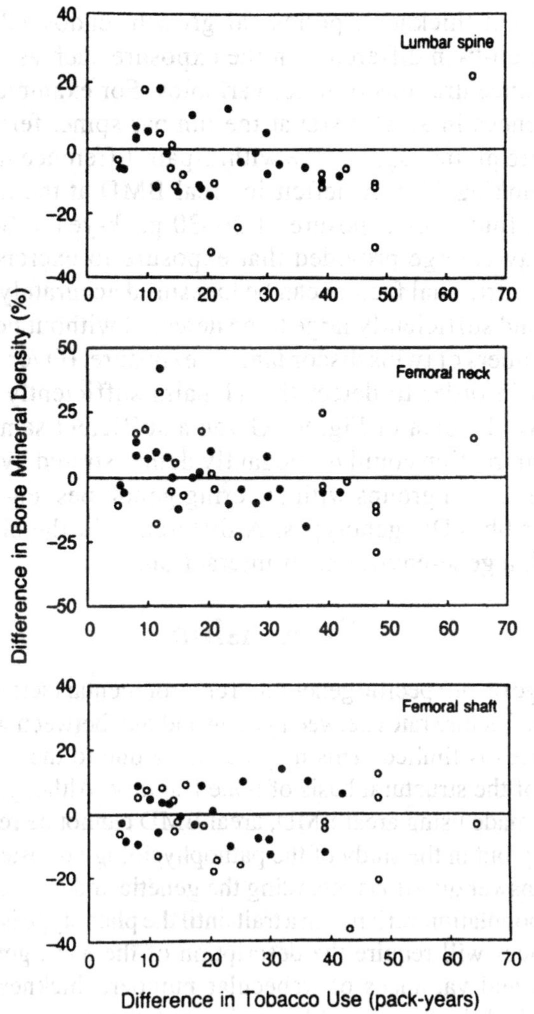

Fig. 9. The co-twin difference (greater minus lesser smoker) in areal bone density expressed as a percentage vs the co-twin difference in pack-years of exposure for the lumbar spine, femoral neck, and femoral shaft. Monozygotic twins (closed circles) and dizygotic twins (open circles).

3. The effects of the environmental factor may be small and difficult to measure, yet important if the exposure is common.

Greater insight into the effect of an environmental factor can be obtained by controlling for genetic variation by using the co-twin control design, plotting the dependent variable — the co-twin difference in areal BMD, and preferably more specific the structural endpoints such as bone size, trabecular number, thickness, cortical thickness, periosteal growth, endosteal growth—as a function of the co-twin difference in the exposure such as calcium intake, sex hormone concentrations or other variables. For example, in Fig. 9, the co-twin differences in areal BMD at the lumbar spine, femoral neck, and femoral shaft are plotted against the within-pair difference in pack-years of exposure to smoking *(71)*. A deficit in areal BMD at the lumbar spine of about 9 % was found for exposure of 20–30 pack-years. Some important information may emerge provided that exposure to exercise, dietary calcium, or other nutritional factors can be measured accurately, and the effect is cumulative and sufficiently large to be detected without needing prohibitively large numbers of twins discordant for exposure. (Over 1000 twin pairs were surveyed in order to detect the 41 pairs sufficiently discordant for smoking to give the data of Fig. 9.) Given a sufficient sample size, gene-environment interaction could be elegantly demonstrated by comparing the co-twin differences in groups with differing genotypes; e.g., subjects with the BB, Bb, or bb VDR genotypes. A difference in the slopes would be consistent with a gene-environment interaction.

Conclusion

Knowledge of the specific genetic and environmental factors that contribute to differences in fracture rates between young and old, between women and men, and between races is limited. This may be partly due to the lack of a detailed understanding of the structural basis of bone fragility. Although some progress may have been made using areal BMD, areal BMD cannot be relied upon as the phenotypic endpoint in the study of the pathophysiology of osteoporosis. It will be difficult to answer questions regarding the genetic and environmental factors explaining the population variance in a trait until the phenotype is unambiguously defined. Advances will require the description of the age-, gender-, and race-specific means and variances of trabecular number, thickness, spacing, and orientation, cortical thickness, and bone size and shape in women and men of different racial groups. The purported genetic and modifiable environmental determinants hypothesized to explain the variances can then be investigated to determine whether these factors partly account for gender and racial differences in fracture rates.

References

1. Melton, L. J. III, Atkinson, E. J., and Madhok, R. (1996) Downturn in hip fracture incidence. *Public Health Rep.* **111,** 146–150.
2. Gullberg, B., Johnell, O., and Kanis, J. A. (1997) World-wide projections for hip fracture. *Osteoporosis Int.* **7,** 407–413.
3. Seeman, E. (1997) From density to structure: growing up and growing old on the surfaces of bone. *J. Bone Miner. Res.* **12(4),** 1–13.

4. Lu, P. W., Cowell, C. T., Lloyd-Jones, S. A., Brody, J. N., and Howman-Giles, R. (1996) Volumetric bone mineral density in normal subjects aged 5–27 years. *J. Clin. Endocrinol. Metab.* **81,** 1586–1590.
5. Garn, S. M. (1970) *The Earlier Gain and Later Loss of Cortical Bone.* Charles C. Thomas Publishers, Springfield, IL.
6. Bass, S., Pearce, G., and Seeman, E. Regional heterogeneity in growth of the axial and appendicular bone mass, bone size and bone density: implications regarding the pathogenesis and epidemiology of fractures (submitted).
7. Seeman, E., Tsalamandris, C., Formica, C., Hopper, J. L., and McKay, J. (1994) Reduced femoral neck bone density in the daughters of women with hip fractures: the role of low peak bone density in the patho-genesis of osteoporosis. *J. Bone Miner. Res.* **9,** 739–743.
8. Hopper, J. L. (1993) Variance components for statistical genetics: applications in medical research to characteristics related to human diseases and health. *Stat. Methods Med. Res.* **2,** 199–223.
9. Seeman, E., Hopper, J., Bach, L., Cooper, M., McKay, J., and Jerums, G. (1989) Reduced bone mass in the daughters of women with osteoporosis. *N. Engl. J. Med.* **320,** 554–558.
10. Gilsanz, V., Loro, M. L., Roe, T. F., Sayre, J., Gilsanz, R., and Schulz, E. E. (1995) Gender differences in vertebral size in adults: biomechanical implications. *J. Clin. Invest.* **95,** 2332–2337.
11. Vega, E., Ghiringhelli, G., Mautalen, C., Valzacchi, G. Rey, Scaglia, H., and Zylberstein, C. (1998) Bone mineral density and bone size in men with primary osteoporosis and vertebral fractures. *Calcif. Tissue Int.* **62,** 465–469.
12. Duan, Y. and Seeman, E. The differing contributions of bone mass and size to the deficit in volumetric bone density in men and women with spinal or hip fractures (submitted).
13. Kelly, P. J., Twomey, L., Sambrook, P. N., and Eisman, J. A. (1990) Sex differences in peak adult bone mineral density. *J. Bone Miner. Res.* **5,** 1169–1175.
14. Aaron, J. E., Makins, N. B., and Sagreiy, K. (1987) The microanatomy of trabecular bone loss in normal aging men and women. *Clin. Orthop.* **215,** 260–271.
15. Zamberlan, N., Radetti, G., Paganini, C., Gatti, D., Rossini, M., Braga, V., and Adami, S. (1996) Evaluation of cortical thickness and bone density by roentgen microdensitometry in growing males and females. *Eur. J. Pediatr.* **155,** 377–382.
16. Butz, S., Wuster, C., Scheidt-Nave, C., Gotz, M., and Ziegler, R. (1994) Forearm BMD as measured by peripheral quantitative computed tomography (pQCT) in a German reference population. *Osteoporosis Int.* **4,** 179–184.
17. Zanchetta, J. R., Plotkin, H., and Alvarez Filgueira, M. L. (1995) Bone mass in children: normative values for the 2–20-year-old population. *Bone* **16(Suppl),** 393–399S.
18. Garn, S. M., Nagy, J. M., and Sandusky, S. T. (1972) Differential sexual dimorphism in bone diameters of subjects of European and African ancestry. *Am. J. Phys. Anthrop.* **37,** 127–130.
19. Rupich, R. C., Specker, B. L., Lieuw-A-Fa, M., and Ho, M. (1996) Gender and race differences in bone mass during infancy. *Calcif. Tissue Int.* **58,** 395–397.
20. Preece, M. A. (1981)The development of skeletal sex differences at adolescence, in: *Human Adaptation*, vol. 2 (Russo, P. and Gass, G., eds.), Department of Biological Sciences Conference, Cumberland College of Health Sciences, Sydney, Australia, pp. 1–13.
21. Preece, M. A., Pan, H., and Ratcliffe, S. G. (1992) Auxological aspects of male and female puberty. *Acta. Paediatr.* **383,** 11–13.

22. Zhang, X. Z., Kalu, D. N., Erbas, B., Hopper, J. L., and Seeman, E. (1999) The effect of gonadectomy on bone Size, mass and volumetric density in growing rats may be gender-, site-, and growth hormone-dependent. *J. Bone Miner. Res.* **14,** 802–809.
23. Kleerekoper, M., Nelson, D. A., Peterson, E. L., Flynn, M. J., Pawluszka, A. S., Jacobsen, G., and Wilson, P. (1994) Reference data for bone mass, calciotropic hormones, and biochemical markers of bone remodeling in older (55–75) postmenopausal white and black women. *J. Bone Miner. Res.* **9,** 1267–1276.
24. Davis, J. W., Novotny, R., Ross, P. D., and Wasnich, R. D. (1994) The peak bone mass of Hawaiian, Filipino, Japanese, and white women living in Hawaii. *Calcif. Tissue Int.* **55,** 249–252.
25. Bell, N. H., Gordon, L., Stevens, J., and Shary, J. R. (1995) Demonstration that bone mineral density of the lumbar spine, trochanter, and femoral neck is higher in black than in white young men. *Calcif. Tissue Int.* **56,** 11–13.
26. Wright, N. M., Papadea, N., Willi, S., Veldhuis, J. D., Pandey, J. P., Key, L. L., and Bell, N. H. (1996) Demonstration of a lack of racial difference in secretion of growth hormone despite a racial difference in bone mineral density in premenopausal women: a clinical research center study. *J. Clin. Endocrinol. Metab.* **81,** 1023–1026.
27. Ettinger, B., Sidney, S., Cummings, S. R., Libanati, C., Bikle, D. D., Tekawa, I. S., Tolan, K., and Steiger, P. (1997) Racial differences in bone density between young adult black and white subjects persist after adjustment for anthropometric, lifestyle, and biochemical differences. *J. Clin. Endocrinol. Metab.* **82,** 429–434.
28. Daniels, E. D., Pettifor, J. M., Schnitzler, C. M., Moodley, G. P., and Zachen, D. (1997) Differences in mineral homeostasis, volumetric bone mass and femoral neck axis length in black and white South African women. *Osteoporosis Int.* **7,** 105–112.
29. Nelson, D. A., Jacobsen, G., Barondess, D. A., and Parfitt, A. M. (1995) Ethnic differences in regional bone density, hip axis length, and lifestyle variables among healthy black and white men. *J. Bone Miner. Res.* **10,** 782–787.
30. Ross, P. D., He, Y.-F, Yates, A. J., Couland, C., Ravn, P., McClung, M., Thompson, D., Wasnich, R. D., for the EPIC Study Group. (1996) Body size accounts for most differences in bone density between Asian and Caucasian women. *Calcif. Tissue Int.* **59,** 339–343.
31. Hamill, P. V. V., Johnston, F. E., and Lemeshow, S. (1973) Body weight, stature and sitting height: white and Negro youths 12–17 years. DHEW Publications No. (HRA) 74–1608. Vital and Health Statistics, Series 11, No. 126. (US Department of Health, Education and Welfare, Rockville, MD) .
32. Malina, R. M. and Brown, K. H. (1987) Relative lower extremity length in Mexican American and in American black and white youth. *Am. J. Phys. Anthropol.* **72,** 89–94.
33. Tanner, J. M., Hayashi, T., Preece, M. A., and Cameron, N. (1982) Increase in length of leg relative to trunk in Japanese children and adults from 1957 to 1977: comparison with British and with Japanese Americans. *Ann. Human Biol.* **9,** 411–423.
34. Cameron, N., Tanner, J. M., and Whitehouse, R. H. (1982) A longitudinal analysis of the growth of limb segments in adolescence. *Ann. Human Biol.* **9,** 211–220.
35. Garn, S. M., Sandusky, S. T., Nagy, J. M., and McCann, M. B. (1972) Advanced skeletal development in low-income negro children. *J. Paediatr.* **80,** 965–969.
36. Bakwin, H. (1964) Secular increase in height: Is the end in sight? *Lancet* **2,** 1195–1196.
37. Meredith, H. V. (1978) Secular change in sitting height and lower limb height of children, youths, and young adults of Afro-black, European, and Japanese ancestry. *Growth* **42,** 37–41.

38. Tanner, J. M., Hayashi, T., Preece, M. A., and Cameron, N. (1982) Increase in length of leg relative to trunk in Japanese children and adults from 1957 to 1977: comparison with British and with Japanese Americans. *Ann. Human Biol.* **9(5),** 411–423.
39. Han, Z.-H., Palnitkar, S., Rao, D. S., Nelso, D., and Parfitt, A. M. (1996) Effect of ethnicity and age or menopause on the structure and geometry of iliac bone. *J. Bone Miner. Res.* **11,** 1967–1975.
40. Schnitzler, C. M., Pettifor, J. M., Mesquita, J. M., Bird, M. D. T., Schnaid, E., and Smith, A. E. (1990) Histomorphometry of iliac creast bone in 346 normal black and white South African adults. *Bone Miner.* **10,** 183–199.
41. Weinstein, R. S. and Bell, N. H. (1988) Diminished rates of bone formation in normal black adults. *N. Engl. J. Med.* **319,** 1698–1701.
42. Parisien, M., Cosman, F., Morgan, D., Schnitzer, M., Liang, X., Nieves, J., Forese, L., Luckey, M., Meier, D., Shen, V., Lindsay, R., and Dempster, D. W. (1997) Histomorphometric assessment of bone mass, structure, and remodeling: a comparison between healthy black and white premenopausal women. *J. Bone Miner. Res.* **12,** 948–957.
43. Meunier and Boivin. (1997) Bone mineral density reflects bone mass but also the degree of mineralization of bone: therapeutic implications. *Bone* **21**, 373–377.
44. Harris, S. S., Eccleshall, T. R., Gross, C., Dawson–Hughes, B., and Feldman, D. (1997) The vitamin D receptor start codon polymorphism (FokI) and bone mineral density in premenopausal American black and white women. *J. Bone Miner. Res.* **12,** 1043–1048.
45. Rosen, C. J., Dimai, H. P., Vereault, D., Donahue, L. R., Beamer, W. G., Farley, J., Linkhart, S., Linkhart, T., Mohan, S., and Baylink, D. J. (1997) Circulating and skeletal insulin–like growth factor–I (IGF–I) concentrations in two inbred strains of mice with different bone mineral densities. *Bone* **21,** 217–223.
46. Flicker, L., Faulkner, K. G., Hopper, J. L., Green, R. M., Kaymakci, B., Nowson, C. A., Young, D., and Wark, J. D. (1996) Determinants of hip axis length in women aged 10–89 years: a twin study. *Bone* **18,** 41–45.
47. Slemenda, C. W., Turner, C. H., Peacock, M., Christian, J. C., Sorbel, J., Hui, S. L., and Johnston, C. C. (1996) The genetics of proximal femur geometry, distribution of bone mass and bone mineral density. *Osteoporosis Int.* **6,** 178–182.
48. Arden, N. K., Baker, J., Hogg, C., Baan, K., and Spector, T. D. (1996) The heritability of bone mineral density, ultrasound of the calcaneus and hip axis length: a study of postmenopausal twins. *J. Bone Miner. Res.* **11,** 530–534.
49. Faulkner, K. G., Cummings, S. R., Black, D., Palermo, L., Gluer, C. C., and Genant, H. K. (1993) Simple measurement of femoral geometry predicts hip fracture in the study of osteoporotic fractures. *J. Bone Miner. Res.* **8,** 1211–1217.
50. Boonen, S., Koutri, R., Dequeker, J., Aerssens, J., Lowet, G., Nijs, J., Verbeke, G., Lesaffre, E., and Geusens, P. (1995) Measurement of femoral geometry in type I and type II osteoporosis: differences in hip axis length consistent with heterogeneity in the pathogenesis of osteoporotic fractures. *J. Bone Miner. Res.* **10,** 1908–1912.
51. Cummings, S. R., Cauley, J. A., Palermo, L., Ross, P. D., Wasnich, R. D., Black, D., and Faulkner, K. G. (1994) Racial differences in hip axis lengths might explain racial differences in rates of hip fracture. *Osteoporosis Int.* **4,** 226–229.
52. Mikhail, M. B., Vaswani, A. N., and Aloia, J. F. (1996) Racial differences in femoral dimensions and their relationship to hip fractures *Osteoporosis Int.* **6,** 22–24.
53. Nakamura, T., Turner, C. H., Yoshikawa, T., Slemenda, C. W., Peacock, M., Burr, D. B., Mizuno, Y., Orimo, H., Ouchi, Y., and Johnston, C. C., Jr. (1994) Do varia-

tions in hip geometry explain differences in hip fracture risk between Japanese and white Americans? *J. Bone Miner. Res.* **9,** 1071–1076.
54. Chin, K., Evans, M. C., Cornish, J., Cundy, T., and Reid, I. R. (1997) Differences in hip axis and femoral neck length in premenopausal women of Polynesian, Asian and European origin. *Osteoporosis Int.* **7,** 344–347.
55. Reid, I. R., Chin, K., Evans, M. C., and Jones, J. G. (1994) Relation between increase in length of hip axis in older women between 1950s and 1990s and increase in age specific rates of hip fracture. *Br. Med. J.* **309,** 508–509.
56. Ravn, P., Hetland, M. L., Overgaard, K., and Christiansen, C. (1994) Premenopausal and postmenopausal changes in bone mineral density of the proximal femur measured by dual-energy X-ray absorptiometry. *J. Bone Miner. Res.* **9,** 1975–1980.
57. Tsai, K. S., Cheng, W. C., Sanchez, T. V., Chen, C. K., Chieng, P. U., and Yang, R. S. (1997) Bone densitometry of proximal femur in Chinese subjects: gender differences in bone mass and bone areas. *Bone* **20,** 365–369.
58. Kuiper, J. W., van Kuijk, C., Grashuis, J. L., Ederveen, A. G. H., and Schotte, H. E. (1996) Accuracy and the influence of marrow fat on quantitative CT and dual-energy X-rayabsorptiometry measurements of the femoral neck in vitro. *Osteoporosis Int.* **6,** 25–30.
59. Looker, A. C., Wahner, H. W., Dunn, W. L., Calvo, M. S., Harris, T. B., Heyse, S. P., Johnston, C. C., Jr., and Lindsay, R. L. (1995) Proximal femur bone mineral levels of US adults. *Osteoporosis Int.* **5,** 389–409.
60. Ruff, C. B. and Hayes, W. C. (1988) Sex differences in age–related remodeling of the femur and tibia. *J. Orthop. Res.* **6,** 886–896.
61. Heaney, R. P., Barger-Lux, M. J., Davies, K. M., Ryan, R. A., Johnson, M. L., and Gong, G. (1997) Bone dimensional change with age: interactions of genetic, hormonal, and body size variables. *Osteoporosis Int.* **7,** 426–431.
62. Ensrud, K. E., Palermo, L., Black, D. M., Cauley, J., Jergas, M., Orwoll, E. S., Nevitt, M. C., Fox, K. M., and Cummings, S. R. (1995) Hip and calcaneal bone loss increase with advancing age: longitudinal results from the study of osteoporotic fractures. *J. Bone Miner. Res.* **10,** 1778–1787.
63. Greenspan, S. L., Maitland, L. A., Myers, E. R., Krasnow, M. B., and Kido, T. H. (1994) Femoral bone loss progresses with age: a longitudinal study in women over age 65. *J. Bone Miner. Res.* **9,** 1959–1965.
64. Jilka, R. L., Weinstein, R. S., Takahashi, K., Parfitt, A. M., and Manolagas, S. C. (1996) Linkage of decreased bone mass with impaired osteoblastogenesis in a murine model of accelerated senescence. *J. Clin. Invest.* **97,** 1732–1740.
65. Bergman, R. J., Gazit, D., Kahn, A. J., Gruber, H., McDougall, S., and Hahn, T. J. (1996) Age-related changes in osteogenic stem cells in mice. *J. Bone Miner. Res.* **11,** 568–577.
66. Eisman, J. A. (1995) Vitamin D receptor gene alleles and osteoporosis: an affirmative view. *J. Bone Miner. Res.* **10,** 1289–1293.
67. Peacock, M. (1995) Vitamin D receptor gene alleles and osteoporosis: a contrasting view. *J. Bone Miner. Res.* **10,** 1294–1297.
68. Hopper, J. L., Green, R. M., Nowsen, C. A., Young, D., Sherwin, J., Kaymacki, B., Larkins, R. G., and Wark, J. D. (1998) Genetic, common environment and individual specific components of variance for age- and lean-mass adjusted bone mineral density in 10 to 26 year old females: a twin study. *Am. J. Epidemiol.* **147,** 17–29.
69. Flicker, L., Hopper, J. L., Rodgers, L., Kaymakci, B., Green, R. M., and Wark, J. D. (1995) Bone density determinants in elderly women: a twin study. *J. Bone Miner. Res.* **10,** 1607–1613.

70. Seeman, E., Hopper, J. L., Young, N. R., Formica, C., Goss, P., and Tsalamandris, C. (1996) Do genetic factors contribute to associations between muscle strength, fat-free mass and bone density? A twin study. *Am. J. Physiol.* **270 (33),** E320–E327.
71. Hopper, J. L. and Seeman, E. (1994) Bone density in twins discordant for tobacco use. *N. Engl. J. Med.* **330,** 387–392.

CHAPTER 2

How to Determine If, and by How Much, Genetic Variation Influences Osteoporosis

John L. Hopper

Genetic Variation: Within and Between Populations

Discussion of nature vs nurture, or "genes vs environment," is often obscured by a failure to understand that what is being considered is the *variation* in genetic make-up of individuals, and how it relates to differences between them in the characteristic or trait of interest. Therefore, a clear distinction needs to be made between genetic differences *within* a population, and genetic differences *between* populations (e.g., between different races, or between blacks and whites). For example, genetic factors may explain much of the difference in a characteristic between two racial groups, but within any such group, the variation may be entirely due to nongenetic factors. Consequently, discussion about the roles of genes and environment in explaining variation in a trait must depend on, first, whether one is considering within or between population comparisons.

Historically, discussion has been in terms of the *relative* roles of genetic and environmental factors in explaining trait variation across a given population, as reflected by the often cited but little understood concept of heritability (see below). However, in order to understand and quantify properly the impact of genetic factors, the critical concept is not the proportion but the *absolute* size of genetic variation. This is because the amounts of variation caused by genetic and nongenetic factors are not universal constants; rather, they can vary both within and across populations according to age, sex, lifestyle, and a multitude of factors that cannot be controlled for, at least not in studies of humans. It is easier to understand that there can be different environmental factors, but genetic factors also can be expressed at different stages of life, or only when the individual is subject to particular environmental challenges. The effect of genes may also depend on exposures or lifestyle, i.e., there may be gene-environment interactions or covariations. Consequently, the size of the genetic variance may differ for different populations and for subgroups within a population.

Therefore, if the ratio of genetic to total variance (heritability) differs between populations or subgroups, one cannot conclude that it is due to differences in the genetic component alone. There could be differences in the nongenetic component, or in both the genetic and the nongenetic components. That is, a trait does not have a unique "heritability"; its heritability may depend on the ethnicity and environmental milieu of the population, and also may differ according to the characteristics used to describe the average of the population under consideration (see the next two sections).

To Study the Causes of Variation, the Mean Must First Be Specified

One cannot define variation, let alone study its causes, without specifying the mean, or "expected value," of the trait in question. The mathematical definition of the variance of a trait is the sum, over all possible values the trait can take, of the squared deviation of each value from its mean, weighted by the probability of that value. That is, for a trait Y that can take at most a finite number of values, by definition:

$$\text{variance (Y)} = S\ (y_i - m)^2 p\ (y_i) \qquad (1)$$

where y_i represents an observed value of Y, $p(y_i)$ represents its probability, summation is over all possible values of i, and $m = \Sigma y_i p(y_i)$ is the mean. (For a continuously distributed trait, the summation is replaced by integration, and the probabilities by a probability density function.)

The term $(y_i{-}m)$ is called the residual of Y about its mean, for individual i. The residuals, not the trait values, are the focus of attention in analyses that aim to determine the role of genetic and environmental factors in explaining the causes of variation in a trait.

Suppose a trait varies, on average, according to factors such as age, sex, lifestyle, environmental exposures, body characteristics, and so forth. The variance of the residuals will then differ according to which of these factors are taken into account in specifying the trait mean, m.

In practice, the mean of a trait can be modeled in terms of the effects of measured factors. These are called "fixed effects." The remaining variation in residuals can then be modeled in terms of the effects of unmeasured factors (both genetic and environmental). These are called "random" effects. This statistical modeling process is a well-established application of linear regression and analysis of variance.

The random effects modeling of unmeasured factors must do more than take into account genetic factors as causes of similarities between blood relatives. It must also allow for environmental factors shared by relatives. The strength of these factors could depend on whether the relatives are currently living together—and if so, for how long and how intensely—and if not, how long since they cohabited, and how often they are in contact with one another.

If genetic factors cause variation in a trait, then genetically related individuals will be more similar. Just as the variance of trait residuals depends on which factors are used to model the trait mean, the covariance between two traits also depends on their trait means. For example, for discretely distributed traits Y_1 and Y_2, by definition:

$$\text{Covariance}(Y_1,Y_2) = \Sigma\,\Sigma\,(y_1 - m_1)\,(y_2 - m_2)p(y_1, y_2) \quad (2)$$

(Y_1 and Y_2 could be two realizations of the same trait, such as when they represent the trait values of the first- and second-born twins of a pair.) Here y_1 and y_j represent the observed values of Y_1 and Y_2, respectively, $p(y_i,y_j)$ represents the probability of the joint occurrence, $m_1 = \Sigma\, y_1 p(y_1)$ is the mean of Y_1 and $m_2 = \Sigma\, y_2 p(y_1)$ is the mean of Y_2, and the double summation is over all values of 1 and 2. The correlation is a measure of how similar traits are. It can take any value from –1 to 1, and is defined as

$$\text{Correlation}(Y_1,Y_2) = \text{covariance}(Y_1,Y_2) / [\text{variance}(Y_1)\ \text{variance}(Y_2)]^{1/2} \quad (3)$$

As discussed in a later section, the process of modeling unmeasured genes as random effects works by matching, for pairs of individuals, the similarity of their trait residuals against their genetic relatedness. The amount of variance in the residuals that can be explained by the covariance between relatives appearing to fit the pattern expected under a genetic model is called the genetic variance. If genetic factors are measured, and are modeled as fixed effects, the total variance will be reduced. This should result in a reduction in the genetic variance, provided the model of genetic and environmental causes of variation across the population, and of covariation within families, is a close approximation to reality.

An Example

When considering height, what factors determine variations in height from individual to individual; i.e., what are the "causes of variation"? The age and sex of an individual are of primary importance. Other critical factors might be nutrition—especially during early childhood—developmental diseases, and variables related to socioeconomic status and lifestyle, and these effects could be confounded with one another. Some of these factors, such as age and sex, and possibly even the occurrence of any developmental diseases, can be measured. Some can be assessed by a surrogate measure; e.g., socioeconomic status is often inferred from measures of income, occupation, and/or residential location. Others, such as childhood nutrition, can be very difficult to determine, yet may be quite similar in genetically related individuals such as siblings, especially twins, and even more especially, within monozygotic (MZ) twin pairs.

There are also genetic factors to consider. There may be (if not now, perhaps sometime in the near future) known genes for which different variants are predictors of height, in both the statistical and biological meaning of the word. There are likely to be, however, a large number of genetic loci involved in the expression of height. How are we to find out if such loci exist, given that they are as yet unidentified and therefore not measured?

First, we have to take into account the nongenetic, or environmental, risk factors. Those that are measured can be incorporated as fixed effects when modeling the mean. The residual height of an individual, after adjusting for age, sex, and any other relevant measured factors of that individual, becomes the focus of attention. It is the correlation or covariation between related individuals in these residuals that forms the basis of analyses that aim to determine the role of genetic and environmental factors in explaining the causes of variation in height. Note that if height was not adjusted for age, the residual variance would be larger, and relatives of the same or similar age (such as twins and siblings) would appear to be more strongly correlated. This could have a substantial effect on the outcome of genetic modeling.

Defining Osteoporosis: Fractures vs Risk Factors

Distinction needs to be made between a fracture (i.e., an event which is represented by a binary trait and can take only two possible values), and a risk factor for that event. The latter could include variables such as bone mineral density (BMD), bone geometry, propensity to fall, and so forth; *see* Chapter 1. These risk factors may also be binary variables (e.g., sex), but are more often scalar variables distributed along a continuum. Moreover, distinction must be made between fractures at different sites, and there is the possibility that different risk factors may be operating at different sites.

There are numerous risk factors for fractures, and these may be interrelated (i.e., correlated within a population). Depending on what factors are taken into account in specifying the mean of these risk factors, some genetic factors may cause variation, and some of the genes involved in causing variation in one risk factor may also cause variation in other risk factors.

The extent to which genes causing variation in a risk factor for fracture explain the incidence of fractures in the population will depend on: (1) The strength of association between the risk factor and fracture risk, and (2) The proportion of the population at different levels of genetic risk (allele frequencies). Therefore, although variation in a risk factor may be strongly genetically determined, it may have little consequence for the disease in question in terms of explaining cases, and why it runs in families. This latter issue will be quantified in a later section.

Making Inference about Possible Genetic Causes of Variation: Biometric Modeling of Twin and Family Data

In trying to infer a role for genes in causing variation, distinction must be made between whether genes are measured or not measured. As discussed earlier, the effect of measured genetic variation can be assessed by modeling the mean, while the effect of unmeasured genes can be assessed by modeling variation about the mean.

For the latter case, inference is made by developing models based on assumptions about the action of genes, and then testing the extent to which the data are compatible with the different models. This process has been referred to as biometric modeling. Note that biometric modeling cannot prove that genetic factors are causing variation, it can only be used to demonstrate that the data are consistent with one or more genetic causes of variation. It has very limited ability to discern how many genetic loci are involved *(1)*. Furthermore, the utility of this process depends critically on the extent to which the design, sample size, and methods of analysis allow the effects of nongenetic causes of variation to be discriminated from those of genetic causes.

Historically, biometric modeling has been focused on fitting more and more elaborate genetic models, trying to interpret variations from simple genetic descriptions in terms of sophisticated modes of action of the genes (e.g., sex-limited expression, or nonadditive effects such as dominance and epistasis). This process is unconvincing, however, to the skeptic.

It is important to realize that familial aggregation does not necessarily imply genetic causation. In theory, familial aggregation in a trait can always be fully explained by an environmental model, simply making the postulated effect of sharing the environment match the observed correlations. For example, monozygotic (MZ) twin pairs might be more similar for a trait than dizygotic (DZ) twin pairs simply because:

1. They live or lived more similar lifestyles, especially during their formative years;
2. They meet with each other more often; and/or
3. They are being or were treated more alike when children.

Similar arguments might explain why first-degree relatives are more similar for a trait than second-degree relatives, and so on. The extent to which this issue is important varies from trait to trait. For example, a large difference in sibling correlation for blood lead levels was observed between adolescent pairs living together ($r = 0.5$) and adult pairs living apart for 20 or more years ($r = 0.1$) *(2)*. On the other hand, for body mass index (BMI = weight/[height]^2) we observed a small decrease in the correlation, about 2,000 DZ pairs, from 0.6 for those who were cohabiting to 0.5 for those living apart (unpublished data). Moreover, that decrease occurred over an age range of less than 5 yr, suggesting that the effects of shared environment on BMI variation dissipate rapidly. For bone density, a similar rapid dissipation of the effects of shared adolescent environment appears to occur *(3)*.

Unfortunately, little attention has been placed on trying to disprove or falsify genetic hypotheses. On the other hand, classic biometric models make simplistic assumptions about the roles of nongenetic factors. Accordingly, only major and specific types of environmental effects can be detected by the statistical approaches typically used, and even then large samples are needed for there to be reasonable statistical power to detect such effects. Designs that allow for contrasts between the effects of shared genes and those of shared environments, measures of environmental exposure, and large data sets ascertained by unbiased sampling are needed if the modeling process is to have credibility in teasing apart the roles and genes from those of the environment. In practice, this is not easy to do and tends to have been the exception, rather than the rule *(4)* .

Genes Measured

Suppose a genetic marker, such as a polymorphism at a candidate gene hypothesized on biological grounds to be involved in the trait of interest, can be measured, and takes the values m_i, for i =1,…,n, say. To test that hypothesis, a simple test would be to select individuals of genotype m_j and compare their trait values against those of genotype m_k, for all pairs of j and k not equal to each other. If these individuals are unrelated, careful consideration needs to be given to how the subjects were sampled, and to the possibility that there could be other factors (such as race and ethnicity) associated with genotype at this marker, and with the trait itself. These are called "potential confounders." If all such potential confounders are known, and measured on all individuals, a statistical adjustment can be made for their effect(s) on the mean of the trait of interest using, e.g., linear regression techniques. In practice, one never knows all the confounders, and it is impossible to adjust for unmeasured or unknown confounders. In particular, care should be taken if the study sample contains different racial or ethnic groups. It is well known that these genetic association studies can give misleading conclusions due to such confounding, or population-stratification as it is referred to in the genetics literature.

Another approach is to select related individuals who differ in genotype. Dizygotic twin pairs of the same sex are perhaps the most useful design. Twins within a same-sex pair are perfectly matched for age and sex, typically among the most important determinants of the mean of a human characteristic. They are also matched, at least to some extent, for a range of nongenetic factors related to their shared environment during gestation and upbringing. Whereas the latter matching may reduce within-pair trait differences, with a consequent loss of statistical power to detect effects associated with the genotyping, it will not bias results if matching is taken into account in the analysis.

An appropriate method of statistical analysis would be to consider within-pair trait differences as a function of within-pair differences in genotype. If there are n different genotypes possible, there will be n(n–1)/2 combinations of differences between genotypes, and it is likely there may be some combinations with few or no pairs. Analyses that suggest differences between some combinations, but not others, are difficult to interpret.

Because each genotype is a combination of two alleles, one from the mother and the other from the father, it is useful to consider the within-pair difference in the number of shared alleles: it can take the values 0, 1, or 2. The first group of pairs, who are concordant for genotype, is uninformative for association studies, and can be excluded from the analysis. The within-pair trait differences of the second and third groups can each be compared with zero, using e.g., a paired Student's t-test, or with each other. Again, the analyses may be difficult to interpret if, e.g., pairs differing by one allele are different, but those differing by two are no different, or differ in the opposite direction.

It might make biological sense to presume that the within-pair trait difference increases linearly as the difference in the number of a certain disease allele (or subgroup of alleles) increases. The trait difference can then be modeled as a linear function of the difference in number of disease alleles, in which case it is presumed that pairs differing in both alleles are twice as different (and in the same direction!) as those differing by only one allele. Again, linear regression techniques can be used for the modeling, making sure that the line of best fit is constrained to pass through the origin. Care must be taken, however, if there are only a few pairs differing by two disease alleles, as they will have a strong influence on the fitted line. Robust regression methods designed to be insensitive to influential points should also be used. Remember that for these *association* studies, the dependent variable is the actual within-pair trait difference, not the absolute or squared difference. There is an implied order within members of a pair, which could be based on an exposure or covariate of interest *(5)*, or may be arbitrary. The independent variable is the ordered difference in the number of disease alleles, and can take the values –2, –1, 0, 1 or 2. The fitted lie should be constrained to pass through the origin; *see* Fig. 1. Note that pairs with the same number of disease alleles have no influence on this fitted line. They will, however, contribute information on the variation about the fitted line, and hence may improve statistical inference.

If multiple regression techniques are used, statistical adjustment for within-pair differences in other measured factors likely to explain trait variation—either genetic or environmental—can be made while concurrently estimating the effect, if any, of the measured genetic markers on the mean; i.e., estimating a genetic association *(6)* . The formula is:

$$\Delta Y = Y_1 - Y_2 = (m_1 - m_2) + (x_{11} - x_{12}) + \ldots = \Delta m + \Delta x_1 + \Delta x_2 + \ldots \quad (4)$$

where the x_{ij} are the observed values for trait i in twin j, $\Delta x_i = x_{i1} - x_{i2}$, and Δx_1 could be the difference in number of disease alleles at the genetic locus of interest.

Another way the effect of a measured genetic marker on a trait can be assessed is in terms of possible genetic linkage. This can be done by testing if related individuals who share 2 alleles are more similar for a trait (in the sense defined below) than those who share 1 allele, and if the latter are more similar than those who share 0 alleles. This is called identity-by-state *(6)*. The parents each

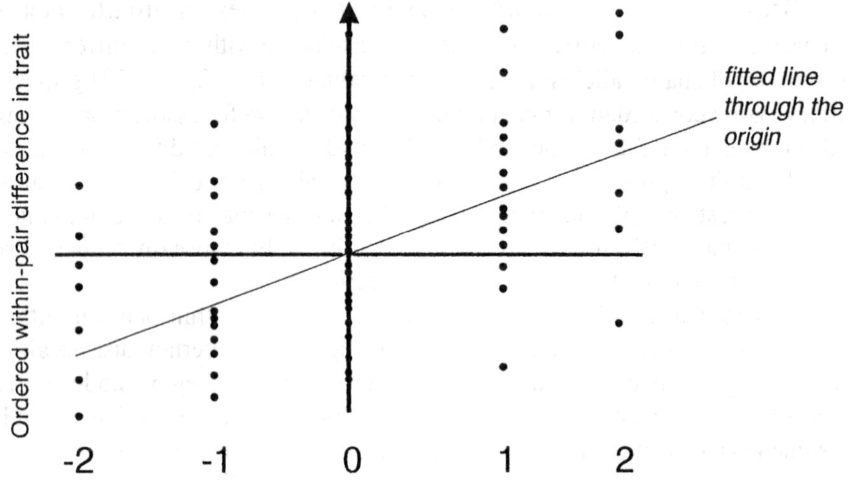

Fig. 1. Best-fitting straight line through the origin, for data from ordered twin pairs plotting their within-pair difference in the trait vs their within-pair difference in number of disease alleles.

have two alleles, although they may not be distinct, and each offspring inherits a copy of one allele from the father and one from the mother. Therefore two offspring can share exactly the same two alleles, just one of the alleles, or neither. This is referred to as identity-by-descent. To conduct an identity-by -decent analysis, parental genotypes must be known or inferred probabilistically. Analysis of whether similarity in such measures of identity at a locus predicts similarity in a trait can be incorporated using the method of analysis described in the next section *(7)*. For further discussion on aspects of genetic linkage *see* Chapter 20.

Genes Not Measured

In 1918, the Royal Society in Edinburgh published a seminal paper in the history of genetics and statistics *(8)*, written by the then 28-year-old Ronald Aylmer Fisher. (The paper had been rejected by the Royal Society in London 2 yr earlier.) Fisher derived the expected pattern of correlations one would observe in a trait if its variance (about its mean) was due to genetic variation at one or more loci, under the assumption that genetic status was transmitted from generation to generation under the rules of Mendelian inheritance. The paper itself is long and not easy, but the basic ideas have been summarized and interpreted many times *(9–13)*.

In brief, suppose the effect of alleles at each loci are additive and independent of one another, in that the trait mean for an individual who has two copies of an allele differs from that for an individual who has no copies of that allele by twice as much as for an individual who has one copy of the allele. Fisher showed that the correlation will be 0.5 between first-degree relatives, 0.25 between second-degree relatives, 0.125 between third-degree relatives, and so on. MZ twin pairs would be identical under this model which assumes additive genetic factors, A, only. There are, however, numerous prenatal factors that could cause MZ pairs to be less than identical for a given trait *(1)*.

Allowing then for nongenetic factors, E, which are assumed to be independent between relatives in the same family—such as random environmental effects and random measurement error—the correlation between MZ twins within a pair will be reduced depending on the relative amount of variation explained by E. That is, if the variance of A is σ_a^2 and that of E is σ_e^2, the MZ correlation will be $\sigma_a^2/(\sigma_a^2+\sigma_e^2) = \rho_{MZ}$. In this case, the correlation between first-, second-, and third-degree relatives will become 1/2 ρ_{MZ}, 1/2 ρ_{MZ}, and 1/8 ρ_{MZ}, and so on.

The model can be extended to allow for nongenetic factors shared by, or common to, members of the same family *(7,14)*. These cohabitation effects, C, that result from sharing or having shared a "common" environment, will result in a perturbation of the pattern of ratios above that should occur when genetic factors only are causing trait correlations. For example, if first-degree but not second-degree relatives share a common environment effect with variance σ_c^2, the ratio of first- to second-degree trait correlations will be greater than 2:1.

Fisher allowed for nonadditive effects at a genetic locus (i.e., for the effect of having two alleles to differ from twice the effect of having one allele), and in doing so introduced the concept of dominance variance, σ_d^2. If there are such nonadditive effects within one or more loci, the MZ pair and sibling correlations will be differentially increased relative to correlations between other pairs of relatives. Fisher also derived the expected correlations under other forms of genetic nonadditivity, such as interactions between the effects of alleles at different loci. There is strong confounding, however, between additive and nonadditive components of variance, and dominance components can mimic common environment effects *(7)*.

Whereas there is a theoretical basis on which genetic models can be based, cohabitation or common environment effects can take virtually any structure. Some examples of plausible models have been derived and fitted *(2,7,13)*. In practice, however, it is very difficult to clearly distinguish the effects of shared genes from those of shared environment. Designs which have the potential to overcome this problem include those using twins reared apart, adoptees and their biological and adopted families, and migrant and nonmigrant families.

The classic twin model purports to allow estimation of the effects of shared genes and shared environment, but does so only by making the very strong assumption that the effects on the trait in question of sharing environment are the same for MZ pairs as they are for DZ pairs. This assumption is difficult to test using twin data alone, unless detailed information is collected on the amount and extent of cohabitation that has or is occurring within the pairs *(15)*. Also, the modeling process is biased toward concluding that genetic factors alone are causing twin correlations *(4)*. Large sample sizes are needed to detect even modest proportions of variance attributable to σ_c^2, the variance attributable to shared, or common environments during or as a result of cohabitation *(16)*. Nevertheless, application to adolescent and young adult female twins has suggested plausible cohabitation effects on bone mineral density, at the spine and the hip, that abate rapidly as the twins begin to live apart *(3)*.

Fisher's theory is best expressed in terms of variance components. For example, suppose a model allows for additive genetic effects, and for a zygosity-independent effect of common environment as in the classic twin model. For a given trait mean, the (residual) variance can be expressed as the sum of variance components $\sigma_a^2 + \sigma_c^2 + \sigma_e^2 = \sigma^2$. The covariance between a pair of relatives will be: $\sigma_a^2 + \sigma_c^2$ for MZ pairs; $1/2\, \sigma_a^2 + \sigma_c^2$ for DZ pairs; $1/4\, \sigma_a^2$ for parent-offspring pairs, and for non-twin sibling pairs; $1/4\, \sigma_a^2$ for second-degree pairs, etc.

Note that the effects of measured genes can be incorporated either in modeling the mean, as fixed effects, or as random effects by including additional component(s) of variance. For example, the covariance between a pair of individuals could be modeled as σ_M^2 if they share two alleles (IBD), or $1/2\, \sigma_M^2$ if they share one allele (IBD) *(7)*. That is, detection of "quantitative trait loci" by variance components modeling can be carried out within the usual framework for fitting genetic and environmental models.

If the variance, σ^2, is the same for all individuals, the difference between the MZ and DZ pair correlations, ρ_{MZ} and ρ_{DZ} respectively, will be $1/2\, \sigma_a^2/\sigma^2$. This has led historically to the simplistic formula: $2(\rho_{MZ} - \rho_{DZ}) = \sigma_a^2/\sigma^2$. The latter term is referred to as the narrow-sense heritability, the proportion of variance attributed to additive genetic factors. This formula is problematic, if only because values greater than unity can occur (i.e., it could lead to the implausible conclusion that more than 100% of the variance is attributable to heritable factors).

The statistical fitting of genetic and environmental models has changed considerably over the last few decades due principally to improvements in computational resources. The underpinning of the statistical approaches, however, is in likelihood theory derived by the young Fisher way back in 1912. They almost always rely on the assumption that families have been sampled at random. This is, of course, not usually true, but small sampling biases may not have a major effect on results. Sampling through related traits, however, can have a major impact. Methods for adjusting for some forms of nonrandom ascertainment exist.

Either the raw data, or summary measures in terms of correlations between relative-pairs, are fitted to variance components or path analytic models. Statistical packages, such as FISHER *(17)* and M_X *(18)*, are available for analysis of continuous traits, and the latter handles categorical traits under some stringent assumptions; see the next section. Newer robust statistical methods have also been developed and compared *(19)*. Standard errors, confidence intervals, correlations between estimates based on large-sample theory are available. Some tests of lack of fit which generally have little power, yet are often mistakenly used to infer a "good fit", are also available with these packages.

It must not be forgotten, however, that no matter how sophisticated the modeling, how good the fit or how elegant the method of statistical analysis, a fitted model is just that. Especially when trying to make inference about unmeasured genes and unmeasured environmental factors, there may be many quite dissimilar models that provide equally good—or bad—descriptions of the data, and it is not possible to discriminate between them.

A significant genetic component of variance in the most parsimonious model does not prove that genes exist *(20)*. For example, although under the classic twin model MZ pairs will be more correlated than DZ pairs, finding that MZ pairs are more correlated does not prove that the classic twin model is correct! In the parlance of mathematical logic, that "statement A implies statement B" is true does not mean that "statement B implies statement A" is also true. If genetic factors exist (statement A), MZ pairs will be more correlated than DZ pairs (statement B). The observation of statement B, however, does not definitively prove the veracity of statement A.

Evidence for Genetic Variation Influencing Fractures

A fracture is an event that either happens or doesn't. Inference about the possible roles of genetic and environmental factors in explaining variation in binary traits (i.e., traits that divide individuals into two groups, such as affected versus unaffected) can be made by a similar approach to that outlined previously.

Association in a binary trait can be measured and modeled a number of ways, such as by a correlation coefficient, odds ratio, or tetrachoric correlation. The latter was first used in this context by Karl Pearson, around the start of the 20th century. It supposes that there is an underlying, normally distributed, but unmeasured "latent" trait. In medical applications, it is referred to as a "liability." For a given 2×2 table of association in a pair of individuals for the binary trait, a unique bivariate normal distribution of the latent liability trait can be derived, with appropriate cut-off points — one horizontal and one vertical — so that the proportion of the distribution in each of the four regions equals the observed numbers in the 2×2 table. The tetrachoric correlation is then defined as the correlation in the bivariate normal distribution that is needed to achieve this fit.

For whatever measure of association is used, its strength can be compared across different categories of relatives, and between cohabiting and noncohabiting pairs. The same issues discussed previously, to do with confounding and the ability of the design and sample size to discriminate between different models, apply. Typically, very large samples in the order of hundreds if not thousands of pairs are needed to have reasonable power.

The tetrachoric correlation modeling has become popular in some disciplines, perhaps because it allows calculation of heritability. There are many problems, however, with this approach. It presumes there is an underlying, but unmeasurable liability, that both predicts the binary trait status and is correlated in relatives. Inference is made about the proportion of variance in liability statistically attributed to genetic or nongenetic factors, along the same arguments as used for continuous traits in 5(ii) above. However, the strength of the quantitative estimates rely implicitly on the assumption that the liability distribution in families is multivariate normal, and it is often impossible to test this assumption, at least not with any substantial statistical power.

Furthermore, the heritability of liability is a difficult concept to understand intuitively . It is usually, and mistakenly, referred to as "heritability of the trait." When the trait is a disease state (affected vs unaffected), the slip is often made of interpreting heritability as the proportion of disease due to genetic factors, when in fact it is the proportion of the variance of liability that is due to genetic factors *(21)*. Unfortunately, judging by the frequency with which this false implication is made even in professional circles, this point is not well-appreciated.

Comparison of twin disease concordance between MZ pairs and DZ pairs is often used to infer a genetic aetiology for the disease in question, but again this inference is predicated by the strong shared environment assumption of the classic twin method.

There has been considerable confusion about the concepts of pairwise, casewise, and probandwise concordance. Pairwise concordance is the probability that a given twin is affected, given that at least one member of the pair is affected. The pairwise estimator is the number of pairs in which both twins are affected, divided by this number plus the number of discordant pairs. Casewise concordance is the probability that one twin is affected, given that the other is also. The casewise estimator is twice the number of pairs in which both are affected, divided by the twice the number of pairs in which both are affected plus the number of pairs in which twins are disease discordant. The decision of which concordance to work with depends on the question(s) being asked. For example, if as is the case in genetic counseling when one wants to predict a twin's disease status from knowledge of the other pair's status, the casewise concordance is indicated. On the other hand, if one is interested in predicting the pair disease status when all one knows is that at least one twin is affected, the pairwise concordance is indicated.

If twin pairs are sampled nonrandomly, e.g., because at least one of the pairs is known to be affected, proper adjustment must be made *(22)*. In this case, it is possible that a pair could be sampled because it is known that both members are affected; this is called a doubly-ascertained pair. It is also possible that a pair will be sampled because one particular member is known to be affected, but once the pair is sampled it is found out that the other twin is also affected; this is called a singly-ascertained pair. "Incomplete ascertainment" is said to occur if the probability of singly ascertained pairs is greater than zero. Otherwise, ascertainment is said to be "complete," although this expression can be confusing, because it does not necessarily mean that all pairs are sampled!

Although reference is often made in the twin literature to the "probandwise concordance rate," "probandwise concordance" actually refers to an estimator, not a concordance, and it certainly is not a rate. The probandwise estimator is defined as the ratio of a numerator to a denominator. The numerator is twice the number of pairs in which both twins are affected and doubly ascertained, plus the number of singly-ascertained pairs both affected. The denominator is equal to the numerator plus the number of disease discordant pairs.

The estimates and large sample standard errors for pairwise and casewise concordance have been derived, and the distinctions above between concordances and estimators clarified, using a likelihood theory approach *(22–23)*. For large samples and under random or complete ascertainment, the casewise estimator is unbiased for the casewise concordance, and the pairwise estimator is unbiased for the pairwise concordance. Under incomplete ascertainment, the casewise estimator is biased for the casewise concordance, and the pairwise estimator is biased for the pairwise concordance. The probandwise estimator, however, is unbiased for the casewise concordance.

Interpreting Genetic Variation in a Risk Factor in Terms of How Much Familial Aggregation in the Disease Is Explained

Finally the question arises: if genetic factors explain a proportion of variation in a risk factor, how much of the familial aggregation for the disease is explained by this source of genetic variation? To address this, suppose that X is a risk factor measured on a continuous scale. Suppose the conditional probability of being affected, p(x), given a value of the risk factor, x, can be represented by the linear logistic model

$$p(x) = \Pr(D = 1 \mid X = x) = \exp\{\alpha + \beta x\}/[1 + \exp\{\alpha + \beta x\}] \qquad (5)$$

where D = 1 signifies the disease is present, and the parameters α and β describe the dependence of the probability of disease on the observed value of X. Assume also, without loss of generality, that X has a standard normal distribution with mean 0 and variance 1, and that for a pair of related individuals, (X_1, X_2) has a bivariate normal distribution with correlation parameter ρ.

On a population-basis, the correlated risks within pairs of relatives translates into clustering of disease. A measure of disease association between relatives is the odds ratio, OR, the ratio of the odds of being affected when a relative is affected to that when the relative is unaffected. The value of OR depends on the correlation, ρ, and the strength of the risk factor on probability of disease. The latter is conveniently represented by the inter-quartile risk ratio, RR, which is the risk for individuals at the upper-quartile level of X divided by the risk for individuals at the lower-quartile level. Hopper and Carlin (*see* ref. *24)* give tables for these relationships.

Bone density at the hip is a risk factor for hip fractures that is itself correlated between first degree relatives. The correlation, ρ, is about 0.4, while the inter-quartile risk ratio, RR, is about 2.5. From Table 1 of Hopper and Carlin *(24)* this translates into an odds ratio, OR, of about 1.1. Given that the increased risk for a daughter consequent upon her mother having had hip fracture is roughly twofold, it is seen that whatever causes bone density at the hip to be correlated in first-degree relatives explains about 10% of familial aggregation for hip fractures. Simple twin models suggest that all of the familial aggregation for hip bone density in adult women is attributable to genetic factors.

Therefore, even if the heritability of hip bone density is 80%, the genes causing variation in hip bone density are not responsible for most of familial aggregation in hip fractures. Similar arguments apply to lumbar spine bone density and spinal fractures. Furthermore, genes involved in causing variation in other risk factors, such as hip axis length, may explain just as much familial aggregation in hip fractures *(25)*. Nevertheless, identifying genes that influence variation in bone density could have important implications for prevention and treatment, for example by providing molecular targets for altering bone density. Finding these genes may provide insight into molecular pathways that are important in regulating osteoclast or osteoblast activity, for example, and this knowledge could be used to manipulate the pathway so as to increase osteoblast activity without increasing bone resorption.

Summary

"Familial aggregation" is the tendency for a trait to be more similar, or positively correlated, in family members. This applies both to the occurrence of disease in an individual—often expressed as a binary trait representing the two states, being or not being affected—and to indices of morbidity and risk factors which are measured on continuums, often referred to as continuous traits. Depending on the strength of association between risk factors and disease, and on the strength of familial aggregation in the risk factors, this can result in familial aggregation in the disease itself. Therefore, familial aggregation in risk factors could in part explain why family history is a risk factor for osteoporosis. Knowing how genetic and environmental factors explain familial associations in risk factors will help understand the causes of osteoporosis.

A theory under which correlations between relatives in a continuous trait can be explained in terms of Mendelian inheritance at one or more genetic loci was published by R. A. Fisher in 1918. Application of this theory has since provided much insight into the design and analysis of studies to resolve the relative contributions of, and interactions between, genetic and environmental factors, and has identified the following statistical and design issues:

1. Prior to genetic and environmental modeling the data should be carefully explored, and relationships between trait mean and covariates examined. To be able to understand properly the genetic determinants of a trait, it is important to first account for the effects of major nongenetic determinants.

2. Descriptive measures of familial aggregation should be explored, and tendencies for the associations between individuals to vary according to the genetic or cohabitational relationship between individuals should be noted. Empirical evidence has shown that genetic and environmental factors can produce a variety of patterns among the trait correlations between pairs of individuals.
3. As mentioned previously, theory shows that if genetic factors determine variations in a continuous trait, certain patterns will be evident among the correlations between relatives. It is therefore possible, in a rigorous statistical manner, to test if observations from independent groups of related individuals are consistent with a proposed genetic model. Note, however, that this does not prove that genetic factors are a cause of variation, let alone the only cause of covariation within a family.
4. For there to be statistical power to discriminate between causes of familial aggregation, first the confounding between genetic and environmental factors needs to be addressed in the design of a study. Second, the sample sizes must be large enough for discrimination and precise estimation of different effects. Third, the families need to be sampled in an unbiased manner, or else a correct statistical adjustment for their ascertainment must be made.
5. Analytical methods should be able to incorporate measurements from covariates, which may include measured genetic markers, in addition to modeling unmeasured genetic and environmental sources of variation.
6. Fitting a model is not an end in itself. Biological and statistical assumptions underlying models should be addressed before and during the modeling process. Selection of a "best" model from among a range of alternatives, even if shown not to provide a bad fit to the data, does not prove that the components of that model are true causes of variation.
7. The genes involved in causing variation in bone density only partially explain the familial aggregation in fractures.

References

1. Martin, N., Boomsma, D., and Machin, G. (1997) A twin-pronged attack on complex traits. *Nat. Genet.* **17,** 387–392.
2. Hopper, J. L. and Mathews, J. D. (1983) Extensions to multivariate normal models for pedigree analysis. II. Modeling the effect of shared environment in the analysis of blood lead levels. *Am. J. Epidemiol.* **117,** 344–355.
3. Hopper, J. L., Green, R. M., Nowson, C. A., Young, D., Sherwin, A. J., Kaymakci, B., Larkins, R. G., and Wark, J. D. (1998) Genetic, common environment, and individual specific components of variance for bone mineral density in 10- to 26-year-old females, a twin study. *Am. J. Epidemiol.* **147,** 17–29.
4. Hopper, J. L. (1999) On why "common environment effects" are so uncommon in the literature, in *Advances in Twin Sub-Pair Analysis* (Spector, T., Sneider, H., and MacGregor, A. J., eds.), Greenwich Medical Media, London, pp. 15–165.
5. Hopper, J. L. and Seeman, E. (1994) The bone density of twins discordant for tobacco use. *N. Engl. J. Med.* **330,** 37–92.

6. Lange, K. (1997) *Mathematical and Statistical Methods for Genetic Analysis.* Springer, New York.
7. Hopper, J. L. and Mathews, J. D. (1982) Extensions to multivariate normal models for pedigree analysis. *Ann. Hum. Genet.* **46,** 373–383.
8. Fisher, R. A. (1918) Correlations between relatives on the supposition of Mendelian inheritance. *Trans. Roy. Soc. (Edinburgh)* **52,** 399–433.
9. Bulmer, M. G. (1980) *The Mathematical Theory of Quantitative Genetics.* Clarendon Press, Oxford, UK.
10. Falconer, D. S. (1989) *Introduction to Quantitative Genetics.* Wiley, New York.
11. Ewens, W. J. (1979) *Mathematical Population Genetics.* Springer-Verlag, Berlin, pp. 5–9.
12. Neale, M. C. and Cardon, L. R. (1992) *Methodology for Genetic Studies of Twins and Families.* Kluwer Academic Publishers, Dordrecht, The Netherlands.
13. Hopper, J. L. (1993) Variance components for statistical genetics, applications in medical research to characteristics related to human diseases and health. *Statist. Methods Med. Res.* **2,** 199–223.
14. Hopper, J. L. and Mathews, J. D. (1994) Amultivariate normal model for pedigreee and longitudinal data and the software FISHER. *Aust. J. Stat.* **36,** 153–176.
15. Clifford, C. A., Hopper, J. L., Fulker, D. W., and Murray, R. M. (1984) A genetic and environmental analysis of a twin family study of alcohol use, anxiety and depression. *Genet. Epidemiol.* **1,** 63–79.
16. Christian, J. C., Norton, J. A., Sorbel, J., and Williams, C. J. (1995) Comparison of analysis of of variance and maximum likelihood based path analysis of twin data, partitioning genetic and environmental sources of covariance. *Genet. Epidemiol.* **12,** 27–35.
17. Lange, K., Boehnke, M., and Weeks, D. (1987) Programs for pedigree analysis. Department of Biomathematics, University of California, Los Angeles, CA.
18. Neale, M. C. (1997) *M: Statistical Modeling.* 4th ed. Box 980126 MCV, Richmond, VA.
19. Huggins, R. M., Loesch, D. Z., and Hoang, N. H. (1998) A comparison of methods of fitting models to twin data. *Aust. N. Z. J. Stat.* **40,** 129–140.
20. Hopper, J. L. (1996) Commentary. Genes for osteoarthritis, interpreting twin studies. *Br. Med. J.* **312,** 943–944.
21. Hopper, J. L. (1998) Heritability, in *Encyclopedia of Biostatistics,* vol. 3, Wiley, London, pp. 1905–1906.
22. Hopper, J. L. (1998) Twin concordance, in *Encyclopedia of Biostatistics,* vol. 6, Wiley, London, pp. 4626–4629.
23. Witte, J., Carlin, J. B., and Hopper, J. L. (1999) A likelihood-based approach to estimating twin concordance for dichotomous traits. *Genet. Epidemiol.* **16,** 290–304.
24. Hopper, J. L. and Carlin, J. C. (1994) Familial aggregation of a disease consequent upon correlation between relatives in a risk factor measured on a continuous scale. *Am. J. Epidemiol.* **136,** 1138–47.
25. Flicker, L., Faulkner, K. G., Hopper, J. L., et al. (1996) Determinants of hip axis length in women aged 10–89 years, a twin study. *Bone* **18,** 41–45.

CHAPTER 3

Vitamin D Receptor Gene Polymorphisms and Bone Mineral Homeostasis

Serge Ferrari, René Rizzoli, and Jean-Philippe Bonjour

Introduction

Osteoporosis is a systemic skeletal disease characterized by a reduced bone mineral mass and a deterioration of bone tissue microarchitecture, with a consequent increased bone fragility and a higher risk of fracture *(1)*. The latter also depends on factors unrelated to bone mineral mass itself. In the search for "osteoporosis genes," it is important to keep in mind that bone mineral mass is a complex notion that may be variably appreciated by different techniques. Actually, various parts of the skeleton are characterized by different proportions of spongious and compact bone, and thereby by different turnover rates. Whole body bone mineral mass can be measured. For this purpose, a variety of techniques based on the attenuation by bony tissue of either a photon radiation (dual X-ray absorptiometry [DXA], single photon absorptiometry [SPA] or ultrasonic energy) have been used. X-ray attenuation-based methods provide information on bone mineral content (BMC, in grams of hydroxyapatite equivalent) and areal bone mineral density (aBMD, in grams of hydroxyapatite equivalent per unit of bone scanned area). The latter integrates the notion of bone mineral mass and an adjustment for outer bone dimensions as determined in a plan perpendicular to the radiation beam direction *(2)*. Besides, volumetric bone mineral density (grams per cubic square of bone tissue) can be assessed by quantitative computerized tomography (QCT), or indirectly estimated from results obtained with the DXA technology. Consequently, although it is presently unknown whether the same set of genes influences both cortical and spongious bone, the association of a single gene locus, which can by essence determine only one bone mineral mass constituent, with any of the measures of "bone mass" defined previously, will be burdened by

The Genetics of Osteoporosis and Metabolic Bone Disease
Ed.: M. J. Econs © Humana Press Inc., Totowa, NJ

a degree of imprecision proportional to the number and magnitude of genetic effects on the other constituents of bone mineral mass.

Bone mineral mass is mainly determined by the amount of bone accumulated during skeletal growth, and by the loss occurring after menopause and with aging. The maximal mass of bone, the so-called peak bone mineral mass, is virtually achieved at most skeletal sites by the end of the second decade of life *(3,4)*. It has long been recognized that peak bone mineral mass is under strong genetic determination, since both twins and parents-offspring comparisons have suggested that heredity accounted for as much as 60–80% of areal bone mineral density and bone mineral content variance in the population (*5–7*; *see* Chapters 1 and 2). Most recent studies however questioned the actual magnitude of direct genetic effects on peak bone mass, due to similarities in environmental covariates *(8,9)* and in lean body mass *(10)* among relatives. Besides, it has become evident that the genetic determination of bone mineral mass is detectable well before pubertal growth spurt, with however notable differences in heritability estimates among various bone sites and traits *(7)*.

Recent characterization of polymorphic loci in genes coding for molecules implicated in bone metabolism or structure has given hope that genetic susceptibility to osteoporosis might be readily unraveled. This chapter will primarly focus on molecular epidemiology studies about the association of aBMD with vitamin D receptor (VDR) gene alleles located in the vicinity of the 3'-end region *(11)* as well as in the 5'-start codon region *(12)*. In keeping with some recent observations emphasized above, the influence of age and environmental interactions on the relationship between bone mineral mass and VDR gene polymorphisms will be also discussed.

Human DNA Polymorphisms

Singlebase variations in DNA sequence occurring in at least 1% of the general population are defined as allelic polymorphisms. Short nucleotide sequence repeats which are scattered throughout the human genome have also been more recently found to be another rich source of polymorphisms *(13)*. Singlebase polymorphisms can be situated either in DNA coding or noncoding regions (exons and introns, respectively), and are detectable as DNA fragments of different lengths after digestion by the appropriate restriction enzyme. Identification of such restriction fragment length polymorphisms (RFLP) initially relied on Southern blot hybridization, but PCR-based methods now allow rapid characterization on large scale populations.

DNA polymorphisms have mostly been useful as proximity markers for tracking down mutated genes through affected families and extended pedigrees. Linkage analysis thus has allowed the mapping of mutations responsible for numerous inherited disorders such as cystic fibrosis, retinoblastoma, and adenomatous polyposis coli *(13)*. More recently, technical improvements and probably also the impetus brought by the human genome project, let polymorphisms be considered as essential tools in identifying genetic predisposition to polygenic disorders as well *(14)*, particularly to common conditions such as hypertension or osteoporosis. In this case, polymorphic markers may be associated either with the presence or absence of the condition in the population, or with values of a continuous variable, for instance blood pressure or aBMD *(15)*. Noteworthy, the former kind of study (case-control) is more vulnerable to selection bias than studies performed in randomly selected populations. Recent attempts to link polymorphic markers to a number of polygenic disorders have brought results sometimes of questionable interest. This particularly concerns situations in which there is a considerable overlap in the distribution of genotypic values among alleles *(16)*. However, this approach has also been sometimes remarkably informative with regard to disease pathophysiology and possibly treatment *(17)*.

Concerning common conditions such as hypertension or osteoporosis, which are defined as extreme deviations from the normal distribution of complex quantitative traits, a single polymorphic locus cannot be expected to explain more than a fraction of the trait variance (or disease susceptibility) across the population and should in essence not be regarded as a disease-causing mutation, whether or not they are located within gene coding regions.

Accordingly, a number of limitations have to be recognized regarding molecular epidemiology studies. First, peculiar alleles may be markers for the condition of interest but not be causal to the condition. Otherwise specific molecular and pathophysiological mechanisms should be able to be demonstrated in direct relation to these polymorphisms. Second, results from a study cohort should be extrapolated to other populations with caution, since strength of the association between allelic polymorphisms and complex quantitative traits will vary as genetic background heterogeneity and environmental influences vary among different populations *(18,19)*. Finally, population-based risks and individual predictions in clinical settings must be clearly distinguished: while mean genotypic values or relative risks of disease may significantly differ among allelic polymorphisms, these markers may not be immediately informative with regard to individual diagnosis or prognosis.

The Vitamin D Endocrine System

Physiology of Vitamin D

The importance of the vitamin D endocrine system for the development and maintenance of bone mineral mass is most apparent during states of either deficiency or resistance to vitamin D. Thus, vitamin D deficiency during growth causes the typical bone deformations depicted as rickets, whereas similar deficiency in adulthood, as it is commonly encountered in the elderly, causes osteomalacia.

Although 1,25(OH)2 D3, the active hormonal metabolite of vitamin D, appears to have pleotropic actions, including on cell growth and differentiation, its role is primarily to maintain serum calcium and phosphate levels to allow adequate bone matrix mineralization *(20)*. Furthermore, the vitamin D system, probably by its effects on calcium bioavailability, could indirectly be implicated in the prevention and treatment of osteoporosis. Indeed, recent studies have demonstrated that in vitamin D replete elderly calcium supplementation significantly increased aBMD and decreased the incidence of osteoporotic fracture *(21–23)*, and that calcium supplements enhanced aBMD gain in growing children *(24,25)*. In other words, the positive influence of calcium appears to require the presence of a normal vitamin D status.

Molecular Endocrinology of Vitamin D

The effects of 1,25(OH)2 D3 are mediated by its nuclear vitamin D receptor (VDR), a phosphorylated zinc-finger molecule which is encoded on the long arm of chromosome 12. Upon binding of 1,25(OH)2 D3, VDR forms a heterodimeric complex with the retinoic acid receptor (RXR) capable to targeting specific responsive elements (VDRE) present upstream to a number of genes (*see* Table 1 and Chapter 6). Following interaction with other transcription factors, such as TFIIB, activity of RNA polymerase II is then upregulated (*see* refs. *26* and *27* for review). Noteworthy with regard to the potential molecular mechanisms by which common VDR 3'-end allelic polymorphisms might affect bone metabolism is the recent suggestion that VDR's homodimers (i.e., VDR × VDR) rather than VDR × RXR heterodimers might regulate osteocalcin gene expression as opposed to osteopontin gene expression for instance *(28)*. These observations however have been disputed (*see* refs.*26* and *27*, for review).

VDR Gene Polymorphisms

Characteristics of 3'- and 5'-End VDR Gene Polymorphisms

Taking a candidate gene approach, Morrison et al. identified a number of common allelic polymorphisms in the 3'-end region of the VDR gene, among which three can be recognized after PCR amplification of the DNA region of interest upon endonuclease restriction by *Bsm*1, *Taq*1, and *Apa*1, respectively *(11,29)*. Thus, genotypes at these sites are defined as BB, Bb, and bb (*Bsm*1); AA, Aa, or aa (*Apa*1) and TT, Tt, or tt (*Taq*1), with capital letters usually used to designate the absence of a cleavage site for a specific endonuclease. Since these polymorphisms are all situated in intron 8 and the proximal region of exon 9 (Fig. 1), they are in strong linkage disequilibrium. Thus, *Bsm*1 and *Taq*1 alleles B and t or, alternatively, b and T show less than 1% recombination frequency, whereas the B allele is always associated with A. The prevalence of the three most common VDR 3'-end alleles, namely baT (50%), BAt (40%) and bAT (10%) and their predicted genotypes BbAaTt (37%), bbaaTT (26%), BBAAtt (15%), bbAaTT (11%), BbAATt (9%), and bbAATT (1%) [these frequencies are averaged from three large cohorts *(30–31)*] appears to be similar among Western populations, but to notably differ among Asians, in whom the BAt allele is much less frequent (10%) whereas the baT allele is more abundant (65%) *(32)*. Although most studies have

Table 1
VDRE-Bearing Genes Involved in Bone and Calcium Metabolism [a]

	Transcriptional activation	Transcriptional inhibition
Bone-osteoblasts	Osteocalcin	Collagen I
	Osteopontin	Bone sialo-protein
	Alkaline phosphatase	
Bone-osteoclasts	Integrin (αv and β3)	
Intestine	Calbindin	
	24-hydroxylase	
Kidney	24-hydroxylase	
Parathyroid gland		PTH
Ubiquitous		PTH-related protein

[a] Other vitamin-D regulated genes exist both in relation to bone and calcium metabolism as well as in "nonclassical" target tissues, such as the immune system, but the presence of VDRE in these cases has not yet been established. (Adapted with permission from ref. *27*).

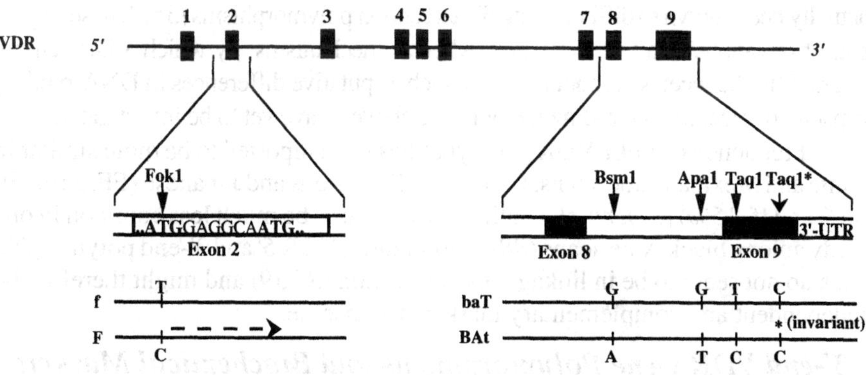

Fig. 1. Structure of the vitamin D receptor (VDR) gene showing the nine exons and intervening introns, the coding sequence at the translation initiation site (exon 2) and the 3'-untranslated region (UTR). Restriction sites for endonucleases (*Bsm*1, *Apa* 1 and *Taq* 1) in the 3'-UTR and (*Fok*1) in the start codon region are indicated by an arrow. Single-base variants responsible for allelic polymorphisms at these sites (*see* text) are shown below, as well as corresponding alleles (baT vs BAt and F vs f). Capital letters in alleles nomenclature indicate absence of a restriction site. Dashed arrow indicates shifting of the translation initiation point (F allele). Short arrow shows an invariant *Taq*1 restriction site in the 3'-UTR (*).

used only one polymorphic marker (mostly *Bsm*1*)*, it is not yet clear whether combination of *Bsm*1 and *Apa*1 polymorphisms or direct haplotyping across the entire VDR 3'-end polymorphic region *(31)* may be more informative.

By using minigene reporter constructs, Morrison et al. suggested that alternate homozygotes for the alleles baT and BAt might differ with regard to VDR gene transcriptional efficiency and/or mRNA stability *(11)*, but this has not been confirmed. The hypothesis that subtle differences in the amount of VDR molecules synthesized in osteoblasts might change the equilibrium between homo- and heterodimeric receptor complexes and hence the effects of 1,25(OH)2 D3 on bone metabolism is appealing *(33)*. However, VDR mRNA amounts have not been demonstrated to differ among VDR 3'-end alleles *(34)*. To date therefore, the molecular mechanisms which might link VDR 3'-end polymorphisms to aBMD differences are not elucidated.

Albeit VDR 5'-end polymorphisms at the translation initiation codon which can be identified by the restriction enzyme *Fok*1 *(12)* have not yet been as extensively investigated in relation to bone mineral mass as VDR 3'-end alleles, they have been known for longer *(35)* and also have been better characterized at the molecular level. Indeed, a unique T/C transition polymorphism in the first ATG codon (exon 2, Fig. 1) predicts delayed transcription initiation until the second ATG codon and a resulting three amino-acid shorter VDR molecule. Very recently, VDR's molecular weight as well as the level of transcriptional activation of a VDRE-containing reporter construct have actually been shown to differ among 5'-start codon polymorphisms *(36)*. These important observations await confirmation, whereas mechanisms by which VDR activity might differ between start codon alleles, such as putative differences in DNA-binding capacity or receptor heterodimerization (see above), have yet to be investigated.

Frequency of *Fok*1 VDR genotypes has been reported to be quite similar in white and Mexican Americans, Caucasian-Europeans and Japanese (FF, 35%, Ff, 50% and ff, 15%) *(37)*, but the f allele was found to be much less common in one study among black Americans *(38)*. Importantly, VDR 5' and 3'-end polymorphic sites do not seem to be in linkage disequilibrium *(37,39)* and might therefore be independent and complementary markers for disease.

3'-end VDR Gene Polymorphisms and Biochemical Markers of Bone Metabolism

Definite momentum for the search of a relationship between bone mineral mass and VDR alleles came from observations by Morrison et al, who found that mean osteocalcin levels were higher among BB (alternatively, AA) normal subjects *(29)*, suggesting increased bone turnover. There was however a prominent overlap of individual osteocalcin values across VDR 3'-end polymorphisms, as well as an excess ratio of postmenopausal women over men among BB subjects as compared to the other genotypes. Nevertheless, subgroup analysis of postmenopausal women showed very distinct differences in osteocalcin levels among VDR genotypes, although the number of subjects in each group was low. In contrast, later studies based on large numbers of observations in homogeneous cohorts of either pre- or postmenopausal women, failed to detect any significant osteocalcin differences among VDR 3'-end alleles *(40–42)*, nor in the level of several different markers of bone resorption *(40,41)*.

Thus, there is no biochemical evidence that VDR 3'-end genotypes have a direct and substantial influence on bone metabolism. Although most currently available bone markers may lack sensitivity to detect subtle bone turnover variations between VDR alleles, the absence of differences in osteocalcin levels, the regulation of which is under straight VDRE control, does not support the contention of differentiated molecular effects on bone cells among VDR 3'-end gene polymorphisms.

3'-End VDR Gene Polymorphisms in Linkage and Association Studies

Osteoporosis studies using segregation analysis of VDR alleles through affected pedigrees have not been reported, probably because so-called primary osteoporosis is unlikely to be simultaneously diagnosed in elderly probands and their younger descendants, and mostly because of the potential for noncommon forms of osteoporosis, such as osteogenesis imperfecta, within these families. In contrast, linkage analysis for quantitative traits have been extensively performed in relation to VDR 3'-end polymorphisms, looking at within-pairs bone mineral mass differences among twins as well as at the population level *(15)*.

Morrison et al. observed a marked reduction of aBMD variance among dizygotic twins sharing identical VDR 3'-end alleles *(11)*, which was suggestive of their major contribution to the genetic determination of aBMD, but the authors later acknowledged some technical and analytical errors *(43)*. In fact, two other linkage studies in twins did not confirm a significant association of VDR 3'-end gene polymorphisms and aBMD heritability *(44,45)*. However, despite the fact that twin models have been very useful to demonstrate overall genetic effects on bone mineral mass (see above), they may have limited power to identify single loci contribution to complex diseases *(46)*.

Association analysis by Morrison et al. also showed significantly lower aBMD at the lumbar spine and proximal femur associated with the B allele in adult twins of both sexes as well as in unrelated pre- and postmenopausal women, both of European descent *(11)*. In agreement with these results, Bb Japanese women were later shown to have lower aBMD as compared to bb women *(32,47)*. In contrast, large scale studies in several Western populations as well as a meta-analysis failed to detect a significant association between aBMD and VDR 3'-end alleles *(Bsm*1*)* before or after menopause *(30,40,48,49)*. Furthermore, others found lower aBMD values in homozygous subjects with the common bb or the rare bbAA genotypes rather than in BB subjects *(31,50)*. Noteworthy, no single VDR 3'-end allele has been shown to be more prevalent in osteoporotic patients (defined by aBMD less than 2.5 standard deviations below the mean peak aBMD or by the presence of a low-energy fracture) than in normals. Thus, discordant findings raised an important controversy upon the reliability of VDR 3'-end gene polymorphisms as susceptibility markers for osteoporosis *(51,52)*. The conclusion is that VDR 3'-end alleles per se are unlikely to predict low bone mineral mass at the time of menopause and cannot therefore be considered useful screening or diagnostic tools for osteoporosis.

On the other side, association between bone mineral mass and VDR 3'-end alleles has been so far somewhat more consistent in growing children *(30,53)* as well as in young people who had recently achieved peak bone mineral mass *(54–56)*. Indeed, VDR 3'-end gene polymorphisms have appeared to explain 5–10% of the bone mineral mass variance in such cohorts. The reasons why bone mineral mass and VDR 3'-end allelic polymorphisms appeared to be better related in young as compared to older subjects cannot be simply explained by variable degrees of genetic background homogeneity between the cohorts. Indeed, it has been clearly demonstrated that bone mineral mass differences among VDR 3'-end genotypes which were present in prepubertal girls were no more detectable in their premenopausal mothers *(30)*. Therefore, interactions with environmental factors have been suggested.

VDR 3'-End Gene Polymorphisms/Dietary Calcium Interactions

Gene-environment interactions, particularly those involving nutrients intake, are well-known modulators of the apparent heritability of quantitative traits, as life span for instance *(57)*. An interaction between VDR 3'-end allelic polymorphisms and dietary calcium was first suggested by two independent analyses of calcium-supplementation trials in vitamin D replete elderly patients *(58,59)*. In these studies, mean rate of lumbar spine aBMD loss was higher in BB than bb or Bb subjects. Moreover, a significant positive correlation between calcium intake and aBMD changes was observed only in Bb subjects, suggesting that the range of dietary calcium intake affecting aBMD may differ among VDR 3'-end genotypes *(58)*. In agreement with this hypothesis, it was later shown that BB postmenopausal women who had more prominent bone loss than females with other VDR genotypes, also had a better response in terms of aBMD changes to calcium supplements *(59)*. Although there have been some discordant findings about a possible association between postmenopausal bone loss and VDR 3'-end alleles *(41,48)*, which were probably related to differences in the time since menopause between the various study cohorts *(59,60)*, a majority of published studies that carefully looked at dietary calcium and/or vitamin D intake and VDR 3'-end gene polymorphisms after the menopause reported significant interactions *(61–63)*.

Two recent investigations indicate that such interactions may also occur in younger subjects. This appears crucial in order to explain the lack of detectable aBMD differences between VDR 3'-end alleles in premenopausal women. Thus, among 470 premenopausal women from the Healthy Lifestyle Project, aBMD was significantly higher in Bb and BB whose dietary calcium intake was above 1036 mg/d (23% of the cohort) as compared to those who had less calcium, whereas bb aBMD was unaffected by the dietary calcium intake *(64)*. On the other hand, a randomized, placebo-controlled trial in prepubertal girls showed that aBMD gain in response to calcium supplements (800 mg/d) was increased at several skeletal sites in Bb and BB subjects receiving calcium supplements. In contrast, calcium did apparently not affect aBMD gain in bb girls, who actually had a trend for higher aBMD accumulation on their usual calcium diet as compared to the other genotypes *(30)*.

In conclusion, a scheme illustrates the potential influence of dietary calcium-VDR 3'-end gene polymorphisms interactions on aBMD accumulation and its consequences on age-adjusted aBMD (Fig. 2). This model predicts that aBMD differences among VDR genotypes can be blunted in subjects whose calcium intake is either relatively low or relatively high for their pubertal stage, growth rate, or level of physical activity. Moreover, the model takes into account other potential gene-environmental as well as gene-gene interactions which may modulate aBMD-VDR 3'-end genotypes relationships independently of dietary calcium intake. The net result of this intricate play of genetic and environmental factors is that intrinsic aBMD differences among VDR 3'-end alleles may become undetectable with increasing age. Very importantly then, the absence of measurable aBMD differences among VDR 3'-end genotypes does not necessarily mean that this polymorphic locus is unrelated to aBMD levels. On the contrary, the interaction between VDR 3'-end genotypes and calcium bioavailability might appear more clearly when aBMD changes are considered, whereas an association between aBMD and VDR 3'-end genotypes would be much less detectable in cross-sectional studies.

VDR 3'-End Gene Polymorphisms and Calcium Metabolism

An interaction between dietary calcium and VDR 3'-end alleles has initially been suggested to affect the level of intestinal calcium absorption. A significantly decreased fractional 45Ca absorption has been found in BB as compared to bb late postmenopausal women on a low calcium intake, but such differences were not detectable on a high calcium intake *(65)*. Decreased intestinal calcium absorption has also been found in BB black American postmenopausal women *(42)*, as well as in BBAA vs bbaa healthy premenopausal women *(66)*. In contrast, no differences in intestinal calcium absorption, duodenal VDR concentrations or serum 1,25 (OH)2 D3 levels were observed in another study including both young adult and postmenopausal women *(67)*, although dietary calcium intake might have been somewhat higher than in the former cohorts. Similar investigations have not yet been reported in children, but differences in intestinal calcium absorption among VDR 3'-end alleles depending on the level of dietary calcium intake would be compatible with the interaction model presented before.

A small dynamic study in young healthy Caucasian males has attempted to further characterize calcium and phosphate metabolism in relation to VDR 3'-end alleles *(68)*. At baseline, these males had a spontaneously elevated intake of calcium and phosphate (i.e., above 1000 mg/d). As compared to bb subjects, BB had significantly lower intestinal calcium absorption (as assessed by the ratio of daily urinary excretion to total intake), higher renal phosphate excretion, bone turnover (as assessed by osteocalcin measurements) as well as PTH levels. When dietary calcium and phosphate were restricted, 1,25 (OH)2 D3 increased more in BB as compared to bb subjects, without however proportional changes in intestinal calcium absorption or PTH levels.

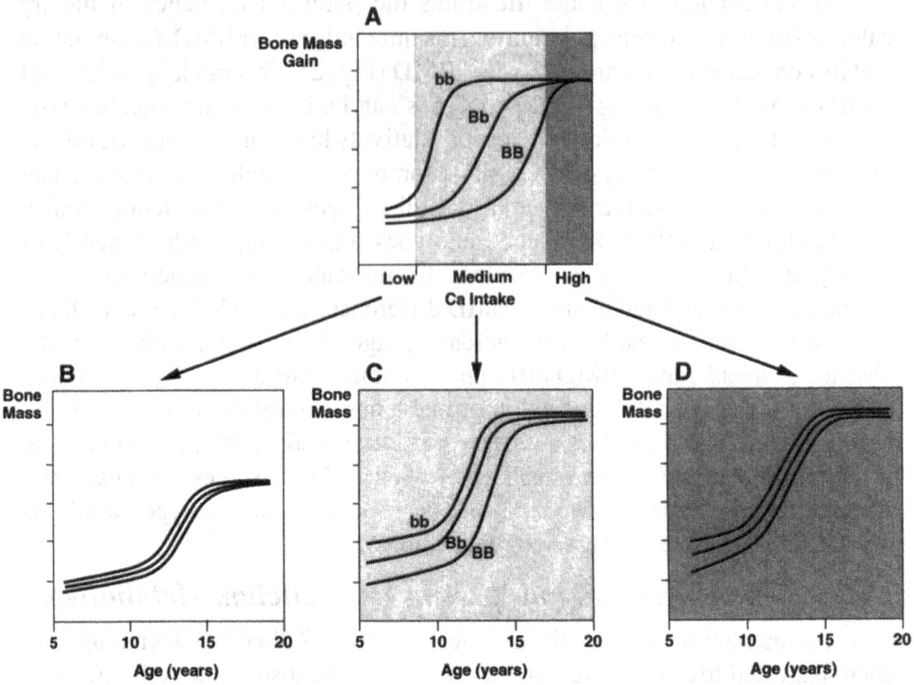

Fig. 2. Schematic illustration of the interaction between dietary calcium and VDR gene polymorphisms on bone mass acrual **(A)**, and its consequences on the association between VDR genotypes and bone mass **(B–D)**. **(A)** Bone mass accrual differs among VDR genotypes only when calcium intake is in the medium range. **(B)** On a low calcium intake, bone mass differences are not detectable among VDR genoypes, due to the longstanding low bone mass accrual in the three genotypes. **(C)** When calcium intake is in the medium range, bone mass differences among VDR genotypes are detectable before puberty, but may then be blunted by other constitutive and environmental factors. **(D)** On a high calcium intake, potential bone mass differences among VDR genotypes disappear before puberty, because maximal bone mass accrual is achieved in all genotypes.

Hence, these observations might be compatible with a decreased sensitivity to calcitriol in BB subjects.

Interestingly, sparse observations seem to corroborate the possibility of a relatively lower sensitivity of the parathyroid glands to calcitriol in BB subjects as compared to the other genotypes, both in normal postmenopausal women *(69)* as well as in patients with primary hyperparathyroidism *(70)*.

VDR 5′-End Gene Polymorphisms and Bone Mineral Mass

Gross et al. reported lower lumbar spine, but not femoral neck, aBMD in ff as compared to FF postmenopausal Mexican-American women *(12)*. The same group also found lower femoral neck, but not lumbar spine aBMD in white premenopausal American women *(38)*. In the latter study, however, association was not detected in blacks. No differences were found in osteocalcin, PTH, or 1,25 (OH)2D3 levels among VDR 5'-end genotypes. A recent report from Japan also found decreased aBMD in ff subjects *(36)*. Similarly, a trend for a lower aBMD ($p = 0.06$) has been found in 124 postmenopausal osteoporotic French women (G. Lucotte, personal communication). In contrast, one European study in healthy premenopausal women *(37)* and another in young adult women as well as prepubertal girls *(39)* did not confirm significant relationships between aBMD and VDR start codon polymorphisms. Interestingly however, the latter study suggested a possible interaction with calcium intake as well as gene-gene interaction involving VDR 3'-end polymorphic loci.

Conclusions

It is well established that a familial history of osteoporotic fractures increases the risk of finding low aBMD among relatives. Molecular epidemiology research in this field, however, is still at an early stage. 3'- and 5'-end VDR allelic polymorphisms have been among the first candidate loci to be investigated, but appear to be unlikely genetic markers for the disease. Nevertheless, they might play a role in the development of bone mineral mass during childhood. Most importantly, it should be remembered that quantitative traits and related complex diseases are affected by a large number of loci as well as by environmental factors acting together. Indeed, other genes are likely to influence the association between VDR gene polymorphisms and bone mineral mass. For instance, two polymorphic genes among the hundreds of potential polymorphic loci scattered across the human genome (virtually one every 200–500 base pairs) *(13)* have been investigated in relation to bone mineral mass, namely estrogen-receptor and type 1 collagen alleles. They are presented elsewhere in this book. Although models for interactions involving multiple genes have not yet been proposed in molecular epidemiology analysis of osteoporosis, it is likely that the few polymorphic genes explored in these chapters as well as several other candidate genes currently under investigation will eventually merge to provide a comprehensive, although extremely complex, picture of bone mineral mass determination.

At the present time, the mechanisms linking genotypes to the osteoporotic phenotype remain to be elucidated.

Acknowledgments

We thank Mrs. M. Perez for her secretarial assistance. The papers by our group quoted in this chapter were supported by the Swiss National Science Research Foundation (grant no. 31–40758.94).

References

1. Peck, W. A., Burckhardt, P., Christiansen, C., Fleisch, H. A., Genant, H. K., Gennari, C. et al. (1993) Consensus Development Conference—Diagnosis, prophylaxis, and treatment of osteoporosis. *Am. J. Med.* **94,** 646–650.
2. Rizzoli, R., Slosman, D., and Bonjour, J. P. (1995) The role of dual energy X-ray absorptiometry of lumbar spine and proximal femur in the diagnosis and follow-up of osteoporosis. *Am. J. Med.* **98,** 2A–33S–36S.
3. Bonjour, J. P., Theintz, G., Buchs, B., Slosman, D., and Rizzoli, R. (1991) Critical years and stages of puberty for spinal and femoral bone mass accumulation during adolescence. *J. Clin. Endocrinol. Metab.* **73,** 555–563.
4. Theintz, G., Buchs, B., Rizzoli, R., Slosman, D., Clavien, H., Sizonenko, P. C., and Bonjour, J. P. (1992) Longitudinal monitoring of bone mass accumulation in healthy adolescents: evidence for a marked reduction after 16 years of age at the level of lumbar spine and femoral neck in female subjects. *J. Clin. Endocrinol. Metab.* **75,** 1060–1065.
5. Pocock, N. A., Eisman, J. A., Hopper J. L., Yeates, M. G., Sambrook, P. N., and Ebert, S. (1987) Genetic determinants of bone mass in adults. A twin study. *J. Clin. Invest.* **80,** 706–710.
6. Kelly, P. J., Morrison, N. A., Sambrook, P. N., Nguyen, T. V., and Eisman, J. A. (1995) Genetic influences on bone turnover, bone density and fracture. *Eur. J. Endocrinol.* **133,** 265–271.
7. Ferrari, S., Rizzoli, R., Slosman, D., and Bonjour, J. P. (1998) Familial resemblance for bone mineral mass is expressed before puberty. *J. Clin. Endocrinol. Metab.* **83,** 358–361.
8. Slemenda, C. W., Christian, J. C., Williams, C. J., Norton J. A., and Johnston, C. C., Jr. (1991) Genetic determinants of bone mass in adult women: a reevaluation of the twin model and the potential importance of gene interaction on heritability estimates. *J. Bone Miner. Res.* **6,** 561–567.
9. Krall, E. A. and Dawson-Hughes B. (1993) Heritable and life-style determinants of bone mineral density. *J. Bone Miner. Res.* **8,** 1–9.
10. Seeman, E., Hopper, J. L., Young, N. R., Formica, C., Goss, P., and Tsalamandris C. (1996) Do genetic factors explain associations between muscle strength, lean mass, and bone density? A twin study. *Am. J. Physiol.* **270,** E320–E327.
11. Morrison, N. A., Qi, J. C., Tokita, A., Kelly, P. J., Crofts, L., Nguyen, T. V., Sambrook, P. N., and Eisman, J. A. (1994) Prediction of bone density from vitamin D receptor alleles. *Nature* **367,** 284–287.
12. Gross, C., Eccleshall, T. R., Malloy, P. J., Villa M. L., Marcus, R., and Feldman, D. (1996) The presence of a polymorphism at the translation initiation site of the vitamin D receptor gene is associated with low bone mineral density in postmenopausal Mexican-American women. *J. Bone Miner. Res.* **11,** 1850–1855.
13. White, R. (1997) Mapping markers and genes in the human genome, in *Exploring Genetic Mechanisms* (Singer, M. and Berg, P., ed.), University Science Books, Sausalito, CA, pp. 271–300.
14. Housman, D. (1995) Human DNA polymorphism. *N. Engl. J. Med.* **332,** 318–320.
15. Weiss, K. M., ed. (1993) *Genetic Variation and Human Disease. Principles and Evolutionary Approaches.* Cambridge University Press, Cambridge, UK.
16. Hall, I. P., Wheatley, A., Wilding, P., and Liggett, S. B. (1995) Association of Glu 27 β2-adrenoceptor polymorphism with lower airway reactivity in asthmatic subjects. *Lancet* **345,** 1213–1214.

17. Hyman, B. T. and Tanzi, R. (1995) Molecular epidemiology of Alzheimer's disease. *N. Engl. J. Med.* **333,** 1283–1284.
18. Lindpaintner, K., Pfeffer, M. A., Kreutz, R., Stampfer, M. J., Grodstein, F., LaMotte, F., Buring, J., and Hennekens, C. H. (1995) A prospective evaluation of an angiotensin-converting-enzyme gene polymorphism and the risk of ischemic heart disease. *N. Engl. J. Med.* **332,** 706–711.
19. Econs, M. J. and Speer, M. C. (1996) Genetic studies of complex diseases: let the reader beware. *J. Bone Miner. Res.* **11,** 1835–1840.
20. Reichel, H., Koeffler, H. P., and Norman, A. W. (1989) The role of the vitamin D endocrine system in health and disease. *N. Engl. J. Med.* **320,** 980–991.
21. Chapuy, M. C., Arlot, M. E., Duboeuf, F., Brun, J., Crouzet, B., Arnaud, S., Delmas, P. D., and Meunier, P. J. (1992) Vitamin–D_3 and calcium to prevent hip fractures in elderly women. *N. Engl. J. Med.* **327,** 1637–1642.
22. Chevalley, T., Rizzoli, R., Nydegger, V., Slosman, D., Rapin, C. H., Michel, J. P., Vasey, H., and Bonjour, J. P. (1994) Effects of calcium supplements on femoral bone mineral density and vertebral fracture rate in vitamin-D-replete elderly patients. *Osteoporos. Int.* **4,** 245–252.
23. Dawson-Hughes, B., Harris, S. S., Krall, E. A., and Dallal, G. E. (1997) Effect of calcium and vitamin D supplementation on bone density in men and women 65 years of age or older. *N. Engl. J. Med.* **337,** 670–676.
24. Johnston, C. C., Jr., Miller J. Z., Slemenda, C. W., Reister, T. K., Hui, S., Christian J. C., and Peacock, M. (1992) Calcium supplementation and increases in bone mineral density in children. *N. Engl. J. Med.* **327,** 82–87.
25. Bonjour, J. P., Carrié, A. L., Ferrari, S., Clavien, H., Slosman, D., Theintz, G., and Rizzoli, R. (1997) Calcium-enriched foods and bone mass growth in prepubertal girls: a randomized, double-blind, placebo-controlled trial. *J. Clin. Invest.* **99,** 1287–1294.
26. Haussler, M. R., Haussler, C. A., Jurutka, P. W., Thompson, P. D., Hsieh, J. C., Remus, L. S., Selznick, S. H., and Whitfield, G. K. (1997) The vitamin D hormone and its nuclear receptor: molecular actions and disease states. *J. Endocrinol.* **154,** S57–S73.
27. Christakos, S., Raval-Pandya, M., Wernyj, R. P., and Yang, W. (1996) Genomic mechanisms involved in the pleiotropic actions of 1,25-dihydroxyvitamin D_3. *Biochem. J.* **316,** 361–371.
28. Carlberg, C., Bendik, I., Wyss, A., Meier, E., Sturzenbecker, L. J., Grippo, J. F., and Hunziker, W. (1993) Two nuclear signalling pathways for vitamin D. *Nature* **361,** 657–660.
29. Morrison, N. A., Yeoman, R., Kelly, P. J., and Eisman, J. A. (1992) Contribution of trans-acting factor alleles to normal physiological variability: vitamin D receptor gene polymorphism and circulating osteocalcin. *Proc. Natl. Acad. Sci. U. S. A.* **89,** 6665–6669.
30. Ferrari, S., Rizzoli, R., Slosman, D., and Bonjour, J. P. (1998) Do dietary calcium and age explain the controversy surrounding the relationship between bone mineral density and vitamin D receptor gene polymorphisms. *J. Bone Miner. Res.* **13,** 363–370.
31. Uitterlinden, A. G., Pols, H. A. P., Burger, H., Huang, Q., Van Daele, P. L. A., Van Duijn, C. M., et al. (1996) A large-scale population-based study of the association of vitamin D receptor gene polymorphisms with bone mineral density. *J. Bone Miner. Res.* **11,** 1241–1248.
32. Tokita, A., Matsumoto, H., Morrison, N. A., Tawa, T., Miura, Y., Fukamauchi, K., et al. (1996) Vitamin D receptor alleles, bone mineral density and turnover in premenopausal Japanese women. *J. Bone Miner. Res.* **11,** 1003–1009.

33. White, C. P., Morrison, N. A., Gardiner, E. M., and Eisman, J. A. (1994) Vitamin D receptor alleles and bone physiology. *J. Cell Biochem.* **56,** 307–314.
34. Mocharla, H., Butch, A. W., Pappas, A. A., Flick, J. T., Weinstein, R. S., De Togni, P., et al. (1997) Quantification of vitamin D receptor mRNA by competitive polymerase chain reaction in PBMC: lack of correspondence with common allelic variants. *J. Bone Miner. Res.* **12,** 726–733.
35. Sajito, T., Ito, M., Takeda, E., Huq, A. H. M. M., Naito, E., Yokota, I., et al. (1991) A unique mutation in the vitamin D receptor gene in three Japanese patients with vitamin D-dependent rickets type II: utility of single–strand conformation polymorphism analysis for heterozygous carrier detection. *Am. J. Hum. Genet.* **49,** 668–673.
36. Arai, H., Miyamoto, K. I., Taketani, Y., Yamamoto, H., Iemori, Y., Morita, K., et al. (1997) A vitamin D receptor gene polymorphism in the translation initiation codon: effect on protein activity and relation to bone mineral density in Japanese women. *J. Bone Miner. Res.* **12,** 915–921.
37. Eccleshall, T. R., Garnero, P., Gross, C., Delmas, P.D., and Feldman, D. (1998) Lack of correlation between start codon polymorphism of the vitamin D receptor gene and bone mineral density in premenopausal French women: the OFELY study. *J. Bone Miner. Res.* **13,** 31–35.
38. Harris, S. S., Eccleshall, T. R., Gross, C., Dawson–Hughes, B., and Feldman, D. (1997) The vitamin D receptor start codon polymorphism (*Fok*I) and bone mineral density in premenopausal American black and white women. *J. Bone Miner. Res.* **12,** 1043–1048.
39. Ferrari, S., Rizzoli, R., Manen, D., Slosman, D., Bonjour, J. P. (1998) Vitamin D receptor gene start codon polymorphisms (*Fok*I) and bone mineral density: interaction with age, dietary calcium and 3'-end region polymorphisms. *J. Bone Miner. Res.* **13,** 925–930.
40. Garnero, P., Borel, O., Sornay-Rendu, E., and Delmas P. D. (1995) Vitamin D receptor gene polymorphisms do not predict bone turnover and bone mass in healthy premenopausal women. *J. Bone Miner. Res.* **10,** 1283–1288.
41. Garnero, P., Borel, O., Sornay-Rendu, E., Arlot, M. E., and Delmas P. D. (1996) Vitamin D receptor gene polymorphisms are not related to bone turnover, rate of bone loss, and bone mass in postmenopausal women: the OFELY study. *J. Bone Miner. Res.* **11,** 827–834.
42. Zmuda, J. M., Cauley, J. A., Danielson, M. E., Wolf, R. L., and Ferrell, R. E. (1997) Vitamin D receptor gene polymorphisms, bone turnover, and rates of bone loss in older African-American women. *J. Bone Miner. Res.* **12,** 1446–1452.
43. Morrison, N. A., Qi, J. C., Tokita, A., Kelly, P. J., Crofts, L., Nguyen, T. V., Sambrook, P. N., and Eisman, J. A. (1997) Prediction of bone density from vitamin D receptor alleles. *Nature* **387,** 106.
44. Huystmyer, F. G., Peacock, M., Hui, S., Johnston, C. C., and Christian, J. (1994) Bone mineral density in relation to polymorphism at the vitamin D receptor gene locus. *J. Clin. Invest.* **94,** 2130–2134.
45. Spector, T. D., Keen, R. W., Arden, N. K., Morrison, N. A., Major, P. J., Nguyen, T. V., et al. (1995) Influence of vitamin D receptor genotype on bone mineral density in postmenopausal women: a twin study in Britain. *BMJ.* **310,** 1357–1360.
46. Rogers, J., Mahaney, M. C., Beamer, W. G., Donahue, L. R., and Rosen, C. J. (1997) Beyond one gene-one disease: alternative strategies for deciphering genetic determinants of osteoporosis. *Calcif. Tissue Int.* **60,** 225–228.
47. Yamagata, Z., Miyamura, T., Iijima, S., Asaka, A., Sasaki, M., Kato, J., and Koizumi, K. (1994) Vitamin D receptor gene polymorphism and bone mineral density in healthy Japanese women. *Lancet* **344,** 1027.

48. Jørgensen, H. L., Schøller, J., Sand, J. C., Bjuring, M., Hassager, C., and Christiansen, C. (1996) Relation of common allelic variation at vitamin D receptor locus to bone mineral density and postmenopausal bone loss: cross–sectional and longitudinal population study. *Br. Med. J.* **313,** 586–590.
49. Cooper, G. S. and Umbach, D. M. (1996) Are vitamin D receptor polymorphisms associated with bone mineral density? A meta-analysis. *J. Bone Miner. Res.* **11,** 1841–1849.
50. Houston, L. A., Grant, S. F. A., Reid, D. M., and Ralston, S. H. (1996) Vitamin D receptor polymorphism, bone mineral density, and osteoporotic vertebral fracture: studies in a UK population. *Bone* **18,** 249–252.
51. Peacock, M. (1995) Vitamin D receptor gene alleles and osteoporosis: a constrasting view. *J. Bone Miner. Res.* **10,** 1294–1297.
52. Eisman, J. A. (1995) Vitamin D receptor gene alleles and osteoporosis: an affirmative view. *J. Bone Miner. Res.* **10,** 1289–1293.
53. Sainz, J., Van Tornout, J. M., Loro, M. L., Sayre, J., Roe, T. F., and Gilsanz, V. (1997) Vitamin D–receptor gene polymorphisms and bone density in prepubertal American girls of Mexican descent. *N. Engl. J. Med.* **337,** 77–82.
54. Fleet, J. C., Harris, S. S., Wook, R. J., and Dawson–Hughes, B. (1995) The *Bsm*I vitamin D receptor restriction fragment length polymorphism (BB) predicts low bone density in premenopausal black and white women. *J. Bone Miner. Res.* **10,** 985–990.
55. Riggs, B. L., Nguyen, T. V., Melton III, L. J., Morrison, N. A., O'Fallon, W. M., Kelly, P. J., et al. (1995) The contribution of vitamin D receptor gene alleles to the determination of bone mineral density in normal and osteoporotic women. *J. Bone Miner. Res.* **10,** 991–996.
56. Viitanan, A. M., Kärkkälnen, M., Laitinen, K., Lamberg-Allardt, C., Kainulainen, K., Räsänen, L., et al. (1996) Common polymorphism of the vitamin D receptor gene is associated with variation of peak bone mass in young Finns. *Calcif. Tissue Int.* **59,** 231–234.
57. Finch, C. E. and Tanzi, R. E. (1997) Genetics of aging. *Science.* **278,** 407–411.
58. Ferrari, S., Rizzoli, R., Chevalley, T., Slosman, D., Eisman, J. A., and Bonjour, J. P. (1995) Vitamin-D-receptor-gene polymorphisms and change in lumbar-spine bone mineral density. *Lancet* **345,** 423–424.
59. Krall, E. A., Parry, P., Lichter, J. B., and Dawson-Hughes, B. (1995) Vitamin D receptor alleles and rates of bone loss: influences of years since menopause and calcium intake. *J. Bone Miner. Res.* **10,** 978–984.
60. Ferrari, S., Rizzoli, R., Chevalley, T., Eisman, J. A., and Bonjour, J. P. (1995) Vitamin-D-receptor-gene polymorphisms and change in lumbar-spine bone mineral density—Reply. *Lancet* **345,** 1239.
61. Matsuyama, T., Ishii, S., Tokita, A., Yabuta, K., Yamamori, S., Morrison, N. A., and Eisman, J. A. (1995) Vitamin D receptor genotypes and bone mineral density. *Lancet* **345,** 1238–1239.
62. Kiel, D. P., Myers, R. H., Cupples, A., Kong, X. F., Zhu X. H., Ordovas, J., et al. (1997) The *Bsm*I vitamin D receptor restriction fragment length polymorphism (bb) influences the effect of calcium intake on bone mineral density. *J. Bone Miner. Res.* **12,** 1049–1057.
63. Graafmans, W. C., Lips, P., Ooms, M. E., van Leeuwen, J. P. T. M., Pols H. A. P., and Uitterlinden, A. G. (1997) The effect of vitamin D supplementation on the bone mineral density of the femoral neck is associated with vitamin D receptor genotype. *J. Bone Miner. Res.* **12,** 1241–1245.

64. Salamone, L. M., Glynn, N. W., Black, D. M., Ferrell, R. E., Palermo, L., Epstein, R. S., et al. (1996) Determinants of premenopausal bone mineral density: the interplay of genetic and lifestyle factors. *J. Bone Miner. Res.* **11,** 1557–1565.
65. Dawson-Hughes, B., Harris, S. S., and Finneran, S. (1995) Calcium absorption on high and low calcium intakes in relation to vitamin D receptor genotype. *J. Clin. Endocrinol. Metab.* **80,** 3657–3661.
66. Wishart, J. M., Horowitz, M., Need, A. G., Scopacasa, F., Morris, H. A., Clifton, P. M., and Nordin B. E. C. (1997) Relations between calcium intake, calcitriol, polymorphisms of the vitamin D receptor gene, and calcium absorption in premenopausal women. *Am. J. Clin. Nutr.* **65,** 798–802.
67. Kinyamu, H. K., Gallagher, J. C., Knezetic, J. A., DeLuca, H. F., Prahl, J. M., and Lanspa, S. J. (1997) Effect of vitamin D receptor genotypes on calcium absorption, duodenal vitamin D receptor concentration, and serum 1,25 dihydroxyvitamin D levels in normal women. *Calcif. Tissue Int.* **60,** 491–495.
68. Ferrari, S. L., Rizzoli, R., Eisman, J. A., and Bonjour, J. P. (1996) Relationship between vitamin D-receptor gene polymorphisms and calcium and phosphate metabolism in young healthy males. *J. Bone Miner. Res.* **11(Suppl. 1),** S209.
69. McClure, L., Eccleshall, T. R., Gross, C., Villa, M. L., Lin, N., Ramaswamy, V., et al. (1997) Vitamin D receptor polymorphisms, bone mineral density, and bone metabolism in postmenopausal Mexican-American women. *J. Bone Miner. Res.* **12,** 234–240.
70. Carling, T., Kindmark, A., Hellman, P., Lundgren, E., Ljunghall, S., Rastad, J., et al. (1995) Vitamin D receptor genotypes in primary hyperparathyroidism. *Nat. Med.* **1,** 1309–1311.

CHAPTER 4

Type I Collagen Polymorphisms and Osteoporosis

Stuart H. Ralston

Introduction

Type I collagen is the most abundant of the vertebrate collagens and is the major protein of bone. The genes that encode collagen type I are candidates for the genetic regulation of bone mass not only because collagen is an important constituent of bone matrix, but also because mutations in the type I collagen genes are the cause of osteogenesis imperfecta (OI), a disease characterized by severe osteoporosis and multiple fractures. This chapter reviews the function of collagen type I, its structure, and the mechanisms by which transcription of the collagen type I genes are regulated. We then go on to discuss collagen type I mutations in osteogenesis imperfecta and try to highlight some of the parallels that exist between this disease and osteoporosis. Finally, recent association studies on the role polymorphisms of the collagen type I genes play as predictors of bone mass and osteoporotic fracture are reviewed.

Bone Formation and Composition of Bone Matrix

Collagen type I constitutes 65% of the organic component of bone tissue. During bone formation, osteoblasts lay down organized lamellae of uncalcified bone matrix (osteoid) which comprises about 90% type I collagen and small amounts of other matrix proteins and growth factors. After a lag phase of about 10 d, the matrix becomes mineralized, as hydroxyapatite crystals are deposited in the spaces between collagen fibrils. Although mineralization confers upon bone the important properties of mechanical rigidity and resistance to compressive forces, the tensile strength of bone and its resistance to torsional forces are mainly derived from bone collagen. The importance of collagen structure as a determinant

The Genetics of Osteoporosis and Metabolic Bone Disease
Ed.: M. J. Econs © Humana Press Inc., Totowa, NJ

of bone's mechanical strength is reflected by the fact that under conditions of increased bone turnover such as Paget's disease, where collagen is laid down in a disorganized and random fashion, the bone is mechanically weak and subject to pathological fracture even though it is denser than normal. This illustrates the important principle that collagen structure is equally as important as collagen content (or bone mineral content) in determining the mechanical strength of bone and hence the risk of fracture.

Collagen Structure and Assembly

The structure and assembly type I collagen is summarized diagramatically in Fig. 1. Type I procollagen is composed of three separate peptide chains encoded by two different genes (*see* Prockop and Kivirikko for review *[1]*). Each mature collagen molecule comprises two alpha (I) I chains and one alpha (I) 2 chain, which are encoded by the COLIA1 and COLIA2 genes which lie on chromosomes 17q21-22 and 7q22, respectively. The COLIA1 gene spans 18Kb and contains 51 exons, whereas the COLIA2 gene spans 35Kb and contains 52 exons. During transcription, each gene produces a monocistronic primary RNA transcript, which is then processed to yield multiple mRNA transcripts of between ~4.4– 6.0 Kb, due to differing patterns of polyadenylation *(2)*. In common with the other interstitial collagens, the collagen type 1 genes have three structurally distinct domains: an N-propeptide domain, a central triple helix domain, and a C-propeptide domain. The triple helix domain is highly conserved between species and has the generic sequence Gly-X-Y where Gly is glycine, and X and Y are other amino acids. This region of the molecule contains a high percentage of proline residues in the X and Y positions. Following translation, the individual collagen chains undergo extensive modification within the Golgi apparatus; the proline and lysine residues are hydroxylated and many of the hydroxylysine residues undergo further glycosylation. The three chains form a triple helix before secretion onto the extracellular space, where the N-propeptide and C-propeptide domains are cleaved off. The resulting truncated molecule (comprising mainly of the triple helix domain and short N-telopeptide and C-telopeptide domains) then further self assembles into compact collagen fibrils. As collagen matures, the fibrils undergo further modification during which individual triple helices are cross linked to one another by specialized covalent bonds (pyridinium cross-links) that enhance the stability and tensile strength of mature collagen.

Transcriptional Regulation of the Collagen Genes

Expression of the COLIA1 and COLIA2 genes is closely coordinated such that the ratio of mRNA for COLIA1 to COLIA2 approaches 2:1, mirroring exactly the ratio of alpha (I) 1 and alpha (I) 2 chains in the collagen protein. It is currently

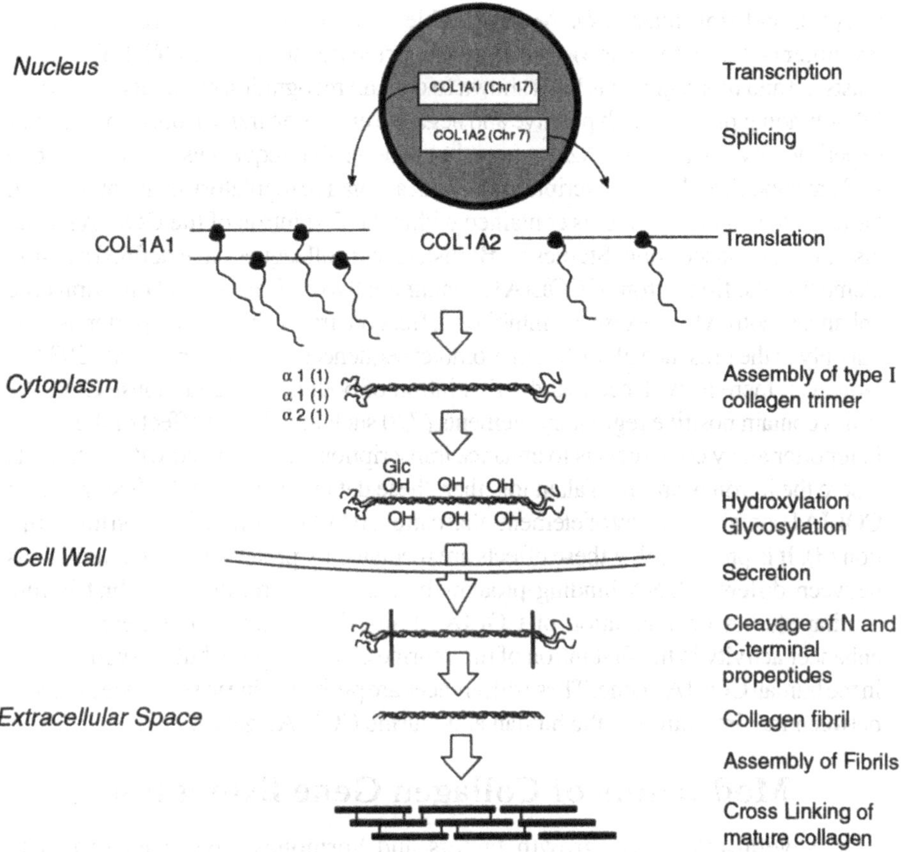

Fig. 1. Structure and assembly of type I collagen. Collagen type I is a triple helical protein composed of three peptide chains derived from two distinct genes. The collagen molecule undergoes extensive posttranslational modification before being secreted into bone matrix, where in undergoes further proteolytic modification with cleavage of the N- and C- terminal propeptides. Subsequently, the triple helical domain of the collagen molecules self assemble into collagen fibrils and these are crosslinked by pyridinium bonds to produce mature collagen.

unclear how the transcription of the collagen genes is coordinated in this way *(3)*. Although both collagen genes contain classical TATA and CCAAT sequences upstream of the transcription start site, there is limited sequence homology between the promoters apart from this. Indeed, the only factor so far identified which could bind to sequences common to both promoters is the CCAAT box binding factor. Deletion studies have shown that between –300bp and +100bp of the human COLIA1 promoter is required to drive reporter transcription in Xenopus oocytes, and fibroblasts *(4)*. A comparable amount of sequence of the murine promoter (–220bp to +16bp) is sufficient to drive transcription in NIH-3T3 fibroblasts *(5)* and this region has been shown to contain recognition elements for several DNA binding proteins with positive and negative effects on transcription *(5)*. Similar experiments with the COLIA2 promoter have shown that sequences between –376 to +58 are enough to drive transcription *(4)*, with a negative regulatory element between bases –376 to –772. Elements contained within the first intron of the COLIA1 gene also affects transcription. Studies by Bornstein and colleagues have defined a 274bp element in the first intron of COLIA1, containing two Sp1 motifs and one viral core enhancer motif which exerts an inhibitory effect on transcription in reporter assays, but only in the presence of upstream promoter sequences between –625 and –293 *(6)*. However, there is evidence that the first intron of both human and mouse COLIA1 genes contain positive regulatory elements *(7,8)* such that the net effect of the intron in reporter assay constructs is to enhance transcription, as compared with constructs where the intron is absent. Taken together, these data indicate that the first intron of COLIA1 contains an array of elements that can exert bidirectional effects on transcription *(3)*. It is probable that these effects are mediated by protein–protein interactions between different DNA binding proteins bound to the promoter and first intron. Similar studies on regulation of COLIA2 transcription have shown evidence of enhancer activity in the first intron of the murine COLIA2 gene, but no such activity in the human COLIA2 gene. These differences are probably due to sequence diversity between the first intron of the human and murine COLIA1 genes.

Modulators of Collagen Gene Expression

Several cytokines, growth factors and hormones have been shown to modulate type I collagen synthesis in vitro and the effects of those relevant to the pathogenesis of osteoporosis are reviewed here. Transforming growth factor (TGF) beta is potent stimulator of type I collagen production in many cell types and is likely to be an important local regulator of collagen synthesis in vivo *(3)*. Since TGF beta is thought to be released from bone matrix during the process of bone remodeling, this could have relevance to mechanisms of coupling between bone resorption and bone formation. Pro-inflammatory cytokines such as interleukin 1 and tumor necrosis factor alpha have complex effects on collagen production depending on the cell type studied and concentrations used. Both cytokines seem to stimulate collagen production by fibroblasts, whereas inhibitory effects on collagen production have been found in bone explants *(3,9)*, which would be in keeping with the depression of bone formation that accompanies inflammatory diseases such as rheumatoid arthritis. Glucocorticoids have inhibitory effects on type I collagen production, due to decreased stability of both procollagen transcripts and down-regulation of gene expression at a transcriptional level. It is probable that these effects on type I collagen are partly responsible for the inhibitory effect of glucocorticoids on bone formation in vivo *(10)*.

Collagen Mutations, Osteogenesis Imperfecta, and Osteoporosis

Osteogenesis imperfecta (OI) is the collective name given to a rare and heterogeneous group of inherited conditions which are characterized by severe osteoporosis and multiple fragility fractures. Various subtypes of OI have been described depending on clinical features, patterns of inheritance, and the underlying molecular lesions (reviewed in Chapter 5 and by Rowe *[11]*), but most arise in association with mutations in the COLIA1 or COLIA2 genes. In severe cases, these mutations result in disruption of the collagen protein chain, due to an amino acid substitution, deletion, or insertion. Most milder cases of OI however are due to under expression of the mRNA for one Collagen type I allele (so-called "null allele"), resulting in under production of one of the collagen protein chains. Some instances of "null alleles" have been shown to be due to splice site mutations which result in nuclear retention of unspliced collagen RNA, with failure of the spliced RNA to appear in the cytoplasm, and under production of the collagen protein *(12)*. In other cases however, nonsense or frameshift mutations which predict premature termination of the protein have also been found to reduce steady-state levels of mRNA resulting in under expression of the mutant allele *(13)*.

The classical picture of OI consists of osteoporosis, multiple fractures during childhood, blue sclerae, deafness, and opalescent teeth. The frequency of fractures and presence of accompanying features are extremely variable, such that there is the potential for considerable clinical overlap between patients with mild OI and those with severe osteoporosis. Proof of this was demonstrated by Spotila et al. *(14)*, who investigated a woman who was initially diagnosed as having post-menopausal osteoporosis, but who turned out to have mild osteogenesis imperfecta due to a glycine-serine mutation at codon 661 of the alpha2 -(1) collagen chain *(14)*. Prompted by the possibility that other individuals with severe "osteoporosis" might harbor similar mutations in the Collagen type I genes, Spotila and colleagues performed extensive sequencing of both collagen type I genes in a multicenter study of 26 patients with osteoporosis *(15)*. These patients were selected on the basis of low bone mass, a family history of osteoporosis, and failure to meet the clinical criteria for OI. The studies revealed the presence of proline-alanine mutations at codon 27 in the COLIA1 gene in two cases (7.6%) and an alanine to proline mutations at codon 459 of the COLIA2 gene in 9 cases (34%). Although both substitutions caused amino acid changes, their role in the pathogenesis of the osteoporosis remains uncertain. The father of the patient with the codon 27 substitution shared the same substitution, but had no obvious bone disease, whereas his brother had severe osteoporosis but did not harbor the substitution. The codon 459 mutation, while common in the osteoporotic population studied was equally common (21%) in a series of 12 control subjects. Other neutral sequence variants of COLIA2 which were observed at equal frequencies in the osteoporotic and control subjects included a T/C change in codon 3; an A/C change in codon 392 and a T/C change in codon 955 *(15)*. Spotila et al. were also able to address the possibility that the osteoporosis may have arisen as the result of null alleles using exonic restriction fragment length polymorphism's (RFLPs) to assess allele-specific transcription. Each individual in the study was found to be heterozygous for at least one exonic polymorphism in the COLIA2 gene, and it was found that both COLIA2 alleles were expressed in all cases. Allele-specific transcription of the COLIA1 gene could only be assessed in 12/26 individuals who were heterozygous for a C/T substitution in the 3' untranslated region. In all cases expression of both COLIA1 alleles was found.

These studies do not support the view that protein coding mutations or null alleles are a common cause of osteoporosis.

Regulatory Polymorphisms of the Collagen Genes and Osteoporosis

In view of the negative results reported by Spotila, Grant, and colleagues investigated the hypothesis that polymorphisms or mutations affecting the regulatory regions of the collagen type I genes may be responsible for osteoporosis *(16)*. Initial investigations focused in the COLIA1 gene, where PCR-SSCP was used to screen for mutations in the proximal promoter (–751 to +38) and first intron (+174 to +1805), two regions of the gene which are thought to be important in regulating transcription *(3)*. These studies showed evidence of 3 polymorphisms, all of which were situated in the first intron. The first was a T insertion at base +498, the second, a C/G substitution at base +811, and the third a G/T substitution at base +1480. The frequency of each polymorphism was studied in a series of 50 healthy women. For the T +498 insertion, two individuals were heterozygous and one homozygous, giving an allele frequency of 4%; for the C/G +811 substitution, 3 C/G heterozygotes were detected, giving an allele frequency of 2% and for the G/T +1480 substitution 17 G/T heterozygotes, and 3 T/T homozygotes were detected giving an allele frequency of 20%.

Grant and colleagues further investigated the G/T polymorphism in more detail, not only because it was relatively common, but also because it lay at the first base of a recognition site for the transcription factor Sp1—a DNA binding protein which is known to be important as a regulation of basal gene transcription. Gel shift studies confirmed that the polymorphic site was recognized by DNA binding proteins in gel shift assays and specificity of binding was confirmed by abrogation of binding by an Sp1 specific antibody *(16)*. Although the consequences of the polymorphisms for regulation of collagen type I transcription and collagen protein production remain unclear as yet, preliminary experiments have shown that the G/T substitution significantly affects the affinity of the recognition site to bind Sp1 in gel shift assays (Grant and Ralston, unpublished data), raising the possibility that it may have functional relevance.

COLIA1 Sp1 Polymorphism and Osteoporosis

The relationship between the COLIA1 Sp1 polymorphism and osteoporosis fracture has now been investigated in several populations, but so far many of these studies have been reported only in abstract form. The first published study was that of Grant and colleagues who initially described the Sp1 polymorphism. Grant investigated the relationhip between the Sp1 polymorphism, bone mass, and osteoporotic fracture in a two-center, UK-based study of predominantly postmenopausal women *(16)*. One study population was drawn from the North East of Scotland, and comprised 205 women, approx 53% of whom had been referred for clinical evaluation and 47% of whom were drawn at random from the local community by postal register. The London population comprised a consecutive series of 94 healthy perimenopausal volunteers who had attended for bone densitometry. A significant effect of COLIA1 genotype on spinal bone mass was observed in both study populations. Individuals with the G/G genotype (termed "SS") were found to have significantly higher bone mineral density (BMD) values than the G/T genotype (termed "Ss") who in turn had higher values than the rare T/T genotype (termed "ss"). A similar trend was observed for BMD values at the femoral neck, but this did not reach statistical significance. An interesting feature of the association between the COLIA1 polymorphism and bone mass was that the effect seemed to increase with age, distinguishing this polymorphism from polymorphisms of other candidate genes such such as VDR and IL-6 which seem to predominantly affect peak bone mass. Thus, when BMD was plotted against age or menopausal age, in relation to COLIA1 genotype, those with the Ss and ss genotypes had a similar intercept on the *Y*-axis to those with the SS genotypes (reflecting similar peak bone mass), but had a significantly different slope of BMD upon age, suggesting that the COLIA1 polymorphism may act as a marker for increased age-related bone loss. (Fig. 2). In the same study, Grant compared distribution of genotypes in 55 vertebral fracture cases when compared with 55 matched controls and found over representation of the Ss and ss genotypes in patients with vertebral fractures (54%) as compared with controls (27%) equivalent to a relative risk of 2.97 in individuals carrying the "s" allele. This observation again is unique among polymorphisms of candidate genes which have been thought to regulate bone mass and suggests that the COLIA1 polymorphism may be of value in predicting the clinically important end-point of osteoporotic fracture risk.

Population-Based Studies of COLIA1 Sp1 Polymorphism

The largest population-based study of COLIA1 Sp1 genotype in relation to bone mass comes from the Netherlands, where Uitterlinden et al. studied 1778 postmenopausal women aged 55–80 yr from the Rotterdam study—a population-based cohort study of diseases in the elderly. Uitterlinden confirmed the association between COLIA1 genotype and spinal bone mass reported by Grant and found a similar association with bone mass at the hip, with an overall effect that accounted for a difference of approx 0.2–0.3 z score units between the extreme

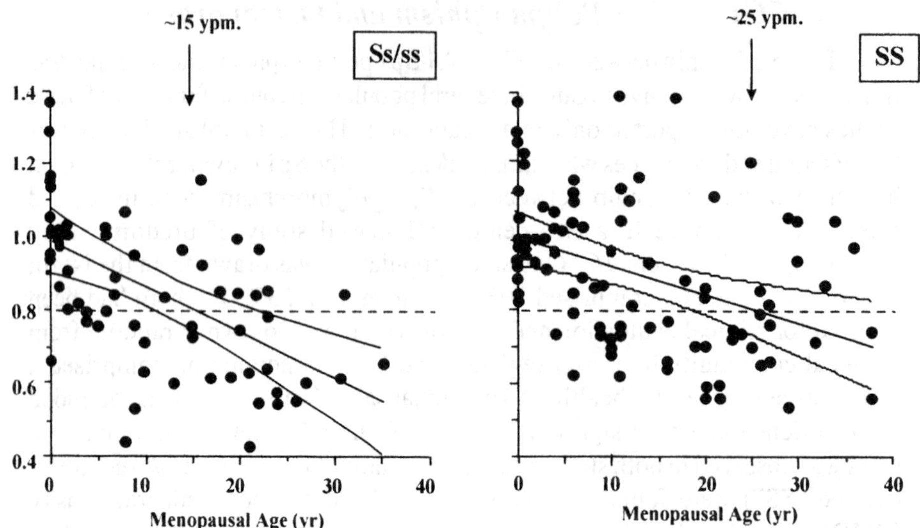

Fig. 2. Relationship between COLIA1 Sp1 polymorphism and bone loss. When BMD is plotted against menopausal age, individuals with the Ss/ss genotypes have evidence of an increased rate of bone loss when compared with the SS genotype as reflected by the steeper slope of the regression line in the Ss/ss genotype group. The regression line in the "Ss/ss" group crosses the notional "fracture threshold" (horizontal interrupted line corresponding to T score of –3.0) 15 yr postmenopause as compared with 25 yr postmenopause for the SS group ($p < 0.05$). Note that the intercept on the *Y*-axis is similar, suggesting that COLIA1 polymorphism may act as a marker for increased age-related bone loss rather than peak bone mass. [/Data from the Aberdeen study population studied by Grant et al. *(16)*/].

genotypes *(17)*. Interestingly, the Rotterdam study also showed a significant association between COL1A1 genotype and body weight, such that weight was lower in individuals who carried the low bone mass associated "s" alleles—a trend that had also been observed in the original study. In agreement with the data of Grant, Uitterlinden found the "Ss" and "ss" genotypes to be significantly over-represented in patients with fractures. Studies in 111 patients who suffered incident nonvertebral fractures during a 5 yr follow-up showed that 42% had the "Ss" or "ss" genotypes as compared with 32% of 1667 individuals without fractures ($p < 0.01$), equivalent to an odds ratio for fracture of 1.54 per copy "s" allele. An interesting feature of this association was that the increased risk of fracture persisted even after correction for confounding factors such weight, age, and BMD, suggesting that COLIA1 genotype may influence fracture risk by mechanisms that are independent of bone mass.

Garnero et al. studied the relationship between COLIA1 Sp1 genotype, bone mass, and biochemical indices of bone turnover in the OFELY study—a population-based cohort study of determinants of bone mass in healthy French women *(18)*.

Analysis of 220 premenopausal women showed a positive association between spinal bone mass and COLIA1 genotype and an association between genotype and total body BMD, total bone mineral content, and height. While femoral neck BMD values showed the same trend as spine BMD values, the difference between genotypes was not significant and there was no significant difference between genotypes with regard to wrist BMD. In addition to the differences in bone mass, Garnero also found significantly reduced circulating PICP values (an index of collagen formation) in the "ss" genotype group when compared with the other genotype groups. When a codominant effect was assumed, COLIA1 genotype was an independent predictor of spine BMD, total body BMD, and serum PICP in multiple regression analysis.

McCloskey and colleagues investigated the relationship between the Sp1 plymorphism and bone mass in a series of 317 elderly women of mean age 80 yr from Sheffield (UK) *(19)*. Although this was a random population sample, recruitment to the study was low, which probably led to over-representation of the "healthy elderly" from the study sample. Possibly reflecting this fact, the genotype distribution differed significantly in the Sheffield population from previous studies of Caucasian individuals, with relative under-representation of the "s" alleles (Ss 20%; ss 2%). Analysis of BMD in relation to genotype in this population showed highest BMD values in the SS group, intermediate values in the Ss group, and lowest in the ss group, with an overall difference of approx 0.4 z-score units between genotypes, but these differences were not significant.

Case-Control Studies of COLIA1 Sp1 Polymorphism

Keen and colleagues related COLIA1 genotype to bone mass and prevalent vertebral fractures in a series of 185 individuals drawn from a population based cohort study in Northern London, fifty-five of whom had suffered fractures in the preceeding 10 yr *(20)*. Keen found that individuals with the Ss and ss genotypes had significantly lower BMD at the spine than those with the SS genotype and a similar, but nonsignificant trend was noted for hip bone density. In keeping with the differences in BMD, the "Ss" and "ss" genotypes were significantly over-represented in patients with fractures (49%) as compared with controls (33%) equivalent to an odds ratio of 1.95 for fracture in those with the "s" allele. Langdahl and colleagues looked at the relationship between COL1A1 genotype and osteoporotic fracture in a case-control study of Danish men and women *(21)*. The study group comprised 249 individuals, with 105 osteoporotic vertebral fracture patients and 144 matched normal controls. As in the studies cited previously, Langdahl found the "Ss" and "ss" genotypes to be associated with vertebral fracture in both men and women such that 47 % of fracture cases carried the "s" allele, compared with 34% of the controls ($p = 0.0003$), equivalent to an odds ratio for fracture of 1.71 in those who carried the "s" allele. Subgroup analysis showed that the effect was similar in men and women. A further case-control study of patients with osteoporotic fracture by de Vernejoul *(22)* looked at allele distribution in 97 postmenopausal French women with crush fractures and 137 controls who were on average 5 yr younger than the fracture cases (65 yr vs 69 yr). This study showed an excess of ss genotypes in the fracture patients (5%) compared with the controls (1%), but the distribution of the Ss genotype was similar in fracture cases, controls, and overall, the difference between the groups failed to reach significance ($p = 0.07$). A further study by McLellan et al. looked at the relationship between the COL1A1 polymorphism, bone mass, and osteoporotic fracture in a series of 606 women from Glasgow (UK) *(23)*. The study population comprised a mix of clinic referrals (~60%) and women who had answered newspaper advertisements calling for volunteers to undergo bone densitometry (~40%). Approx 18% of the population had been treated with HRT and another 10% with the bisphosphonate disodium etidronate. BMD values at the spine and femoral neck were approx 0.2 z-score units lower in the Ss genotype as compared with the SS genotype, but these differences were not significant. BMD values were highly variable in the small number of "ss" individuals studied ($n = 15$), who were on average, 6 yr older than the other genotype groups, possibly reflecting the nonrandom method of patient selection. A nested case-control study was performed looking at allele distribution in 81 patients with osteoporotic fractures as compared with a series of 114 controls, who were on average, about 14 yr younger than the fracture cases. Although the controls and cases were not aged matched, there was significant over-representation of the Ss and ss genotypes in the fracture cases (43%) as compared with the controls (28%) ($p < 0.04$).

Twin Studies of COLIA1 Sp1 Polymorphism

The relationship between COLIA1 genotype and bone mass has been investigated in two twin studies. Grant et al. *(24)* looked for evidence of linkage between COLIA1 Sp1 alleles and bone mass in 113 female Australian twins of mean age 53 yr (55 nonidentical (DZ)/58 identical (MZ). In this study, intra-pair differences in femoral neck BMD were significantly greater among DZ twin pairs who shared one COLIA1 allele identical by descent than those who shared two alleles, providing evidence of linkage between COLIA1 alleles and hip bone mass ($p = 0.01$). A similar trend was seen at the spine but this was not significant ($p = 0.20$). A similar study of 79 premenopausal female twins of average age 35 years (38 MZ/41 DZ) was conducted by Hustmyer et al. *(25)*, but here no evidence of linkage between COLIA1 genotype and bone mass was found. Although the studies used similar methods and were of similar size, they differed significantly in terms of the twins age. This is relevant since data from the Aberdeen study and Rotterdam study indicate that the effect of COLIA1 genotype on bone mass increases with age, which could account for the positive effect in the Australian twins and negative effect in the U S twins

Ethnic Differences in COLIA1 Sp1 Polymorphism

The polymorpism has also been studied in COLIA1 Sp1 genotype noncauscasian populations. In one study, Beavan reported that the "s" allele was rare in Africans and absent from 200 Chinese individuals *(26)*. In another study, Lim et al. looked at the COLIA1 Sp1 polymorphism in 152 Korean individuals *(27)*. Lim found no individuals with the "Ss" or "ss" genotype. These data suggest that the "s" allele is rare or absent from Asian (Oriental) populations. This observations is of interest in relation to ethnic differences in incidence of osteoporotic fracture *(28)*. Asians have a lower incidence of osteoporotic fractures than Caucasians and these differences are not completely explained by differences in bone mass. Factors such as difference in hip axis length have been invoked as a possible explanation for these differences *(28)*, but another factor might be differences in genetic makeup of the different populations.

Other Polymorphisms at the COLIA1 and COLIA2 Loci

Vandervyver investigated the relationship between Msp1 and Rsa1 polymorphisms at the COLIA1 and COLIA2 loci in relation to bone mass and osteoporotic fracture in 335 healthy postmenopausal Belgian women *(29)*. No significant difference in ditribution of the polymorphisms was observed between osteoporotic, osteopaenic, or normal women and there was no difference between the genotype groups in terms of BMD at the spine, hip, or wrist. These polymorphisms were also investigated by Spotila et al. in a linkage study of osteoporotic families. In this study Spotila classified individuals as affected, partially affected, or unaffected according to Z-score and analyzed the relationhip between affection status and genetic markers at candidate loci including COLIA1 and COLIA2. No evidence of linkage between bone mass and polymorphisms at the collagen loci was found in these families *(30)*.

Conclusions

Several polymorphisms have been described at the COLIA1 and COLIA2 loci, but few have been studied in relation to bone mass and osteoporotic fracture. The most extensively studied and potentially most important is the polymorphic Sp1 binding site in the COLIA1 gene. Data from several studies suggests that this polymorphism acts as a genetic marker for BMD and osteoporotic fracture, although the molecular mechanisms which underlie this association are at present unclear. Six case-control studies have been performed, looking at the distribution of COLIA1 Sp1 alleles in fracture patients and five of these have shown a significant over-representation of the "Ss" and "ss" genotypes in patients with fracture cases as compared with controls. In the sixth a similar trend was observed which failed to reach significance. When data from all the studies are combined there is significant over-representation of the "s" allele in osteoporotic fracture cases as compared with controls with an overall relative risk of about 1.65 (Fig. 3). Studies on bone density in relation to COLIA1 genotyping have shown that BMD values are generally lower in those with the Ss /ss genotypes than those with the SS genotype although the effect on BMD is modest and in most studies has been equivalent to 0.2–0.3 z score units. This is not sufficient to account for the increased risk of fracture associated with the "s" allele and suggests that the

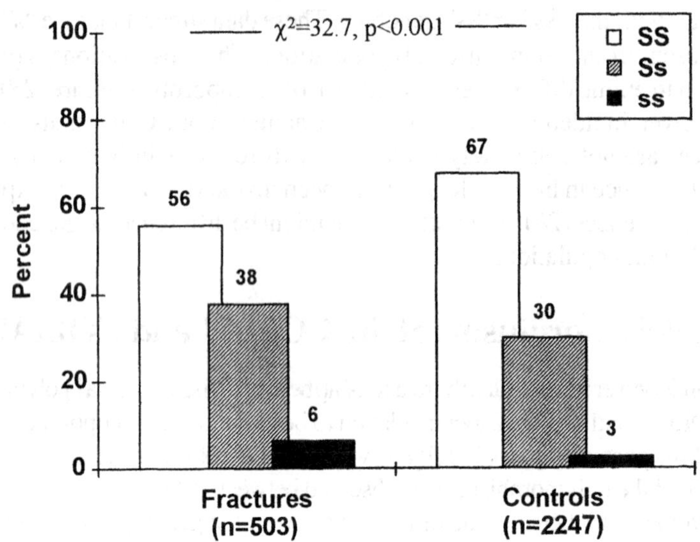

Fig. 3. Relationship between COLIA1 Sp1 polymorphism and osteoporotic fracture. The figure shows cumulative data from six studies where COLIA1 genotype has been investigated in case control studies of patients with osteoporotic fractures *(16,20–23,25)* (see text for details). Although cases were not aged matched with controls in two of these studies *(23,25)*, there was a highly significant over representation of the "Ss" and "ss" genotypes in fracture cases as compared with controls. ($\chi^2 = 23.9$, $p < 0.0001$), equivalent to an odds ratio for fracture of 1.65 (95% CI = 1.36–1.96) in individuals who carry the "s" allele. Percentage values for each genotype group in cases and controls are shown above each column.

COLIA1 Sp1 polymorphism may act as a marker for increased fracture risk by mechanisms which are partly independent of differences in bone mass. Further studies, using techniques such as ultrasound in relation to COLIA1 genotype will be of interest to investigate this observation further.

The COLIA1 Sp1 polymorphism is the only polymorphism of a candidate gene so far identified to predict the clinically important endpoint of fracture raising the possibility that it may have a role in risk assessment. Although the COLIA1 polymorphism has predictive value in population terms, it is likely to be of limited predictive value in individual terms, since many osteoporotic fractures occur in individuals who do not carry the "s" allele and vice-versa. This reflects the fact that COLIA1 is only one of the genes which regulate bone mass and predisposition to the development of osteoporosis. When other candidate genes are defined, it is possible that we shall be able to combine information from several polymorphisms to give better prediction of those at risk of osteoporotic fracture, and to combine this information with other means of risk assessment such as bone mass measurements and biochemical markers.

Acknowledgment

I wish to thank Dr. S. Grant, Dr. B. Langdahl, Dr. A. McLellan, Dr. P. Garnero, Dr. A. Uitterlinden, and Dr. M.-C. de Vernejoul, for sharing information in advance of publication, and the Wellcome Trust and the Arthritis and Rheumatism Council for Grant Support.

References

1. Prockop, D. J. and Kivirikko, K. I. (1984) Heritable diseases of collagen. *N. Engl. J. Med.* **311,** 376–386.
2. Chu, M. L., de Wet, W., Bernard, M., and Ramirez, F. (1985) Fine structural analysis of the human pro-alpha-1(I) collagen gene. *J. Biol. Chem.* **260,** 2315–2320.
3. Slack, J. L., Liska, D. J., and Bornstein, P. (1993) Regulation of expression of the type I collagen genes. *Am. J. Med. Genet.* **45,** 140–151.
4. Boast, S., Su, M., Ramirez, F., Sanchez, M., and Avvedimento, E. V. (1990) Functional analysis of cis-acting sequences controlling transcription of the human type I collagen genes. *J. Biol. Chem.* **265,** 13,351–13,356.
5. Karsenty, G. and de Crombrugghe, B. (1990) Two different negative and one positive regulatory factors interact with a short promotor segment of the alpha-1(I) collagen gene. *J. Biol. Chem.* **265,** 9934–9942.
6. Bornstein, P., McKay, J., Morishima, J. K., Devarayalu, S., and Gelinas, R. E. (1987) Regulatory elements in the first intron contribute to transcriptional control of the human collagen alpha 1 (I) collagen gene. *Proc. Natl. Acad. Sci. USA* **84,** 8869–8873.
7. Bornstein, P. and McKay, J. (1988) The first intron of the alpha 1(I) collagen gene contains several transcriptional regulatory elements. *J. Biol. Chem.* **263,** 1603–1606.
8. Rippe, R. A., Lorenzen, S. I., Brenner, D. A., and Breindl, M. (1989) Regulatory elements in the 5'-flanking region and the first intron contribute to transcriptional control of the mouse alpha 1 type I collagen gene. *Mol. Cell. Biol.* **9,** 2224–2227.
9. Canalis E. (1986) Interleukin-1 has independent effects on deoxyribonucleic acid and collagen synthesis in cultures of rat calvariae. *Endocrinology* **118,** 74–81.
10. Reid, I. R. and Grey, A. B. (1993) Corticosteroid osteoporosis, in *Bailliere's Clinical Rheumatology,* 7th ed. (Reid, D. M., ed.), Bailliere Tindall, London, pp. 573–587.
11. Rowe, D. W. (1991) Osteogenesis imperfecta, in *Bone and Mineral Research,* (Heersche, J. N. M. and Kanis, J. A., eds.), Elsevier, Amsterdam, pp. 209–241.
12. Stover, M. L., Primorac, D., Liu, S. C., McKinstry, M. B., and Rowe, D. W. (1993) Defective splicing of mRNA from one COL1A1 allele of type I collagen in nondeforming (type I) osteogenesis imperfecta. *J. Clin. Invest.* **92,** 1994–2002.
13. Willing, M. C., Pruchno, C. J., and Byers, P. H. (1993) Molecular heterogeneity in osteogenesis imperfecta type I. *Am. J. Med. Genet.* **45,** 223–227.
14. Spotila, L. D., Constantinou, C. D., Sereda, L., Ganguly, A., Riggs, B. L., and Prockop, D. J. (1991) Mutation in the gene for type I procollagen (COL1A2) in a woman with postmenopausal osteoporosis, evidence for a phenotypic and genotypic overlap with mild osteogenesis imperfecta. *Proc. Natl. Acad. Sci. USA* **88,** 5243–5427.
15. Spotila, L. D., Colige, A., Sereda, L., et al. (1994) Mutation analysis of coding sequences for type I procollagen in individuals with low bone density. *J. Bone Miner. Res.* **9,** 923–932.

16. Grant, S. F. A., Reid, D. M., Blake, G., Herd, R., Fogelman, I., and Ralston, S. H. (1996) Reduced bone density and osteoporosis associated with a polymorphic Sp1 site in the collagen type I alpha 1 gene. *Nat. Genet.* **14,** 203–205.
17. Uitterlinden, A. G., Burger, H., Huang, O., Yue, F., McGuigan, F. E. A., Grant, S. F. A., Hofman, A., van Leeuwen, J. P. T. M., Pols, H. A. P., and Ralston, S. H. (1998) Relation of alleles of the collagen type I α 1 gene to bone density and risk of osteoporotic fractures in postmenopausal women. *N. Engl. J. Med.* **338,** 1016–1022.
18. Garnero, P., Borel, O., Grant, S. F. A., Ralston, S. H., and Delmas, P. D. (1998) Collagen I α 1 polymorphism, bone mass and bone turnover in healthy French premenopausal women: the OFELY study. *J. Bone Miner. Res.* **12,** 813–818.
19. McCloskey, E. V., Gray, R. L., Grant, S. F. A., et al. (1997) COL1A1 polymorphism and bone mass in elderly women. *J. Bone Miner. Res.* **12(suppl),** S547.
20. Keen, R. W., Woodford-Richens, K. L., Grant, S. F. A., Lanchbury, J. S., and Ralston, S. H., and Spector, T. D. (1999) Polymorphism at the type I collagen (COLIA1) locus is associated with reduced bone mineral density, increased fracture risk and increased collagen turnover. *Arth. Rheum.* 42**,** 285–290.
21. Langdahl, B. L., Ralston, S. H., Grant, S. F. A., and Eriksen, E. F. (1998) An Sp1 binding site polymorphism in the COLIA1 gene predicts osteoporotic fractures in men and women. *J. Bone Miner. Res.* **13,** 1384–1389.
22. de Vernejoul, M., Haguenauer, D., Cohen-Solal, M. E., and Beaudreuil, J. (1997) Polymorphism of collagen I and vertebral osteoporosis, no association. *J. Bone Miner. Res.* **12(suppl),** S549(Abstract).
23. McLellan, A. R., Jagger, C., Spooner, R., Sutcliffe, R., Harrison, J., and Shapiro, D. (1997)Are COLIA1 polymorphisms important determinants of bone mineral density and osteoporosis in postmenopausal women in the UK? *J. Bone Miner. Res.* **12(suppl),** S119(Abstract).
24. Grant, S. F. A., Nguyen, T. V., Howard, G. M., et al. (1997) Genetic linkage between a polymorphism in the collagen I alpha 1 gene and bone mineral density, a twin study. *Bone* **20(suppl),** 7S(Abstract).
25. Hustmyer, F. G., Lui, G., Christian, J. C., Johnston, C. C., and Peacock, M. (1999) Polymorphism at an Sp1 binding site of COLIA1 and bone mineral density in premenopausal female twins and elderly fracture patients. *Osteoporosis Int.* **9,** 346–350.
26. Beavan, S., Prentice, A., Dibba, B., Yan, L., Cooper, C., and Ralston, S. H. (1998) Polymorphism of the collagen type I alpha 1 gene and thenic differenced in hip-fractue rates. *N. Engl. J. Med.* **339,** 351–352.
27. Lim, S., Li, S. Z., Won, Y. J., Shin, W., Lee, H. C., and Huh, K. B. (1997) Lack of association between a polymorphic Sp1 binding site in collagen type 1 alpha 1 gene and osteoporosis in Korean women. *J. Bone Miner. Res.* **12(suppl),** S491(abstract).
28. Cummings, S. R., Cauley, J. A., Palermo, L., et al. (1994) Racial differences in hip axis lengths might explain racial differences in rates of hip fracture. Study of Osteoporotic Fractures Research Group. *Osteoporosis Int.* **4**, 226–229.
29. Vandevyer, C., Philipparts, L., Cassiman, J., Raus, J., and Guesens, P. (1997) Bone mineral density in post-menopausal women is not associated with type I collagen (COL1A1 and COL1A2) dimorphisms. *J. Bone Miner. Res.* **12(suppl),** S490(Abstract).
30. Spotila, L. D., Caminis, J., Devoto, M., et al. (1996) Osteopenia in 37 members of seven families, analysis based on a model of dominant inheritance. *Mol. Med.* **2,** 313–324.

Chapter 5

Osteogenesis Imperfecta

Paul A. Dawson and Joan C. Marini

Introduction

Osteogenesis imperfecta (OI) is a genetic disorder of connective tissue which includes a spectrum of phenotypes ranging from perinatal-lethal to mild, virtually asymptomatic conditions *(1)*. The most significant clinical feature that defines all OI types is the susceptibility to bone fracture from mild trauma. OI is the most common disorder causing fractures in childhood and occurs in all races with a prevalence of about 1 in 10–20,000. The clinical features of OI are caused by structural or quantitative defects in type I collagen, the predominant component of bone and skin extracellular matrix. Thus, the "brittle bone" feature of OI can be accompanied by other connective tissue abnormalities including short stature, joint laxity, blue sclerae, dentinogenesis imperfecta (DI), fragile skin, and hearing loss.

Most of our knowledge related to this disease has come from studies on OI patients within the last two decades. However, the earliest example of an OI phenotype is preserved in the skeletal remains of a 4-yr-old Egyptian child of the second century BC *(2)*. Early accounts of the OI phenotype which describe crippling skeletal distortion and familial transmission were documented from the late eighteenth and nineteenth centuries *(3)*. By the early 1900s, Looser described both the severe early onset infantile (OI congenita) and a later childhood and early adult form (OI tarda) *(4)*. More than a decade later, Bell formally described the autosomal dominant inheritance in mild OI *(5)*. However, it was not until recently that the classification of OI expanded and the molecular basis of its pathogenesis was revealed. This chapter reviews the different types of OI with emphasis on the clinical, biochemical, and molecular aspects of the disease. In addition, issues on OI management and future prospects for therapeutic treatments is discussed.

The Genetics of Osteoporosis and Metabolic Bone Disease
Ed.: M. J. Econs © Humana Press Inc., Totowa, NJ

Clinical

The full clinical spectrum of OI is described by the Sillence classification (*see* Table 1) and ranges from neonatal death to individuals without childhood fractures who are identified only because of a positive family history or physical signs. Most OI patients can be grouped into one of the four Sillence classifications, which are based on clinical, physical, and radiographic findings and mode of inheritance *(1)*. In general, the degree of bone fragility is most severe in type II OI, less severe in type III OI, moderate in type IV OI, and least severe in type I OI (Fig. 1). Although some patients show a phenotypic overlap of these groups, the Sillence classification has proved valuable for clinical and biochemical discussion on the topic of OI *(6)*.

Type I OI is the mildest and most common form of OI with an estimated frequency of between 1 in 15,000 and 1 in 20,000. However, the prevalence of type I OI may be underestimated due to its mild clinical presentation. Individuals with this mild form of the disease are usually diagnosed on the basis of blue sclerae and mild to moderate bone fragility prior to puberty. Fractures rarely occur *in utero* or in the perinatal period, although mild osteopenia or femoral bowing may be present in some newborns. Fractures may occur in any bone and are usually related to moderate trauma while changing diapers or when the child begins to walk. Fracture frequency usually remains constant throughout childhood but sharply declines with the onset of puberty. The height of individuals with type I OI is usually within normal limits, although affected individuals are often shorter than their unaffected family members. Vertebral bone compression ("codfish" vertebrae) frequently accompanies loss of height in later decades. An increase in fracture frequency often occurs following the menopause in women and the sixth to eighth decades in men.

OI type I is subclassified as IA if the teeth are normal or IB if dentinogenesis imperfecta is present. About one half of patients with type I OI have premature hearing loss, beginning in the late teens and progressing to severe loss by the fourth decade. Additional clinical findings frequently present in individuals with type I OI include mitral valve prolapse, hyperextensibility of large joints, and easy bruising. Overall, the life span for individuals with type I OI is near normal.

The moderately severe type IV form of OI also has A and B subtypes based on the absence or presence of dentinogenesis imperfecta. Type IV OI is characterized by mild to moderate bone fragility and short stature which is generally below the 5th percentile for age. Although birth length is often normal, the height of affected individuals drops below the 25th percentile by 2 yr of age, and in most cases below the 5th percentile. Most infants with type IV OI can be identified in the perinatal period or immediately following birth based on the presence of bone fractures. In occasional cases, type IV OI infants have only mild femoral bowing. Fractures in type IV OI patients are quite variable but are common during the first few months after birth. Fracture frequency usually increases

Table 1
Modified Sillence Classification of the Four Types of OI

Classification	Clinical features	Inhertance
Type I	Mild bone fragility Blue sclerae in most cases Premature hearing loss in some families Dentinogenesis imperfecta (type IB)	Autosomal dominant
Type II	Extremely severe bone fragility Blue or black sclerae Lethal in fetal or perinatal period Rare cases of survival up to 1 yr	Autosomal dominant Recurrence risk in sibs is about 7% due to parental mosaicism
Type III	Progressively severe bone fragility Normal, blue or gray sclerae in infancy, progressing to normal in adolescence Dentinogenesis imperfecta and/or hearing loss may be present in some cases	Autosomal dominant Rare autosomal recessive
Type IV	Moderate bone fragility Normal, blue or gray sclerae in infancy, progressing to normal in adolescence Hearing loss in some families Dentinogenesis imperfecta (type IVB)	Autosomal dominant

following ambulation but declines with the onset of puberty. Although fractures are uncommon in the 20–40-yr-old age group, there is a dramatic increase in the later decades, especially in postmenopausal women. Hearing loss also occurs in some cases of type IV OI and is consistent within pedigrees. Scoliosis may occur in individuals with type IV OI and ranges from mild to severe. The presence of kyphoscoliosis may compromise cardiopulmonary function. However, the prognosis of affected individuals following surgery is significantly improved. In the absence of cardiovascular problems, the life span for individuals with type IV OI is near normal.

The severe and progressively deforming variety of osteogenesis imperfecta is classified as type III OI. Affected individuals are recognized in the perinatal period or immediately following birth because of long bone fractures and cranial abnormalities. Radiographs of newborns generally reveal an undermineralized calvarium with a large anterior fontanelle and Wormian bones, thin ribs, and gracile long bones which usually show signs of fractures or bowing. Many type III OI individuals die in infancy or during childhood and adolescence as a result

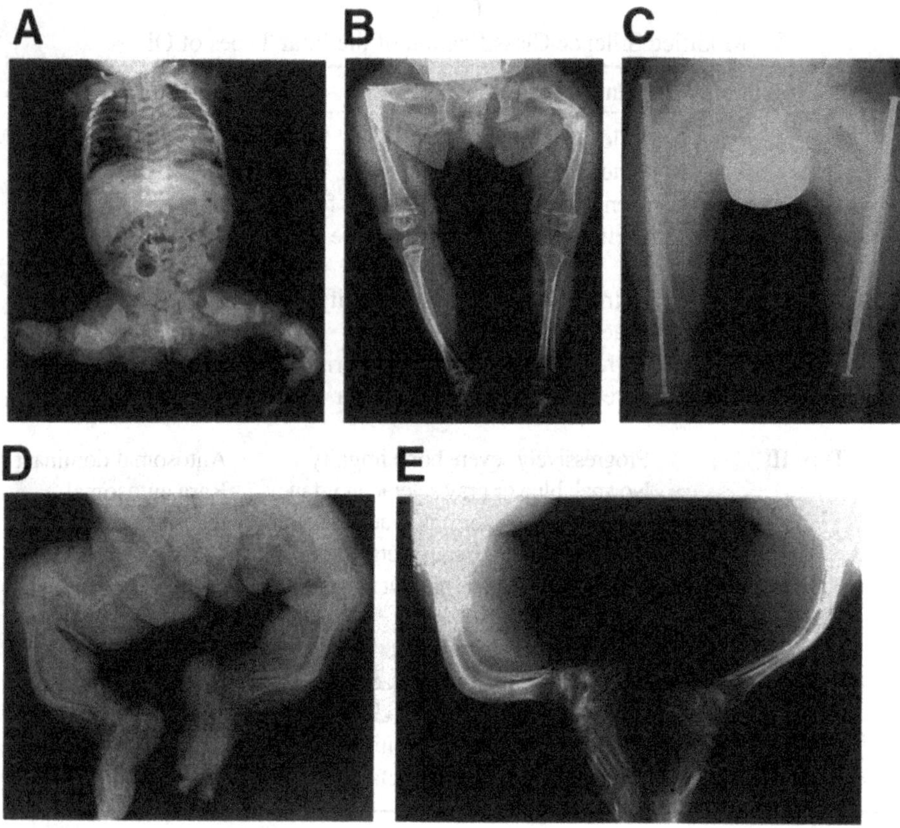

Fig. 1. Radiographs of individuals with **(A)** type II, **(B** and **C)** type IV, and **(D** and **E)** type III OI.

of respiratory problems, cardiac decompensation, or basilar impression with compression of the brain stem. However, longterm survival is not infrequent. In those individuals who survive, there is a gradual deformity of the long bones and spine as a result of fractures and gravitational stress. The thin cortex of the long bones predisposes to angulation deformities, which in turn leads to fractures. Individuals with type III OI have the highest fracture frequency of all OI types and it is not uncommon for affected individuals to have more than 100 fractures throughout life. Additional clinical findings include DI, blue sclerae in infancy which become white in late childhood, and chest wall deformities, either pectus excavatum or carinatum. In occasional cases of type III OI, hyperplastic callus formation may be observed at the site of fractures. These sites of hyperplastic callus have been associated with osteosarcoma in a small proportion of affected children. Almost all affected individuals have relative macrocephaly and many have absolute macrocephaly. There may be ventricular enlargement and sulcal prominence. However, there is no evidence for decreased intellectual function. Type III OI children usually develop a characteristic triangular facies, with a broad and bossed forehead and small chin.

Type II OI is the perinatal lethal form of osteogenesis imperfecta and affects between 1 in 20–60,000 infants. Affected individuals are often delivered prematurely or are stillborn, and some are hydropic. Rare cases of survival beyond a year have been reported. Birth weight and length are often small for gestational age. The type II OI phenotype has a characteristic triangular facies, flat midface, small beaked nose, dark sclerae and extremely soft calvarium. The thoracic cavity is small and the ribs are generally beaded because of callus formation associated with healing *in utero* fractures. Type II OI individuals have either broad or gracile ribs. The extremities are short and bowed, and the legs are usually flexed and abducted at right angles to the body in the "frog-leg" position. Radiographs at birth generally demonstrate severely decreased calvarial mineralization, crumpled femurs, and bowed tibias. Affected individuals are extremely fragile and vaginal delivery may result in avulsion of body parts or intracranial hemorrhage. Pulmonary insufficiency, congestive heart failure, or infection are the usual causes of death for those infants surviving delivery.

Biochemical Mechanisms of OI

Type I collagen is the most abundant fibrous protein in the human body, and provides the major mechanical strength of several connective tissues including bone. Type I procollagen, the precursor of type I collagen, consists of a triple helix of two proα1(I) chains and one proα2(I) chain (Fig. 2). The chains consist of approximately 1000 amino acids with uninterrupted repeats of the Gly-X-Y sequence in the triple helical domain, where Gly is glycine and X and Y are often proline and hydroxyproline, respectively. Glycine residues normally occupy the sterically restricted position in the center of the triple helix. Substitution of glycine at this position with a bulkier amino acid interferes with the normal formation of the triple helix *(7)*.

In normal fibroblasts and osteoblasts, the proα(I) chains are synthesized in the rough endoplasmic reticulum (ER). These chains are secreted into the ER lumen where they assemble in the correct proportion and alignment. Chain nucleation begins within a specific 15 amino-acid alignment region in the carboxyl-terminal extensions *(8)*. Helix formation then proceeds spontaneously from the carboxyl end to the amino terminal end with simultaneous hydroxylation of proline and lysine residues *(9)*. Hydroxylysine residues are then glycosylated by sugar transferases *(10)*. These modifications occur only on the portion of the α-chains that have not assumed a helical conformation. Substitutions for glycine residues produce overmodification because they cause a delay in helix formation at the site of the alteration which results in a longer time of exposure of proα-

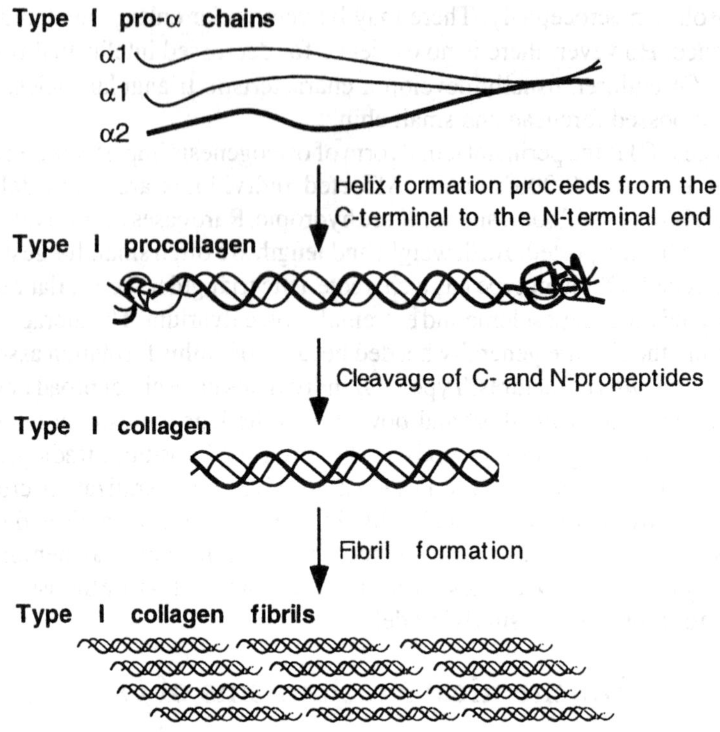

Fig. 2. Two pro-α1(I) chains and one pro-α2(I) chain assemble to form type I procollagen, which is then processed to type I collagen.

chains to the modifying enzymes. Because of the unidirectional folding of the triple helix, the overmodification is generally amino terminal to the alteration *(7)*.

Newly formed procollagen molecules are secreted into the pericellular space where they undergo further processing by specific proteinases which cleave off the N- and C-propeptides. The type I collagen molecules then assemble into the crosslinked collagen fibrils of the extracellular matrix. The fibrils are stabilized by intermolecular cross-links formed by oxidative deamination of lysine and hydroxylysine residues. The fibrillar array of type I collagen owes its strength to the precise chain alignment, thermostable helix, and proper modifications. Thus, disruptions to these structural properties would be predicted to have significant functional consequences. Indeed, collagen-stained bone sections from all OI phenotypes show abnormalities ranging from matrix depletion in type I or IV OI, to severe disorganization of severely depleted bone matrix in types II and III OI.

Most cases of the mild type I form of OI result from a quantitative defect of type I collagen. In these situations, only half the normal amount of collagen is synthesized. This type of defect is usually the consequence of a mutation in the

COL1A1 gene that introduces a premature stop codon, producing either unstable mRNA or the synthesis of truncated unstable collagen. Analysis of α1(I) chains from type I OI individuals usually reveals an increased α1(III):α1(I) ratio as a result of reduced levels of α1(I) chains. Glycine substitutions and exon skipping in α1(I) and α2(I) chains have also been reported in cases of type I OI. Most of these defects are clustered toward the amino-terminal end, presumably reducing their effect on helix formation and structure *(11)*.

The clinically significant types II, III and IV OI are associated with structurally abnormal collagens which are incorporated into the extracellular matrix. Substitutions of amino acids with charged, polar, or bulky side groups for single glycine residues in the triple helix domain of either pro-α chain are the most common (80%) form of structural defect in type I collagen. The functional consequences of glycine substitutions in any of the repeating Gly-X-Y triplets of the helical domain of the α-chains depend on the α-chain involved, the nature and site of the substitution and the surrounding amino acid sequence. Single exon splicing errors account for about 11% of structural defects and the remainder comprises deletions, duplications, and insertions.

The production of structurally abnormal α-chains has a variety of effects on the function of type I collagen. Defects in either chain of type I collagen can give rise to decreased thermal stability, increased intracellular degradation (termed 'procollagen suicide'), and impaired secretion of procollagen molecules incorporating one or more mutant chains. In some cases, the cleavage of the N- and C-propeptides may be prevented, leading to the failure of fibril assembly. Most of the severe OI phenotypes occur when abnormal collagen polymerizes with normal collagen in the extracellular matrix to produce fibrils with irregular shape, slow assembly, and abnormal mineralization. Structural defects in the α1(I) chain might have been expected to be more deleterious than those at equivalent positions of the α2(I) chain because of the stoichiometry of type I collagen molecules. In the heterozygous state, mutations in the α2(I) chain would be expected to result in equal amounts of normal and mutant helices. Defects in the α1(I) chain would be expected to result in 25% normal helices, while 75% of the molecules would contain either 1 or 2 mutant chains. However, approximately equal proportions of all clinical types occur in each chain. A gradient of severity has been observed with substitutions of cysteine for glycine in the α1(I) chain(11). Amino terminal cysteine substitutions produce mild type I OI phenotypes, central substitutions produce type III and IV OI, and carboxyl terminal substitutions produce the lethal type II form of OI. The presence of a cysteine substitution in α1(I) results in the formation of reducible cysteine dimers which are distinct on polyacrylamide gels (Fig. 3C). Gradients are not apparent with other amino acid substitutions in either chain of type I collagen. However, alternating clusters of lethal and nonlethal phenotypes have been mapped to the COL1A2 gene and this has led to a Regional Model for the α2(I) chain *(12,13)*.

In most cases, biochemical testing can distinguish structurally abnormal type I collagen from normal type I collagen (Fig. 3). The abnormal collagen chains

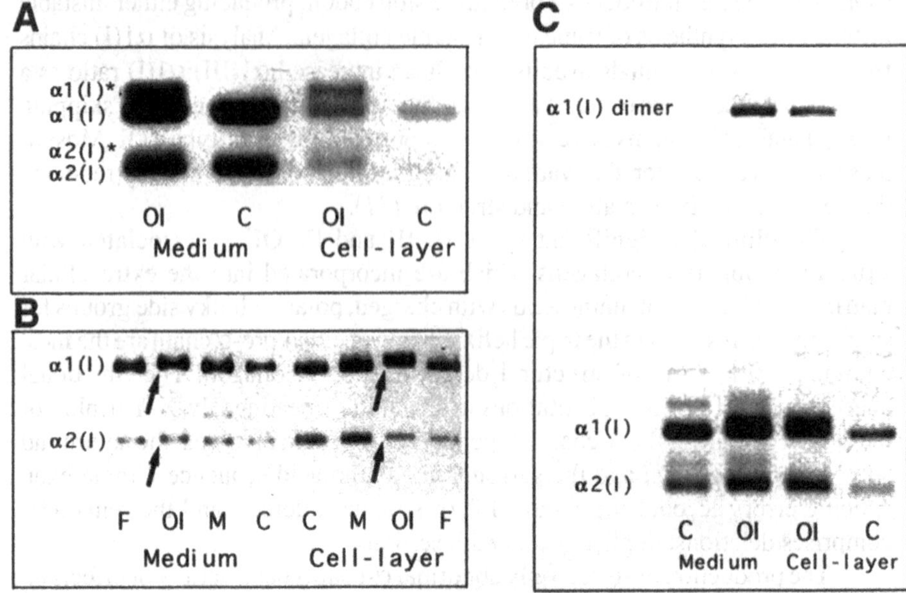

Fig. 3. SDS-urea-polyacrylamide gel analysis of collagen synthesized by fibroblasts derived from OI individuals (OI) and their father (F) and mother (M) and a control (C). Mutant collagens are detected as a doublet **(A)**, slight baseline shift **(B)**, and α1(I) dimers as a result of a cysteine for glycine substitution **(C)**.

appear on polyacrylamide gels as additional bands with faster or slower migration (Fig. 3A), or as bands with a diffuse back-streaking appearance. In some instances, the biochemical alteration is very slight and causes only a small baseline shift on gel electrophoresis (Fig. 3B). Digestion of intact α chains of type I collagen with cyanogen bromide (cleaves at methionine) yields smaller peptides whose order is known. Analysis of the smaller peptides can identify the extent of chain overmodification and suggest the helical location of the glycine substitution. This knowledge can then be used to screen for the underlying defect in complementary segments of both type I collagen genes. Some cases display an unequivocal clinical diagnosis of OI, but do not show any biochemical abnormality in type I collagen. Thus, it is difficult to predict the severity of clinical phenotype, based on the biochemical abnormality. Other factors also modify the severity of phenotype, as different phenotypes have been described with the same mutation. For example, the substitution of glycine352 and 415 in the α1(I) chain by serine can produce the type II, III, or IV OI phenotypes *(14)*.

Biochemical differences between osteoblast and fibroblast type I collagen from patients with OI suggest that the metabolism of collagen is cell-specific. OI osteoblast collagen is more modified than fibroblast collagen derived from the same individual *(15)*. These differences would appear to have significant implications for understanding why type I collagen mutations affect bone more than skin.

Genetics

The familial incidence of OI has been documented since 1788 *(16)*. By the early 1900s, accounts of familial transmission were grouped into either the severe early onset infantile "congenita" or a later childhood OI "tarda" form *(4)*. Renewed interest in the inheritance of OI came from studies of Sillence and colleagues in the 1970s *(1)*. Since then, interest in the molecular mechanisms and genetics of OI has expanded. We now know that virtually all OI cases (>90%) are inherited in an autosomal dominant manner, with mutations in the genes (*COL1A1* or *COL1A2*) encoding the α1(I) and α2(I) subunits of type I procollagen *(17)*. Almost 200 mutations have been reported in the *COL1A1* and *COL1A2* genes that are located on chromosomes 17q21.3-q22 and 7q21.3-q22, respectively *(18)*. Most of these mutations (92%) are scattered throughout the helical coding domains of both genes and cause the disruption of triple helix formation or introduction of a premature-termination codon. All classes of mutation are represented, with missense mutations causing the substitution of glycine being the most common (80%), splicing-defects less common (11%), and the remainder comprising insertions, deletions, and duplications. Rare occurrences of mutations in the C-propeptide and C-telopeptide of both genes have also been described in cases of type II and III OI. These mutations cause the substitution or deletion of amino acids in the α-chain alignment region which is an absolute requirement for initiating triple helix formation *(8)*.

The mildest forms of OI are usually caused by premature-termination codons or out-of-frame RNA-splicing defects which lead to a reduction in the level of type I collagen α1 mRNA *(19)*. Such defects are also known as "null-allele" mutations. Recent investigations have demonstrated that null-allele mutations which convert the arginine codon CGA to the premature-termination codon TGA tend to occur in a common 9 nucleotide sequence context *(20)*. This sequence context is present six times in the COL1A1 gene, whereas the COL1A2 gene has none. This finding is consistent with a lack of COL1A2 null-allele mutations in the literature. However, the 2:1 ratio of α1:α2 chains in collagen should also be considered as a factor for an absence of COL1A2 null-alleles in OI patients. Additional studies are warranted to further our understanding of why null-alleles exist in the COL1A1 gene but may not in the COL1A2 gene. Null-allele α1(I) genotypes have the most predictable effect on the OI phenotype. Genotype-phenotype correlations in the type II, III, and IV forms of the disease are more difficult to predict. Nonetheless, clusters of lethal and nonlethal mutations have been mapped in the COL1A2 gene which have led to the α2(I) Regional Model *(13)*.

In most cases, OI occurs sporadically as a consequence of a new type I collagen mutation which presumably occurs in the germinal cells or in the very early embryonic stages of development. Molecular studies have established that type II OI cases almost always result from a new dominant mutation in type I collagen and that the recurrence in a subsequent pregnancy results from germline or mixed germline and somatic mosaicism in one of the parents *(21)*. Mosaicism in a known carrier can be detected by molecular techniques which identify both normal and mutant sequences on the same allele derived from leukocyte genomic DNA. Depending on the percentage and tissue distribution of the mutation, the mosaic carrier may show some signs of the disease or appear clinically normal. Before these studies, some type II OI babies were considered to have an autosomal recessive inheritance of a type I collagen mutation with a 25% chance of recurrence in subsequent pregnancies. However, a number of recent studies have demonstrated that babies with type II OI are heterozygous for the mutation and that the empiric recurrence risk is about 7% rather than the 25% expected for recessive inheritance *(7)*. In an individual family, the actual recurrence risk depends on the proportion of germ cells carrying the mutation. As a result of these investigations, families have elected to have more children when previously they would have avoided it. Similarly, type III and IV OI siblings with clinically normal parents usually result from parental mosaicism for a dominant type I collagen mutation. Thus, recurrence of OI in siblings identifies a family in which there is very likely to be germline mosaicism for the mutation. Interestingly, the ratio of male:female germline mosaic carriers is approx 2:1, presumably due to a higher rate of mutagenesis in the male germ cell lineage.

Individuals with homozygous type I collagen defects are extremely rare and only 3 cases have been documented at both the biochemical and molecular level. In each case, homozygous COL1A2 mutations were detected in children with the severe type III form of OI. In two of these cases, the mildly affected parents were heterozygous for either a missense mutation causing a glycine substitution (G751S) *(22)*, or a 4 nucleotide frame-shift deletion in the $\alpha 2$(I) C-propeptide which prevented the incorporation of the pro-$\alpha 2$ chain into the type I collagen molecule *(23)*. The third case was due to maternal isodisomy of a fragment of chromosome 7 which contained a single base mutation in the COL1A2 gene *(24)*. This mutation caused the substitution of serine for glycine (G661S). In this family, the mildly affected mother was heterozygous for the mutation. The phenotype of her son resembled two previously reported cases with uniparental isodisomy of chromosome 7. Additional clinical findings in this OI case included slightly blue sclerae and low bone mineral density which were consistent with the COL1A2 mutation. These homozygous cases, although rare, show that genetic counseling for OI must take into account that transmission of two mutant alleles does occur and that heterozygous carriers can show mild expression of the disease.

Prenatal diagnosis of OI can be made using ultrasound, biochemical, and DNA testing and is largely dependent on the prior study of an affected individual in the family. In families with no history of the disease, only the severe phenotypes of type II and III OI are accurately detected by ultrasound, usually at 15–16 and 19–20 wk of gestation, respectively. In those families with a history of OI, direct mutational or biochemical analysis can be performed to identify abnormal collagen in chorionic villus (CV) cells. However, chorionic villi are not useful for the accurate identification of the amounts of type I collagen synthesized and thus, have limited value in the diagnosis of type I OI. Prenatal diagnosis of type I OI is usually performed by linkage analysis of the COL1A1 gene or screening for a known mutation. Amniocytes are not suitable for biochemical studies of type I collagen but are useful for direct molecular detection of known mutations. In a recent study, 120 couples with a family history of type II, III, or I OI were screened for type I collagen defects using biochemical or DNA based assays *(25)*. Twenty-six affected fetuses were identified from this screening and there were neither false-negative nor false-positive results.

The differential diagnosis of OI includes a number of disorders with overlapping phenotype but lacking in linkage to collagen *(7)*. Recessive cases of a condition with a type III OI phenotype have been documented in the black population of South Africa *(26)*, and in one Pakistani consanguineous pedigree *(27)*. The cause is presumably due to defects in another extracellular matrix component involved in bone morphogenesis or metabolism. A number of metabolic disorders including homocystinuria, thanatophoric dysplasia, and hypophosphatasia are also in the differential diagnosis of OI.

Clinical Management

The mainstay of OI clinical management is aggressive rehabilitation medicine intervention to facilitate the attainment of gross motor skills, including ambulation when possible, and to maximize skills for independent living. In infancy, children with OI should be handled with appropriate precautions rather than having contact minimized for fear of fractures. Physical therapy will usually be necessary for type III and some type IV children to attain head control, because of relative macrocephaly. Custom molded seating may be required to maintain proper alignment of head, spine, and trunk before severely affected infants attain postural control. For children who initially hold their legs in the abducted “frog-legs” position, stretching and extension exercises are effective in bringing the lower extremities into proper alignment for motor development *(28)*.

Children at the more severe end of the Type III OI phenotypic range often cannot attain ambulation despite optimum intervention. For these individuals, mobility will be by electric wheelchair and therapy should aim at transfer and independent living skills. Children at the milder end of the Type IV OI range will attain ambulation spontaneously and will require orthopedic management of fractures to maintain community ambulation status. For children between these phenotypic extremes, ambulation may be attained by an assisted program of long-leg braces and an exercise program aimed at strengthening quadriceps and gluteal muscles *(29)*. Children initially ambulate in braces plus a walker for balance and weight distribution. They progress to lightweight crutches, then to braces alone. Eventually, most type IV and some type III individuals can be weaned from braces, especially as bone density rises with puberty.

Orthopedic care should be obtained from a surgeon with experience in the management of OI. Hairline or microfractures may be managed with splinting and ace wraps. All significant fractures should be cast for proper alignment and maximum function. To minimize the osteoporosis of immobilization, casts should be replaced by splints as soon as allowed by healing. Lower limb long bones which are bowed more than 45° are at increased fracture risk. Intramedullary rod placement may be required to correct bowing or alignment or to stabilize a particularly severe fracture *(30)*. Bailey-Dubow rods have the advantage of extensibility. Their disadvantages are high incidence of migration from the bone and increased osteoporosis due to the diameter and stiffness of the rod. Rush and Enders rods are thinner and somewhat more flexible and have a lower incidence of migration but do not telescope. Unfortunately, the scoliosis of OI is not amenable to correction or stabilization by bracing. Fixation and stabilization by rods and wires will be more successful if performed before the curvature reaches 60°.

Short stature is the second most prevalent and significant feature of OI. All type III OI patients have extreme short stature with final adult height less than that of an unaffected late-prepubertal child of the same gender *(31)*. Type IV patients have significant short stature with heights always below the 2nd percentile and type I patients are usually shorter than unaffected family members *(32)*. The loss of stature is disproportionately in the lower limbs, with better preservation of trunk height and armspan. A pilot treatment study with standard dose growth hormone (0.1–.2 u/kg/d, 6 d/wk) has shown that the majority of type IV children are responsive and can attain substantial increases in linear growth rate. Responders also show improved bone histology after 1 yr of treatment and a modest, but statistically significant, increase in bone mineralization compared to nonresponders.

The morbidity and mortality of OI is predominantly cardio-pulmonary, with recurrent pneumonias in infancy and childhood and development of cor pulmonale in middle age. Respiratory infections should be treated promptly and aggressively in children. Convention management of cor pulmonale, guided by pulmonary function tests, is appropriate. An additional significant secondary feature of OI is the development of basilar invagination (BI) *(33)*. The incidence of BI is greater than previously appreciated, although progression to brain stem compression in childhood or teen years occurs in a minority of cases. Initial detection of BI may be done by spiral CT; progression to compression of neural tissue is best followed by MRI at annual intervals. Changes in long track signs may be detected; symptoms such as headache occur relatively late and require consultation for neurosurgical management.

Recently, there have been several studies suggesting that the bisphosphonates may be a useful therapeutic agent in OI, with potential to increase bone density and reverse osteopenia. The bisphosphonates are synthetic analogs of pyrophosphate, a natural inhibitor of osteoclastic bone resorption. Although the members of the bisphosphonate family, especially pamidronate and alendronate, would not be expected to decrease the synthesis or matrix incorporation of mutant collagen, they may be beneficial to OI patients by decreasing the high bone turnover state. It is not yet clear whether bisphosphonate-treated bone will have improved biomechanical properties.

Future Prospects for Gene Therapy of OI

The clinical phenotypes of severely affected OI patients continue to challenge pediatric care. Because of the limited response of severely affected patients to conventional therapies, it is important to develop new therapeutic approaches that can be applied either separately or in conjunction with current treatments. Gene therapy represents a promising approach to ameliorate the severity of the disease. In general, gene therapy involves the augmentation of a missing or defective gene. Gene augmentation therapy can be helpful in recessive disorders. However, augmentation therapy alone will not be of much benefit when a mutation yields a protein with a dominant negative effect, as is the case of mutant type I collagen in OI. In order to correct the dominant negative effect in OI, therapy would have to selectively inactivate the mutant type I collagen gene without affecting the expression of the normal allele. Because the mildest form of OI is usually associated with a null alpha chain, suppression of mutant mRNAs would be predicted to modulate the severity of the disease from the moderate and severe forms to a biochemical equivalent of mild type I OI.

One strategy involves the inactivation of mutant mRNA using antisense technologies. Antisense oligonucleotides have been used to inhibit the expression of a mutant α2(I) allele in cultured fibroblasts derived from a patient with type IV OI *(34)*. That study used OI cells which harbor a single nucleotide change (G^{+1}->A) at the exon 16 splice donor site in one α2(I) collagen allele. Antisense, and control (sense and missense) 20-mer phosphorothioates were designed to target both the abnormal mRNA exon 15/17 junction and the nuclear level point mutation. This investigation demonstrated the antisense suppression of mutant protein to approx 50% and mutant α2(I) mRNA to about 40% of their levels in control cells. However, the antisense oligonucleotides also suppressed the normal allele mRNA to 80% of its level in untreated cells. Unfortunately, the level and specificity of mutant allele suppression observed in the cell culture system appears to be insufficient for therapeutic trials.

Ribozymes represent an alternative to antisense oligonucleotides for the inactivation of mutant mRNAs *(35)*. Hammerhead ribozymes are the smallest form of catalytic RNA which can be designed to cleave almost any RNA. The basic structure of the hammerhead ribozyme consists of a small catalytic core domain plus 5'- and 3'-flanking sequences (Fig. 4). The flanking sequences are designed to bind to a particular RNA. Another major requirement for ribozyme action is on the target sequence and consists of a three nucleotide cleavage site which is most often GUC in nature, although other trinucleotides can be cleaved as well. The binding arms position the ribozyme on the target so that the catalytic core cleaves after the third nucleotide in the cleavage sequence. The combination

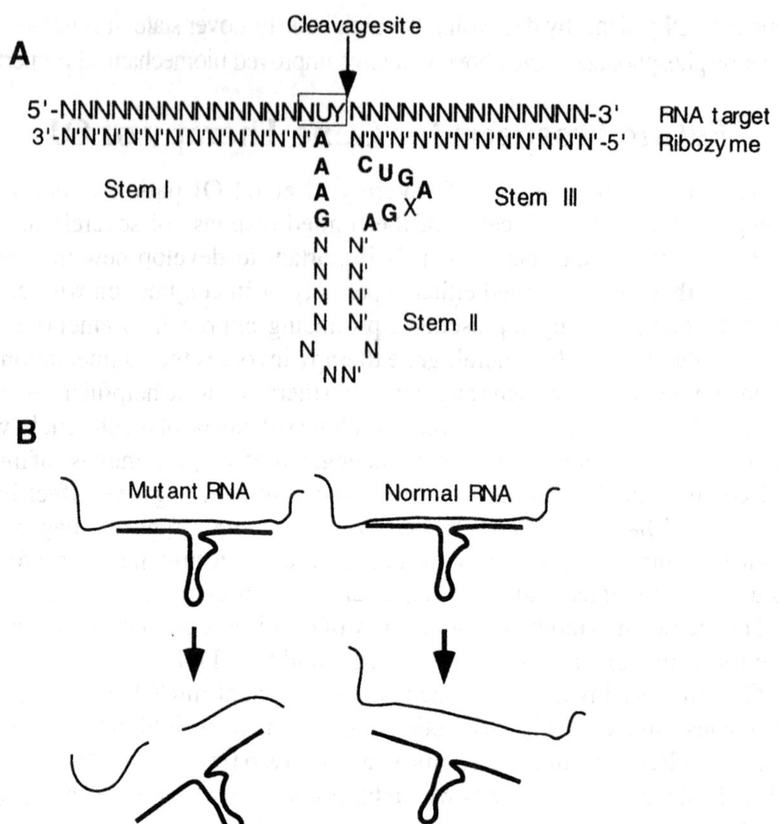

Fig. 4. **(A)** Secondary structure of the hammerhead ribozyme. Conserved sequences are bolded and the cleavage site is shown. **(B)** Ribozymes can be designed to bind to a specific target site which is present on both mutant and normal RNAs. However, since the mutation on the mutant RNA creates a ribozyme cleavage site, only mutant RNA is cleaved.

of requirements for both a binding site and a cleavage site provide ribozymes with specificity capabilities for point mutations that cannot be achieved with linear antisense oligonucleotides. In addition, the catalytic capability of the ribozyme provides the potential for increased efficiency and stability. Hammerhead ribozymes have been used to cleave viral (HIV, influenza) and cellular RNAs in vitro and in vivo *(36–39)*. Recent studies on Marfan syndrome, another dominant negative genetic disorder, demonstrated that ribozymes efficiently cleaved fibrillin RNA in cultured fibroblasts *(40)* and osteosarcoma cells *(41)*. However, cleavage in these situations was not allele specific. Mutation-specific cleavage of N-*ras* transcripts in HeLa cells *(42)* suggests that ribozymes can be used to selectively suppress the expression of one allele. Approx 25% of the collagen point mutations that cause OI also generate a novel ribozyme cleavage site. Thus, the mutation itself provides the target for mutant mRNA suppression *(35)*.

Recently, hammerhead ribozymes were employed to selectively cleave mutant type I collagen mRNAs in cell-free assays *(43)*. Hammerhead ribozymes were designed to cleave synthetic transcripts of two naturally occurring human collagen mutations and a point mutation introduced into a murine knock-in construct. Only mutant targets were cleaved, whereas normal allele targets remained intact despite the presence of the complete binding site. However, a high ratio of ribozyme:substrate (5–10:1) was required to achieve a 50% ribozyme saturation, suggesting a low catalytic efficiency of ribozymes in vitro. This study also investigated the competitive effects of both total RNA and normal synthetic RNA on ribozyme cleavage activity. Cleavage was unaffected by the presence of total RNA in vast excess (500× ratio). However, the efficiency of cleavage was linearly inhibited by a noncleavable competitor substrate containing the same binding site present in the cleavable target. This competitive effect was eliminated by introducing a mismatch between one binding arm and the target, at some cost to cleavage efficiency of the mutant mRNA. These findings on the selective in vitro cleavage of mutant type I collagen RNAs are encouraging for future gene therapy approaches to OI.

To further develop a gene therapy system for OI, a suitable animal model is required. Several murine models for OI have been reported *(44–48)*. However, none of these models have the same molecular and biochemical characteristics as the typical human OI cases which harbor a nonlethal glycine substitution that occurs in a single copy in each cell under the control of the endogenous promoter. Investigations are currently underway to generate knock-in mice with various glycine substitutions (G160C, G211C and G349C) in the α1(I) collagen chains. In humans, these changes cause the clinically mild type I, moderate/severe type IV/III, and moderate type IV forms of OI, respectively. In addition to the OI-causing mutation, the murine alleles each contain a closely positioned silent base change which creates a ribozyme cleavage site *(49)*.

Future studies will test the efficiency and specificity of ribozyme cleavage in these OI mouse models. Khillan and co-workers demonstrated the partial rescue of a lethal OI mouse phenotype using an antisense strategy *(50)*. In mice that expressed both an OI mini-gene and the antisense gene, the lethal phenotype was reduced from 92% to 27%. These findings are promising for a gene therapy approach to OI and highlight the potential of transgenic systems for testing antisense technologies in vivo. Transgenic expression systems bypass the problem of vector delivery and should produce a therapeutic effect in all of the target cells. To date, three studies have demonstrated successful transgenic expression of ribozymes in mouse models *(51–53)*. Although transgenic systems are useful for testing the effectiveness of cleavage in cells, they are not practical in the human situation. Delivery of ribozymes to patients will require either a direct delivery or an ex vivo approach. For the ex vivo system, pre-osteoblast cells will need to be transduced with a ribozyme vector and then reintroduced back into the patient. Mesenchymal stem cells can differentiate into marrow stromal cells (MSCs) which in turn can become osteoblasts *(54)*. Thus, mesenchymal stem cells and MSCs are reasonable targets for the gene therapy of OI. In one study, MSCs were detected in bone following injection into the distal abdominal aorta of mice *(55)*. However, the efficiency of directly injected viral vectors to target bone has not been demonstrated.

Gene therapy of OI is in its early stages of development and much more needs to be determined about such technology, its delivery and effectiveness in reducing bone fragility in OI patients. Nevertheless, potential gene therapy approaches such as the ribozyme systems have been initiated and should prove valuable for determining the short and long term effects of gene suppression on the OI phenotype.

Summary

Osteogenesis imperfecta is a heterogeneous group of inherited disorders with phenotypes ranging from perinatal-lethal to mild. Defects in type I collagen are responsible for all forms of the disease. Qualitative defects alter the structure of type I collagen and cause all forms of OI, whereas quantitative defects of type I collagen are associated with the mild forms of the disease. Based on this knowledge, future gene therapy approaches which suppress mutant allele expression are expected to convert the severe forms of the disease to a biochemically equivalent of the mild type I form. Such treatments, in conjunction with conventional therapies, may ameliorate the severity of the disease.

References

1. Sillence, D. O. (1979) Genetics and heterogeneity in osteogenesis imperfecta. *J. Med. Genet.* **16,** 101–116.
2. Gray, P. H. K. (1969) A case of osteogenesis imperfecta, associated with dentinogenesis imperfecta, dating from antiquity. *Clin. Radiol.* **20,** 106–108.
3. Lobstein, J. F. (1835) Von der Knochenbreichigkeit oder Osteopsathyrose, in *Lehrbuch der Pathologischen Anatomie* (Neurohr, A., ed.), Brodhag, Stuttgart, p. 179.
4. Looser, E. (1906) Zur kenntis der osteogenesis imperfecta congenita et tarda. *Mitt. Grenzeb. Med. Chir.* **15,** 161–165.
5. Bell, J. (1928) Blue sclerotics and fragility of bone, in *Treasury of Human Inheritance*, vol. 2 (III), (Pearson, K., ed.), Cambridge University Press, Cambridge, UK.
6. Marini, J. C. (1988) Osteogenesis imperfecta: comprehensive management. *Adv. Pediatr.* **35,** 391–426.
7. Byers, P. H. (1993) Osteogenesis imperfecta, in *Connective Tissue and its Heritable Disorders* (Royce, P. M. and Steinmann, B., eds.) Wiley-Liss, New York, pp. 317–350.
8. Lees, J. F., Tasab, M., and Bulleid, N. J. (1997) Identification of the molecular recognition sequence which determines the type–specific assembly of procollagen. *EMBO J.*.**16,** 908–916.

9. Kivirikko, K. I. and Myllyea, R. (1980) Hydroxylation of prolyl and lysyl residues, in *The Enzymology of Post-translational Modification of Proteins* (Freedman, R. B. and Hawkins, H. C., eds.), Academic Press, London, p. 53.
10. Kivirikko, K. I. and Myllyea, R. (1979) Collagen glycosyltransferases. *Int. Rev. Connect. Tissue* **18,** 23.
11. Byers, P. H., Wallis, G. A., and Willing, M. C. (1991) Osteogenesis imperfecta: Translation of mutation to phenotype. *J. Med. Genet.* **28,** 433–442.
12. Wang, Q., Orrison, B., and Marini, J. C. (1993) Two additional cases of osteogenesis imperfecta with substitutions for glycine in the alpha-2(I) collagen chain—a regional model relating mutation location with phenotype. *J. Biol. Chem.* **268,** 25,162–25,167.
13. Marini, J. C., Lewis, M. B., Wang, Q., Chen, K. J., and Orrison, B. M. (1993) Serine for glycine substitutions in type I collagen in two cases of type IV osteogenesis imperfecta (OI). Additional evidence for a regional model of OI pathophysiology. *J. Biol. Chem.* **268,** 2667–2673.
14. Mottes, M., Lira, M. M. G., Valli, M., Scarano, G., Lonardo, F., Forlino, A., Cetta, G., and Pignatti, P. F. (1993) Paternal mosaicism for a COL1A1 dominant mutation (α1 Ser-415) causes recurrent osteogenesis imperfecta. *Hum. Mutat.* **2,** 196–204.
15. Sarafova, A. P., Choi, H., Forlino, A., Gajko, A., Cabral, W. A., Tosi, L., Reing, C. M., and Marini, J. C. (1998) Three novel type I collagen mutations in osteogenesis imperfecta type IV probands are associated with discrepancies between electrophoretic migration of osteoblast and fibroblast collagen. *Hum. Mutat.* **11,** 395–403.
16. Ekman, O. (1788) Dissertatio medica descriptionem et casus aliquot osteomalaciae sistens.
17. Sykes, B., Ogilvie, D., Wordsworth, P., Wallis, G., Mathew, C., Beighton, P., et al. (1990) Consistent linkage of dominantly inherited osteogenesis imperfecta to the type I collagen loci: COL1A1 and COL1A2. *Am. J. Hum. Genet.* **46,** 293–307.
18. Kuivaniemi, H., Tromp, G., and Prockop, D. J. (1997) Mutations in fibrillar collagens (types I, II, III, and XI), fibril-associated collagen (type IX), and network-forming collagen (type X) cause a spectrum of diseases of bone, cartilage, and blood vessels. *Hum. Mutat.* **9,** 300–315.
19. Willing, M. C., Deschenes, S. P., Scott, D. A., Byers, P. H., Slayton, R. L., Pitts, S. H., Arikat, H., and Roberts, E. J. (1994) Osteogenesis imperfecta type I: molecular heterogeneity for COL1A1 null alleles of type I collagen. *Am. J. Hum. Genet.* **55,** 638–647.
20. Korkko, J., Ala-Kokko, L., De Paepe, A., Nuytinck, L., Earley, J., and Prockop, D. J. (1998) Analysis of the COL1A1 and COL1A2 genes by PCR amplification and scanning by conformation-sensitive gel electrophoresis identifies only COL1A1 mutations in 15 patients with osteogenesis imperfecta type I: identification of common sequences of null-allele mutations. *Am. J. Hum. Genet.* **62,** 98–110.
21. Lund, A. M., Nicholls, A. C., Schwartz, M., and Skovby, F. (1997) Parental mosaicism and autosomal dominant mutations causing structural abnormalities of collagen I are frequent in families with osteogenesis imperfecta type III/IV. *Acta Paediatr.* **86,** 711–718.
22. De Paepe, A., Nuytinck, L., Raes, M., and Fryns, J.-P. (1997) Homozygosity by descent for a COL1A2 mutation in two sibs with severe osteogenesis imperfecta and mild clinical expression in the heterozygotes. *Hum. Genet.* **99,** 478–483.
23. Pihlajaniemi, T., Dickson, L. A., Pope, F. M., Korhonen, V. R., Nicholls, A., Prockop, D. J., and Myers, J. C. (1984) Osteogenesis imperfecta: Cloning of a pro-α2(I) collagen gene with a frameshift mutation. *J. Biol. Chem.* **259,** 12,941–12,944.

24. Spotila, L. D., Constantinou, C. D., Sereda, L., Ganguly, A., Riggs, B. L., and Prockop, D. J. (1991) Mutation in a gene for type-I procollagen (COL1A2) in a woman with postmenopausal osteoporosis—evidence for phenotypic and genotypic overlap with mild osteogenesis imperfecta. *Proc. Natl. Acad. Sci. USA* **88,** 5423–5427.
25. Pepin, M., Atkinson, M., Starman, B. J., and Byers, P. H. (1997) Strategies and outcomes of prenatal diagnosis for osteogenesis imperfecta: a review of biochemical and molecular studies completed in 129 pregnancies. *Prenat. Diagn.* **17,** 559–570.
26. Wallis, G., Sykes, B., Byers, P. H., Mathew, C. H., Viljoen, D. and Beighton, P. (1986) Osteogenesis imperfecta type III: mutations in the type I collagen structural genes, COL1A1 and COL1A2, are not necessarily responsible. *J. Med. Genet.* **34,** 492–496.
27. Aitchison, K., Ogilvie, D., Honeyman, M., Thompson, E., and Sykes, B. (1988) Homozygous osteogenesis imperfecta unlinked to collagen I genes. *Hum. Genet.* **78,** 233–236.
28. Binder, H., Hawks, L., Graybill, G., Gerber, N. L., and Weintrob, J. C. (1984) Osteogenesis imperfecta: rehabilitation approach with infants and young children. *Arch. Phys. Med. Rehab.* **65,** 537.
29. Gerber, L. H., Binder, H., Berry, R., Mizell, S., and Marini, J. C. (1998) Effects of withdrawal of bracing in matched pairs of children with osteogenesis imperfecta. *Arch. Phys. Med. Rehab.* **79,** 46–51.
30. Reing, C. M. (1995) Report on new types of intramedullary rods and treatment effectiveness data for selection of intramedullary rodding in osteogenesis imperfecta. *Conn. Tissue Res.* **31,** 1–10.
31. Marini, J. C., Bordenick, S., and Chrousos, G. P. (1995) Endocrine aspects of growth deficiency in OI. *Conn. Tissue Res.* **31,** S55–S57.
32. Marini, J. C., Bordenick, S., Heavner, G., Rose, S. R., Rosenfeld, R. G., Hintz, R. L., and Chrousos, G. (1993) Evaluation of hormones related to growth in short children with osteogenesis imperfecta. *J. Clin. Endocrinol. Metab.* **76,** 251–256.
33. Charnas, L. R. and Marini, J. C. (1995) Neurologic profile in osteogenesis imperfecta. *Conn. Tissue Res.* **31,** S23–S26.
34. Wang, Q. and Marini, J. C. (1996) Antisense oligodeoxynucleotides selectively suppress expression of the mutant $\alpha 2(I)$ collagen allele in type IV osteogenesis imperfecta fibroblasts. *J. Clin. Invest.* **97,** 448–454.
35. Grassi, G. and Marini, J. C. (1996) Ribozymes: structure, function and potential therapy for dominant genetic disorders. *Trends Mol. Med.* **28,** 499–510.
36. Rossi, J. (1995) Controlled, targeted, intracellular expression of ribozymes: progress and problems. *Trends Biotechnol.* **13,** 301–306.
37. Sun, L., Pytati, J., Smythe, J., Wang, L., MacPherson, J., Gerlach, W., and Symonds, G. (1995) Resistance to human immunodeficiency virus type I infection conferred by transduction of human peripheral blood lymphocytes with ribozyme, antisense, or polymeric transactivation response element constructs. *Proc. Natl. Acad. Sci. USA* **92,** 7272–7276.
38. Zhou, C., Bahner, I., Larson, G., Zaia, J., Rossi, J., and Kohn, D. (1994) Inhibition of HIV-1 in human T-lymphocytes by retrovirally transduced anti-TAT and REV hammerhead ribozymes. *Gene* **149,** 3–39.
39. Tang, X., Hobom, G. and Lao, D. (1994) Ribozyme mediated destruction of influenza A virus in vitro and in vivo. *J. Med. Virol.* **42,** 385–395.
40. Kilpatrick, M., Phylactou, L., Godfrey, M., Wu, C., Wu, G., and Tsipouras, P. (1996) Delivery of a hammerhead ribozyme specifically down-regulates the production of fibrillin-1 by cultured dermal fibroblasts. *Hum. Mol. Genet.* **5,** 1939–1944.

41. Montgomery, R. A. and Dietz, H. C. (1997) Inhibition of fibrillin 1 expression using U1 snRNA as a vehicle for the presentation of antisense targeting sequence. *Hum. Mol. Genet.* **6,** 519–525.
42. Scherr, M., Grez, R., Ganser, A. and Engels, J. W. (1997) Specific hammerhead ribozyme-mediated cleavage of mutant N-ras mRNA *in vitro* and *ex vivo*: oligoribonucleotides as therapeutic agents. *J. Biol. Chem.* **272,** 14,304–14,313.
43. Grassi, G., Forlino, A. and Marini, J. C. (1997) Cleavage of collagen RNA transcripts by hammerhead ribozymes *in vitro* is mutation-specific and shows competitive binding effects. *Nucleic Acids Res.* **25,** 3451–3458.
44. Bonadio, J., Saunders, T., Tsai, E., Goldstein, S., Morris–Wiman, J., Brinkley, L., Dolan, D., Altschuler, R., Hawkins Jr, J., Bateman, J., Mascara, T., and Jaenish, R. (1990) Transgenic mouse model of the mild dominant form of osteogenesis imperfecta. *Proc. Natl. Acad. Sci. USA* **87,** 7145–7148.
45. Schnieke, A., Harbers, K., and Jaenish, R. (1983) Embryonic lethal mutation in mice induced by retrovirus insertion into the α1(I) collagen gene. *Nature* **304,** 315–320.
46. Chipman, S. D., Sweet, H. O., McBride Jr, D. J., Davisson, M. T., Marks Jr, S. C., Shuldiner, A. R., et al. (1993) Defective proα2(I) collagen synthesis in a recessive mutation in mice: a model of human osteogenesis imperfecta. *Proc. Natl. Acad. Sci. USA* **90,** 1701–1705.
47. Khillan, J. S., Olsen, A. S., Kontusaari, S., Sokolov, B., and Prockop, D. J. (1991) Transgenic mice that express a mini–gene version of the human gene for type I procollagen (COL1A1) develop a phenotype resembling a lethal form of osteogenesis imperfecta. *J. Biol. Chem.* **266,** 23,373–23,379.
48. Pereira, R., Khillan, J. S., Helminen, H. J., Hume, E. L., and Prockop, D. J. (1993) Transgenic mice expressing a partially deleted gene for type I procollagen (COL1A1). *J. Clin. Invest.* **91,** 709–716.
49. Forlino, A., Porter, F. D., and Marini, J. C. (1998) Osteogenesis imperfecta murine models: Use of the cre/lox recombination system to create the first knock-in OI mouse. *Eur. J. Hum. Genet.* **6,** C803.
50. Khillan, J., Li, S., and Prockop, D. J. (1994) Partial rescue of a lethal phenotype of fragile bones in transgenic mice with a chimeric antisense gene directed against a mutated collagen gene. *Proc. Natl. Acad. Sci. USA* **91,** 6298–6302.
51. Efrat, S., Leiser, M., Wu, Y., Fusco-DeMane, D., Emran, O., Surana, M., et al. (1994) Ribozyme-mediated attenuation of pancreatic beta-cell glucokinase expression in transgenic mice results in impaired glucose-induced insulin-secretion. *Proc. Natl. Acad. Sci. USA* **91,** 2051–2055.
52. L'Huiller, P. J., Soulier, S., Stinnakre, M. G., Lepourry, L., Davis, S. R., Mercier, J. C., and Vilotte, J. L. (1996) Efficient and specific ribozyme-mediated reduction of bovine alpha–lactalbumin expression in double transgenic mice. *Proc. Natl. Acad. Sci. US A* **93,** 6698–6703.
53. Larsson, S., Hotchkiss, G., Andang, M., Nyholm, T., Inzunza, J., Jansson, I., and Ahrlund-Richter, L. (1994) Reduced β2-microglobulin mRNA levels in transgenic mice expressing a designed hammerhead ribozyme. *Nucleic Acids Res.* **22,** 2242–2248.
54. Bruder, S. P., Fink, D. J., and Caplan, A. I. (1994) Mesenchymal stem cells in bone development, bone repair, and skeletal regeneration therapy. *J. Cell. Biochem.* **56,** 283–294.
55. Mankani, M., Satomura, K., Kuznetsov, S., Krebsbach, P., Taylor, R., and Robey, P. (1997) Engraftment of marrow stromal fibroblasts. *J. Bone Miner. Res.* **12,** S205.

CHAPTER 6

Vitamin D-Dependent Rickets Type I and Type II

Sachiko Kitanaka and Shigeaki Kato

Introduction

Vitamin D is one of the fat-soluble vitamins, and the most biologically active form, calcitriol (1α,25-Dihydroxyvitamin D_3[1α, 25$(OH)_2D_3$]) plays a role in a variety of biological actions such as calcium homeostasis, cell proliferation, and cell differentiation in many target tissues *(1–4)*. Calcitriol is a prime regulatory factor in bone formation and metabolism *(3)*. Vitamin D deficiency causes rickets, osteomalacia, and impaired calcium and phosphorous homeostasis *(5)*.

1α,25$(OH)_2D_3$ is biosynthesized from cholesterol, or from vitamin D taken in from the diet. At the final steps of the vitamin D biosynthesis, two hydroxylations (hepatic 25-hydroxylation and renal 1α-hydroxylation) occur for its metabolic activation into a hormonal form *(1,3,6)*. Renal 1α-hydroxylation of 25$(OH)D_3$ is crucial for the biosynthesis of the active hormone, 1α,25$(OH)_2D_3$, and is conducted by 25$(OH)D_3$ 1α-hydroxylase [1α(OH)ase] in the proximal tubule of the kidney *(7)*. 1α,25$(OH)_2D_3$ specifically binds to the vitamin D receptor (VDR), and activates its transactivation function to regulate the expression of a particular set of the target genes.

Mutations in the 1α(OH)ase gene are recently shown to result in vitamin D-dependent rickets type I (VDDR I), also known as pseudovitamin D-deficient rickets(PDDR) *(8)*. Mutations in the vitamin D receptor (VDR) result in vitamin D-dependent rickets type II (VDDR II), also known as hypocalcemic vitamin D-resistant rickets (HVDRR) *(9)*.

Phenotypic Manifestations of VDDR I and VDDR II

VDDR I is an autosomal recessive disorder, and the clinical course is similar to that of nutritional rickets due to simple vitamin D deficiency *(10)*. Affected children appear normal at birth, and the first symptoms usually appear within the

The Genetics of Osteoporosis and Metabolic Bone Disease
Ed.: M. J. Econs © Humana Press Inc., Totowa, NJ

first to second year of life. Muscle weakness, growth retardation, and bone deformity are common manifestations. In some patients, the initial event is convulsions or tetany. Laboratory findings include hypocalcemia, secondary hyperparathyroidism, and aminoaciduria. Levels of 25(OH)D are normal or elevated, whereas levels of 1,25(OH)2D are low *(5)*. Although pharmacologic doses of vitamin D or 25(OH)D can be used to treat the disorder, physiological doses of calcitriol are sufficient to treat the disorder *(11)*. These laboratory and therapeutic findings on vitamin D metabolites suggested that 25(OH)D_3 1α-hydroxylase is defective in VDDR I patients.

VDDR II is also inherited as an autosomal recessive trait, and the clinical features are almost identical to those in VDDR I with the exception that VDDR II has been associated with alopecia in about two-thirds of the kindreds. VDDR II is distinguished from VDDR I in that serum levels of 1,25(OH)2D are high, and that they do not respond to physiological doses of calcitriol *(5)*. These findings lead to the hypothesis that these individuals are resistant to calcitriol. This hypothesis was supported by the findings that cells isolated from VDDR II patients exhibit lack of physiological response to calcitriol *(12)*.

The clinical presentation and therapeutic response in VDDR II show a marked heterogeneity. The onset of their symptoms are usually before 2 yr of age, however, late onset (in their teens to adults) was reported in several sporadic cases *(13)*. Alopecia varies from sparse hair to total alopecia without eyelashes, and this seems to be a marker of a more severe form of the disease. Patients with normal hair usually respond to pharmacological doses of vitamin D or calcitriol, however, only about half of the patients with alopecia have shown calcemic response even to higher doses of calcitriol. Most severe patients who are refractory to treatment with high doses of calcitriol require long-term intravenous calcium infusions *(14)*. Life-long therapy is usually required, although sporadic cases of remissions maintained off therapy have been described *(15)*. Even if osteomalacia and the biochemical parameters in patients with alopecia respond to the treatments, none has shown improvement of hair growth.

Molecular Mechanism of Vitamin D Actions

25-Hydroxyvitamin D_3 1α-Hydroxylase Acting as Key Enzyme in Vitamin D Synthesis

The precursor of vitamin D, 7-dehydrocholesterol, is biosynthesized from cholesterol, then converted into vitamin D_3 by UV light in the skin. Vitamin D is also ingested from the diet, as vitamin D_2 (ergocalciferol) mainly from plants, and vitamin D_3 (cholecalciferol) from animals *(16)*. A hormonal form of vitamin D, 1α,25$(OH)_2D_3$, is metabolically formed through two steps of hydroxylation at the final stage (Fig. 1). First, vitamin D is hydroxylated in the liver to 25-dihydroxyvitamin D3 [25(OH)D_3], which is subsequently hydroxylated in the kidney to 1α,25$(OH)_2D_3$ *(1,3,6,7)*. For metabolic inactivation of 25(OH)D_3, or

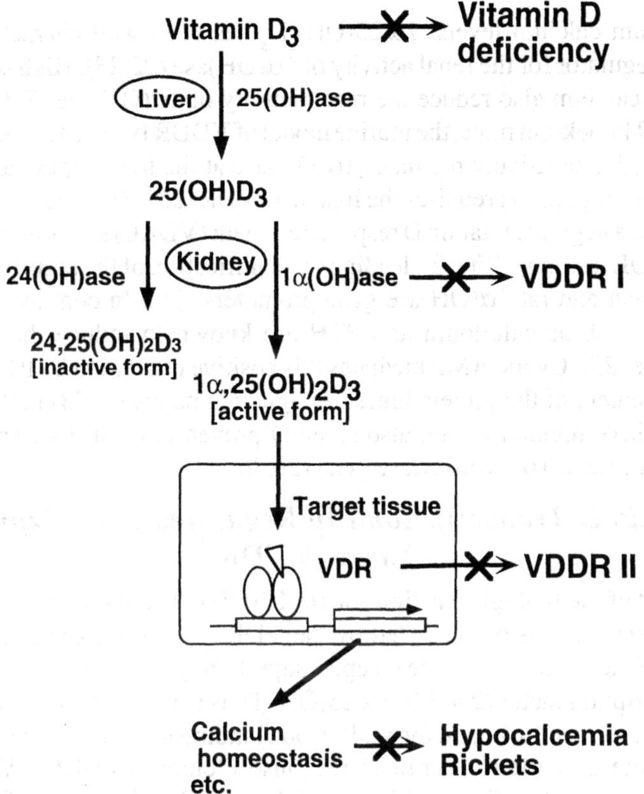

Fig. 1. Rickets related to vitamin D. The biosynthesis pathway of $1\alpha,25(OH)_2D_3$ and the mode of $1\alpha,25(OH)_2D_3$ action are illustrated. The defects in these process cause rickets. Nutritional vitamin D deficiency, and the defect of the renal 1α(OH)ase activity by genetic mutations(vitamin D-dependent rickets type I; VDDRI patients) result in short supply of active vitamin D. The mutated VDR in the vitamin D dependent rickets type II(VDDRII) patients is unable to respond to $1\alpha,25(OH)_2D_3$, resulting in the rickets.

1α,25(OH)2D3, the 24-hydroxylation to form $24,25(OH)_2D_3$ or $1\alpha,24,25(OH)_3D_3$, is the first step in degradation of vitamin D *(17)*. The serum level of $1\alpha,25(OH)_2D_3$ is kept constant in the normal state, and is regulated in response to factors controlling calcium homeostasis. The regulation of $1\alpha,25(OH)_2D_3$ and 24, $25(OH)_2D_3$ production by these factors is conducted by altering the activities of the enzymes that hydroxylate vitamin D derivatives. Vitamin D_3-25-hydroxylase(CYP27) catalyzes hepatic 25-hydroxylation *(18,19)*, and renal 1-hydroxylation is catalyzed by 25-hydroxyvitamin D_3 1α-hydroxyla se[1α(OH)ase]. 24-Hydroxylation of vitamin D metabolites is catalyzed by $25(OH)D_3$-24-hydroxylase (CYP24) *(20,21)*.

As $1\alpha,25(OH)_2D_3$ plays a primary role in calcium homeostasis, the renal activity of 1α(OH)ase is positively regulated by calcitropic hormones, responding to serum calcium levels. 1α,25(OH)$_2$D$_3$ has been well characterized as a negative regulator for the renal activity of 1α(OH)ase *(22,23)*. High serum phosphate and calcium also reduce the renal activity of 1α(OH)ase *(7,24)*. A study using VDR knock-out mice, the murine model of VDDR type 2, demonstrated that 1α,25(OH)$_2$D$_3$ negatively regulates 1α(OH)ase at the transcriptional level, and this negative regulation requires the liganded-VDR *(25)*. These findings led us to suspect that a negative vitamin D response element (VDRE) exists in the promoter of the 1α(OH)ase gene (Fig. 2), leading to identification of the regulatory regions in the human and rat 1α(OH)ase gene promoters *(26)*. In contrast, calcitropic hormones such as calcitonin and PTH are known to induce the activity of 1α(OH)ase *(27)*. Cyclic AMP mediates this positive regulation by PTH, suggesting involvement of the protein kinase A signaling pathway *(28)* in this process. These positive regulations are also recently proved to occur by transcriptional induction of renal 1α-hydroxylase gene *(29,30)*.

Vitamin D Transcriptionally Regulates Gene Expression Through VDR

Most of the biological actions of 1α, 25(OH)$_2$D$_3$ are thought to be exerted through gene expression mediated by the VDR (Fig. 3) *(2,4,31,32)*. VDR is a member of the nuclear hormone receptor superfamily and acts as a ligand-inducible transcription factor *(2,4,33)*. 1α,25(OH)$_2$D$_3$ is a most potent form of vitamin D and acts as a specific ligand for VDR. Upon binding to a specific DNA enhancer element, the so-called vitamin D response element (VDRE), VDR forms homodimer or heterodimer with one of three RXRs (RXRa, RXRb, RXRg). These RXRs derived distinct genes are functionally identical to act as a partner receptor for many nuclear receptors in heterodimerization. Though 9-*cis* retinoic acid binds to RXRs, the physiological role of its RXR binding is unclear in most heterodimers (Fig. 4) *(34)*. Several types of naturally occurring VDREs have been found in the promoters of vitamin D target genes. Systematic sequence analysis of these VDREs and the comparison of VDREs with the response elements for the other members of nuclear receptors led us to identify a consensus VDRE (cVDRE) *(31,35)*. Like the response elements for all-trans retinoic acid receptor(RAR), RXR, thyroid receptor (TR), peroxisome proliferator-activator receptor (PPAR), cVDRE is composed of two AGGTCA core motifs. The space between two motifs in cVDRE is 3 bp (the 3bp sequence is not specific), and this space appears to discriminate VDR/RXR heterodimer from the other heterodimers in DNA binding. For the transactivation function of VDR, both the ligand binding and DNA binding, is prerequisite. In the nucleus, VDR forms a transcriptional unit with the basal transcription machinery and putative cotranscriptional mediators (Fig. 3). As the transactivation function of VDR is ligand-dependent, two classes of transcriptional mediators, coactivator and corepressors, are speculated to be involved in transactivation, and indeed several coactivators for VDR, like the SRC-1/TIF2 family proteins and CBP/p300, have recently been identified *(32,36)*.

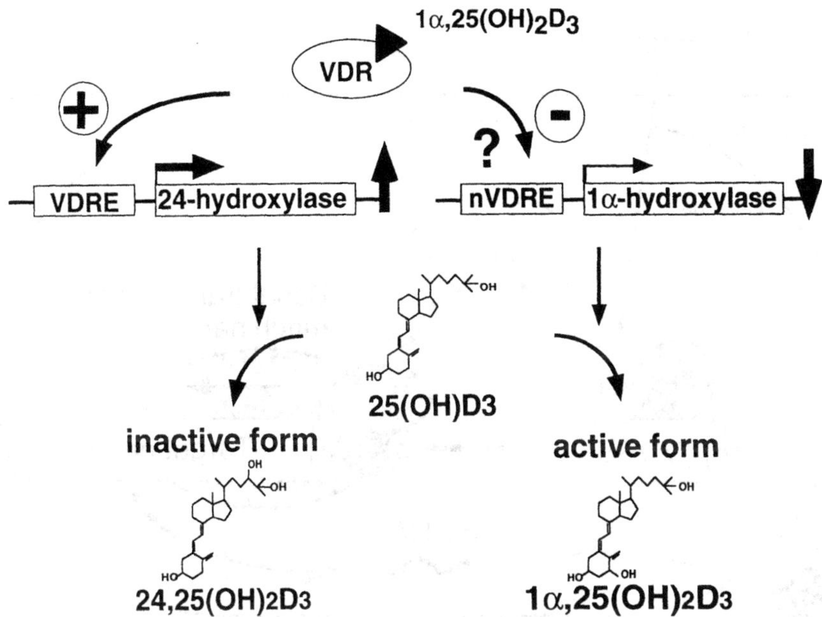

Fig. 2. A proposed molecular mechanism of regulations of 1α,25$(OH)_2D_3$ biosynthesis by 25-hydroxyvitamin D_3 1α-hydroxylase and 25(OH)D_3-24-hydroxylase. A negative VDRE has been identified in the promoter of the human 1α(OH)ase gene. The positive VDRE has been identified in the promoter of the 25(OH)D_3-24-hydroxylase gene.

Most of vitamin D actions are considered through VDR-mediated genomic actions. In addition, a nongenomic action is also postulated to be exerted through an unknown cell membrane receptor(s), which induces rapid cellular biological events in response to vitamin D *(1,3,37)*. Systematic studies have demonstrated that there are structure-function differences of vitamin D derivatives in their genomic actions and nongenomic actions *(1,3,37)*. However, the physiological significance of the nongenomic action remains unknown in the biological actions of vitamin D.

Molecular Bases of Vitamin D-Dependent Rickets

Mutations in the 1α-Hydroxylase Gene Cause Vitamin D-Dependent Rickets Type I

Genetic defects in the enzymes responsible for biosynthesis of 1α,25$(OH)_2D_3$ evoke vitamin D deficiency due to lack of 1α,25$(OH)_2D_3$ production. 1α(OH)ase plays a crucial role in 1α,25$(OH)_2D_3$ biosynthesis, so that mutation in the 1α(OH)ase gene resulting in loss of its enzymatic activity is a cause of hereditary rickets. A group

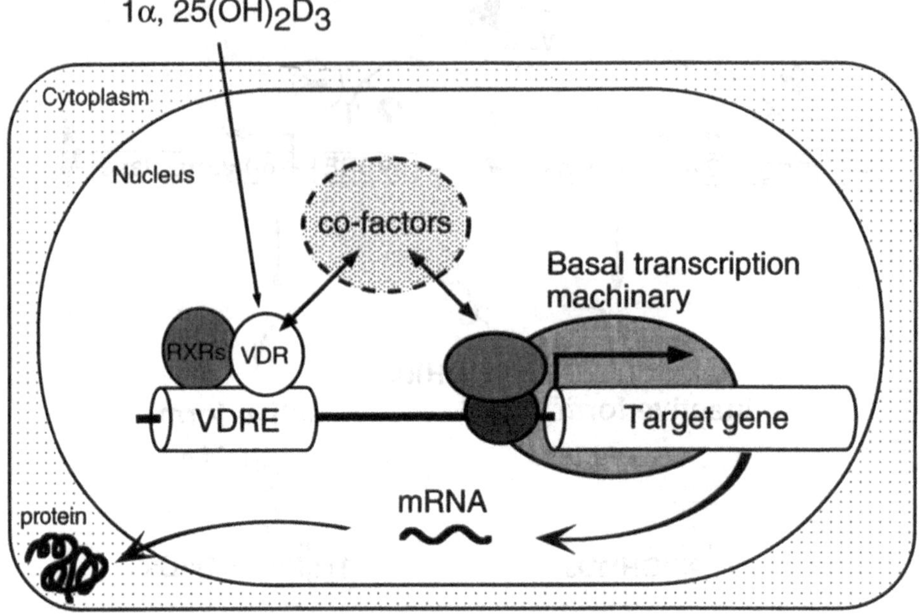

Fig. 3. Schema of molecular mechanism of vitamin D actions through VDR-mediated gene expression.

of hereditary rickets patients exhibiting low serum levels of 1α,25$(OH)_2D_3$, referred to as vitamin D dependency type I(VDDR I) *(5,10,11)*, have been considered to be caused by mutation in the 1α(OH)ase gene. Indeed, inactivating mutations in the 1α(OH)ase gene have been identified in the VDDR I patients by us *(8)* and others *(38)*. It was thus established at the molecular level that the 1α(OH)ase gene is responsible for VDDR I. To date, various mutations in this gene have been identified spreading over all exons (Fig. 5) *(8,38–40)*.

Mutations inVDR Gene Cause Hereditary Type II Rickets

In contrast to type I hereditary rickets, the other group of hereditary rickets patients(vitamin D dependency type II : VDDR II) do not respond to physiological doses of 1α,25$(OH)_2D_3$. The genetic analysis of VDDR II patients identified mutations in the human VDR gene causing loss of the VDR function as a ligand-inducible transcriptional factor *(41,42)*.

Several missense mutations in the DNA binding domain (DBD) of the VDR are reported and these mutations, which do not affect binding of 1,25$(OH)_2D_3$, cause decreased receptor affinity for DNA. Such mutant proteins are found to be totally transcriptionally inactive. Alternatively, mutations in the ligand binding

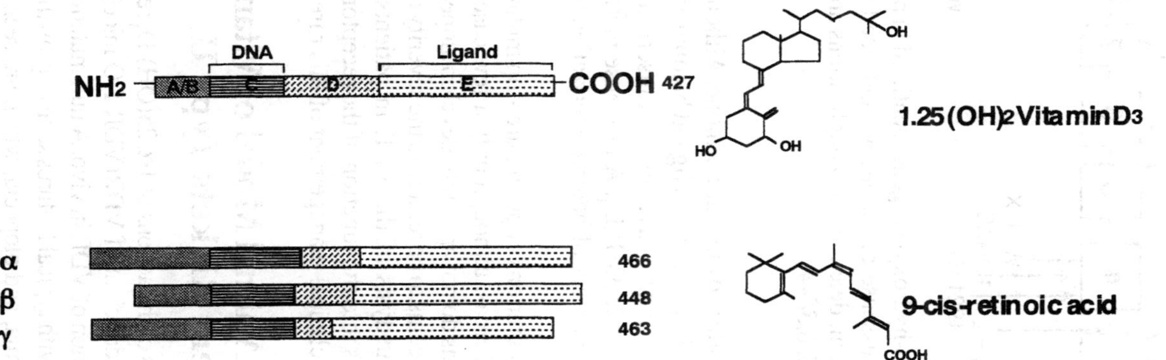

Fig. 4. Schematic structure of VDR. Schematic structure of VDR and RXRs, and their ligands are illustrated.

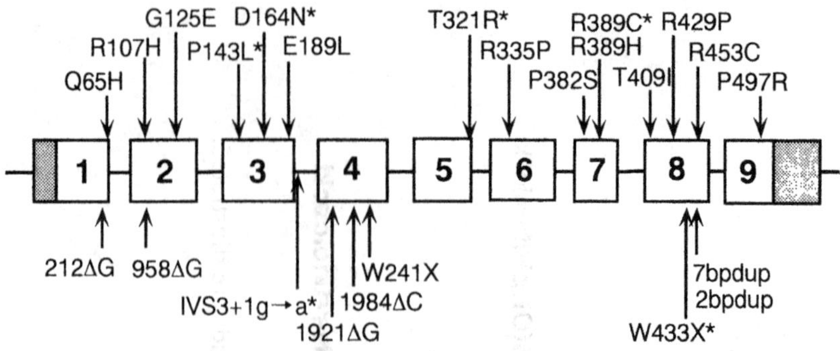

Fig. 5. Mutation in the 1α-hydroxylase gene identified in patients with VDDR I. The exons are numbered missense mutations are indicated above, and nonsense mutations, a splicing mutation, deletions, and duplications are indicated below the diagram. (Adapted from ref. *8,38–40.*)

domain (LBD) result in inability to bind the hormone. Although the most common nonsense mutation, Tyr295Stop, shows no ligand binding and is transcripionally inactive, some missense mutants have some transcriptional activity to the increased concentration of 1α25$(OH)_2D_3$. A missense mutation in the hormone binding domain resulting in defect of heterodimerization with RXR have been also reported *(43)*.

It appears that DBD mutations or premature stop mutations generally result in alopecia or hair loss, whereas, although only a few cases have been studied, patients with LBD mutations do not appear to develop alopecia. Thus, the type of mutation in the VDR gene seems to be related to the severity of the phenotype. The biochemical and genetic analysis of the VDR in patients with VDDR II has provided important insights into the function of the receptor and useful information on the diagnostic and clinical management of this rare disease.

VDR KO Mice as Animal Model of Vitamin D-Dependent Rickets Type II

As the molecular basis of the actions of 1α, 25$(OH)_2D_3$ remained only partially known, we generated mice deficient of VDR(VDR KO mice) by gene targeting in order to investigate the function of VDR in vivo. A null mutation of the VDR gene in mice indeed caused rickets with typical features such as growth retardation, impaired bone formation, hypocalcemia, and alopecia, which are seen in VDDR II patients *(44,45)*. The VDR KO mice are animal models of VDDR II.

Phenotype of the VDR KO Mice

The VDR KO(VDR–/–) mice did not differ from the heterozygous(VDR+/–) or wild-type(VDR+/+) littermates in growth rate (Fig. 6A) or behavior, and seemed

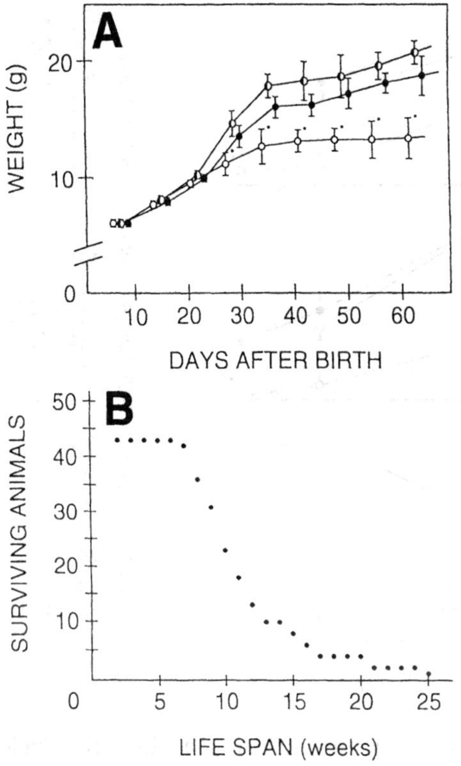

Fig. 6. Phenotypes of the VDR–/– mice: **(A)** Representative growth curve of wild-type (shaded circles), heterozygote (half shaded circles), and homozygote (open circles) littermates; **(B)** Survival rate of 43 VDR–/– mice.

functionally normal after birth until weaning. No bone malformation or overt phenotypic abnormalities were seen in the VDR–/– fetuses. However, after weaning (about 3 wk), the VDR KO mice showed marked growth retardation, and the body weight of the null mutant mice at 6 wk was about 50 % of those of the heterozygous and wild-type mice (Fig. 6A). After weaning the VDR KO mice developed rickets, and most of them died by 15 wk due to an unknown reasons (Fig. 6B). However, no overt abnormalities were found in the heterozygotes even at 6 mo. In addition to rickets by 7 wk, all of the VDR KO mice developed alopecia and poor whiskers and most of them displayed flat face with shorter nose. In the KO mice at 7 and 13 wk, no apparent abnormalities were found by histological analysis in the VDR-expressing tissues other than bone and skin, including the intestine, kidney, brain, and spleen. Most interestingly, dietary supplementation of calcium and phophorus recovered the abnormalities except alopecia in the VDR KO mice, and they survived more than 6 mo.

The observations in the VDR KO mice by us and the others *(44,45)* are similar to a VDDR type II *(10)*. These patients exhibit rickets with hypocalcemia,

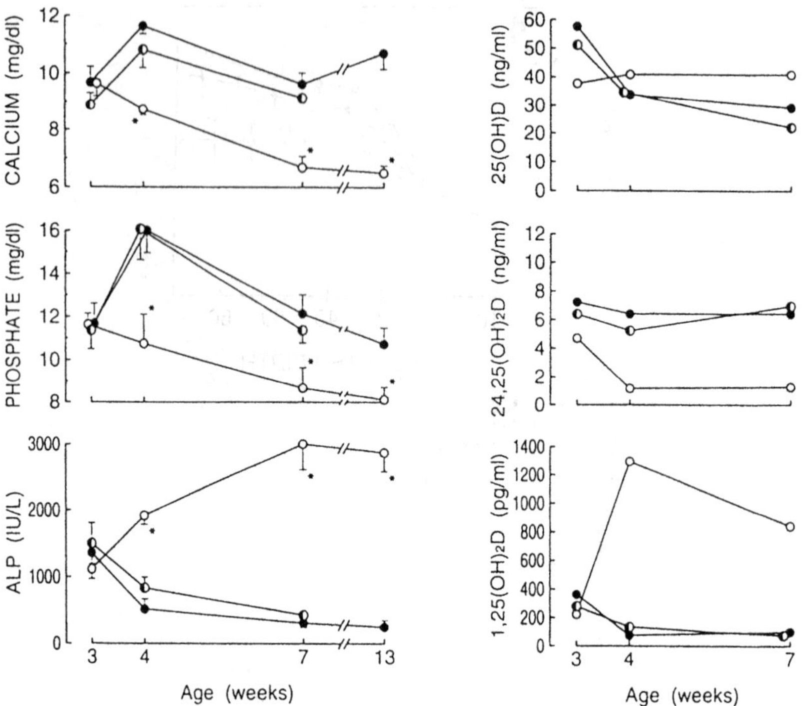

Fig. 7. Analyses of endocrine indicators in wild-type (shaded circles), heterozygote (half shaded circles), and homozygote (open circles) mice. Serum levels of Calcium, Phosphate and Alkaline phosphatase (ALP) in the left panel. Results are expressed as means ±SE for 4 samples. *Significantly different from the wild-type mice. Concentrations of serum vitamin D metabolites in the right panel. Results are the means for two determinations.

hypophosphatemia, and elevated serum alkaline phosphatase (ALP). In the VDR KO mice, such typical features of the rickets in serum parameters were seen only after weaning, but not before it (Fig. 7).

The serum level of 1α, 25(OH)2D3 is strictly regulated. Several enzymes, which are regulated by several factors including 1α, 25(OH)2D3, are involved in synthesis and metabolism of 1α, 25(OH)2D3 *(7)*. The activities of 25(OH)D 1α-hydroxylase and 24-hydroxylase are regulated negatively and positively, respectively, by 1α, 25(OH)2D3. In the VDR KO mice at 3 wk, the serum levels of 1α, 25(OH)2D, 24, 25(OH)2D, and 25(OH)D were the same as those in the heterozygous and wild-type mice (Fig. 7). However, a marked increase in serum 1α, 25(OH)2D, and a clear reduction in serum 24, 25(OH)2D developed in the VDR KO mice at 4 wk and persisted at 7 wk. These changes in serum vitamin D are comparable to the VDDR II patients. These findings also predicted increased activity of 25(OH)D 1α-hydroxylase and reduced activity of 24-hydroxylase.

Indeed, from the VDR KO mice, we cloned the cDNA encoding mouse 25(OH)D 1α-hydroxylase by a newly developed expression cloning method *(25)*. These observations establish that the 1α, 25(OH)2D3-VDR system plays a critical role only after weaning.

Loss of VDR Affected Cell Numbers of Chondrocytes, but Not Those of Osteoblasts or Osteoclasts, in VDR KO Mice

After weaning, severe malformation induced by loss of VDR was detected in bone. Radiographic analysis of the VDR KO mice at 7 wk revealed growth retardation with loss of bone density. In gross appearance and on X-ray analysis of tibia and fibula, typical features of advanced rickets were observed including widening of epiphyseal growth plates, thinning of the cortex, fraying, cupping, and widening of the metaphysis (Fig. 8). In addition, the normal orderly columns of hypertrophic chondrocytes were lost and the layers of cartilage were widened with inadequate mineralization. In cancellous bone adjacent to the growth plates, marked increases in the extent and the width of osteoid seams were noted (consistent with osteomalacia), and bone surfaces were surrounded by numerous osteoblastic cells (Fig. 8). Interestingly, the numbers of osteoclasts and osteoblasts appeared to be normal in the bone from the VDR null mutant mice. Dietary supplement of calcium to the VDR KO mice significantly rescued the impaired mineralizaion in bone, however, the malformation in the cartilage was not recovered (N. Yagishita et al., unpublished results). These findings indicate that 1α, $25(OH)_2D_3$ can stimulate, but is not essential for osteoclast formation in vivo, and that another factor(s) can induce the osteoclast formation in the absence of the 1α, $25(OH)_2D_3$ actions. Mineralization in bone appears to depend on the levels of serum calcium and the other minerals. In contrast to oestoblasts and osteoclasts, chondrocytes may be one of direct target cells for 1α, $25(OH)_2D_3$.

Lessons from VDR KO Mice

Molecular Basis for Hereditary Rickets Type II

By generating the VDR KO mice, we showed here that the 1α, $25(OH)_2D_3$-VDR system is essential for growth, bone formation, and hair development only after weaning. The phenotype of the VDR KO mice was similar to a human recessive genetic disease, VDDR II, providing experimental evidence that the VDR gene is responsible for VDDR II.

Actions of Vitamin D on Bone Formation and Metabolism

As previously reported in rickets patients and animals in a vitamin D deficiency, loss of VDR caused impaired bone formation. However, it is notable that the onset of the rickets is only after weaning in the VDR KO mice, unlike in the hereditary type II patients. The fact may indicate a possible presence of the substitute for vitamin D in milk. One possible substitute could be calcium, which is abundant especially in rodent milk. In this respect, it is interesting that dietary

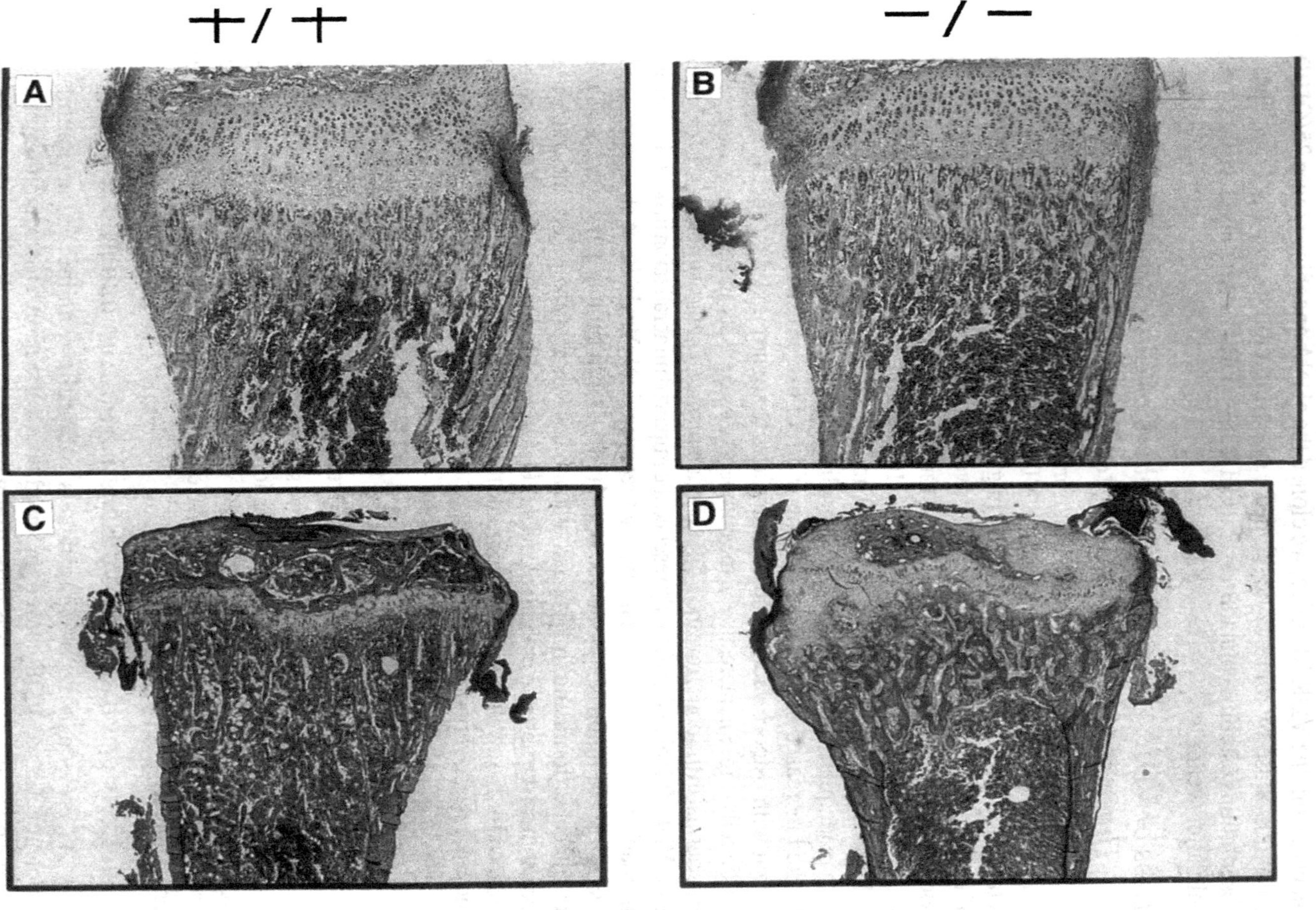

Fig. 8. Histological analysis of the bone of VDR knockout mice and normal control littermate. a, Villaneuva-Goldner staining of proximal tibia metaphysis in mice at 3 wk (upper panels) and 7 wk (lower panels). Wild-type, +/+, homozygote, –/–.

supplementation of calcium to VDR KO mice significantly recovers the impaired mineralization in bone. However, the disordered proliferation and differentiation of chondrocyte in the VDR KO mice could not be significantly restored by this dietary calcium supplementation (N.Yagishita, et al., unpublished result). Such responses to dietary calcium in the skeletal tissue are also seen in the hereditary type II patients. Thus, it is most likely that action of vitamin D on the mineralization in the bone tissue is indirect, possibly mediated through serum minerals. Thus, from these findings, we speculate that the 1α, $25(OH)_2D_3$-VDR system is more important for the cell proliferation and differentiation of chondrocyte, than osteoclasts and osteoclast differentiation.

In contrast to the bone, alopecia in the VDR KO mice was not recovered by the dietary calcium, suggesting that the action of vitamin D in the hair follicle is direct, and not mediated through serum calcium. To better understand the actions of vitamin D in such target tissues, and the pathogenesis of the hereditary type II patients, tissue-specific inactivation of VDR in bone, intestine, skin, and the major target tissues is clearly required. These studies by means of the conditional KO system are currently underway in our laboratory.

Summary

Vitamin D plays a role in a wide variety of biological events such as calcium homeostasis, bone formation, and cellular differentiation. The active form of vitamin D, 1α,$25(OH)_2D_3$, is biosynthesized from cholesterol. The final, critical step in this biosynthesis is conversion from 25-hydroxyvitamin D_3 to 1α,$25(OH)_2D_3$ by the enzyme 25-hydroxyvitamin D_3 1α-hydroxylase, which will be referred to as 1α(OH)ase. 1α,$25(OH)_2D_3$ transcriptionally controls the expression of a particular set of target genes through VDR, thereby exerting its biological actions. Two kinds of vitamin D dependent hereditary rickets are known to be caused by genetic mutations. Mutations of the 1α(OH)ase gene and the VDR gene have been identified as causes of vitamin D dependent rickets type I and type II, respectively. Both of the diseases display an autosomal recessive trait, but clinical features and response to administrated 1α,$25(OH)_2D_3$ are distinct. The phenotypes of the VDR KO mice, an animal model of the type II rickets, are also described to understand the defects in the hereditary rickets type II patients.

References

1. Bouillon, R., Okamura, W. H., and Norman, A. W. (1995) Structure–functional relationships in the vitamin D endocrine system. *Endocr. Rev.* **16,** 200–257.
2. Studzinski, G. P., McLane, J. A., and Uskokovic, M. R. (1993) Signaling pathways for vitamin D–induced differentiation: implications for therapy of proliferative and neoplastic diseases. *Crit. Rev. Eukaryot. Gene Exp.* **3,** 279–312.
3. Walters, M. R. (1992) Newly identified actions of the vitamin D endocrine system. *Endocr. Rev.* **13,** 719–764.

4. Darwish, H. and DeLuca, H. F. (1993) Vitamin D-regulated gene expression. *Crit. Rev. Eukaryot. Gene Exp.* **3,** 89–116.
5. Scriver, C. R., Reade, T. M., DeLuca, H. F., and Hamstra, A. J. (1978) Serum 1,25-dihydroxyvitamin D levels in normal subjects and in patients with hereditary rickets or bone disease. *N. Engl. J. Med.* **299,** 976–979.
6. Kato S., Yanagisawa J., Murayama A., Kitanaka S., and Takeyama K. (1998) The importance of 25-hydroxyvitamin D3 1α–hydroxylase gene in vitamin D-dependent rickets. *Curr. Opin. Nephrol. Hypertens.* **7,** 377–383.
7. Fraser, D. R. (1980) Regulation of the metabolism of vitamin D. *Physiol. Rev.* **60,** 551–613.
8. Kitanaka, S., Takeyama, K., Murayama, A., Sato, T., Okumura, K., Nogami, M., et al. (1998) Inactivating mutations in the human 25-hydroxyvitamin D3 1α-hydroxlase gene in patients with pseudovitamin D-deficient rickets. *N. Engl. J. Med.* **338,** 653–661.
9. Hughes, M. R., Malloy, P. J., Kieback, D. G., Kesterson, R. A., Pike, J. W., Feldman, D., and O'Malley, B. W. (1988) Point mutations in the human vitamin D receptor associated with hypocalcemic rickets. *Science* **242,** 1702–1705.
10. Demay, M. B. (1995) Hereditary defects in vitamin D metabolism and vitamin D receptor defects, in *Endocrinology.* Vol. 2., 3rd ed. (DeGroot, L. J., Besser, M., Burger, H. G., et al. eds.), pp. 1173–1178 .
11. Fraser, D., Kooh, S. W., Kind, H. P., et al. (1973) Pathogenesis of hereditary vitamin D-dependent rickets: An inborn error of vitamin D metabolism involving defective conversion of 25-hydroxyvitamin D to 1α,25-dihydroxyvitamin D. *N. Engl. J. Med.* **289,** 817–822.
12. Gamblin, G. T., Liberman, U. A., Eil, C., et al. (1985) Vitamin D-dependent rickets type II: Defective induction of 25-hydroxyvitamin D3-24-hydroxylase by 1,25-dihydroxyvitamin D in cultured skin fibroblasts. *J. Clin. Invest.* **75,** 954–960.
13. Brooks, M. H., Bell, N. H., Love, L., Stern, P. H., Ordei, E., Queener, S. J., Hamstra, A. J., and Deluca, H. F. (1978) Vitamin D dependent rickets type II, resistance of target organs to 1,25-dihydroxyvitamin D. *N. Engl. J. Med.* **293,** 996–999.
14. Balsan, S., Garabedian, M., Larchet, M., et al. (1986) Long-term nocturnal calcium infusions can cure rickets and promote normal mineralization in hereditary resistance to 1,25-dihydroxyvitamin D. *J. Clin. Invest.* **77,** 1661–1667.
15. Takeda, E., Yokota, I., Kawakami, I., et al. (1989) Two siblings with vitamin D-dependent rickets type II: no recurrence of rickets for 14 years after cessation of therapy. *Eur. J. Pediatr.* **149,** 54–57.
16. DeLuca, H. F. and Schnoes, H. K. (1976) Metabolism and action of vitamin D. *Annu. Rev. Biochem.* **45,** 631–666.
17. Holick, M. F., Schnoes, H. K., DeLuca, H. F., Gray, R. W., Boyle, I. T., and Suda, T. (1972) Isolation and identification of 24,25-dihydroxycholecalciferol, a metabolite of vitamin D3 made in the kidney. *Biochemistry* **11,** 4251–4255.
18. Su, P., Rennert, H., Shayiq, R. M., Yamamoto, R., Zheng, Y. M., Addya, S., Strauss, J. F. 3d., and Avadhani, N. G. (1990) A cDNA encoding a rat mitochondrial cytochrome P450 catalyzing both the 26–hydroxylation of cholesterol and 25-hydroxylation of vitamin D3: gonadotropic regulation of the cognate mRNA in ovaries. *DNA Cell Biol.* **9,** 657–667.
19. Usui, E., Noshiro, M., and Okuda, K. (1990) Molecular cloning of cDNA for vitamin D3 25-hydroxylase from rat liver mitochondria. *FEBS Lett.* **262,** 135–138.

20. Ohyama, Y. and Okuda, K. (1991) Isolation and characterization of a cytochrome P-450 from rat kidney mitochondria that catalyzes the 24-hydroxylation of 25-hydroxyvitamin D3. *J. Biol. Chem.* **266,** 8690–8695.
21. Chen, K.-S. and DeLuca, H. F. (1995) Cloning of the human 1α,25-dihydroxyvitamin D-3 24-hydroxylase gene promoter and identification of two vitamin D-responsive elements. *Biochim. Biophys. Acta* **1269,** 1–9.
22. Henry, H. L., Midgett, R. J., and Norman, A. W. Studies on calciferol metabolism (1974) Regulation of 25-hydroxvitamin D3-1α-hydroxlase, in vivo. *J. Biol. Chem.* **249,** 7584–7592.
23. Henry, H. L. (1979) Regulation of the hydroxylation of 25-hydroxvitamin D3 in vivo and in primary cultures of chick kidney cells. *J. Biol. Chem.* **254,** 2722–2729.
24. Portale, A. A., Halloran, B. P., and Morris, Jr. R. C. (1989) Physiologic regulation of the serum concentration of 1,25-dihydroxyvitamin D by phosphorus in normal men. *J. Clin. Invest.* **83,** 1494–1499.
25. Takeyama, K., Kitanaka, S., Sato, T., Kobori, M., Yanagisawa, J., and Kato, S. (1997) 25-Hydroxyvitamin D3 1α-hydroxlase and vitamin D synthesis. *Science* **277,** 1827–1830.
26. Murayama, A., Takeyama, K., Kitanaka, S., Kodera, Y., Hosoya, T., and Kato, S. (1998) The promoter of the human 25-hydorxyvitamin D3 1α-hydroxylase gene confers positive and negative responsiveness to PTH, calcitonin, and 1α,25(OH)2 D3. Bioche. *Biophys. Res. Commun.* **249,** 11–16,
27. Booth, B. E., Tsai, H. C., and Morris, R. C. (1985) Vitamin D status regulates 25- hydroxvitamin D3-1-alpha-hydroxlase and its responsiveness to parathyroid hormone in the chick. *J. Clin. Invest.* **75,** 155–161.
28. Henry, H. L. and Luntao, E. M. (1989) Interactions between intracellular signals involved in the regulation of 25-hydroxvitamin D3 metabolism. *Endocrinology* **124,** 2228–2234.
29. Murayama, A., Takeyema, K., Kitanaka, S., Kodera, Y., Kawaguchi, Y., Hososya, T., and Kato, S. (1999) Positive and negative regulations of the renal 25-hydroxyvitamin D3 1α–hydroxylase gene by parathyroid hormone, calcitonin and 1α,25(OH)2D3 in intact animals. *Endocrinology* **140,** 2224–2231.
30. Brenza, H., Kimmel-Jehan, C., Jehan, F., Shinki, T., Wakino, S., Anazawa, M., Suda, T., and DeLuca H. F. (1998) Parathyroid hormone activation of the rat 25-hydroxyvitamin D3-1α-hydroxylase gene promoter. *Proc. Natl. Acad. Sci. USA* **95,** 1387–1391.
31. Ebihara, K., Masuhiro, Y., Kitamoto, T. et al. (1996) Intron retention generates a novel isoform of the murine vitamin D receptor that acts in a dominant negative way on the vitamin D signaling pathway. *Mol. Cell. Biol.* **16,** 3393–3400 .
32. Yanagisawa, J., Yanagi, Y., Masuhiro, Y., Suzawa, M., Toriyabe, T., Kashiwagi, K., Watanabe, M., Kawabata, M., Miyazono, K., Kato, S. (1999) Convergence of TGFb and vitamin D signaling pathways on SMAD proteins acting as common transcriptional co-activators. *Science* **283,** 1317–1321.
33. Mangelsdorf, D. J. and Evans, R. M. (1995) The RXR heterodimers and orphan receptors. *Cell* **83,** 841–850 .
34. Kato, S., Sasaki, H., Suzawa, M., Masushige, S., Tora, L., Chambon, P., and Gronemeyer, H. (1995) Widely spaced, directly repeated PuGGTCA elements act as promiscuous enhancers for different classes of nuclear receptors. *Mol. Cell. Biol.* **15,** 5858–5867.

35. Freedman, L. P., Arce, V., and Fernandez, R. P. (1994) DNA sequences that act as high affinity targets for the vitamin D3 receptor in the absence of the retinoid X receptor. *Mol. Endocrinol.* **8,** 265–273 .
36. Horwitz, K. B., Jackson, T. A., Bain, D. L., Richer, J. K., Takimoto, G. S., and Tung L. (1996) Nuclear receptor coactivators and corepressors. *Mol. Endocrinol.* **10,** 1167–1177.
37. Norman, A. W., Roth, J., and Orchi, L. (1982) The vitamin D endocrine system:steroid metabolism, hormone receptors, and biological response (calcium binding proteins). *Endocr. Rev.* **3,** 331–366.
38. Fu, G. K., Lin, D., Ahang, M. Y. H. et al. (1997) Cloning of human 25–hydroxyvitamin D-1α-hydroxylase and mutaitons causing vitamin D–dependent rickets type I. *Mol. Endocrinol.* **11,** 1961–1970.
39. Wang, J. T., Lin, D., Burridge, S. M., et al. (1998) Genetics of vitamin D 1α–hydroxylase deficiency in 17 families. *Am. J. Hum. Genet.* **63,** 1694–1702.
40. Kitanaka, S., Murayama, A., Sakai, T., Inouye, K., Seino, Y., Fukumoto, S., et al. (1999) No enzyme activity of 25-hydroxyvitamin D3 1α-hydroxylase gene product in pseudovitamin D deficiency rickets, including that with mild clinical manifiestation. *J. Clin. Endocrinol. Metab.* **84,** 4111–4117.
41. Malloy, P. J., Hochberg, Z., Tiosano, D., Pike, J. W., Hughes, M. R., and Feldman, D. (1990) The molecular basis of hereditary 1,25-dihydroxyvitamin D3 resistant rickets in seven related families. *J. Clin. Invest.* **86,** 2071–2079.
42. Malloy, P. J., Pike, J. W., and Feldman, D. (1997) Hereditary 1,25-dihydroxyvitamin D resistant rickets, in *Vitamin D* (Feldman, D., Glorieux, F. H., and Pike, J. W. eds.) Academic Press, San Diego, CA, pp. 765–787.
43. Whitefield, G. K., Selznick, S. H., Haussler, C. A., et al. (1996) Vitamin D receptors from patients with resistance to 1,25-dihydroxyvitamin D3: point mutations confer reduced transactivation in response to ligand and impaired interaction with the retinoid X receptor heterodimeric partner. *Mol. Endocrinol.* **10,** 1617–1631.
44. Yoshizawa, T., Handa, Y., Uemasu, Y., Takeda, S., Sekine, K., Yoshihara, Y., Kawakami, T., Arioka, K., Sato, H., Uchiyama, Y., Masushige, S., Fukamizu, A., Matsumoto, T., and Kato, A. (1997) Impaired bone formation and uterine hypoplasia with growth retardation after weaning in mice lacking the vitamin D receptor. *Nat. Genet.* **16,** 391–396.
45. Li, Y.C., Pirro, A. E., Amling, M., Delling, G., Baron, R., Bronson, R., and Demay, M.B. (1997) Targeted ablation of the vitamin D receptor: an animal model of vitamin D-dependent rickets type II with alopecia. *Proc. Natl. Acad. Sci. USA* **94,** 9831–9835.

Chapter 7

Inherited Phosphate Wasting Disorders

Michael J. Econs and Kenneth E. White

Introduction

There are several hereditary disorders of isolated phosphate wasting that have been described. These include X-linked hypophosphatemic rickets (XLH); autosomal dominant hypophosphatemic rickets (ADHR); hypophosphatemic bone disease (HBD), and hereditary hypophosphatemic rickets with hypercalciuria (HHRH). Phosphate wasting is also a predominant feature of disorders that result from mutations in the CLCN5 gene, however, these disorders are covered in Chapter 8. The large number of hereditary renal phosphate wasting disorders indicates that control over renal phosphate homeostasis is a complex process. Investigators are starting to find genes that when mutated result in renal phosphate wasting. The discovery of these genes provides insights into phosphate homeostasis and helps to elucidate the pathophysiology of these disorders. Additionally, in some instances, the isolation of a disease gene allows clinicians to combine what were previously thought to be distinct disorders into one disorder.

X-Linked Hypophosphatemic Rickets

X-linked hypophosphatemic rickets (XLH) is the most common form of hereditary renal phosphate wasting with a prevalence of approx 1:20,000 *(1)*. The hallmark of this disease is isolated renal phosphate wasting with inappropriately normal calcitriol concentrations. An osteoblast defect has also been proposed to contribute to impaired mineralization in the disorder (*see* below). Classically, patients present with lower extremity deformities, rickets, growth retardation, bone pain, tooth abscesses, enthesopathy (calcification of tendons, ligaments, and joint capsule), and osteomalacia *(2,3)*. Severely affected individuals may also display cranial abnormalities *(4)* and spinal stenosis *(5–7)*. However, the severity of the disease is variable and affected members of the same family, who have the same genetic defect, may have markedly different phenotypes. Despite hypophosphatemia, weakness is not a predominant feature of the disease although patients do complain of weakness more than controls *(8)*. XLH is an X-linked dominant disorder *(9)*, and although controversy exists regarding whether there is a gene dosage effect, the available evidence suggests that males and females are affected equally *(10)*.

Much of our understanding of the pathophysiology of XLH has been derived from the two mouse models, the Hyp and Gy mice. In accord with the human disease, these mice have renal phosphate wasting, impaired mineralization and growth retardation *(11,12)*. The Gy mouse also has inner ear abnormalities, deafness, hyperactivity, and circling behavior *(12)*. Linkage studies mapped the two mutations to a region of the mouse X chromosome that is syntenic to the human HYP locus *(13,14)*. As with the human disease there does not appear to be a marked difference in severity between male and female Hyp mice *(15)*, however, less data is available for the Gy.

The etiology of the phosphate wasting defect has been examined in the Hyp mouse. This defect has been directly demonstrated in the brush border membrane of the renal proximal tubule *(16)*. More recent studies demonstrate that the phosphate wasting in the proximal tubule is due to a defect in the high affinity/low capacity sodium dependent phosphate cotransport system *(17)*. This transporter (Npt-2) has been cloned for both the human [/NPT-2, *(18)* /] and mouse [/Npt-2 *(19)* /]. The murine Hyp and Gy mutations result in an approx 50% decrease in NPT-2 mRNA and protein *(20,21)*. Since human NPT-2 is located on chromosome 5q35 it is not a candidate gene for HYP *(22)*. However, the data suggest that the HYP gene is involved in regulation of NPT-2 expression and/or turnover.

Despite these results is was unclear as to whether the phosphate wasting results from a primary renal defect or whether the phosphate wasting is the result of elaboration of a humoral factor that alters phosphate transport in the renal proximal tubule. In this regard, Meyer et al. performed parabiosis experiments using Hyp and normal mice *(23)*. In these experiments mice are surgically joined together and vascular channels are allowed to develop between the animals, resulting in cross circulation between them. Normal mice joined to Hyp mice had a progressive reduction in plasma phosphate over three weeks and a greater renal phosphate excretion index than normal mice joined to other normal mice. Furthermore, after separating the normal/Hyp pairs, plasma phosphate returned to normal in the normal mouse within 24 hr and after 2 and 7 d these normal mice had "rebound hyperphosphatemia" as compared to mice separated from normal/normal pairs *(23)*. These results were not dependent on PTH since similar results were obtained in thyro-parathyroidectomized mice *(24)*.

Since parabiosis experiments have significant limitations, Nesbitt et al. *(25)* performed renal cross transplantation between Hyp and normal mice. They found that when normal kidneys were transplanted into nephrectomized Hyp mice the kidneys wasted phosphorus. When Hyp kidneys were transplanted into nephrectomized normal mice the kidneys retained phosphorus normally. Thus, the defect in the Hyp mouse is neither corrected nor transferred by renal cross transplantation indicating that the phosphate transport defect in the Hyp mouse is not due to an intrinsic renal abnormality.

The aforementioned studies demonstrate that the defect in the Hyp mouse, and probably in the human disease, is not in the kidney. However, they do not establish which tissues are defective. Some investigators have focused on the osteoblast since there is a mineralization defect in the Hyp mouse. Ecarot et al. *(26,27)* transplanted periostea and osteoblasts from normal and Hyp mice into the gluteal muscles of normal and Hyp mice. As anticipated, when normal cells were transplanted into Hyp mice mineralization was impaired. However, when Hyp cells were transplanted into normal mice, reduction, but not normalization of the defect was observed leading these investigators to conclude that there is an intrinsic osteoblast defect in the Hyp mouse. Although these studies supported the hypothesis that there is a primary osteoblast defect in the Hyp mouse, they did not exclude the possibility that the putative circulating factor in the Hyp mouse could have led to an irreversible developmental defect in the Hyp osteoblast. Such a situation would be analogous to the permanent developmental defects that are produced in developing neural tissue by lack of sufficient thyroid hormone at a critical stage of development *(28)*.

An intrinsic osteoblast defect was also postulated by Lajeunesse et al. *(29)* who studied the effects of Hyp serum and Hyp osteoblast conditioned media on phosphate transport in primary mouse proximal tubule cultures (MPTC). They found that Hyp serum, when added to the culture media for at least 24 hr, impaired phosphate transport in MPTC in a dose dependent fashion. Furthermore, conditioned media from Hyp osteoblasts, compared to conditioned media from normal osteoblasts, also inhibited phosphate transport. These data suggest that the Hyp osteoblast is responsible for the release and/or modification of a humoral factor(s) that inhibits phosphate reabsorption *(29)*. Additional preliminary studies by this group *(30)* support the notion that the Hyp osteoblasts may modify a factor rather than directly produce this factor. Whether the osteoblast is solely responsible for the production and/or modification of this factor or whether another cell type plays an important role in the pathogenesis of the phosphate wasting has not been determined. However, these studies do implicate the osteoblast as a potentially important cell in maintenance of phosphate homeostasis.

The possibility that a hormonal factor plays a role in phosphate wasting is supported by existence of tumor induced osteomalacia. These tumors, which are frequently of mesenchymal origin, result in renal phosphate wasting and inappropriately low serum calcitriol concentrations *(3,19,31–33)*. Both the phosphate wasting and low calcitriol concentrations resolve when the tumor is removed. Since tumors frequently secrete, in abnormal amounts and in an unregulated fashion, substances that have a role in normal physiology, it is plausible that the phosphate wasting observed in patients who have tumor induced osteomalacia is due to over production of a factor(s) that normally controls renal phosphate reabsorption. We have referred to this factor as "phosphatonin" *(31)*. Unfortunately, this factor has only been partially purified *(32,34)* and its role in the phosphate wasting seen in XLH has yet to be determined.

Vitamin D Metabolism

In the setting of hypophosphatemia, increased calcitriol (1,25OH vitamin D) concentrations are anticipated since this is one of the homeostatic mechanisms that is present to return serum phosphate concentrations to normal. However, several investigators have found normal serum calcitriol concentrations in XLH patients *(35–37)*. Thus, XLH patients have a relative insufficiency of calcitriol. Studies in the Hyp mouse confirm and expand the human observations. 25(OH)D-1α-hydroxylase, the enzyme that converts 25OH vitamin D into 1,25OH vitamin D, plays a critical role in determining serum calcitriol concentrations. Lobaugh and Drezner *(38)* studied the activity of this enzyme in Hyp mice and compared it to normal mice on control and phosphate deplete diets. Normal mice on phosphate deplete diets profoundly increased 1α-hydroxylase activity compared to normal mice on the control diet while Hyp mice had a much lesser increment in 1α-hydroxylase despite having serum phosphorus concentrations that were similar to the phosphate deplete mice. Moreover, other investigators have found that the catabolism of 1,25(OH)2D3 is increased in Hyp mice as compared to controls *(39,40)*.

Unfortunately, studies of 1α-hydroxylase activity in the Gy mouse are more controversial. Davidai et al. *(41)* found that activity of renal 25(OH)D-1α-hydroxylase in the Gy mouse was similar to that of normal mice on phosphate depleted diets, but much greater than that of normal mice on control diets. They concluded that, unlike the Hyp mouse, 1α-hydroxylase activity is appropriately regulated in the Gy mouse. Tenenhouse et al. *(42)* were unable to detect a statistically significant difference in calcitriol concentrations between Gy and normal mice on control diets, although there was a trend for Gy mice to have higher calcitriol concentrations. However, when Gy and normal mice were placed on phosphate restricted diets normal mice appropriately increased their calcitriol concentration, but the calcitriol concentration in phosphate deplete Gy mice paradoxically dropped substantially below that of Gy mice on the control diet. Meyer et al. *(43)* postulated that some of the observed differences between the Hyp and Gy models were due to differences in genetic background since the Gy mouse is bred on the B6C3H background and the Hyp mouse is bred on the C57BL/6J background. Of note, the male Gy mouse does not survive on the C57BL/6J background *(44)*. When both mutations were bred on the B6C3H background there were no differences in calcitriol concentrations between Hyp and Gy mice. However, both Hyp and Gy mice calcitriol concentrations were substantially effected by calcium concentrations in the diet. Thus, it is possible that much of the observed difference in vitamin D metabolism between Gy and Hyp mice was secondary to differences in background strain and diet. These findings are important since several investigators have asserted that the Hyp and Gy mice arose from mutations in two different genes, particularly in light of the occurrence of a recombination event between the two mutations *(12)*. However, a definitive answer to this question required cloning the gene and characterizing the mutations.

Positional Cloning of the PHEX Gene

Despite extensive study, as outlined previously, the pathophysiology of XLH has not been fully elucidated. To gain a better understanding of the disorder we used the positional cloning approach to map and clone the gene responsible for the disorder (reviewed in refs. *45* and *46*). The positional cloning approach has two major advantages: 1. it does not require the investigator to make any assumptions about the gene's function and 2. knowledge of tissue expression, although helpful, is not required. As outlined in Chapters 20–22, this approach is becoming more common-place and it has been used to clone a wide variety of disease genes *(47)*.

To locate a gene by the positional cloning approach investigators first use linkage analysis to determine the chromosomal location of the gene. Once a general location is known they perform additional linkage analysis with multiple genetic markers from the region to find two markers that closely flank the disease gene. Subsequently, the investigators construct a "contig" map of human DNA between the flanking genetic markers. They use this contig to identify genes contained within the contig and test these genes for mutation in affected individuals.

Early linkage studies by Machler et al. and Thakker et al. placed the HYP gene on Xp22 *(48,49)* between the markers DXS41 and DXS43, but the distance between these markers was far too great to consider creating a contig map with the available technology. Over the course of several investigations *(50–53)* members of the HYP consortium refined the genetic map determined that the markers DXS365 (telomeric) and DXS274 (centromeric) flanked the disease gene. These flanking markers were now close enough to try to bridge the distance between them with yeast artificial chromosomes (YAC). As detailed in Chapter 21, YACs are yeast vectors that contain large pieces of human DNA (up to 1 MB) and can be propagated in yeast *(54)*. DXS365 and DXS274, and/or cosmids that contained these probes, were used to screen YAC libraries *(55)*. This screening identified 4 nonchimeric YACs on the centromeric side and 2 nonchimeric YACs on the telomeric side. To complete the contig we isolated a cosmid from the telomeric end of one of the centromeric YACs and used this cosmid to rescreen the YAC library. This "walking" technique allowed us to isolate several new YAC clones. One of these YAC clones overlapped with one of the YACs that was obtained by the initial library screen with DXS365, the telomeric marker. Thus, the distance between the two flanking markers DXS365, on the telomeric side, and DXS274 on the centromeric side was spanned by a 3 YAC contig which covered approx 1.5 MB of genomic DNA *(55)*.

To further define the region we developed new microsatellite markers, DXS1683 and DXS7474, from two of the YACs *(56,57)*. These markers were physically mapped to lie on opposite ends of the YAC in the center of the contig *(55)*. We tested these markers in 20 large HYP kindreds. Two recombinants were seen between DXS1683 and HYP. Both of these matings placed DXS1683 on the centromeric side of the HYP gene *(50)*. Similarly, there were two recombination events between DXS7474 and HYP which placed DXS7474 telomeric to HYP *(51)*. These results allowed us to place the HYP gene on one YAC between DXS1683 and DXS7474 in a physical distance of approx 350kb *(51)*.

Since the distance between the new flanking markers is relatively short and since cosmids have several advantages over YACs, we constructed a cosmid contig *(58)* across the region. The cosmid contig allowed us to change our approach to mutation detection. In addition to trying to isolate cDNAs from the region and test them for mutation in our 20 large kindreds, we used the cosmids to screen large numbers of affected individuals for deletions. These affected individuals were either members of small kindreds that were not suitable for linkage studies or were isolated cases. Through the collaborative efforts of the five laboratories that make up the HYP consortium *(58)* we obtained DNA samples from approx 150 unrelated affected individuals. We looked for deletions by hybridizing whole cosmids to Southern blots of restriction enzyme digested genomic DNA from these individuals. Although we did not think that deletions would be common in this disease, the detection of even one deletion with a cosmid would be a strong indication that the cosmid contained the HYP gene.

We found three affected individuals who demonstrated deletions in DNA contained within cosmid 611 and we found a fourth affected individual who demonstrated a small (approx 1kb) deletion within cosmid 1005, which lies immediately centromeric to cosmid 611 *(58)*. This latter deletion does not overlap with the other three deletions. Thus, we focused our efforts on these cosmids.

Cloning the PHEX Gene

To clone the gene the members of the HYP consortium employed three complementary approaches (*see* Chapter 21 for detailed illustrations on how these techniques are used to find genes). We used the cosmids that were identified by patient deletions to screen cDNA libraries made from fetal brain, fetal liver, and adult muscle. We also performed exon trapping *(59)* to detect exons from genes that were contained within the contig. Additionally, we performed automated sequencing of the cosmids and used standard computer programs to search for exons within the genomic sequence. All three lines of investigation revealed the presence of a candidate gene in the region. Sequence analysis of this gene indicated that it contains significant homology at the peptide level to the M13 family of endopeptidase genes, which includes neutral endopeptidase, endothelin-converting enzyme-1 (ECE1), and the Kell antigen. Further analysis revealed that in all four patients who had deletions, the deletions involved at least one exon from this gene *(58)*. We labeled this gene "PEX" for phosphate regulating gene with homologies to endopeptidases on the X chromosome. The name has been subsequently changed to "PHEX" to avoid confusion with genes that are responsible for peroxisomal disorders.

The PHEX gene contains 22 exons, which code for a 749 amino acid protein *(58,60)*. As is typical for the M13 endopeptidases, PHEX has 10 conserved cysteines that are seen in other members of this class, it has a short N-terminal cytoplasmic domain, and a single transmembrane domain. Thus, most of the molecule is in the extracellular space. The PHEX protein contains several highly conserved sequence motifs including a zinc binding domain (HEXXH in exon 17) and an invariant glutamic acid residue in exon 19 *(58,60)*. Cloning the human PHEX gene has led to relatively rapid cloning of the mouse Phex gene, which has high homology to human PHEX *(61,62)*. Of interest, neither the human nor murine PHEX/Phex genes have "classic" Kozak sequences *(63)*. PHEX/Phex is one of only three percent of known genes that does not have a purine at the -3 position before the ATG initiation sequence *(60–62)*. This finding may be significant since, in general, genes that do not have good Kozak sequences tend to be post transcriptionally regulated *(64)*.

Although little is known about the Kell blood group protein, ECE 1 and neutral endopeptidase function as ectoenzymes. Neutral endopeptidase degrades/ inactivates several small peptides including substance P, bradykinin, and enkephalins *(65)*. Endothelin converting enzyme 1, on the other hand, serves to convert Big endothelin to endothelin, the active form *(66)*. Thus, it is likely that PHEX functions to either activate or degrade a peptide hormone.

Expression Pattern

Several investigators have examined PHEX/Phex tissue expression by a variety of techniques *(61,67–69)*. When relative abundance of PHEX/Phex mRNA was determined, the highest level of expression was apparent in bones and teeth *(67,69)*. This is consistent with the fact that XLH patients display abnormalities in bone and teeth and demonstration of an osteoblast defect in the Hyp mouse. However, expression has also been found in lung, brain, muscle, ovary, and testis. In light of these findings there are several tissues that could play a role in phosphate homeostasis and PHEX may have roles in processes unrelated to phosphate homeostasis. Of note, even in bone and tooth PHEX/Phex is a low abundance transcript and concentrations of this 6.6 kb mRNA *(61)* are two orders of magnitude less than that of B actin *(67)*. Surprisingly, preliminary studies using quantitative RT-PCR indicate that PHEX is not up-regulated by dietary phosphate depletion *(70)*.

PHEX Mutations

Although the PHEX deletions that we found in four patients were consistent with PHEX being the gene responsible for XLH, it was possible, although unlikely, that these deletions also involved another gene, which was the "real" gene. To establish with certainty that PHEX was the gene responsible for the disease we looked for point mutations in our XLH patients. In our initial efforts we detected a frameshift mutation caused by the loss of a TC dinucleotide in exon 6. We also found two point mutations in the splice acceptor site of exon 7. These two mutations led to exon skipping *(58)*. More recent efforts by several investigators *(60,71–74)* have allowed detection of over 100 different PHEX mutations. There are deletions, frame shifts, exon splice mutations, and nonsense mutations all of which are inactivating mutations. Additionally, multiple missense mutations have been identified and these mutations may provide information about important regions of the protein *(60,71–74)*. For example, changing the glycine at codon 579, which immediately precedes the zinc binding motif and which is conserved in NEP and ECE-1 and ECE-2, to either arginine *(60,72,73)* or valine *(71)* likely results in the loss of catalytic activity. The multiple reported proline to leucine, leucine to proline, and cysteine to serine missense mutations likely affect protein conformation *(60,71–74)*. Although a few mutations, such as glycine to arginine at codon 579, occur in several different series, no mutation occurs in more than 10% of XLH families. Thus, there are a wide variety of mutations that are scattered throughout the coding region and all the mutations are consistent with loss of function. Although the issue of genotype/phenotype correlations has not been entirely resolved, there does not appear to be strong correlation between type of mutation and severity of disease. When considering genotype/phenotype correlations one should remember that there is a great deal of variation in severity of disease between affected individuals from the same family who have the same mutation. Thus, great caution is necessary when correlating genotype to phenotpye when only a small number of affected individuals with each mutation is available for study.

Recent success in identification of the murine Phex gene and the Hyp and Gy mutations *(61,62,67)* provides an opportunity to interpret previous studies of Gy and Hyp mice in a new light. Since there are phenotypic differences and an alleged biochemical difference between Hyp and Gy mice, several investigators proposed that there were two separate genes that when mutated resulted in phosphate wasting *(41,44,75)*. The occurrence of a single recombinant event *(12)* between these two mutations further misled investigators into concluding that there were two closely linked genes that regulated phosphate transport on the X chromosome. Gy and Hyp mice have deletions in the 5' and 3' ends, respectively, of the murine Phex gene *(62,67)*. The Gy mouse has a contiguous gene syndrome since the deletion involves the first 3 Phex exons, the spermine synthase gene (which lies 35kb upstream from Phex) and all the DNA between these two genes *(76,77)*. Since the Hyp and Gy mutation occur at opposite ends of the gene and the human PHEX gene (and most likely the murine Phex gene) spans a distance of over 220kb of genomic DNA *(60)*, it is not surprising that a recombination event occurred between the two deletions. The fact that the Gy has a contiguous gene syndrome, as well as differences in background strain, probably account for the phenotypic differences between the two mouse models. In any event, identification of the Hyp and Gy mutations provides strong evidence that Phex is the only phosphate regulating gene on this portion of the X chromosome.

Why Is XLH a Dominant Disorder?

XLH is an X-linked dominant disorder with little, if any, gene dosage effect *(10)*. Although many dominant disorders, such as osteogenesis imperfecta (*see* Chapter 5), result from dominant negative effects, where the mutant protein interferes with the function of the normal protein, this does not appear to be the case in XLH for two reasons. First the Gy mutation results in loss of the first 3 Phex exons and all of the upstream DNA between Phex and spermine synthase, which likely includes the Phex promotor region. Thus, it is highly unlikely that any mutant Phex protein is made by the Gy mouse. Second, female XLH patients have a normal X chromosome inactivation pattern *(78)* and only one PHEX/Phex gene should be expressed per cell. Thus, even in cases where mutant protein is made it is unlikely that it could interfere with normal protein. In light of the fact that one of the PHEX gene copies is inactivated in each cell and X-chromosome inactivation is normal in female XLH patients, it is difficult to see why there is no significant gene dosage effect in this disorder since approximately half of the cells express the normal PHEX gene. XLH may be a haploinsufficiency disorder in which having half the normal amount of PHEX gene could result in the disease phenotype. Such a situation might exist if the PHEX enzyme is responsible for catalyzing the rate limiting step in a pathway. An alternative mechanism to either the classic dominant negative mechanism or haploinsufficiency is a "cellular dominant negative" mechanism. As noted previously, there is data that the Hyp osteoblast either secretes or modifies a humoral factor that causes phosphate wasting and, perhaps, impairs mineralization *(29)*. Thus, it is possible that XLH osteoblasts that have the normal PHEX gene turned off secrete or modify a humoral factor that affects osteoblasts that have the mutant PHEX gene turned off. Such a situation, if it exists, would be a new mechanism of how mutations lead to disease.

How Does Loss of Phex/Phex Function Lead to Disease and What Is Its Normal Role in Phosphate Homeostasis?

Although it is clear that PHEX mutations are responsible for XLH, the mechanism whereby loss of PHEX function leads to the disease is not immediately obvious. A few points are noteworthy. First, as noted previously, the Hyp and Gy mouse mutations result in decreased levels of Npt2 mRNA and protein *(20,21)*. Thus, PHEX/Phex may directly or indirectly regulate renal phosphate handling. Second, studies demonstrating PHEX expression in osteoblasts are consistent with the notion of a primary osteoblast defect which is responsible for at least part of the mineralization abnormalities. These studies also indicate that the osteoblast could play an important role in regulating phosphate homeostasis, although there is currently insufficient data to fully support this contention. Third, there is evidence for the secretion of a phosphaturic factor by tumors excised from patients with tumor induced osteomalacia *(32,34,79–81)*. This putative phosphaturic factor, which we termed "phosphatonin" *(31)*, may be related to the putative circulating factor which may be responsible for the renal Pi leak in Hyp mice *(23,25,29)*. Since PHEX mutations, which result in the disease phenotype, are loss of function mutations and not activating mutations, it is clear that PHEX is not "phosphatonin." However, the PHEX gene product may play a role in regulating the concentration of phosphatonin.

There are several possible roles for the normal PHEX protein in phosphate homeostasis. Since PHEX is a member of the neutral endopeptidase family, it is possible that it degrades/inactivates a phosphaturic hormone. Thus, mutations in PHEX would result in excessive concentrations of phosphatonin. However, if this is the case one might predict that parabiosis between a Hyp and normal mouse would rescue the Hyp phenotype (i.e., the normal Phex protein might be expected to degrade excessive phosphatonin originating from the mutant animal). However, parabiosis did not rescue the Hyp phenotype. Instead, normal mice, when parabiosed to Hyp mice, started to waste phosphate *(23)*. Although resolution of this apparent discrepancy awaits additional data, it is possible that the kidney is exposed to high concentrations of phosphatonin before the Phex protein has a chance to degrade it. Alternatively the normal animal may not adequately up-regulate Phex to degrade the excessive amounts of phosphatonin that accumulated in the mutant animal. Another potential mechanism of action that is keeping with an enzymatic role for PHEX is that, under normal circumstances, PHEX could function to activate a phosphate conserving hormone. However, this model would also predict that parabiosis of normal mouse to Hyp mouse would rescue the Hyp phenotype. An alternative possibility is that PHEX protein indirectly functions to influence concentrations of phosphatonin or a phosphate conserving hormone. Finally, it is possible that PHEX mutations result in a compensatory up-regulation of another enzyme and over expression of this enzyme results in the phenotypic manifestations of XLH.

Therapeutic Implications

The pathophysiology of XLH has important implications for treatment of the disease. Current therapy involves the use of high dose calcitriol and phosphate. (For information on the proper use of this therapy, *see* ref. *3*). If the normal function of PHEX protein is to degrade/inactivate "phosphatonin," therapeutic efforts could be directed toward inhibiting phosphatonin action (receptor blockade, etc). If PHEX activates a phosphate conserving hormone, treatment could be initiated with the active hormone. If the disease results from compensatory up-regulation of another endopeptidase, consideration should be given to treatment with an endopeptidase inhibitor. Indeed, if up-regulation of another enzyme resulted in phosphate wasting we would expect that activating mutations in the gene that codes for this enzyme would lead to phosphate wasting.

Adult-Onset Vitamin D-Resistant Hypophosphatemic Osteomalacia

Despite recognition that there is variability in the clinical spectrum of XLH, one group of investigators proposed that there are two forms of X-linked hypophosphatemic rickets. Frymoyer and Hodgkin *(82)* described a 133-person kindred with what they referred to as "adult onset vitamin D resistant hypophosphatemic osteomalacia." The inheritance pattern was consistent with X-linked dominant transmission. Hypophosphatemic young adults had minimal femoral bowing and older adults (defined as over age 40) were "progressively disabled by severe bowing" *(82)*. There were 14 hypophosphatemic children in the kindred. Moderate bowing was observed in one 17-yr-old who had closed epiphyses. Although "mild femoral bowing" was observed in some of the other 13 children, these investigators reported that none of the affected children had radiographic evidence of rickets. Based largely on this lack of radiographically evident rickets, these authors concluded that there are two forms of X-linked hypophosphatemic rickets.

Since the absence of radiographic evidence of rickets was used to define this new disease, we tested the hypothesis that radiographic evidence of rickets is an invariant feature of XLH. To perform these studies we obtained radiographs from affected children who were from several well established XLH families. We found rachitic abnormalities in 5 of 11 wrist radiographs and 13 of 15 knee radiographs. Indeed, two children aged 3.8 and 5.2 yr displayed no radiographic evidence of rickets at either the wrist or knee, although their relatives exhibited rickets *(83)*.

In light of our findings that radiographic evidence of rickets is not an invariant feature of XLH, we felt that it was premature to define new disease entities based largely on the lack of rickets in affected children. However, since Frymoyer and Hodgkin reported that none of the affected children had radiographic evidence of rickets, the possibility still existed that their kindred did have a distinct disorder. The identification of the PHEX gene provided us with an opportunity to examine this question further. In this regard, we obtained DNA samples from many members of this kindred and searched for PHEX mutations in affected members. We found that affected individuals have a missence mutation in PHEX exon 16 that results in an amino acid change from leucine to proline in residue 555 *(74)*. Furthermore, clinical evaluation of individuals from this family indicated that some of these individuals display classic features of XLH, including radiographic evidence of rickets, and we were unable to verify progressive bowing in adults. In light of the variability in the clinical spectrum of XLH and the presence of a PHEX mutation in affected kindred members, we conclude that there is only one form of X-linked dominant phosphate wasting. Thus, identification of the PHEX gene has not only shed light into the pathophysiology of XLH, but has allowed us to demonstrate that two disorders, which were thought to be distinct, are, in fact, the same disorder.

Autosomal Dominant Forms of Renal Phosphate Wasting

In addition to XLH, there are two proposed autosomal dominant forms of isolated renal phosphate wasting: autosomal dominant hypophosphatemic rickets (ADHR) and hypophosphatemic bone disease (HBD). Both of these disorders are less common than XLH and have been less well-studied, although ongoing studies may provide an opportunity to understand the pathogenesis of these disorders.

Autosomal Dominant Hypophosphatemic Rickets (ADHR)

Bianchine et al. described a small family with an autosomal dominant form of renal phosphate wasting *(84,85)*. The father was a markedly affected man who had isolated renal phosphate wasting, short stature, and an impressive windswept deformity (valgus on one side and varus on the other). He had two affected daughters and one affected son. These investigators reported that the father had a marked tendency toward fracture with or without trauma. Otherwise the clinical course in these individuals appeared to be similar to that of XLH patients.

We have recently had the opportunity to evaluate a large ADHR kindred with over 20 affected individuals *(86)*. This kindred provided us with an opportunity to explore the phenotypic variability of this disease in a large number of individuals who all have the same mutation. Affected kindred members have isolated renal phosphate wasting with inappropriately normal serum calcitriol concentrations. In contrast to XLH, ADHR displays variable penetrance. The family contains two subgroups of affected individuals. One subgroup consists of patients who presented with phosphate wasting as adults or adolescents. These individuals complained of bone pain, weakness, and insufficiency fractures, but did not have lower extremity deformities. The second group consists of individuals who presented during childhood with phosphate wasting, rickets, and lower extremity deformity in a pattern similar to the classic presentation of XLH. Surprisingly, some of the children in this group presented with phosphate wasting and rickets, but later lost the phosphate wasting defect after puberty *(86)*. In addition to these two groups there appear to be at least two unaffected individuals who are carriers for the ADHR mutation *(86)*. Thus, the clinical manifestations of ADHR are even more variable than those observed in XLH.

Hypophosphatemic Bone Disease (HBD)

Hypophosphatemic bone disease (HBD) was originally described by Scriver et al. *(87)* who studied five small families in which affected members had isolated renal phosphate wasting, short stature, and lower extremity deformity. In one family (family 4) there was a male to male transmission, indicating an autosomal dominant pattern of inheritance in this family. These investigators stated that HBD differed from ADHR since affected children in their kindreds did not display radiographic evidence of rickets. In other respects the patients appeared to be similar to other patients with phosphate wasting. As noted previously, radiographic evidence of rickets is not always present in XLH *(83)*. By analogy, it is possible that radiographic evidence of rickets may not be universal in children with ADHR. Of note, in the original description of HBD family 4, which was the only family that demonstrated a father to son transmission, contained two members who were said to have a clinical picture consistent with XLH (including rickets in at least one of these individuals) in addition to the two individuals who had HBD *(87)*. The paternal grandmother of the propositus, who was also the aunt of the two individuals who reportedly had XLH, had a serum phosphorus of 3.1mg/dL. In light of the incomplete penetrance that is observed in ADHR and the fact that the occurrence of two different uncommon renal phosphate wasting disorders in the same family is unlikely, this family may have had ADHR. Thus, HBD may not be a distinct clinical entity. However, definitive evidence as to whether ADHR and HBD are distinct entities or forme fruste of one another awaits identification of the gene(s) that cause these disorders. Indeed, even if these diseases result from mutations in the same gene, it will be important to characterize the mutations that cause ADHR and HBD since different mutations in the same gene can give rise to different phenotypes. One example of this phenomenon is the dsytrophin gene in which missense mutations give rise to Beckers muscular dystrophy and nonsense mutations result in Duchenne muscular dystrophy *(88)*. In any case, the weight of the evidence currently favors the hypothesis that ADHR and HBD are the same disorders.

Positional Cloning Efforts in Autosomal Dominant Phosphate Wasting Disorders

We have recently initiated studies aimed at identifying the gene(s) responsible for ADHR. In this regard we are performing linkage studies in the large ADHR kindred described previously. Since the high affinity/low capacity sodium dependent phosphate cotransporter plays an important role in the maintenance of phosphate homeostasis we considered it a strong candidate gene. Kos et al. *(22)* located this transporter to the long arm of chromosome 5 (5q35) so in our initial studies we used markers from this region to look for linkage with ADHR. Our results excluded linkage of the ADHR gene to markers on 5q35 ruling out mutations in NPT-2 as a cause of ADHR in this family *(89)*. Since another phosphate cotransporter has been identified on the short arm of chromosome 6 *(90)*, we extended our study to include markers from this region in the linkage analysis. Our results similarly excluded linkage to this region *(89)*. In absence of further candidate genes, we undertook a genome wide linkage search with markers spaced every 20 centiMorgans across the genome and found linkage to chromosome 12p13 *(89)*. More recent studies place the ADHR gene locus in the approx 6.5MB interval between the markers D12S1685 and D12S397 *(91)*. Studies in additional ADHR kindreds and in kindreds with hypophosphatemic bone disease (HBD, *[87]*), are in progress to determine if there is genetic heterogeneity for the ADHR phenotype and if ADHR and HBD result from mutations in the same gene. More importantly, these studies will further localize the gene(s) that are responsible for ADHR and HBD and eventually lead to their identification.

Since the primary defect in ADHR results in isolated phosphate wasting it is likely that the ADHR gene plays a role in phosphate homeostasis. Current models of phosphate homeostasis indicate that renal phosphate wasting could result from:

1. Mutations in a gene that enables the organism to assess extracellular phosphate concentrations (a phosphate sensor or a phosphate sensing system);
2. Activating mutations in a gene(s) that codes for a renal phosphate wasting hormone ("phosphatonin") or its receptor (including associated G proteins or other effector molecules);

3. Mutations in a gene(s) that codes for a phosphate conserving hormone or its receptor;
4. Mutations in genes that code for repressors or inducers for the above hormones;
5. Mutations in genes that code for enzymes that activate or degrade these hormones (as is likely to be the case with the PHEX gene); and
6. Mutations in genes that code for the phosphate cotransporters.

Isolation of the ADHR gene may result in identifying one of the genes in the above model or, if the ADHR gene codes for a protein that has none of the above functions, isolation of the ADHR gene may result in changes to the current model as well as a better understanding of the pathogenesis of the disorder.

Hereditary Hypophosphatemic Rickets with Hypercalciuria

Hereditary hypophosphatemic rickets with hypercalciuria (HHRH) was first described in a Bedouin tribe *(92)*. In concert with other disorders of phosphate wasting, HHRH results in decreased serum phosphate levels and reduced tubular phosphate reabsorption, with normal serum calcium concentrations. However, in contrast to other phosphate wasting disorders, serum concentrations of 1,25-dihydroxyvitamin D are elevated despite suppressed parathyroid function, and HHRH patients display a marked increase in urinary calcium excretion. Oral calcium and phosphate loading tests show that there is intestinal hyperabsorption of calcium and phosphate. It was suggested that the pivotal HHRH defect consists of renal phosphate depletion which stimulates renal 25-hydroxyvitamin D 1-α hydroxylase followed by an increase of 1,25-dihydroxyvitamin D. This in turn enhances intestinal calcium and phosphate absorption, increases the renal calcium filtered load and suppresses parathyroid gland function, with both events contributing to the hypercalciuria *(92)*.

The accurate diagnosis of HHRH has important therapeutic implications. In contrast to XLH, phosphate supplementation alone can cause a complete remission of the disease whereas the addition of active vitamin D can be harmful and create complications, such as hypercalcemia, kidney stones, and renal damage *(93)*.

Since the original report of HHRH *(92)*, Tieder et al. *(94)* have further characterized this family. Of the 59 family members that they studied there were nine individuals with HHRH and an additional 21 members who had idiopathic hypercalciuria (IH), slightly reduced serum phosphate levels and elevated serum 1,25-dihydroxyvitamin D concentrations *(94)*. The mode of inheritance has not been unequivocally established. It has been suggested that HHRH is inherited in an autosomal recessive mode. The biochemical data from the Bedouin tribe, however, may indicate an autosomal codominant pattern with high, but incomplete penetrance. All of the individuals that had severe hypophosphatemia also had IH, and none of the family members showed signs of hypophosphatemia alone. This finding makes the probability of two defective genes as the cause of HHRH highly unlikely. Of note, an autosomal dominant form of HHRH has been described, where the clinical and biochemical abnormalities are less pronounced *(95)*. Linkage analysis has not been reported for HHRH, however candidate genes, such as NPT1, NPT2, and stanniocalcin, have been mapped by FISH analysis and somatic cell hybrid panels to human chromosomes 6p21.3-p23 *(90)*, 5q35 *(22)*, and 8p21 *(96)*, respectively.

An NPT2 knockout mouse was recently developed by Beck and colleagues *(97)* that resembled the HHRH phenotype in many aspects. The null (NPT2$^{-/-}$) mouse possessed a biochemical profile similar to HHRH individuals and displayed marked skeletal deformities. NPT2$^{-/-}$ mice had significant decreases in serum phosphorus, an increased fractional excretion index for phosphate, as well as hypercalcemia and hypercalciuria when compared to wild-type mice *(97)*. Serum alkaline phosphatase activity was also elevated in NPT2$^{-/-}$ mice, but declined with age. Interestingly, the heterozygous NPT2$^{+/-}$ animal had elevated serum 1,25$(OH)_2$ vitamin D concentrations and an increased fractional excretion index for phosphate when compared to wild-type animals, however showed a normal serum phosphate level. This may indicate that both copies of NPT2 must be deleted to observe the HHRH phenotype and, with heterozygous knockout of transporter function, that an intermediate phenotype is seen, supporting the idea that HHRH may be an autosomal codominant disorder.

Histological analysis of NPT2$^{-/-}$ mice tibiae revealed perturbations in bone remodeling, such as poorly developed metaphyseal trabeculae and slowed secondary ossification in the epiphysis when compared to wild-type mice *(97)*. In contrast to HHRH patients, however, the NPT2$^{-/-}$ animals do not show indications of rickets or osteomalacia. Possible species variations in phosphate handling and vitamin D adaptation were proposed for the differences in bone structure between HHRH patients and NPT2$^{-/-}$ mice *(97)*.

When comparing the phenotype of a knockout mouse to a disorder of unknown origin, the results should be interpreted carefully. Genetic heterogeneity exists in many disorders, therefore inactivating mutations in critical accessory proteins that regulate renal NPT2 expression or function could potentially lead to HHRH. For example, the intracellular proteins Diphor-1 *(98)* and PiUS *(99)*, recently mapped to human chromosomes 1q *(100)* and 3p *(101)*, respectively, were shown to increase phosphate uptake in vitro when co-expressed with NPT2, and therefore could also be considered candidate HHRH genes.

In summary, HHRH is a phosphate wasting disorder in which the etiology is unknown. Current investigation is underway to determine the inheritance pattern and molecular defect causing the disease. The NPT2 knockout mouse shares a similar phenotype with HHRH individuals and this animal model will help to provide insight into the regulation of mineral balance. Finding the gene for HHRH will not only help to determine the pathogenesis of the disorder, but will also provide important answers to questions involving the PTH-vitamin D-phosphate feedback loop.

Conclusion

Phosphate homeostasis is a complex process, but new methods of analysis are shedding light on phosphate homeostasis and the hereditary disorders of phosphate wasting. In several instances, advances in molecular genetics not only help investigators gain a better understanding of the pathogenesis of these diseases, but allow clinicians to understand the variability in the clinical presentation of these disorders.

Acknowledgments

Work in the authors' laboratory was supported by NIH grants #AR42228, AR02095, and AG05793.

References

1. Davies, M. and Stanbury, S. W. (1981) The rheumatic manifestations of metabolic bone disease. *Clin. Rheum. Dis.* **7,** 595–646.
2. Econs, M. J. and Drezner, M. K. (1992) Bone disease resulting from inherited disorders of renal tubule transport and vitamin D metabolism, in *Disorders of Bone and Mineral Metabolism* (Favus, M. J. and Coe, F. L., eds.), Raven Press, New York, pp. 935–950.
3. Tenenhouse, H. S. and Econs, M. J. (2000) Mendelian hypophosphatemias, in *The Metabolic and Molecular Basis of Inherited Disease* (Scriver, C. R., ed) McGraw-Hill, New York, in press.
4. Coleman, E. N. and Foote, J. B. (1954) Craniostenosis with familial vitamin-D-resistant rickets. *Br. Med. J.* 561–562.
5. Bradbury, P. G., Brenton, D. P., and Stern, G. M. (1987) Neurological involvement in X-linked hypophosphatemic rickets. *J. Neurol. Neurosurg. Psychiatr.* **50,** 810–812.
6. Vera, C., Cure, J. K., Naso, W. B., Gelven, P. L., Worsham, F., Roof, B. F., Resnick, D., Salinas, C. F., Gross, J. A., and Pacult, A. (1997) Paraplegia due to ossification of ligamenta flava in X-linked hypophosphatemia. *Spine* **22,** 710–715.
7. Cartwright, D. W., Masel, J. P., and Latham, S. C. (1981) The lumbar spinal canal in hypophosphatemic vitamin D-resistant rickets. *Aust. N. Z. J. Med.* **11,** 154–157.
8. Econs, M. J., Samsa, G. P., Monger, M., Drezner, M. K., and Feussner, J. R. (1994) X–linked hypophosphatemic rickets: a disease often unknown to affected patients. *J. Bone Miner. Res.* **24,** 17–24.
9. Winters, R. W., Graham, J. B., Williams, T. F., McFalls, V. W., and Burnett, C. H. (1958) A genetic study of familial hypophosphatemia and vitamin D resistant rickets with a review of the literature. *Medicine* **37,** 97–142.
10. Whyte, M. P., Schrank, F. W., and Armamento, V. R. (1996) X-linked hypophosphatemia: a search for gender, race, anticipation, or parent of origin effects on disease expression in children. *J. Clin. Endocrinol. Metab.* **81,** 4075.
11. Eicher, E. M., Southard, J. L., Scriver, C. R., and Glorieux, F. H. (1976) Hypophosphatemia: mouse model for human familial hypophosphatemic (vitamin D-resistant) rickets. *Proc. Natl. Acad. Sci. USA* **73,** 4667–4671.
12. Lyon, M. F., Scriver, C. R., Baker, L. R., Tenenhouse, H. S., Kronick, J., and Mandla, S. (1986) The Gy mutation: another cause of X-linked hypophosphatemia in mouse. *Proc. Natl. Acad. Sci. USA* **83,** 4899–4903.

13. Kay, G., Thakker, R. V., and Rastan, S. (1991) Determination of a molecular map position for Hyp using a new interspecific backcross produced by in vitro fertilization. *Genomics* **11,** 651–657.
14. Sonin, N. V., Taggart, R. T., Meyer, M. H., Meyer, R. A., and Meyer, Jr. (1996) Molecular mapping of the mouse Gy mutation on chromosome X. *Mouse Genome* **94,** 491–493.
15. Qiu, Z. Q., Tenenhouse, H. S., and Scriver, C. R. (1993) Parental origin of mutant allele does not explain absence of gene dose in X-linked Hyp mice. *Genet. Res.* **62,** 39–43.
16. Tenenhouse, H. S., Scriver, C. R., McInnes, R. R., and Glorieux, F. H. (1978) Renal handling of phosphate in vivo and in vitro by the X-linked hypophosphatemic male mouse: evidence for a defect in the brush border membrane. *Kidney Int.* **14,** 236–244.
17. Tenenhouse, H. S., Klugerman, A. H., and Neal, J. L. (1989) Effect of phosphonoformic acid, dietary phosphate and the HYP mutation on kinetically distinct phosphate transport processes in mouse kidney. *Biochim. Biophys. Acta* **984,** 207–213.
18. Magagnin, S., Werner, A., Markovich, D., Sorribas, V., Stange, G., Biber, J., and Murer, H. (1993) Expression cloning of human and rat renal cortex Na/Pi cotransport. *Proc. Natl. Acad. Sci. USA* **90,** 5979–5983.
19. Ryan, E. A. and Reiss, E. (1984) Oncogenous osteomalacia: review of the world literature of 42 cases and report of two new cases. *Am. J. Med.* **77,** 501–512.
20. Tenenhouse, H. S., Werner, A., Biber, J., Ma, S., Martel, J., Roy, S., and Murer, H. (1994) Renal Na(+)-phosphate cotransport in murine X-linked hypophosphatemic rickets. Molecular characterization. *J. Clin. Invest.* **93,** 671–676.
21. Tenenhouse, H. S. and Beck, L. (1996) Renal Na(+)-phosphate cotransporter gene expression in X-linked Hyp and Gy mice. *Kidney Int.* **49,** 1027–1032.
22. Kos, C. H., Tihy, F., Econs, M. J., Murer, H., Lemieux, N., and Tenenhouse, H. S. (1994) Localization of a renal sodium-phosphate cotransporter gene to human chromosome 5q35. *Genomics* **19,** 176–177.
23. Meyer, R. A., Jr., Meyer, M. H., and Gray, R. W. (1989) Parabiosis suggests a humoral factor is involved in X-linked hypophosphatemia in mice. *J. Bone Miner. Res.* **4,** 493–500.
24. Meyer, R. A., Jr., Tenenhouse, H. S., Meyer, M. H., and Klugerman, A. H. (1989) The renal phosphate transport defect in normal mice parabiosed to X-linked hypophosphatemic mice persists after parathyroidectomy. *J. Bone Miner. Res.* **4,** 523–532.
25. Nesbitt, T., Coffman, T. M., Griffiths, R., and Drezner, M. K. (1992) Crosstransplantation of kidneys in normal and Hyp mice. Evidence that the Hyp mouse phenotype is unrelated to an intrinsic renal defect. *J. Clin. Invest.* **89,** 1453–1459.
26. Ecarot-Charrier, B., Glorieux, F. H., Travers, R., Desbarats, M., Bouchard, F., and Hinek, A. (1988) Defective bone formation by transplanted Hyp mouse bone cells into normal mice. *Endocrinology* **123,** 768–773.
27. Ecarot, B., Glorieux, F. H., Desbarats, M., Travers, R., and Labelle, L. (1995) Effect of 1,25-dihydroxyvitamin D3 treatment on bone formation by transplanted cells from normal and X-linked hypophosphatemic mice. *J. Bone Miner. Res.* **10,** 424–431.
28. Cao, X. Y., Jiang, X. M., Dou, Z. H., Rakeman, M. A., Zhang, M. L., O'Donnell, K., Ma, T., Amette, K., DeLong, N., and DeLong, G. R. (1994) Timing of vulnerability of the brain to iodine deficiency in endemic cretinism. *N. Engl. J. Med.* **331,** 1739–1744.
29. Lajeunesse, D., Meyer, JR. R. A., and Hamel, L. (1996) Direct demonstration of a humorally mediated inhibition of renal phosphate transport in the Hyp mouse. *Kidney Int.* **50,** 1531–1538.

30. Lajeunesse, D. and Delalandre, A. (1998) Evidence that the putative phophaturic product present in Hyp mouse may be modified, not produced, by osteoblasts and bone marrow stromal cells. *Bone* **23(5),** S546(Abstract).
31. Econs, M. J. and Drezner, M. K. (1994) Tumor-induced osteomalacia-unveiling a new hormone. *N. Engl. J. Med.* **330,** 1679–1681.
32. Cai, Q., Hodgson, S. F., Kao, P. C., Lennon, V. A., Klee, G. G., Zinsmiester, A. R., and Kumar, R. (1994) Brief report: inhibition of renal phosphate transport by a tumor product in a patient with oncogenic osteomalacia. *N. Engl. J. Med.* **330,** 1645–1649.
33. Drezner, M. K. (1996) Tumor-induced rickets and osteomalacia, in *Primer on the Metabolic Bone Diseases and Disorders of Mineral Metabolism* (Favus, M. J., ed), Lippincott–Raven, Philadelphia, pp. 319–325.
34. Rowe, P. S., Ong, A. C., Cockerill, F. J., Goulding, J. N., and Hewison, M. (1996) Candidate 56 and 58 kda protein(s) responsible for mediating the renal defects in oncogenic hypophosphatemic osteomalacia. *Bone* **18,** 159–169.
35. Scriver, C. R., Reade, T. M., DeLuca, H. F., and Hamstra, A. J. (1978) Serum 1,25-dihydroxyvitamin D levels in normal subjects and in patients with hereditary rickets or bone disease. *N. Engl. J. Med.* **299,** 976–979.
36. Drezner, M. K. and Haussler, M. R. (1979) Correspondence. *N. Engl. J. Med.* **300,** 435.
37. Lyles, K. W., Clark, A. G., and Drezner, M. K. (1982) Serum 1,25-dihydroxyvitamin D levels in subjects with X-linked hypophosphatemic rickets and osteomalacia. *Calcif. Tissue Int.* **34,** 125–130.
38. Lobaugh, B. and Drezner, M. K. (1983) Abnormal regulation of renal 25-hydroxyvitamin D-1 alpha-hydroxylase activity in the X–linked hypophosphatemic mouse. *J. Clin. Invest.* **71,** 400–403.
39. Cunningham, J., Gomes, H., Seino, Y., and Chase, L. R. (1983) Abnormal 24-hydroxylation of 25-hydroxyvitamin d in the X-linked hypophosphatemic mouse. *Endocrinology* **112,** 633–638.
40. Tenenhouse, H. S., Yip, A., and Jones, G. (1988) Increased renal catabolism of 1,25-dihydroxyvitamin D3 in murine X–linked hypophosphatemic rickets. *J. Clin. Invest.* **81,** 461–465.
41. Davidai, G. A., Nesbitt, T., and Drezner, M. K. (1990) Normal regulation of calcitriol production in Gy mice. Evidence for biochemical heterogeneity in the X-linked hypophosphatemic diseases. *J. Clin. Invest.* **85,** 334–339.
42. Tenenhouse, H. S., Meyer, R. A., Jr., Mandla, S., Meyer, M. H., and Gray, R. W. (1992) Renal phosphate transport and vitamin D metabolism in X-linked hypophosphatemic Gy mice: Responses to phosphate deprivation. *Endocrinology* **131,** 51–56.
43. Meyer, R. A., Jr., Meyer, M. H., and Morgan, P. L. (1996) Effects of altered diet on serum levels of 1,25-dihydroxyvitamin D and parathyroid hormone in X-linked hypophosphatemic (Hyp and Gy) mice. *Bone* **18,** 23–28.
44. Meyer, R. A., Jr., Meyer, M. H., Gray, R. W., and Bruns, M. E. (1995) Femoral abnormalities and vitamin D metabolism in X-linked hypophosphatemic (Hyp and Gy) mice. *J. Orthop. Res.* **13,** 30–40.
45. Econs, M. J. (1996) Positional cloning of the HYP gene: a review. *Kidney Int.* **49,** 1033–1037.
46. Econs, M. J. and Francis, F. (1997) Positional cloning of the PEX gene: new insights into the pathophysiology of X-linked hypophosphatemic rickets. *Am. J. Physiol.* **273,** F489–F498.

47. Collins, F. S. (1995) Positional cloning moves from perditional to traditional. *Nat. Genet.* **9,** 347–350.
48. Machler, M., Frey, D., Gal, A., Orth, U., Wienker, T. F., Fanconi, A., and Schmid, W. (1986) X-linked dominant hypophosphatemia is closely linked to DNA markers DXS41 and DXS43 at Xp22. *Hum. Genet.* **73,** 271–275.
49. Read, A. P., Thakker, R. V., Davies, K. E., Mountford, R. C., Brenton, D. P., Davies, M., et al. (1986) Mapping of human X-linked hypophosphataemic rickets by multilocus linkage analysis. *Hum. Genet.* **73,** 267–270.
50. Econs, M. J., Rowe, P. S., Francis, F., Barker, D. F., Speer, M. C., Norman, M., et al. (1994) Fine structure mapping of the human X-linked hypophosphatemic rickets gene locus. *J. Clin. Endocrinol. Metab.* **79,** 1351–1354.
51. Rowe, P. S., Goulding, J. N., Francis, F., Oudet, C., Econs, M. J., Hanauer, A., et al. (1996) The gene for X-linked hypophosphataemic rickets maps to a 200–300kb region in Xp22.1–Xp22.2 and is located on a single YAC containing a putative vitamin D response element (VDRE). *Hum. Genet.* **97,** 345–352.
52. Econs, M. J., Barker, D. F., Speer, M. C., Pericak-Vance, M. A., Fain, P. R., and Drezner, M. K. (1992) Multilocus mapping of the X-linked hypophosphatemic rickets gene. *J. Clin. Endocrinol. Metab.* **75,** 201–206.
53. Econs, M. J., Fain, P. R., Norman, M., Speer, M. C., Pericak-Vance, M. A., Becker, P. A., et al. (1993) Flanking markers define the X-linked hypophosphatemic rickets gene locus. *J. Bone Miner. Res.* **8,** 1149–1152.
54. Massry, S. G. (1995) Hypophosphatemia and Hyperphosphatemia, in *Textbook of Nephrology* (Massry, S. G. and Glassock, R. J., eds) William and Wilkins, Baltimore, pp. 398–412.
55. Francis, F., Rowe, P. S. N., Econs, M. J., See, C. G., Benham, F., O'Riordan, J. L. H., Drezner, M. K., Hamvas, R. M. J., and Leharach, H. (1994) A YAC contig spanning the hypophosphatemic rickets gene candidate region. *Genomics* **21,** 229–237.
56. Econs, M. J., Francis, F., Rowe, P. S., Speer, M. C., O'Riordan, J. L., Lehrach, H., and Becker, P. A. (1994) Dinucleotide repeat polymorphism at the DXS1683 locus. *Hum. Mol. Genet.* **3,** 680.
57. Rowe, P. S., Francis, F., and Goulding, J. (1994) Rapid isolation of DNA sequences flanking microsatellite repeats. *Nucleic Acids Res.* **22,** 5135–5136.
58. HYP Consortium (1995) A gene (PEX) with homologies to endopeptidases is mutated in patients with X-linked hypophosphatemic rickets. *Nat. Genet.* **11,** 130–136.
59. Buckler, A. J., Chang, D. D., Graw, S. L., Brook, J. D., Haber, D. A., Sharp, P. A., and Housman, D. E. (1991) Exon amplification: a strategy to isolate mammalian genes based on RNA splicing. *Proc. Natl. Acad. Sci. USA* **88,** 4005–4009.
60. Francis, F., Strom, T. M., Hennig, S., Boddrich, A., Lorenz, B., Brandau, O., et al. (1997) Genomic organization of the human PEX gene mutated in X-linked dominant hypophosphatemic rickets. *Genome Res.* **7,** 573–585.
61. Du, L., Desbarats, M., Viel, J., Glorieux, F. H., Cawthorn, C., and Ecarot, B. (1996) cDNA cloning of the murine Pex gene implicated in X-linked hypophosphatemia and evidence for expression in bone. *Genomics* **36,** 22–28.
62. Strom, T. M., Francis, F., Lorenz, B., Boddrich, A., Econs, M. J., Lehrach, H., and Meitinger, T. (1997) Pex gene deletions in Gy and Hyp mice provide mouse models for X-linked hypophosphatemia. *Hum. Mol. Genet.* **6,** 165–171.
63. Kozak, M. (1987) An analysis of 5'-noncoding sequences from 699 vertebrate messenger RNAs. *Nucleic Acids Res.* **15,** 8125–8148.

64. Kozak, M. (1991) An analysis of vertebrate mRNA sequences: intimations of translational control. *J. Cell Biol.* **115,** 887–903.
65. Welches, W. R., Brosnihan, K. B., and Ferrario, C. M. (1993) A comparison of the properties and enzymatic activities of three angiotensin processing enzymes: angiotensin converting enzyme, prolyl endopeptidase and neutral endopeptidase 24.11. *Life Sci.* **52,** 1461–1480.
66. Xu, D., Emoto, N., Giaid, A., Slaughter, C., Kaw, S., deWit, D., and Yanagisawa, M. (1987) ECE-1: a membrane-bound metalloprotease that catalyzes the proteolytic activation of big endothelin-1. *Cell Nucleic Acids Res.* **15,** 8125–8148.
67. Beck, L., Soumounou, Y., Martel, J., Krishnamurthy, G., Gauthier, C., Goodyer, C. G., and Tenenhouse, H. S. (1997) Pex/PEX tissue distribution and evidence for a deletion in the 3' region of the Pex gene in X–linked hypophosphatemic mice. *J. Clin. Invest.* **99,** 1200–1209.
68. Lipman, M. L., Panda, D., Bennett, H. P., Henderson, J. E., Shane, E., Shen, Y., et al. (1998) Cloning of human PEX cDNA. Expression, subcellular localization, and endopeptidase activity. *J. Biol. Chem.* **273,** 13,729–13,737.
69. Ruchon, A. F., Marcinkiewicz, M., Siegfried, G., Tenenhouse, H. S., DesGroseillers, L., Crine, P., and Boileau, G. (1998) Pex mRNA is localized in developing mouse osteoblasts and odontoblasts. *J. Histochem. Cytochem.* **46,** 459–468.
70. Meyer, M. H. and Meyer, R. A. Jr. (1998) The effect of low phosphate diet on Pex mRNA expression in the normal mouse. *Bone* **23(5),** S545(Abstract).
71. Holm, I. A., Huang, X., and Kunkel, L. M. (1997) Mutational analysis of the PEX gene in patients with X-linked hypophosphatemic rickets. *Am. J. Hum. Genet.* **60,** 790–797.
72. Rowe, P. S., Oudet, C. L., Francis, F., Sinding, C., Pannetier, S., Econs, M. J., et al. (1997) Distribution of mutations in the PEX gene in families with X-linked hypophosphataemic rickets (HYP). *Hum. Mol. Genet.* **6,** 539–549.
73. Dixon, P. H., Christie, P. T., Wooding, C., Trump, D., Grieff, M., Holm, I., et al. (1998) Mutational analysis of PHEX gene in X-linked hypophosphatemia. *J. Clin. Endocrinol. Metab.* **83,** 3615–3623.
74. Econs, M. J., Friedman, N. E., Rowe, P. S. N., Speer, M. C., Francis, F., Strom, T. M., et al. (1998) A PHEX gene mutation is responsible for adult onset vitamin-D-resistant hypophosphatemic osteomalacia: evidence that the disorder is not a distinct entity from X-linked hypophosphatemic rickets (HYP). *J. Clin. Endocrinol. Metab.* **83,** 3459–3462.
75. Scriver, C. R., Tenenhouse, H. S., and Glorieux, F. H. (1991) X-linked hypophosphatemia: an appreciation of a classic paper and a survey of progress since 1958. *Medicine* **70,** 218–228.
76. Lorenz, B., Francis, F., Gempel, K., Boddrich, A., Josten, M., Schmahl, W., et al. (1998) Spermine deficiency in Gy mice caused by deletion of the spermine synthase gene. *Hum. Mol. Genet.* **7,** 541–547.
77. Meyer, R. A.,Jr., Henley, C. M., Meyer, M. H., Morgan, P. L., McDonald, A. G., Mills, C., and Price, D. K. (1998) Partial deletion of both the spermine synthase gene and the PEX gene in the X-linked hypophosphatemic, gyro (Gy) mouse. *Genomics* **48,** 289–295.
78. Orstavik, K. H., Orstavik, R. E., Halse, J., and Knudtzon, J. (1996) X chromosome inactivation pattern in female carriers of X linked hypophosphataemic rickets. *J. Med. Genet.* **33,** 700–703.

79. Nelson, A. E., Namkung, H. J., Patava, J., Wilkinson, M. R., Chang, A. C.-M., Reddel, R. R., Robinson, B. G., and Mason, R. S. (1996) Characteristics of tumor cell bioactivity in oncogenic osteomalacia. *Mol. Cell. Endocrinol.* **124,** 17–23.
80. Miyauchi, A., Fukase, M., Tsutsumi, M., and Fujita, T. (1988) Hemangiopericytoma-induced osteomalacia: tumor transplantation in nude mice causes hypophosphatemia and tumor extracts inhibit renal 25-hydroxyvitamin D 1-hydroxylase activity. *J. Clin. Endocrinol. Metab.* **67,** 46–53.
81. Chalew, S. A., Lovechild, J. C., Brown, C. M., and Sun, C.-C. J. (1996) Hypophosphatemia induced in mice by transplantation of a tumor-derived cell line from a patient with oncogenic rickets. *J. Pediatr. Endocrinol. Metab.* **9,** 593–597.
82. Frymoyer, J. W. and Hodgkin, W. (1977) Adult-onset vitamin D-resistant hypophosphatemic osteomalacia. A possible variant of vitamin D-resistant rickets. *J. Bone Joint Surg. (Am. Vol.)* **59,** 101–106.
83. Econs, M. J., Feussner, J. R., Samsa, G. P., Effman, E. L., Vogler, J. B., Martinez, S., et al. (1991) X-linked hypophosphatemic rickets without "rickets." *Skeletal Radiol.* **20,** 109–114.
84. Bianchine, J. W., Stambler, A. A., and Harrison, H. E. (1971) Familial hypophosphatemic rickets showing autosomal dominant inheritance. *Birth Defects: Original Article Series* **7,** 287–295.
85. Harrison, H. E. and Harrison, H. C. (1979) Rickets and osteomalacia, in: *Disorders of Calcium and Phosphate Metabolism in Childhood and Adolescence* W.B. Saunders Company, Philadelphia, pp. 230–249,
86. Econs, M. J. and McEnery, P. T. (1997) Autosomal dominant hypophosphatemic rickets/osteomalacia: clinical characterization of a novel renal phosphate wasting disorder. *J. Clin. Endocrinol. Metab.* **82,** 674–681.
87. Scriver, C. R., MacDonald, W., Reade, T., Glorieux, R. H., and Nogrady, B. (1977) Hypophosphatemic nonrachitic bone disease: an entity distinct from X-linked hypophosphatemia in the renal defect, bone involvement, and inheritance. *Am. J. Med. Genet.* **1,** 101–117.
88. Koenig, M., Beggs, A. H., Moyer, M., Scherpf, S., Heindrich, K., Bettecken, T., et al. (1989) The molecular basis for Duchenne versus Becker muscular dystrophy: correlation of severity with type of deletion. *Am. J. Hum. Genet.* **45,** 498–506.
89. Econs, M. J., McEnery, P. T., Lennon, F., and Speer, M. C. (1997) Autosomal dominant hypophosphatemic rickets is linked to chromosome 12p13. *J. Clin. Invest.* **100,** 2653–2657.
90. Chong, S. S., Kozak, C. A., Liu, L., Kristjansson, K., Dunn, S. T., Bourdeau, J. E., and Hughes, M. R. (1995) Cloning, genetic mapping, and expression analysis of a mouse renal sodium-dependent phosphate cotransporter. *Am. J. Physiol.* **268,** F1038–F1045.
91. White, K. E., Speer, M. C., Biber, J., Murer, H., and Econs, M. J. (1998) Refining the autosomal dominant hypophosphatemic rickets (ADHR) interval on chromosome 12p13 and localization of two candidate ADHR genes. *Bone* **23 (5),** S379(Abstract).
92. Tieder, M., Modai, D., Samuel, R., Arie, R., Halabe, A., Bab, I., Gabizon, D., and Liberman, U. A. (1985) Hereditary hypophosphatemic rickets with hypercalciuria. *N. Engl. J. Med.* **312,** 611–617.
93. Chen, C., Carpenter, T., Steg, N., Baron, R., and Anast, C. (1989) Hypercalciuric hypophosphatemic rickets, mineral balance, bone histomorphometry, and therapeutic implications of hypercalciuria. *Pediatrics* **84,** 276–280.

94. Tieder, M., Modai, D., Shaked, U., Samuel, R., Arie, R., Halabe, A., et al. (1987) "Idiopathic" hypercalciuria and a hereditary hypophosphatemic rickets. Two phenotypical expressions of a common genetic defect. *N. Engl. J. Med.* **316,** 125–129.
95. Proesmans, W. C., Fabry, G., Marchal, G. J., Gillis, P. L., and Boullian, R. (1987) Autosomal dominant hypophosphataemia with elevated serum 1,25 dihydroxyvitamin D and hypercalciuria. *Pediatr. Nephrol.* **1,** 479–484.
96. Olsen, H. S., Cepeda, M. A., Zhang, Q. Q., Rosen, C. A., and Vozzolo, B. L. (1996) Human stanniocalcin: a possible hormonal regulator of mineral metabolism. *Proc. Natl. Acad. Sci. USA* **93,** 1792–1796.
97. Beck, L., Karaplis, A. C., Amizuka, N., Hewson, A. S., Ozawa, H., and Tenenhouse, H. S. (1998) Targeted inactivation of NPT2 in mice leads to severe renal phosphate wasting, hypercalciuria, and skeletal abnormalities. *Proc. Natl. Acad. Sci. USA* **95,** 5372–5377.
98. Custer, M., Spindler, B., Verrey, F., Murer, H., and Biber, J. (1997) Identification of a new gene product (Diphor-1) regulated by dietary phosphate. *Am. J. Physiol.* **273,** F801–F806.
99. Norbis, F., Boll, M., Stange, G., Markovich, D., Verrey, F., Biber, J., and Murer, H. (1997) Identification of a cDNA/protein leading to an increased Pi-uptake in Xenopus laevis oocytes. *J. Memb. Biol.* **156,** 19–24.
100. White, K. E., Biber, J., Murer, H., and Econs, M. J. (1998) A PDZ domain-containing protein with homology to Diphor-1 maps to human chromosome 1q21. *Ann. Hum. Genet.* **62,** 287–290.
101. White, K. E. and Econs, M. J. (1998) Localization of PiUS, a stimulator of cellular phosphate uptake to human chromosome 3p21.3. *Somat. Cell Mol. Genet.* **24,** 71–74.

CHAPTER 8

X-Linked Nephrolithiasis/Dent's Disease and Mutations in the ClC-5 Chloride Channel

Steven J. Scheinman and Rajesh V. Thakker

Introduction

In the past several years, a number of syndromes have been defined that, though apparently distinct in several ways, all shared features of hypercalciuria, nephrocalcinosis, and evidence of renal proximal tubular reabsorptive failure; clinically significant disease was confined almost exclusively to males. In both X-linked recessive nephrolithiasis (XRN) in North America *(1)* and Dent's disease in the United Kingdom *(2)*, calcium nephrolithiasis was a prominent presenting feature, and renal failure often progressed to end-stage. A family described by Buckalew in 1974 had a similar pattern of clinical abnormalities *(3)*. In X-linked recessive hypophosphatemic rickets, described in two families in Italy and France, the most prominent feature was deforming rickets in childhood *(4,5)*; this occurred in a third of patients with Dent's disease and rarely in XRN. In addition, a syndrome of low-molecular-weight (LMW) proteinuria with hypercalciuria and nephrocalcinosis was described in Japanese schoolchildren without kidney stones, clinical bone disease, or significant renal failure *(6)*. The similarities among all of these syndromes were substantial, particularly the consistent finding of LMW proteinuria which strongly suggested proximal tubular dysfunction, as well as hypercalciuria and nephrocalcinosis. Beyond these phenotypic similarities, a common genetic etiology has been identified, and clearly establishes that these are all variants of a single disease.

The gene responsible for this disease, *CLCN5*, is a member of the voltage-gated chloride channel family of genes, and was identified through a positional cloning approach. The gene, *CLCN5*, encodes a channel protein, ClC-5, and is expressed predominantly in kidney. This chapter will focus on describing the clinical features of this disease, the molecular genetic studies that led to the identification of the disease gene, and our knowledge, as yet incomplete, as to the localization and function of the gene product.

The Genetics of Osteoporosis and Metabolic Bone Disease
Ed.: M. J. Econs © Humana Press Inc., Totowa, NJ

Reports of Clinical Syndromes

A wide variety of syndromes, described over a span of more than three decades, are now known to be connected by the common molecular basis of mutations in *CLCN5*. This section will discuss the syndromes for which mutations in *CLCN5* are now known to be responsible, in the chronologic order in which they were reported. This disease might be given the descriptive name "X-linked nephrolithiasis," or might more simply be called by the name of the one syndrome, "Dent's disease," which encompasses all of the major findings of the other syndromes.

1. Dent and Friedman (1964): "Hypercalciuric rickets associated with renal tubular damage." Dent and Friedman described two unrelated boys who had rickets in the setting of renal calcium loss and evidence of proximal renal tubular dysfunction *(7)*. These patients and others were followed over the subsequent decades by Prof. Oliver Wong, who 30 yr later described a familial syndrome with a marked male predominance that included nephrocalcinosis, nephrolithiasis, and renal failure often progressing to end-stage. They emphasized the important observation that low-molecular-weight proteinuria was the most consistent finding *(2)*.
2. Buckalew et al. (1974): "Hereditary renal tubular acidosis." This large North Carolina kindred with 64 members inherited a disease characterized by hypercalciuria, nephrocalcinosis, nephrolithiasis, LMW proteinuria, aminoaciduria, polyuria, and renal failure. Despite the title of that report, impaired urinary acidification was present in only four patients, while 19 had hypercalciuria and six had nephrocalcinosis. The authors proposed that hypercalciuria was the primary defect, and that the acidification defect was secondary to hypercalciuria *(3)*. Thus, the recent report documenting *CLCN5* mutations in these patients was instead entitled "X-linked renal failure without X-linked recessive hypophosphatemic rickets" *(8)*, serving both to compare and contrast this family with phenotypic variants in other families with the same mutation.
3. Frymoyer et al. (1991): "X-linked recessive nephrolithiasis with renal failure." In this six-generation, 162-member kindred of Irish descent in northern New York State, the presence of disease exclusively in males, the absence of father-to-son inheritance, and the multiple occurrences of inheritance from a maternal grandfather through an unaffected daughter to her sons, established that the disease in this family was X-linked (Fig. 1). Prominent features included recurrent nephrolithiasis, nephrocalcinosis, tubular solute wasting, and progression to renal failure *(1)*. LMW proteinuria and hypercalciuria were common in this family *(9)* as well as in the several subsequent reports of an identical syndrome elsewhere in North America *(10–12)*. Although the absence of rickets in these North American families was once thought to be a defining difference between "X-linked recessive nephrolithiasis" (XRN) and "Dent's disease," the recent reports included *CLCN5* mutations in boys from Canada *(10,12)* and Ohio *(14)* with rickets.

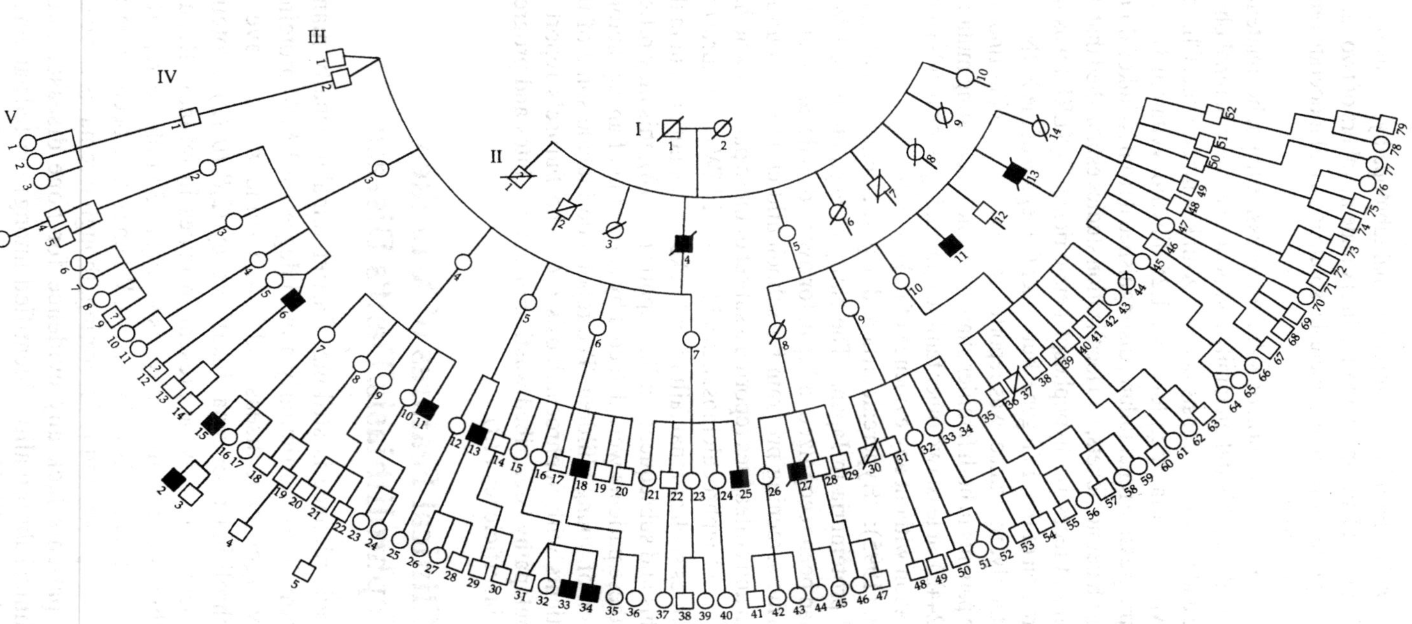

Fig. 1. Pedigree of original North American family with X-linked recessive nephrolithiasis (XRN). (Adapted with permission from ref. *1*) to indicate additional affected males identified since original report. (Copyright © 1991, Massachusetts Medical Society. All rights reserved.)

4. Furuse et al. (1992): "Familial progressive renal tubulopathy." This report described an inherited Fanconi syndrome in six male members of two families, with LMW proteinuria, hypercalciuria, solute loss, and moderate renal insufficiency in two adults *(13)*.
5. Bolino et al. (1993): "A new form of X-linked recessive hypophosphatemic rickets." Five males in this Italian family had bone disease with renal phosphate wasting and a pedigree consistent with X-linked inheritance. Clinical features of hypercalciuria, high levels of 1,25-dihydroxyvitamin D, proteinuria, and progressive renal failure, distinguished it from X-linked dominant hypophosphatemic rickets, and localization studies established that the disease, "X-linked recessive hypophosphatemic rickets" (XLRH) was not linked to the region of the HYP gene, but rather the region of the XRN gene *(4)*. Another family, in France, was reported in 1997 with similar findings *(5)*, and while patients in both families share the same inactivating mutation in *CLCN5* (S244L), at least two other families (including Buckalew's) have the same mutation without any evidence of rickets *(8,10)*.
6. Igarashi et al. (1995): "Hypercalciuria and nephrocalcinosis with idiopathic LMW proteinuria in Japan." The entity of asymptomatic LMW proteinuria had been recognized in Japan for over a decade, as a result of the annual urine screening program for schoolchildren in that country, when Igarashi and colleagues reported a subset of these patients who had hypercalciuria and nephrocalcinosis, in addition to LMW proteinuria *(6)*. Although features such as renal failure and rickets were not present in the children in this and subsequent similar reports *(15–18)*, this may reflect the fact that these patients were detected by screening of an asymptomatic population of young children. The reports do include some of the youngest patients with nephrocalcinosis *(16)*, and Furuse's report of "familial tubulopathy" described wasting of other solutes and progression to renal insufficiency *(13)*.

Clinical Features of X-Linked Nephrolithiasis/Dent's Disease

The male predominance is striking. Carrier females usually manifest biochemical abnormalities, particularly a mild degree of LMW proteinuria, without clinically significant disease, although some women have been reported with nephrolithiasis or renal insufficiency *(2,8,10,12)*. Proteinuria and microscopic hematuria may be present in males in infancy. Recurrent calcium nephrolithiasis can begin in boys as young as 3 yr old, as reported in families in North America and Britain *(1,2,9)*. When rickets occurs it is clinically evident at an early age, and is deforming, though it remains to be elucidated why most patients lack any evidence for bone disease. Table 1 summarizes the clinical abnormalities identified among reported patients with documented mutations in *CLCN5*.

Table 1
Major Features of X-Linked Nephrolithiasis (Dent's Disease)[a]

Abnormality	# Positive/# total	Percent positive
LMW proteinuria	57/57	100
Hypercalciuria	51/54	94
Nephrocalcinosis	42/57	74
Nephrolithiasis	21/43	49
Renal failure	40/59	68
Rickets or osteomalacia	15/62	24
Concentrating defect	15/17	88
Aminoaciduria	26/35	74
Renal glycosuria	9/34	56
Hypophosphatemia	24/48	50
Hypokalemia	12/35	34
Acidification defect	5/35	14
Hypouricemia	1/23	4

[a]Data were taken from published reports of all reported cases that were confirmed by mutation analysis *(1,2,4,5,8–12)*, excluding those identified solely by screening of asymptomatic children *(6,10,15–17)*. Percentages are calculated as the number positive for that abnormality among those for whom any result (positive or negative) is specifically described, and thus these numbers may overestimate the true frequency since reports are more likely to fail to mention features that were absent than those that were present.

Evidence of Renal Tubular Dysfunction

Proximal Tubulopathy and LMW Proteinuria

The most consistent abnormality across all of these reports is LMW proteinuria. Affected males excrete proteins such as retinol-binding protein (RBP) and β2-microglobulin in quantities that exceed normal rates of excretion by as much as 3000-fold (Fig. 2). These proteins, of molecular mass less than 40,000 Daltons, are normally filtered freely at the renal glomerulus and reabsorbed almost completely by the proximal tubule, and excretion of excessive amounts of LMW proteins is evidence of proximal tubular dysfunction. Varying degrees of LMW proteinuria occur in a wide range of tubulointerstitial renal diseases, from pyelonephritis to transplant rejection *(19)*. The literature contains reports of LMW proteinuria in kidney stone disease, though it is unusual in the absence of infection or obstruction from recurrent stones *(20)*. The LMW proteinuria in Dent's disease is remarkable both in the extreme degrees of proteinuria and in the fact that it occurs so consistently in virtually all patients, and at very early ages, before any signs of nephrolithiasis or nephrocalcinosis *(2,9)*. Some patients have been described in whom LMW proteinuria is the only abnormality *(21,22)*.

Carrier females display milder degrees of LMW proteinuria, usually above the normal range but not nearly as excessive as those seen in the affected males

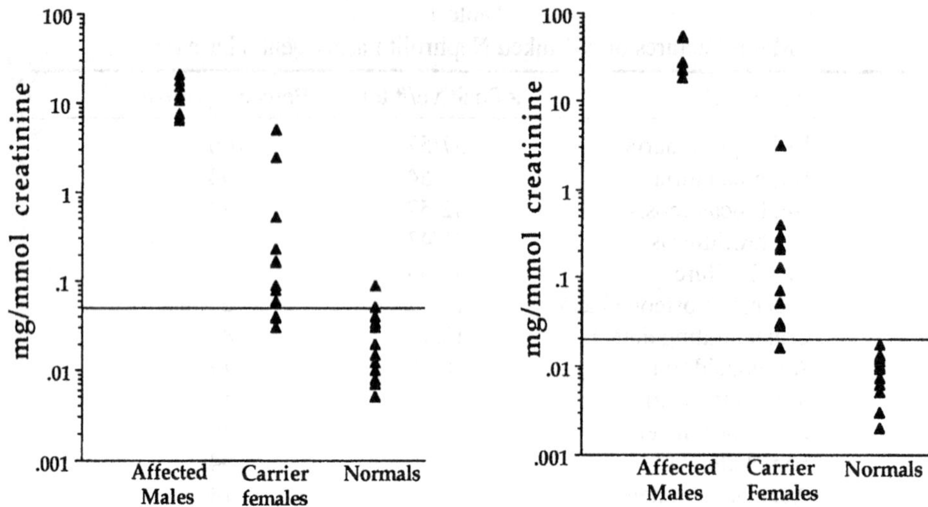

Fig. 2. Left, β2 = microglobulin. Right, retinol = binding protein. Urinary excretion of low-molecular-weight proteins β2-microglobulin (left) and retinol-binding protein (right) in affected males, obligate carrier females, and normal members of the large family with XRN. Horizontal lines indicate the established upper limit of the normal range. (Adapted with permission from ref. *9*.)

(Fig. 2). Since the gene is on the X chromosome, this finding is consistent with random inactivation of the X chromosome in somatic cells (Lyonization).

Other Tubular Functional Defects

Phosphate wasting, renal glycosuria, and aminoaciduria are also seen in this disease and provide further evidence of proximal tubular dysfunction, but no other defect is as consistently present as LMW proteinuria. Hypophosphatemia *(4,5)* or hypokalemia *(1,2)* can be pronounced but overall these occur in fewer than half of patients *(1,2,9)*. Aminoaciduria, glycosuria *(2,6,9)*, and hyperuricosuria *(10)* also occur in a minority of patients. The presence of these abnormalities can be intermittent. Although it has not been studied formally, renal sodium handling appears to be normal in this disease *(9)*. One patient was reported to have a marked natriuretic response to hydrochlorothiazide *(2)*.

In boys the first symptom is often nocturia, and a moderate degree of polyuria occurs in many patients. Urinary concentration responds subnormally to vasopressin *(2,9)*. Most patients are able to acidify the urine normally in response to acid-loading or spontaneously (Table 1), but some patients have impaired acidifying ability *(2,8,9)*. In such cases the acidification defect is consistent with the presence of renal insufficiency or nephrocalcinosis *(2,3,9)*, but recent evidence that ClC-5 is expressed in the acid-secreting intercalated cells of the collecting duct *(23)* may prompt reassessment of this view.

Hypercalciuria and Stones

Kidney stones in this disease are composed of calcium, usually as oxalate but occasionally with phosphate as well *(1)*. The urine is supersaturated with respect to calcium oxalate, reflecting primarily the hypercalciuria, which appears to be the major risk factor for stones in this disease *(24)*. Urinary excretion of citrate is normal *(1,2,9)*, and hyperoxaluria is uncommon *(2,25)*.

Hypercalciuria

In the absence of renal insufficiency, patients with Dent's disease have hypercalciuria with an exaggerated response to oral calcium loading *(6,9)*, while fasting hypercalciuria is seen in only half of patients *(9)*. Consistent with this observation, serum levels of 1,25-dihydroxyvitamin D tend to be near or above the upper limit of the normal range, and serum levels of PTH are normal to low *(1,2,6,9)* (Fig. 3). Serum levels of calcium are normal. Thus, calcium metabolism in this disease resembles one pattern seen in many patients with idiopathic hypercalciuria, in whom there is a tendency to mild hypophosphatemia, excessive production of 1,25-dihydroxyvitamin D, absorptive hypercalciuria, and a component of enhanced bone resorption. To the extent that either hypophosphatemia or excessive 1-hydroxylation of 25-hydroxyvitamin D is a primary event in the hypercalciuria, this is also consistent with a defect in renal proximal tubular function. However, fasting hypercalciuria occurs in half of patients. While this would also be consistent with excessive effect of 1,25-dihydroxyvitamin D on bone, it might alternatively suggest the presence of a renal calcium leak. ClC-5 is expressed in the medullary thick ascending limb of Henle's loop *(26,45)*, a nephron segment involved in active calcium transport. A chloride channel, as yet unidentified, also participates in calcium transport in the cortical distal tubule *(27,28)*.

Renal Failure

Both the occurrence and the severity of renal failure are variable in this disease. Medullary nephrocalcinosis is common in affected males by the teenage years, and often earlier, but the presence of nephrocalcinosis does not correlate with the level of renal function. The degree of albuminuria usually ranges from 1 – 2 g/d, and the nephrotic syndrome does not occur. Nephrolithiasis and nephrocalcinosis have not been observed following renal transplantation among nine transplant recipients followed for up to 12 yr *(25)*.

Histopathology

Nonspecific findings include tubular atrophy and interstitial fibrosis, usually with minimal inflammation. Glomeruli exhibit varying degrees of sclerosis, with some hypertrophic. On electron microscopy the glomerular basement membranes are normal, and immunofluorescence reveals no evidence of antibody deposition. Overall the picture suggests a non-immune focal tubulopathy with secondary glomerular damage.

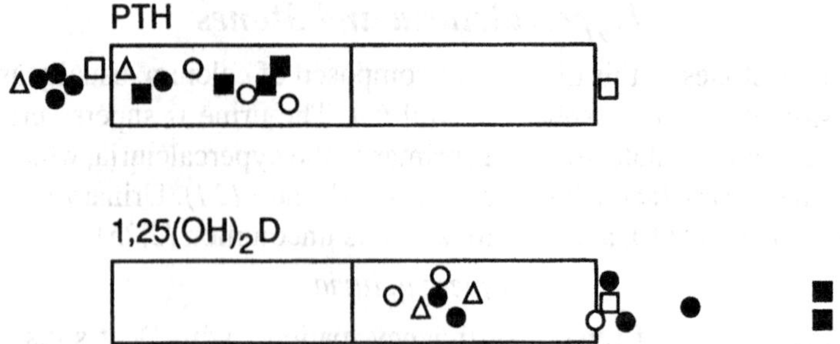

Fig. 3. Serum levels of intact PTH and 1,25-dihydroxyvitamin D in patients with ClC-5-associated syndromes. Boxes indicate the limits and midpoints of the normal ranges for the assays, and values in individual patients are represented relative to the normal limits for that assay. Symbols represent British patients with Dent's disease; (open squares, *[2]*), North American cases of XRN (original report, solid circles *[1]*; other reports, solid squares *[10–12]*); X-linked recessive rickets (open triangles, *[4]*), and Japanese cases of LMW proteinuria with nephrocalcinosis (open circles, *[6]*). (Reprinted with permission from ref. *25*.)

Bone Disease

One of the most puzzling questions in understanding this disease is why rickets or osteomalacia occurs in some patients but not in others, even among patients who share the same mutation in different families or even within the same family. For example, one mutation, S244L, is associated with severe rickets in the Italian and French families with XLRH *(4,5)*, but not in Buckalew's large kindred *(8)* or in a recently reported Ashkenazi family with XRN *(14)*. Hypophosphatemia may contribute to bone disease in some patients, although at least two of the patients with "X-linked recessive hypophosphatemic rickets" were normophosphatemic *(5)*, as were several of the British patients with rickets *(2)*. In patients without clinical bone disease, bone density by dual-energy X-ray absorptiometry was normal *(9)*, as were serum levels of alkaline phosphatase *(1,2,9)*.

Treatment Issues

Until we have a better understanding of how mutations in the gene responsible for this disease explain the clinical findings, treatment recommendations can be only empirical. It seems prudent to attempt to reduce hypercalciuria, which is at least the major factor promoting nephrolithiasis in these patients, although we do not know to what extent if any it is responsible for the progressive renal insufficiency. Although the major component of the hypercalciuria is excessive intestinal absorption, restriction of dietary calcium should not be prescribed. In idiopathic hypercalciuria, lower calcium intakes are associated with an increased risk of stone events *(29,30)* and a higher intestinal oxalate absorption *(31)*. In addition, dietary calcium restriction might exacerbate a tendency to bone demineralization. In contrast, thiazide diuretics should promote a positive calcium balance through their effect to stimulate distal tubular calcium transport. Thus, therapy with thiazides seems reasonable, and amiloride may be an attractive alternative in the hypokalemic patient. One patient had a dramatic natriuretic and kaliuretic response to a large dose of hydrochlorothiazide *(2)*, and patients should be followed closely when starting the diuretic.

Wrong et al. have described healing of rickets in Dent's disease following treatment with vitamin D analogs, and recommend small doses of vitamin D *(2)*. It would seem important to monitor urinary calcium excretion as well as clinical markers of bone disease during this therapy. Bianchi and Bosio reported that phosphorus supplementation corrected the hypophosphatemia, high 1,25-dihydroxyvitamin D levels, hypercalciuria, and bone mineral density in two boys (32) who were subsequently proven to have a nonsense mutation in *CLCN5 (22)*.

Other therapeutic considerations not specific to this disease are also potentially valuable. These include careful attention to urinary tract infection, as in any patient with nephrolithiasis or renal failure, and the possible value of dietary protein restriction or therapy with angiotensin-converting enzyme inhibitors, which are of value in other settings of progressive renal failure.

Molecular Basis of X-Linked Nephrolithiasis/Dent's Disease

Positional Cloning of the Disease Gene

The clinical physiological observations in patients with Dent's disease provided evidence of renal tubular dysfunction particularly affecting the proximal nephron, but did not suggest any likely candidate proteins or pathways. Thus, the gene was sought through a positional cloning approach. The largest pedigree was that reported by Frymoyer et al. *(1)* from the St. Lawrence River valley in New York State, in which it was clear that the inheritance pattern was X-linked recessive (Fig. 1). Thus it was possible to confine the gene mapping strategy to polymorphic DNA markers on the X chromosome.

Figure 4 illustrates the multipoint analysis for markers on the short arm of the X chromosome in this pedigree with XRN. These markers included both restriction fragment length polymorphisms (RFLPs) and PCR-based microsatellite polymorphisms. The highest degree of linkage (LOD = 5.91, recombinant frequency 0.036) was associated with an RFLP identified by the marker M27β at the locus DXS255 near the centromere on the short arm of X *(33)*.

Linkage was also established with this locus in two British families *(34)*. More precise localization using additional markers in the family with XRN appeared initially to indicate a location for XRN distinct from and telomeric to that of Dent's disease *(9)*. However, subsequent cloning of the candidate gene and

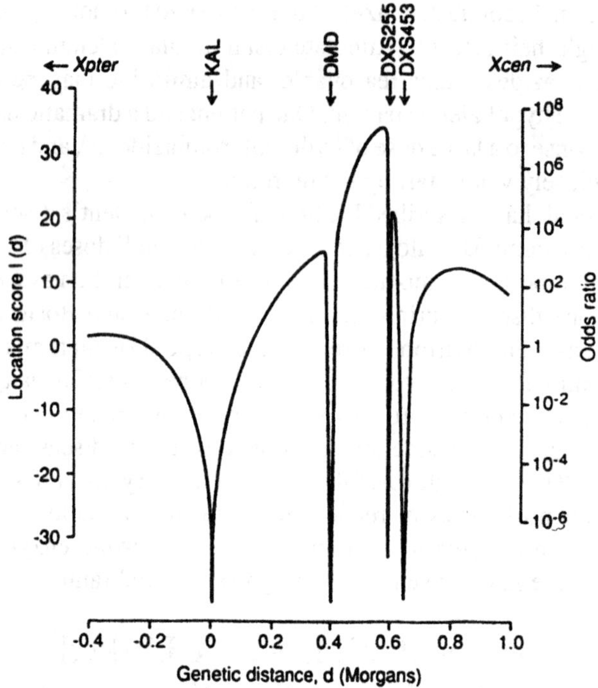

Fig. 4. Location scores of XRN relative to four markers on the short arm of the X chromosome. A location of XRN between DMD and DXS255 was assigned the highest likelihood, with an odds ratio of 2.2 × 107 relative to other localizations. (Reprinted with permission from ref. *33*.)

identification of inactivating mutations in patients with both XRN and Dent's disease established that both disorders are due to mutations in the same gene; the apparent difference in localization was the result of a very mild phenotype in a male with XRN that led to misclassification of his phenotype.

In the largest of the British families with Dent's disease, the absence of a hybridizing band using this marker (M27ß) following restriction digestion of DNA strongly suggested that this region was deleted in affected members of this family (Fig. 5) *(34)*. The size of this deletion was found to be approximately 515 kb, and a yeast artificial chromosome (YAC) contig was established that spanned the deletion. Using these YAC clones to screen a human renal cDNA library, several cDNA clones were identified, and sequencing of these revealed that they represented overlapping sequences of a single expressed gene *(35)*. Analysis of this sequence revealed homology to the ClC family of voltage-gated chloride channels. This family includes ClC-0 which participates in generating electric charge in the marine ray Torpedo marmorata, and ClC-1, the major chloride channel in human muscle. The new gene identified in the deletion from patients with Dent's disease, *CLCN5*, has 11 coding

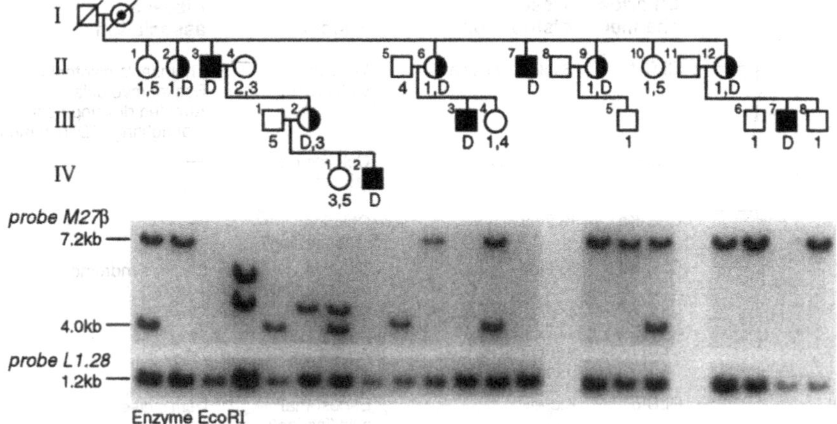

Fig. 5. Family 12/89. Evidence for a microdeletion detected by M27β in affected males and carrier females in the largest of the British families with Dent's disease. Affected males with clinical disease are indicated as solid squares, and carrier females, all of whom had LMW proteinuria (with or without hypercalciuria) are indicated as half-filled circles. In this RFLP the probe M27β hybridizes with fragments of several sizes in normal individuals, but no fragments are identified in any of the affected males, consistent with deletion of the region containing this marker, and only one band for this polymorphic X-chromosome marker is identified in each of the carrier females, consistent with hemizygosity. (Adapted with permission from ref. *34*.)

exons, a transcript of 9.5 kb, and an open reading frame of 2238 bases. It encodes a protein product, designated ClC-5, of 746 amino acids *(36)*.

Structure and Function of CLC-5

Phylogeny and Electrophysiology

The Torpedo ClC-0 channel was isolated by expression cloning by Dr. Thomas Jentsch, and ClC-1, the mammalian homologue, was isolated by the same group by hybridization screening of skeletal muscle libraries using ClC-0 as the probe *(37)*. The homology relationships among members of this channel family are illustrated on Fig. 6. ClC-1 supports the predominant chloride current in mammalian muscle, and is the gene mutated in both the dominant and recessive forms of congenital myotonia (Thomsen's disease) *(38)*. ClC-3 and ClC-4 are expressed in the kidney as well as a wide variety of other tissues. ClC-Ka and ClC-Kb are expressed exclusively in kidney, and are highly homologous to each other; one or both are on the basolateral membrane of the cells of the medullary thick ascending limb of Henle's loop, and ClC-Kb is mutated in a significant number of patients with the Bartter syndrome *(39)*. Thus, three human diseases so far have been found to be explained by inactivating mutations in three members of this gene family.

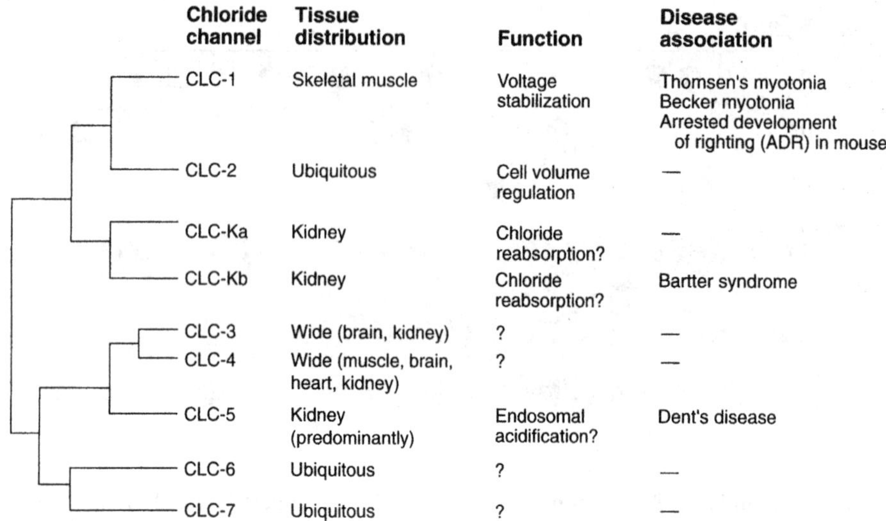

Chloride channel
Tissue distribution
Function
Disease association
CLC-1
Skeletal muscle
Voltage stabilization
Thomsen's myotonia
Becker myotonia
Arrested development of righting (ADR) in mouse
CLC-2
Ubiquitous
Cell volume regulation
—
CLC-Ka
Kidney
Chloride reabsorption?
—
CLC-Kb
Kidney
Chloride reabsorption?
Bartter syndrome
CLC-3
Wide (brain, kidney)
?
—
CLC-4
Wide (muscle, brain, heart, kidney)
?
—
CLC-5
Kidney (predominantly)
Endosomal acidification?
Dent's disease
CLC-6
Ubiquitous
?
—
CLC-7
Ubiquitous
?
—

Fig. 6. Dendrogram representing homology relationships among mammalian members of the ClC family of voltage-gated chloride channels. Not represented is ClC-0, the first member of the ClC family, which was isolated from the electric organ of the eel Torpedo marmorata. (Adapted with permission from ref. *46*.)

Members of the ClC family appear to constitute chloride channels as multimeric complexes. Mutations in ClC-1 occurring in Thomsen's congenital myotonia have a dominant-negative effect on channel function, consistent with this view *(37)*. Dominant-negative mutations have not been identified in ClC-5. Studies of the electrophysiology of the ClC-5 channel reflect the activity of the ClC-5 message expressed alone in Xenopus *(40,41)*, and may or may not reflect the properties of the channel as it occurs in nature. In these studies, the channel has a high selectivity for chloride, is activated at inside-positive membrane voltages, and produces outwardly-rectifying currents *(40)*.

The schematic illustration of the ClC-5 amino-acid sequence shown on Fig. 7 represents a predicted topology based on hydropathy analysis that is similar for all members of the ClC family of chloride channel proteins. Recently, Schmidt-Rose and Jentsch confirmed and clarified this topology in studies using a combination of three complementary techniques: in vitro glycosylation scanning, protease protection assays, and cysteine scanning *(42)*. Thus, the intracellular orientation of both the amino-terminal and carboxy-terminal sequences has been confirmed. The segment following the third transmembrane domain (codons 203 - 242) includes a region that is predicted to be hydrophobic in the sequences of ClC-0 and ClC-1 but not ClC-5, and its extracellular position, as pictured here is supported by some experiments *(42)* but not others *(43)*. The segment from codons 450 to 550 is a broad hydrophobic region in which the number of transmembrane spans is indeterminate *(42)*. Thus, ClC-5 has from 10 to 12 transmembrane domains.

Expression of ClC-5

Our knowledge of ClC-5 expression along the nephron was, until recently, limited to the rat, where it has been studied by reverse-transcriptase PCR amplification from microdissected nephron segments *(26)*, *in situ* hybridization *(23)*, and immunohistochemistry and confocal microscopy *(44)*. In the rat, ClC-5 is expressed particularly in the endosomal membranes of the proximal tubule and the intercalated cells of the connecting tubule and collecting duct, where it colocalizes with the proton-ATPase *(44)*. There is also evidence for ClC-5 expression in the thick ascending limb of Henle's loop *(26)*. These observations have recently been confirmed in the human *(45)*. These findings are consistent with a role for ClC-5 in dissipating charge generated by endosomal acidification, and impairment of this function would explain impaired proximal tubular endosomal reabsorption of LMW proteins. Other physiologic consequences of ClC-5 inactivation, such as hypercalciuria and renal failure, remain unexplained.

Mutations in CLCN5

A total of 32 mutations have been described in 41 families (Fig. 7 and Table 2). In addition, one benign polymorphism has been reported in which a single-base change does not alter the amino-acid sequence. These mutations include 11 missense mutations, each of which alters a single base leading to a change in a single amino acid in a highly conserved sequence, all but one of which are in or near transmembrane domains (Fig. 7). Nine of these have been confirmed by expression in *Xenopus* oocytes to inactivate channel function partially or completely (*see* Table 2 for references). One in-frame insertion of a codon for histidine also reduces channel function in expression studies. Six mutations lead to premature termination of translation through frameshift (*see* Table 2 for references). Two different mutations result in loss of the same 41 amino acids through splice-site disruption; two intragenic deletions lead to loss of 110 and 318 amino acids; and deletions of 180 and 515 kb each result in loss of the entire gene.

When expressed in *Xenopus*, these mutations inactivate the chloride channel *(15,18,22,40)*. There is no correlation between the nature of these mutations and the phenotypic severity of the disease, nor with the presence or absence of variable features such as rickets. For example, the S244L mutation is associated with rickets in all affected males in two families but not in two other families. Phenotypes can range from severe to very mild, and the presence of rickets can vary, even among individuals in a single family sharing the same mutation *(1,40)*.

Conclusion

The clinical features of the several syndromes discussed here shared overlapping features, but were distinct enough to suggest that they might be

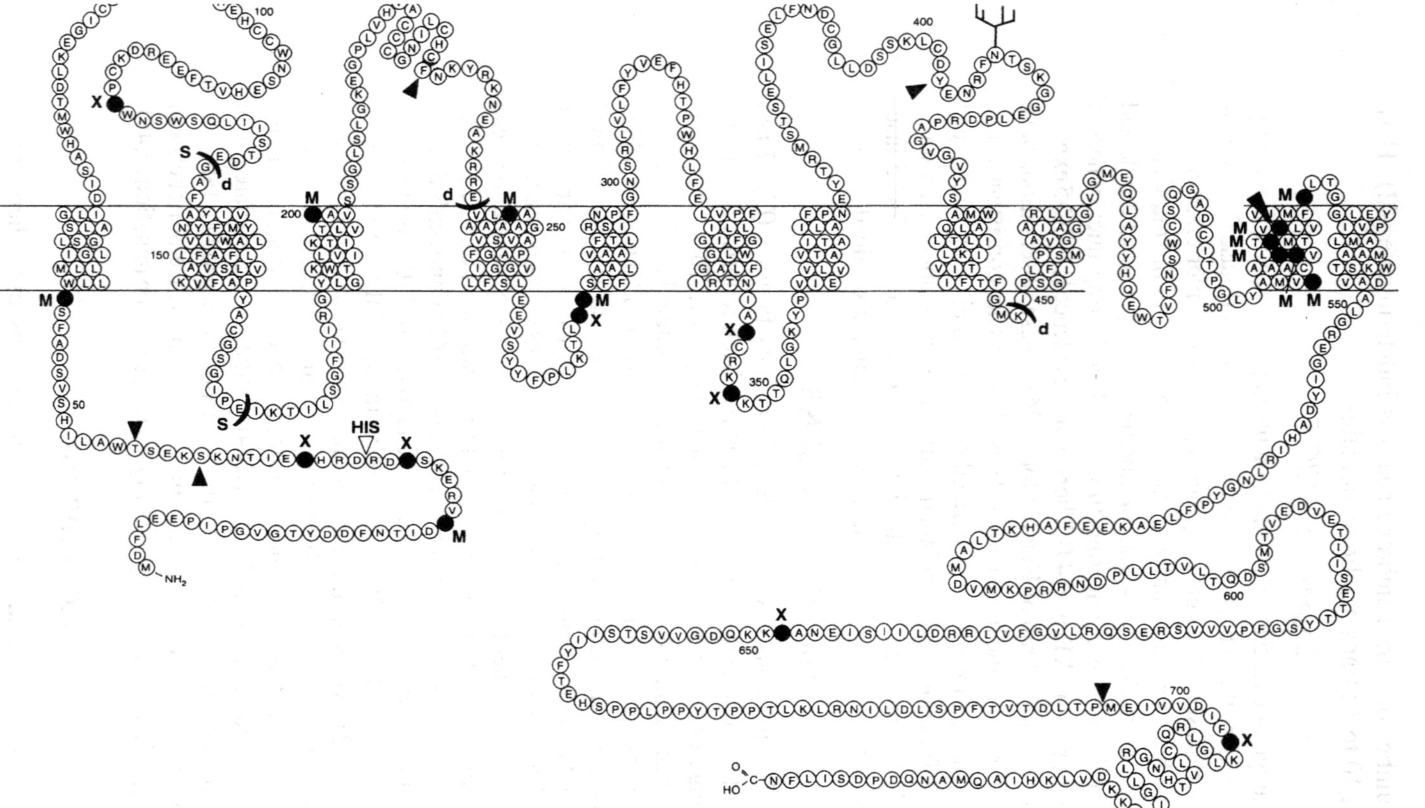

Fig. 7. Schematic representation of the amino-acid sequence of ClC-5 with predicted topology, revised from Lloyd et al. *(40)* to indicate the 32 mutations published to date. Mutations are represented as solid circles indicating the codon affected by missense (M) or nonsense (X) mutations, a solid wedge indicating the position of a frameshift mutation, an open wedge indicating an in-frame insertion of a codon for histidine, and brackets indicating the boundaries of intragenic deletions (d) or splice-site mutations (s). Specific mutations correspond to those listed in Table 2.

Table 2
Published Mutations in *CLCN5* in Patients with X-Linked Dent's Disease Nephrolithiasis

	Codon	Base change	Amino acid change	Predicted effect	Expression	Source	Phenotype[a]	Ref.
Missense								
1	22	TGG→GGG	Trp→Gly	Amino-term. domain	Abolished	Japan	1	*(18)*
2	57	GGC→GTC	Gly→Val	D1 helix	Reduced	US	1, 2, 3, 4	*(22)*
3	200	CTG→CGG	Leu→Arg	D3 charge distribution	Abolished	UK	1, 2, 3, 4, 5	*(40)*
4	244	TCG→TTG	Ser→Leu	D5 helix	Reduced	Italy	2, 3, 4, 5	*(40)*
	244	TCG→TTG	Ser→Leu	D5 helix		France	1, 2, 5	*(5)*
	244	TCG→TTG	Ser→Leu	D5 helix		US	1, 2, 3, 4	*(8)*
	244	TCG→TTG	Ser→Leu	D5 helix		US	1, 2, 3, 4	*(14)*
5	280	CGT→CCT	Arg→Pro	at border of D6	Reduced	Japan	1, 2, 3	*(15)*
6	506	GGG→ GAG	Gly →Glu	D11 charge distrib	Abolished	US	1, 2, 3, 4	*(40)*
7	512	GGT→ CGT	Gly →Arg	D11 charge distrib	Abolished	US	1, 2, 3, 4	*(22)*
8	513	GGG→GAG	Gly→Glu	D11 charge distrib		Japan	1, 2	*(16)*
9	516	CGG→TGG	Arg→Trp	D11 charge distrib		Japan	1, 2, 3	*(16)*
10	520	TCT→CCT	Ser→Pro	D11 helix	Reduced	UK	1, 2, 3, 4, 5	*(40)*
11	527	GAA→GAT	Glu→Asp	? (highly conserved)	Abolished	India	1, 2, 3, 4, 5	*(22)*[b]
Nonsense								
12	28	CGA→TGA	Arg→Stop	Lose 718 aa		US	1, 3, 4	*(10)*
13	34	CGA→TGA	Arg→Stop	Lose 712 aa		Canada	1, 2, 3, 4, 5	*(10)*
14	118	GAG→TAG	Gu→Stop	Lose 628 aa		Japan	1	*(18)*
15	279	TGG→TGA	Trp→Stop	Lose 469 aa	Abolished	UK	1, 2, 3, 4	*(40)*
	279	TGG→TGA	Trp→Stop	Lose 469 aa		Japan	1, 2, 3	*(15)*
	279	TGG→TGA	Trp→Stop	Lose 469 aa		Japan	1, 2	*(16)*
16	343	TGG→TAG	Trp→Stop	Lose 404 aa		Japan	1, 2, 3	*(15)*
	343	TGG→TAG	Trp→Stop	Lose 404 aa		US	1, 2, 3	*(10)*
17	347	CGA→TGA	Arg→Stop	Lose 399 aa		Japan	1	*(18)*

Table 2 (cont.)

	347	CGA→TGA	Arg→Stop	Lose 399 aa		Japan	1	(16)
	347	**CGA**→**TGA**	Arg→Stop	Lose 399 aa	Abolished	Japan	1, 2	*(18)*
18	648	**CGA**→**TGA**	Arg→Stop	Lose 98 aa	Abolished	UK	1, 2, 3, 4, 5	*(40)*
	648	**CGA**→**TGA**	Arg→Stop	Lose 98 aa		Italy	1, 2, 3, 4	*(22)*
19	704	**CGA**→**TGA**	Arg→Stop	Lose 42 aa	Abolished	Canada	1, 3, 4	*(40)*
Insertion								
20	30	ACC in-frame insertion	30:H insertion	? (Charge distrib.)	Reduced	UK	1, 2	*(22)*[b]
Splice-site								
21	132-172 del	gt→**gg**	Lose 41 amino acids	Lose D2	Abolished	UK	1, 2, 3, 4, 5	*(40)*
22	132-172 del	gt→**at**	Lose 41 amino acids	Lose D2	Abolished	UK	1, 2, 3, 4	*(40)*
Frameshift								
23	40	ΔA	Δ40fs→47 Stop	Lose 699 aa		US	2, 3, 4, (5)	*(10)*
24	44	ΔA	Δ44fs→47 Stop	Lose 699 aa		US	1, 2, 3	*(10)*
25	229	ΔC, insert TA	Δ229fs→236 Stop	Lose 510 aa		Japan	1	*(16)*
26	403	T**A**T T-T	Δ403fs→433 Stop	Lose 314 aa		Japan	1	*(17)*
27	520	**T** insertion	Δ520fs→527 Stop	Lose 220 aa		Japan	1, 2	*(17)*
28	695	ΔC	Δ695fs→699 Stop	Lose 47 aa		Japan	1, 2, 3	*(15)*
Deletions								
29	132–241 2(kb)		Lose 110 amino acids	Lose D2–D4	Abolished	UK	1, 2, 3, 4, 5	*(40)*[b]
30	(n.s.) exons 5–8 (>7kb)		Lose 318 amino acids	Lose D2–D9		Japan	1, 5	*(18)*
31	(n.s.) entire gene (180 kb)		Protein absent	No protein		Japan	1, 2, 3	*(16)*
32	(n.s.) entire gene (515 kb)		Protein absent	No protein		UK	1	*(34)*
Polymorphism								
484		ACC ACT	No change			Japan	1	*(16)*

[a] Phenotypic features : 1, LMW proteinuria; 2, hypercalciuria; 3, nephrocalcinosis/stones; 4, renal insufficiency; 5, rickets.
[b] Clinical data from Prof. Oliver Wong, personal communication.
[c] 32 distinct mutations in 41 families.

separate entities. Physiologic findings did not indicate any particularly likely candidates to explain any of these syndromes. However, mapping of three of these syndromes to the same region of Xp, and ultimately the identification in all of these syndromes of mutations in the gene encoding the ClC-5 chloride channel, expressed predominantly in kidney, clarified the relationships among these syndromes and established that they are all variations of a single disease entity, most simply called Dent's disease. Physiologic information about the role of this chloride channel in kidney function is beginning to emerge, and it appears probable that it plays a role in acidification of endocytotic vesicles in proximal tubule and possibly elsewhere in the nephron. The clinical findings of LMW proteinuria and other signs of proximal tubular dysfunction will probably be explained by this mechanism. Many other questions, particularly regarding the mechanism of hypercalciuria and the variable occurrence of rickets, still need to be addressed. This represents a gratifying example of a molecular genetic approach leading not only to clarification of clinical issues regarding disease syndromes, but also identifying a new gene product of physiologic importance in renal function.

Acknowledgments

This work was supported by the National Institutes of Health DK46838 (S.J.S.); the North Atlantic Treaty Organization CGR950114 (S.J.S. and R.V.T.); and the Medical Research Council (U. K.) (R.V.T.).

References

1. Frymoyer, P. A., Scheinman, S. J., Dunham, P. B., Jones, D. B., Hueber, P., and Schroeder, E. T. (1991) X-linked recessive nephrolithiasis with renal failure. *N. Engl. J. Med.* **325,** 681–686.
2. Wong, O., Norden, A. G. W., and Feest, T. G. (1994) Dent's disease: a familial proximal renal tubular syndrome with low-molecular-weight proteinuria, hypercalciuria, nephrocalcinosis, metabolic bone disease, progressive renal failure, and a marked male predominance. *Q. J. Med.* **87,** 473–493.
3. Buckalew, V. M., Purvis, J. L., Shulman, M. G., Herndon, N., and Rudman, D. (1974) Hereditary renal tubular acidosis. *Medicine* **53,** 229–254.
4. Bolino, A., Devoto, M., Enia, G., Zoccali, C., J., W., and Romeo, G. (1993) A new form of X-linked hypophosphatemic rickets with hypercalciuria (HPDR II) maps in the Xp11 region. *Eur. J. Hum. Genet.* **1,** 269–279.
5. Oudet, C., Martin-Coignard, D., Pannetier, S., Praud, E., Champion, G., and Hanauer, A. (1997) A second family with XLRH displays the mutation S244L in the CLCN5 gene. *Hum. Genet.* **99(6),** 781–784.
6. Igarashi, T., Hayakawa, H., Shiraga, H., Kawato, H., Yan, K., Kawaguchi, H., Yamanaka, T., Tsuchida, S., and Akagi, K. (1995) Hypercalciuria and nephrocalcinosis in patients with idiopathic low–molecular–weight proteinuria in Japan: is the disease identical to Dent's disease in United Kingdom? *Nephron* **69(3),** 242–247.
7. Dent, C. E., and Friedman, M. (1964) Hypercaluric rickets associated with renal tubular damage. *Arch. Dis. Childhood* **39,** 240–249.

8. Kelleher, C. L., Buckalew, V. M., Frederickson, E. D., Rhodes, D. J., Conner, D. A., Seidman, J. G., and Seidman, C. E. (1998) CLCN5 mutation Ser244Leu is associated with X-linked renal failure without X-linked recessive hypophosphatemic rickets. *Kidney Int.* **53(1),** 31–37.
9. Reinhart, S. C., Norden, A. G. W., Lapsley, M., Thakker, R. V., Pang, J., Moses, A. M.,et al. (1995) Characterization of carrier females and affected males with X-linked recessive nephrolithiasis. *J. Am. Soc. Nephrol.* **5,** 1451–1461.
10. Hoopes, R. R., Hueber, P. A., Reid, R. J., Braden, G. L., Goodyer, P. R., Melnyk, A. R., et al. (1998) CLCN5 chloride-channel mutations in six new North American families with X-linked nephrolithiasis. *Kidney Int.* **54,** 698–705.
11. Schurman, S. J., Norden, A. G. W., and Scheinman, S. J. (1998) X-linked recessive nephrolithiasis: Presentation and diagnosis in children. *J. Pediatr.* **132,** 859–862.
12. Langlois, V., Chantale, B., Scheinman, S. J., Thakker, R. V., Cox, J. P. D., and Goodyer, P. R. (1998) Clinical features of X-linked nephrolithiasis in childhood. *Pediatr. Nephrol.* **12,** 625–629
13. Furuse, A., Futagoishi, Y., Karashima, S., Hattori, S., and Matsuda, I. (1992) Familial progressive renal tubulopathy. *Clin. Nephrol.* **37,** 192–197.
14. Raja, K., Kenagy, D., and Scheinman, S. J. (1998) Hypomagnesemia associated with an inactivating mutation (S2++L) in *CLCN5* in X-linked recessive nephrolithiasis (Dent's disease). *J. Am. Soc. Nephrol.* **9,** 558A–559A (Abstract).
15. Lloyd, S. E., Pearce, S. H., Gunther, W., Kawaguchi, H., Igarashi, T., Jentsch, T. J., and Thakker, R. V. (1997) Idiopathic low molecular weight proteinuria associated with hypercalciuric nephrocalcinosis in Japanese children is due to mutations of the renal chloride channel (CLCN5). *J. Clin. Invest.* **99(5),** 967–974.
16. Akuta, N., Lloyd, S. E., Igarashi, T., et al. (1997) Mutations of CLCN5 in Japanese children with idiopathic low molecular weight proteinuria, hypercalciuria and nephrocalcinosis. *Kidney Int.* **52(4),** 911–916.
17. Nakazato, H., Hattori, S., Furuse, A., et al. (1997) Mutations in the CLCN5 gene in Japanese patients with familial idiopathic low-molecular-weight proteinuria. *Kidney Int.* 52(4), 895–900.
18. Morimoto, T., Uchida, S., Sakamoto, H., Kondo, Y., Hanamizu, H., Fukui, M., et al. (1998) Mutations in CLCN5 chloride channel in Japanese patients with low molecular weight proteinuria. *J. Am. Soc. Nephrol.* **9(5),** 811–818.
19. Waller, K. V., Ward, K. M., Mahan, J. D., and Wismatt, D. K. (1989) Current concepts in proteinuria. *Clin. Chem.* **35(5),** 755–765.
20. Jaeger, P., Portmann, L., Ginalski, J. M., Jacquet, A. F., Temler, E., and Burckhardt, P. (1986) Tubulopathy in nephrolithiasis: consequence rather than cause. *Kidney Int.* **29(2),** 563–571.
21. Geary, D. F., Dillon, M. J., Gammon, K., and Barratt, T. M. (1985) Tubular proteinuria in children without other defects of renal function. *Nephron* **40(3),** 329–331.
22. Lloyd, S. E., Gunther, W., Pearce, S. H. S., Thomson, A., Bianchi, M. L., Bosio, M., et al. (1997) Characterisation of renal chloride channel, CLCN5, mutations in hypercalciuric nephrolithiasis (kidney stones) disorders. *Hum. Mol. Genet.* **6,** 1233–1239.
23. Obermuller, N., Gretz, N., Kriz, W., Reilly, R. F., and Witzgall, R. (1998) The swelling-activated chloride channel ClC-2, the chloride channel ClC-3, and ClC-5, a chloride channel mutated in kidney stone disease, are expressed in distinct subpopulations of renal epithelial cells. *J. Clin. Invest.* **101(3),** 635–642.
24. Asplin, J. R., Reinhart, S. C., Scheinman, S. J., Nakagawa, Y., and Coe, F. L. (1994) Excessive supersaturation with calcium oxalate and calcium phosphate contributes

to stone formation in X–linked recessive nephrolithiasis. *J. Am. Soc. Nephrol.* **5(3),** 858 (Abstract).
25. Scheinman, S. J. (1998) X-linked hypercalciuric nephrolithiasis: Clinical syndromes and chloride channel mutations. *Kidney Int.* **53,** 3–17.
26. Steinmeyer, K., Schwappach, B., Bens, M., Vandewalle, A., and Jentsch, T. J. (1995) Cloning and functional expression of rat CLC–5, a chloride channel related to kidney disease. *J. Biol. Chem.* **270(52),** 31,172–31,177.
27. Gesek, F. A., and Friedman, P. A. (1992) On the mechanism of parathyroid hormone stimulation of calcium uptake by mouse distal convoluted tubule cells. *J. Clin. Invest.* **90(3),** 749–758.
28. Gesek, F. A., and Friedman, P. A. (1992) Mechanism of calcium transport stimulated by chlorothiazide in mouse distal convoluted tubule cells. *J. Clin. Invest.* **90(2),** 429–438.
29. Curhan, G. C., Willett, W. C., Rimm, E. B., and Stampfer, M. J. (1993) A prospective study of dietary calcium and other nutrients and the risk of symptomatic kidney stones. *N. Engl. J. Med.* **328(12),** 833–838.
30. Curhan, G. C., Willett, W. C., Speizer, F. E., Spiegelman, D., and Stampfer, M. J. (1997) Comparison of dietary calcium with supplemental calcium and other nutrients as factors affecting the risk for kidney stones in women. *Ann. Int. Med.* **126(7),** 497–504.
31. Lemann, J., Jr., Pleuss, J. A., Worcester, E. M., Hornick, L., Schrab, D., and Hoffmann, R. G. (1996) Urinary oxalate excretion increases with body size and decreases with increasing dietary calcium intake among healthy adults. *Kidney Int.* **49(1),** 200–208.
32. Bianchi, M. L., and Bosio, M. (1995) A syndrome characterized by hypophosphatemic hyperphosphaturia, hypercalciuria, microglobinuria, nephrocalcinosis and osteopenia. *J. Bone Miner. Res.* **10 (Suppl),** S509 (Abstract).
33. Scheinman, S. J., Pook, M. A., Wooding, C., Pang, J. T., Frymoyer, P. A., and Thakker, R. V. (1993) Mapping the gene causing X-linked recessive nephrolithiasis to Xp11.22 by linkage studies. *J. Clin. Invest.* **91,** 2351–2357.
34. Pook, M. A., Wrong, O., Wooding, C., Norden, A. G. W., Feest, T. G., and Thakker, R. V. (1993) Dent's disease, a renal Fanconi syndrome with nephrocalcinosis and kidney stones, is associated with a microdeletion involving DXS255 and maps to Xp11.22. *Hum. Mol. Genet.* **2,** 2129–2134.
35. Fisher, S. E., Black, G. C. M., Lloyd, S. E., Wrong, O. M., Thakker, R. V., and Craig, I. W. (1994) Isolation and partial characterization of a human chloride channel gene which is expressed in kidney and is a candidate for Dent's disease (an hereditary nephrolithiasis). *Human Mol. Genet.* **3,** 2053–2059.
36. Fisher, S. E., Van Bakel, I., Lloyd, S. E., Pearce, S. H. S., Thakker, R. V., and Craig, I. W. (1995) Cloning and characterization of CLCN5, the human kidney chloride channel gene implicated in Dent disease (an X-linked hereditary nephrolithiasis). *Genomics* **29,** 598–606.
37. Jentsch, T. J., Gunther, W., Pusch, M., and Schwappach, B. (1995) Properties of voltage-gated chloride channels of the ClC gene family. *J. Physiol.* (London) **482,** 19S–25S.
38. Koch, M. C., Steinmeyer, K., Lorenz, C., Ricker, K., Wolf, F., Otto, M., Zoll, B., Lehmann-Horn, F., Grzeschik, K. H., and Jentsch, T. J. (1992) The skeletal muscle chloride channel in dominant and recessive human myotonia. *Science* **257(5071),** 797–800.
39. Simon, D. B., Bindra, R. S., Mansfield, T. A., Nelson-Williams, C., Mendonca, E., Stone, R., et al. (1997) Mutations in the chloride channel gene, CLCNKB, cause Bartter's syndrome type III. *Nat. Genet.* **17(2),** 171–178.
40. Lloyd, S. E., Pearce, S. H. S., Fisher, S. E., Steinmeyer, K., Schwappach, B., Scheinman, S. J., et al. (1996) A common molecular basis for three inherited kidney stone diseases. *Nature* **379,** 445–449.

41. Lorenz, C., Pusch, M., and Jentsch, T. J. (1996) Heteromultimeric CLC chloride channels with novel properties. *Proc. Natl. Acad. Sci. USA* **93(23),** 13,362–13,366.
42. Schmidt-Rose, T., and Jentsch, T. J. (1997) Transmembrane topology of a CLC chloride channel. *Proc. Natl. Acad. Sci. USA* **94(14),** 7633–7638.
43. Fahlke, C., Yu, H. T., Beck, C. L., Rhodes, T. H., and George, A. L., Jr. (1997) Pore-forming segments in voltage-gated chloride channels. *Nature* **390(6659),** 529–532.
44. Gunther, W., Luchow, A., Cluzeaud, F., Vandewalle, A., and Jentsch, T. J. (1998) ClC-5, the chloride channel mutated in Dent's disease, colocalizes with the proton pump in endocytotically active kidney cells. *Proc. Natl. Acad. Sci. USA* **95(14),** 8075–8080.
45. Devuyst, O., Christie, P. T., Courtoy, P. J., Beauwens, R., and Thakker, R.V. (1999) Intra-renal and subcellular distribution of the human chloride channel, CLC-5, reveals a pathophysiological basis for Dent's disease. *Hum. Mol. Genet.* **8,** 247–257
46. Thakker, R. V. (1997) Chloride channels cough up. *Nat. Genet.* **17(2),** 125–127.

CHAPTER 9

Genetics of Tumoral Calcinosis

Kandaswamy Jayaraj and Kenneth Lyles

Introduction

Tumoral calcinosis is a condition characterized by ectopic periarticular calcifications without the involvement of visceral organs. Five salient features of tumoral calcinosis are:

1. elevated serum phosphorus concentration;
2. elevated serum 1,25 dihydroxy vitamin D (calcitriol) concentration;
3. elevated renal tubular phosphate reabsorbtion;
4. ectopic calcifications; and
5. characteristic dental abnormalities.

Extensive vascular calcifications have been reported in this condition *(1)*. Metastatic calcinosis can occur in other conditions that can cause hypercalcemia such as, chronic renal failure, sarcoidosis, milk alkali syndrome, and vitamin D intoxication, and these conditions should be differentiated from tumoral calcinosis *(2)*. Affected subjects usually have normocalcemia, low normal serum parathyroid hormone levels, and a normal renal function. All five of these features are expressed in varying extent in affected individuals. Approximately one-third of the cases are familial. Two subjects have been described with tumoral calcinosis who develop a multi-infarct type of dementia *(3)*.

Tumoral calcinosis was initially described by Giard *(4)* in 1898 followed by Durret *(5)* in 1899. It was given different names including lipo-calcino-granulomatosis and Teutschlander's disease, until 1943 when Inclan *(6)* gave its name "tumoral calcinosis." There are 2000 reported cases. Initially, tumoral calcinosis was thought to be inherited as autosomal recessive *(7)* disorder. Subsequent study of 27 subjects of a kindred from North Carolina suggests that the mode of inheritance to be autosomal dominant with variable expression *(8)*.

The Genetics of Osteoporosis and Metabolic Bone Disease
Ed.: M. J. Econs © Humana Press Inc., Totowa, NJ

Pathogenesis

Affected subjects are in positive calcium and phosphorus balance with an elevation of the renal tubular phosphate reabsorbtion threshold, even in the face of elevated serum phosphate levels. It is hypothesized that the basic defect lies in the proximal renal tubular cell, which abnormally reabsorbs phosphorus and also produces excessive calcitriol. The elevated calcitriol levels cause an increase in gastrointestinal absorption of calcium and phosphorus. The elevated 1,25 hydroxy vitamin-D levels and the gastrointestinal calcium absorbtion are postulated to suppress parathormone levels *(9)*.

Pathology

Tumor

Macroscopically, tumor can be as large as a football and weigh as much as a kilogram *(10)* (Fig. 1). It is lobular and has a rubbery firm to hard consistency. The tumors have pinkish, grayish-yellow or white cystic areas with a honey comb appearance on cross-section (Fig. 2). The cysts are filled with a gritty, chalky fluid of calcium carbonate or triple phosphate held in suspension with albumin.

Microscopically, the tissue shows examples of foreign body granuloma consisting of calcium with lymphocytes, plasma cells, and multinucleated giant cells. The cystic spaces are separated by fibrous septae that has calcium embedded in it.

Dental Abnormalities

A dental lesion has been reported as a phenotypic abnormality that occurs in affected families *(8)*. The lesion consists of short bulbous roots, formation of pulp stones, and radicular dentin deposition in swirls. This lesion is specific for tumoral calcinosis. Dentin abnormality typically occurs in the later part of root formation with radicular dentin deposition and extensive pulp calcifications and formation of pulp stones. It is not clear whether the primary defect is in the odontoblasts or a secondary defect due to elevated phosphorus and 1,25 (OH) 2D levels.

Genetics

In 1969 investigators in Galveston, TX, reported a group of patients with idiopathic tumoral calcinosis and concluded that this disease may be inherited as an autosomal recessive disorder, since it involved only one generation *(11)*. Subsequent follow-up and investigations of the family led to a total of 7 members of one 15-member generation of kindred were affected with this condition. Though they concurred with the prior investigators, they could not explain the reason for the 1:1 involvement between the affected and unaffected members of the same family and the elevated 1,25-hydroxycalciferol levels in unaffected family members from a different generation. The authors also queried that this disease may be inherited in a mode other than autosomal recessive fashion *(7)*.

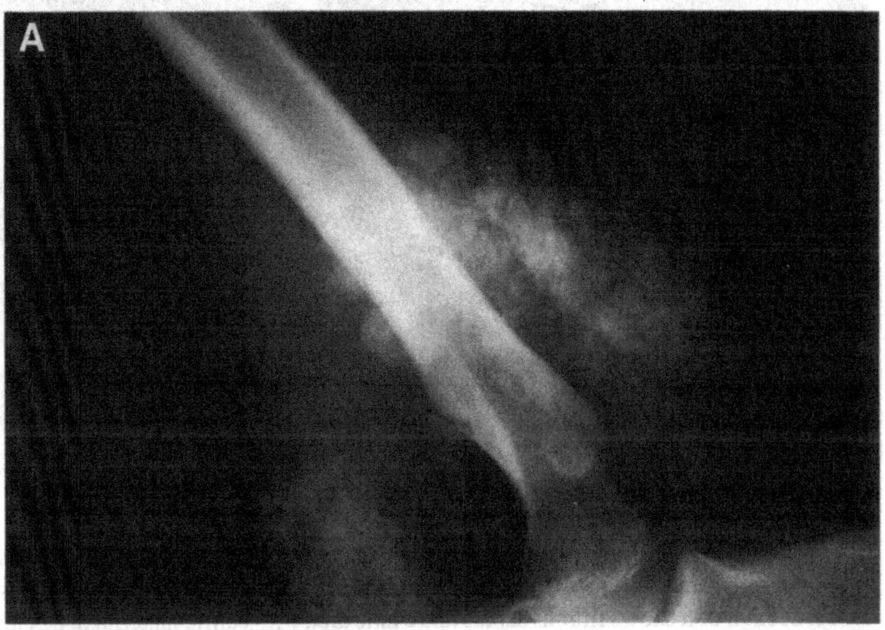

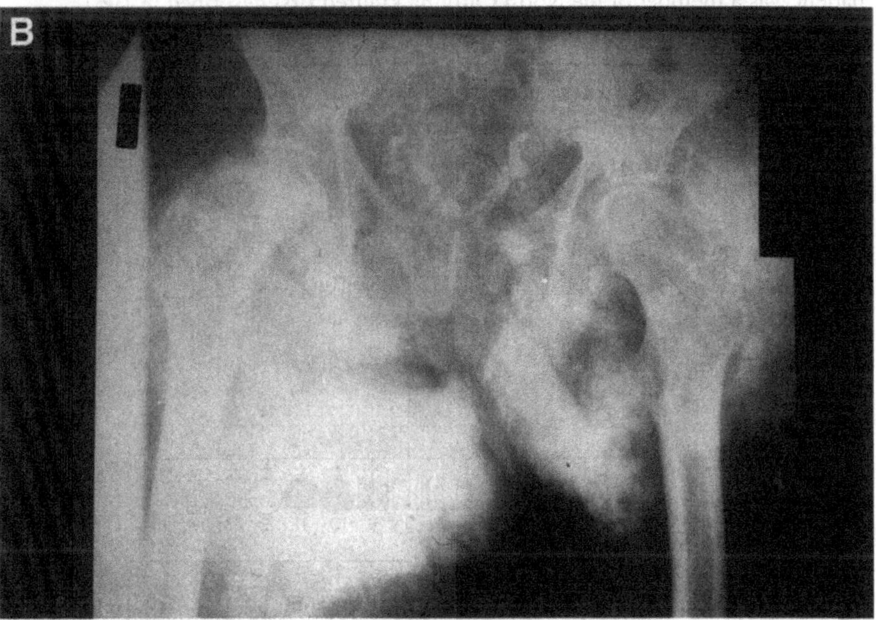

Fig. 1. Pelvis and femurs radiograph of a 77-yr-old Caucasian male who had hyperphosphatemic tumoral calcinosis. Note the calcific masses in each buttock that were easily palpable. The patient had no family history of this disorder.

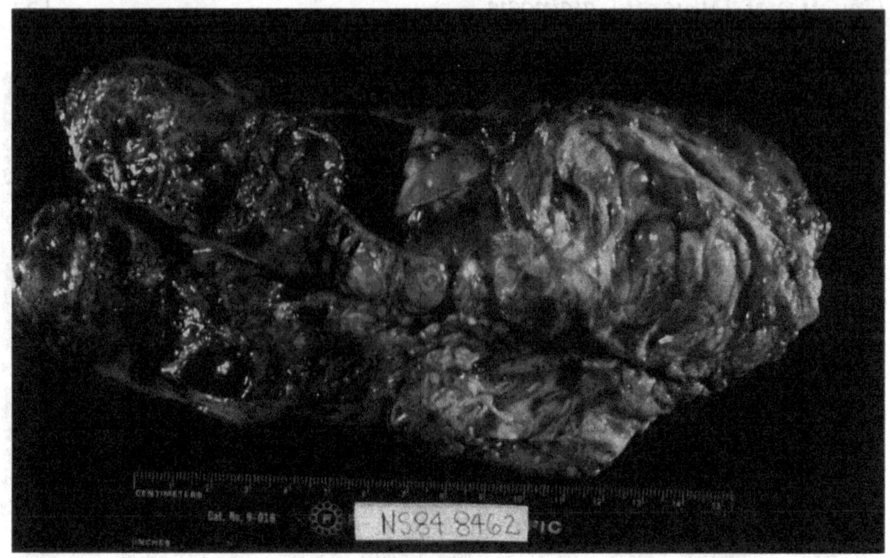

Fig. 2. Right buttock periarticular tumor resected from a 9-yr-old African-American male. The tumor measured 19 × 8 × 4 cm, weighed 400 g, and was enclosed in fibrous tissue. Section of it shows fibrous septae and cystic area with calific material in it. The patient was a member of the North Carolina kindred first described in 1961.

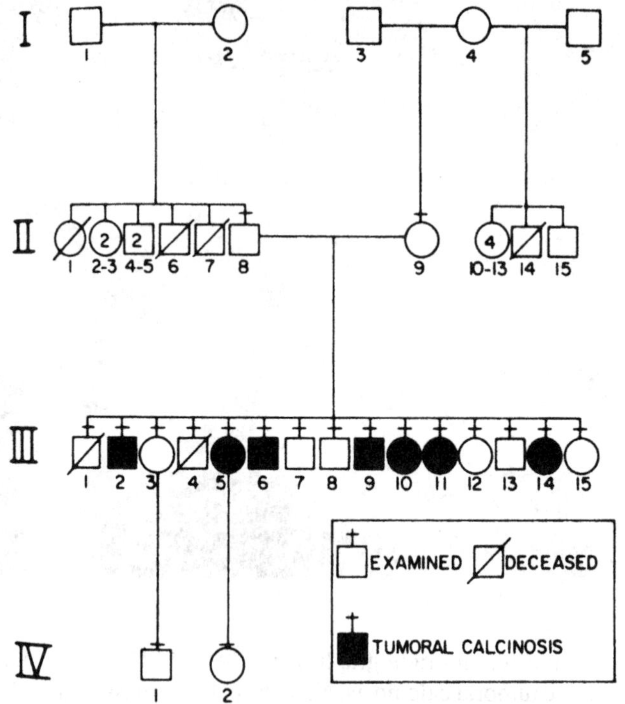

Fig. 3. Family pedigree of family G.

Table 1
Biochemical Parameters of the Studied Individuals of Family G

Pedigree	Age (yr)	Calcium (mg/dL)	Phosphorus (mg/dL)	25-Hydroxycholecalciferol (ng/mL)	1,25-Dihydroxycholecalciferol (pg/dL)
Nonaffected					
II-8	48	10.0	3.7	15.7	36.3
II-9	45	10.0	4.5	16.0	49.4
III-1	25	—	—	—	—
III-3	24	—	—	—	—
III-4	16	—	—	—	—
III-7	17	10.2	4.2	—	55.0
III-8	15	9.9	5.0	14.0	58.7
III-12	9	10.2	4.8	15.1	59.6
III-13	8	10.2	5.4	21.9	57.1
III-15	3	10.1	5.5	—	63.4
IV-1	4	10.4	5.6	14.9	41.8
IV-2	2	10.6	5.0	—	63.9
Mean (± SD)		10.1 ± 0.2	16.3 ± 3.4	53.9 ± 9.6	
Affected					
III-2	25	10.0	6.4	13.3	73.8
III-5	21	9.9	5.9	10.3	75.5
III-6	19	10.2	7.4	4.1	69.8
III-9	14	9.8	6.6	11.5	89.2
III-10	12	9.8	6.8	8.1	80.0
III-11	10	9.4	7.3	—	96.7
III-14	6	9.6	7.0	7.0	96.2
Mean (± 1SD)		9.8 ± 0.3	6.8 ± 0.5	9.0 ± 3.0	83.0 ± 12.6
Normal values (± 1SD)		9.8 ± 0.5	3.9 ± 0.7	27.7 ± 8.8	33.9 ± 7.8

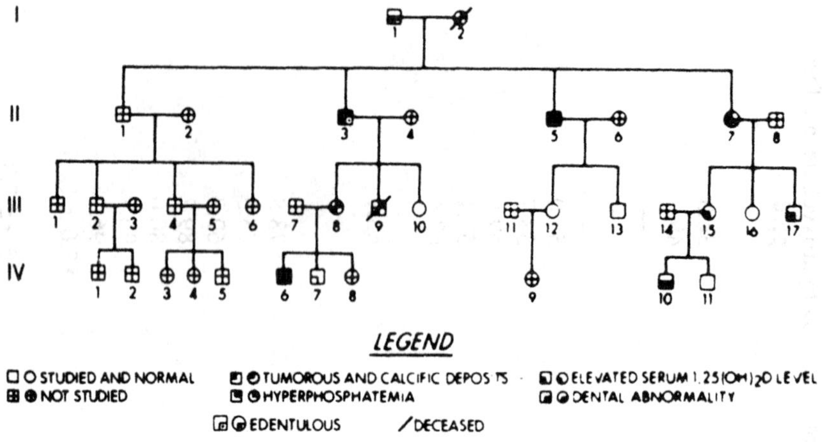

Fig. 4. Family pedigree of family-D.

In 1961, a family from central North Carolina was reported with a syndrome in which two brothers and an unrelated man had hetrotopic calcification as periarticular masses, hyperphosphatemia, and angioid streaks of the retina *(12)*. This kindred led other investigators to speculate that hyperphosphatemic tumoral calcinosis was transmitted in an autosomal recessive mode. Later studies of the same North Carolina kindred showed other phenotypic markers (dental lesion and elevated 1,25 [OH] D levels) in addition to periarticular tumors, that suggested an autosomal dominant mode of inheritance with variable clinical expressivity.

Analysis

We review data from the two kindreds below to gain insight into the possible genetic mode of disease transmission. We label the Galveston family as family G (Fig. 3 and Table 1), and the North Carolina family as family D (Fig. 4 and Table 2). Both the families were African-American families and there was no reported consanguinity in either family.

Analysis of Family G

1. The index generation (III) has affected individuals only in one generation.
2. Affected to unaffected members ratio within the family was approx 1:1.
3. Biochemical profile of the parents of the index generation (II8 and II9) shows that the mother had significant elevation of calcitriol.
4. Similar findings are found in the subsequent generation of family G (IV1 and IV2).
5. Even among the unaffected members of family G had an elevated mean phosphorus (4.9) and 1,25 (OH) Vit. D levels (53.9).

The presence of elevated serum phosphorus and elevated calcitriol levels as disease markers, suggest a variable clinical expressivity of tumoral calcinosis.

Table 2
Biochemical Parameters of the Studied Individuals of Family D

Pedigree	Age (yr)	Sex	Calcium (mg/dL)	Phosphorus (mg/dL)	250HD (ng/mL)	1,25-$(OH)_2$D (pg/mL)	Dental lesion	Clinically apparent tumors
I-1	87	M	8.91	3.11	24.8	72.1	Edentulous	No
II-3	56	M	8.70	5.50	71.4	83.5	Edentulous	Yes
II-5	52	M	10.00	6.10	41.3	59.8	Yes	Yes
II-7	49	F	8.80	4.03	37.9	60.5	Edentulous	Yes
III-8	30	F	9.90	4.90	17.3	87.7	No	No
III-10	20	F	9.08	4.03	18.2	45.6	No	No
III-12	21	F	9.32	3.56	40.9	34.1	No	No
III-13	20	M	8.82	4.04	22.2	25.8	No	No
III-15	30	F	8.72	3.03	36.5	80.6	No	No
III-16	27	F	8.70	2.65	34.5	27.6	No	No
III-17	15	M	8.80	4.83	60.8	73.0	No	No
IV-6	8	M	8.80	7.30	18.2	88.6	Yes	Yes
IV-7	6	M	9.63	4.99	NA	30.2	No	No
IV-10	12	M	8.92	4.35	60.8	73.3	Yes	No
IV-11	8	M	8.88	4.96	29.5	NA[a]	No	No
Normal Range			8.70–10.2	[b]	15–80	19–50		

[a] NA, Not available.

[b] Age-specific normal range: 4.5 –6. 5 (children 2–8 yr); 3.5–6.0 (children 8–16); 2.5 – 4.5 (adults).

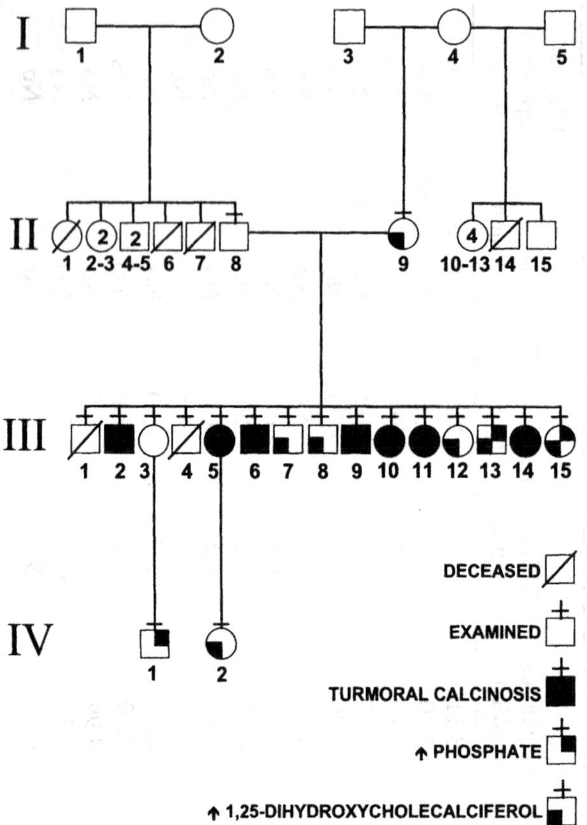

Fig. 5. Re-creation of pedigree of family G.

The 1:1 mode of affection favors an autosomal dominant mode of inheritance. Dental lesions were not documented in the family.

In family D, the disease is present in all generations. The clinical expression varies from a simple dental abnormality, asymptomatic elevations of phosphate and calcitriol to periarticular calcific masses with dental lesions, and biochemical abnormalities. The disease may skip generations. We believe that these findings suggest an autosomal dominant mode of inheritance with variable expression and incomplete penetrance. Figure 5 is a re-creation of the family G with the available data.

Conclusion

We postulate that the mode of inheritance of tumoral calcinosis is autosomal dominant with variable clinical expression and incomplete penetrance. Further studies of affected kindred will be necessary to confirm our hypothesis.

Acknowledgments

We appreciate artistic support from the Durham VAMC medical media service. This work was supported by the VA medical research service, A611268 from NIA, HD 30442 from NICHHD and RR-30 from the division of research resources, General clinical research centers program, NIH.

References

1. White, M. P. (1996) *Tumoral Calcinosis. Primer on the Metabolic and Bone Diseases and Disorders of Mineral Metabolism*, 3rd ed., Lippincott-Raven, Philadelphia.
2. Quarles, L. D., Murphy, G., Econs, M. J., Martinez, S., Lobaugh, B., and Lyles, K. W. (1991) Uremic tumoral calcinosis: a disorder associated with aberrant vitamin D homeostasis. *Am. J. Kidney Dis.* **18 (6),** 760–710.
3. Beck, D. and Lyles, K. W. (1998) Dementia associated with tumoral calcinosis. *Clin. Neurol. Neurosurg.* **100,** 121–125 .
4. Giard, A. (1898) Sur la calcification hibernale. *CR Soc. Biol* . **10,** 1013–1015.
5. Duret, M. H. (1899) Tumers multiples et singulietes des bourses sereuses. *Bull. Soc. Anat. Paris* **74,** 725–733.
6. Inclan, A. (1943) Tumoral calcinosis. *JAMA* **121,** 490–495.
7. Prince, M. J., Schaefer, P. C., Goldsmith, R. S., and Chausmer, A. B. (1982) Hyperphosphatemic tumoral calcinosis. *Ann. Intern. Med.* **96,** 586–591.
8. Lyles, K. W., Burkes, E. J., Ellis, G. J., Lucas, K. J., Dolan, E. A., and Drezner, M. K. (1985) Genetic transmission of tumoral calcinosis; Autosomal dominant with variable clinical expressivity, *J. Clin. Endocrinol. Metab.* **60(6),** 1093–1096.
9. Lyles, K. W., Halsey, D. L., Friedman, N. E., and Lobaugh, B. (1988) Correlations of serum concentrations of 1,25. Dihydroxy vitamin D, Phosphorus and parathyroid hormone in tumoral calcinosis. *J. Clin. Endocrinol. Metab.* **67(1),** 88–92.
10. Ghormley, R. K., Manning, G. F., Power, M. H., and McCrary, W. E. (1941) Multiple calcified bursae and calcified cysts in the soft tissues. *Trans. Western Surg. Assn.* **51,** 292–309.
11. Baldursson, H., Evans, B. E., Dodge, W. F., and Jackson, W. T. (1969) Tumoral calcinosis with hyperphosphaternia. *J. Bone Joint Surg.* **51A(5),** 913–925.
12. Mc.Phaul, J. J. and Engel, F. L. (1961) Heterotopic calcification hyperphosphatemia and angioid streaks of the retina, *Am. J. Med.* **31,** 488–492.

CHAPTER 10

Fibrous Dysplasia and the McCune–Albright Syndrome

Lee S. Weinstein

Introduction

Fibrous dysplasia (FD) was first described over 50 years ago *(1)*. The majority of patients with FD have a single bone lesion (monoostotic fibrous dysplasia, MOFD). The remainder have multiple lesions (polyostotic fibrous dysplasia, POFD) and of these, a small fraction have the McCune–Albright syndrome (MAS), characterized by the coexistence of FD, hyperpigmented café-au-lait skin lesions, and multiple hyperfunctional endocrine abnormalities. Although the relative incidence of these three entities has been reported to be 70% MOFD, 30% POFD, and less than 3% MAS *(2)*, the relative incidence of MAS is higher if one considers the co-occurrence of FD and any other MAS manifestation to be a form-fruste of MAS. The femur, tibia, humerus, ribs, and craniofacial bones are most commonly affected *(2–4)* whereas the bones of the hands, feet, and spine are usually spared. In long bones FD is typically found in the metaphyses and diaphyses, generally sparing the epiphyses *(3,5–7)*.

FD can result in skeletal deformities (leg length discrepancy, shepard's crook deformity, facial assymmetry), recurrent pathological fractures, pain, and nerve compression *(3,4,8)*. Rarely chest wall deformity may lead to restrictive pulmonary disease *(2,3)*. High output cardiac failure due to arteriovenous shunting through bone lesions in patients with extensive disease has been reported *(9)*. In many patients (particularly those with MOFD), FD is asymptomatic and noted as an incidental radiologic finding *(3)*. FD is usually diagnosed in the first decade of life and often progresses until the third decade, at which time it usually becomes quiescent *(4,8)*. In children, FD may be associated with advanced bone age *(6,10)*. In some cases the onset of puberty, pregnancy, or the use of oral contraceptives may be associated with progression of FD *(3,11)*. Active disease is usually asso-

The Genetics of Osteoporosis and Metabolic Bone Disease
Ed.: M. J. Econs © Humana Press Inc., Totowa, NJ

ciated with mildly to moderately increased serum alkaline phosphatase and other biochemical markers of bone turnover *(12)*. FD may undergo malignant degeneration, most often to osteosarcoma and occasionally to chondrosarcoma, fibrosarcomas, or other types of sarcoma *(13–15)*. It is possible, although not proven, that radiotherapy increases the risk of malignant transformation. Some FD patients also have multple intramuscular myxomas, often located in the vicinity of the FD lesions (Mazaboud's syndrome) *(16)*.

McCune–Albright Syndrome (MAS)

MAS *(5,17)* has been generally defined as the co-occurrence of sexual precocity, POFD, and areas of skin hyperpigmentation (café-au-lait spots). However MAS can present with multiple other endocrine abnormalities, including thyroid nodules and hyperthyroidism, adrenal hyperplasia and hypercortisolism, pituitary tumors with acromegaly and hyperprolactinemia, and hypophosphatemic rickets or osteomalacia *(6,8,18)*. Other nonendocrine abnormalities, affecting the liver, heart, thymus, spleen, bone marrow, gastrointestinal tract, and brain, are also occasionally present. *(19,20)*. Therefore some MAS patients may present with only two of the features of the classic triad or one of these features and another endocrine or nonendocrine abnormality *(8,21,22)*.

The café-au-lait spots appear as hyperpigmented flat macules which become more obvious with age *(6,8)*. Café-au-lait spots in MAS generally have irregular borders (''coast of Maine''), in contrast to those in neurofibromatosis (''coast of California'') *(5)*. The café-au-lait spots are often on one side of the body (which corresponds to the side with FD) and generally do not cross the midline. They are usually arranged in a segmental pattern following the developmental lines of Blaschko *(23)*. Histologically the pigmented macules in MAS and neurofibromatosis appear similar. However, the melanocytes within neurofibromatosis lesions develop giant pigmented granules in response to DOPA while those within MAS lesions do not *(10)*.

Sexual precocity in girls usually presents as premature menses followed by breast development *(6,8,24)*. Enlarged ovarian follicles appear and regress in a cyclic manner accompanied by cyclical changes in serum estrogen *(22,24,25)*. There is no evidence of ovulation and sometimes enlarged follicles remain as ovarian cysts. Females with MAS generally undergo normal adolescent development with normal reproduction in adult life. Boys present with precocious puberty less commonly than girls *(6,8)*. In both males and females sexual precocity is gonadotropin-independent *(26)*. Sexual precocity in either sex is usually associated with advanced bone age.

MAS patients may present with thyroid abnormalities at any age, even soon after birth, usually with benign nodular or diffuse goiter detected by physical exam or ultrasound *(6,8,27)*. The nodules usually show increased radioiodine uptake *(28)* and are often associated with hyperthyroidism. Hypercortisolism in

MAS often presents as decreased growth rate in children and can occur very early in life *(6,8)*. MAS patients with hypercortisolism might be more prone to unexplained sudden death after adrenalectomy *(20)*. Patients have adrenal nodular hyperplasia or adrenal adenomas which secrete cortisol in an ACTH-independent manner *(6,8,29)*. Acromegaly and hyperprolactinemia in association with pituitary adenoma or nodular hyperplasia are also present in a small number of patients *(6,8)*. Whereas acromegaly in MAS may be associated with hyperprolactinemia, hyperprolactinemia in the absence acromegaly has not been reported in MAS. Acromegaly in young children will accelerate bone growth and the deformities resulting from craniofacial FD may sometimes appear similar to those of acromegaly. No other pituitary hormones have been reported to be hypersecreted in MAS.

Some patients with MAS or POFD present with hyperphosphaturic hypophosphatemic rickets or osteomalacia in the absence of hyperparathyroidism *(6,8,30–33)*. Some have suggested that hypophosphatemia results from inappropriate secretion of a phosphaturic factor from FD lesions, similar to the mechanism of tumor-associated hypophosphaturic hypophosphatemic rickets *(31,34)*, although others have suggested that there is a primary defect in the renal proximal tubule *(35,36)*. MAS patients with hypophosphatemia were demonstrated to have increased basal urinary cAMP *(33)*, consistent with the presence of a defect in the proximal tubule that leads to abnormal cAMP production. The coexistence of hyperparathyroidism (due to parathyroid adenoma) and FD (primarily MOFD) has been reported *(10,37–39)*. Surgical correction of hyperparathyroidism did not result in regression of the bone lesions. It is possible that most, if not all, of these patients have the autosomal dominant syndrome of hyperparathyroidism and fibro-osseous tumors, a distinct clinical and genetic entity that has been subsequently recognized *(39–41)*. Hyperparathyroidism has not been associated with MAS.

There are a small number of MAS patients who present with one or more nonendocrine abnormalities, which are sometimes associated with increased morbidity and mortality *(20)*. Nonendocrine manifestations occur more frequently in patients with the early development of extensive POFD or hypercortisolism *(4,20)*. These abnormalities may include severe neonatal jaundice, elevated liver enzymes, cardiomegaly, persistent tachycardia and unexplained sudden death, thymic hyperplasia, myelofibrosis with extramedullary hematopoiesis, gastrointestinal polyps, pancreatitis, breast and endometrial cancer, microcephaly, and other neurological abnormalities *(8,20)*.

Genetics

All forms of FD, with very rare exceptions, occur sporadically in a single family member. There is one report of POFD in multiple family members *(42)*. Two other reports suggest the inheritance of disease from mother to daughter *(37,43)*. In one of these families both mother and daughter had hyperparathyroidism and FD *(37)*. It is possible that this latter family has the autosomal dominant syndrome of hyperparathyroidism and fibro-osseous tumors *(40,41)*. Two brothers with POFD were reported to be born from nonconsanguinous unaffected parents *(44)*. There are no reported instances of MAS in more than one family member.

Radiological Findings

Nuclear scintigraphy with 99m-technetium methylene diphosphonate is the most sensitive method to survey the skeleton for FD *(45)*. FD lesions have also been reported to have increased gallium-67 uptake *(46,47)*. One MOFD lesion has been recently demonstrated to have increased peripheral activity on single photon emission compated tomography (SPECT) scanning *(48)*. On standard radiographs FD lesions are typically cystic and appear to originate in the medullary cavity and expand into the surrounding cortical bone *(3,6,7)*. Usually the surrounding cortex is thin but in some cases becomes sclerotic. The lesions are usually radiolucent or exhibit a ground-glass appearance but occasionally may be sclerotic or have a mixed appearance *(7)*. Calcifications may be visible in those lesions with a large cartilagenous component *(49)*. Other bone lesions with a similar radiographic appearance to FD include Paget's disease, osteitis fibrosa cystica, bone cysts, giant cell tumor, fibroma, chondroma, and other types of bone tumors *(3,7)*. Young patients with POFD or MAS may show advanced bone age *(6,10)*. Decreased bone density or radiographic features of rickets or osteomalacia is usually present in patients with accompanying hypophosphatemia or hypercortisolism *(6,8,50)*.

Magnetic resonance imaging (MRI) has recently been shown to be useful in defining the extent of disease, particularly in areas in which standard X-rays are not very sensitive, such as the spine *(51,52)*. Usually the lesions are hypodense on T1-weighted images but may be hypo- or hyperdense on T2- or STIR-weighted images *(51–53)*. It has been suggested that lesions with a large amount of cartilage *(51)*, decreased cellularity, or cystic changes *(53)*, are hyperdense on T2-weighted images whereas those that have more cellularity and bony trabeculae or sclerotic changes are hypodense on T2-weighted images *(51,53)*.

Pathology of FD

FD lesions expand concentrically from the medullary cavity to the cortical bone and are composed primarily of cells which appear like long, spindle-shaped fibroblasts and myofibroblasts arranged in parallel arrays or whirls and embedded in a collagen matrix (Fig. 1)*(54)*. In some areas the matrix may appear myxomatous. The fibroblast-like cells are actually of the osteogenic lineage, since they express alkaline phosphatase and proteins associated with the early stages of osteoblast maturation *(55)*. Embedded within the hypercellular matrix are spicules of immature woven bone mostly lined by flat osteoblasts with retracted cell bodies, forming pseudo-lacunar spaces *(54,55)*. Unlike normal woven bone, collagen bundles are arranged perpendicular to the bone-forming surface *(55)*. Also, these

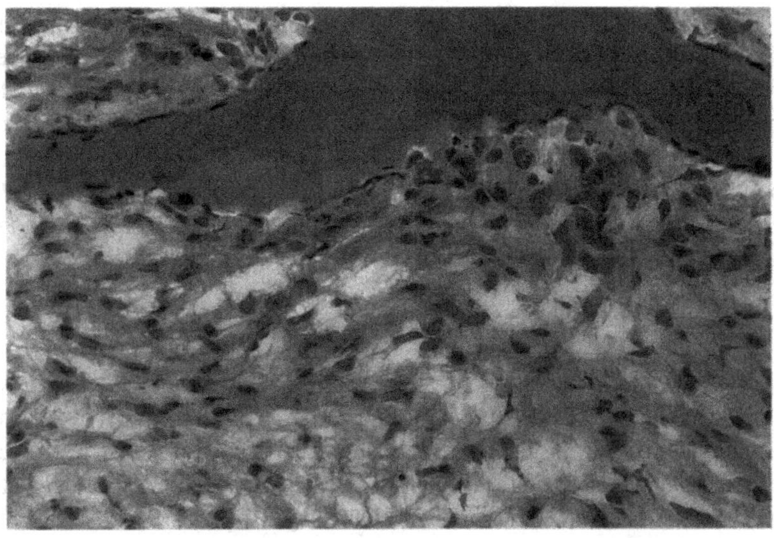

Fig 1. Histological section from a lesion of FD (H & E). Hypercellular tissue containing elongated fibroblast-like cells in a collagenous matrix dominate the section. One spicule of immature woven bone is present. Note that the bone spicule is surrounded in many areas by flattened cells which are morphologically different than normal cuboidal osteoblasts. There are no cartilaginous elements in this section.

trabeculae have large osteocytic lacunae each accommodating multiple osteocytes (hyperosteocytic bone) *(55)*. The cells and matrix of woven bone trabeculae in FD contain osteonectin, but not osteopontin or bone sialoprotein, proteins which are present in normal woven bone *(55)*. Replacement of the woven bone by mature lamellar bone, which normally occurs during bone development, does not occur in FD lesions.

Some FD lesions have islands of hyaline cartilage surrounded by fibroblast-like cells *(54)*. The cartilage generally appears normal and can undergo endochondral ossification. In rare cases the cartilaginous component is the dominant feature (termed fibrocartilaginous dysplasia) *(49)*. Although this can be confused with chondrosarcoma, the presence of surrounding fibro-osseous tissue usually makes the diagnosis of FD straightforward. Endochondral ossification in these lesions may produce stippled or ring-like calcifications on radiographs. Some lesions of FD contain calcified spherules, a typical feature of cemento-ossifying fibroma. These two benign fibrous lesions can be difficult to distinguish histologically and may represent a histological spectrum of a similar process *(56)*. Osteitis fibrosa cystica and Paget's disease also look histologically similar to FD. Paget's disease occurs in later life and osteitis fibrosa cystica is associated with hyperparathyroidism or uremia. Neither of these lesions contain cartiginous islands.

FD expands into the outer cortical bone resulting in cortical thinning and in some cases concentric bulging of the cortex. Peripherally there are increased numbers of osteoclasts which have increased numbers of nuclei per cell *(57)* and spicules of normal lamellar bone undergoing active osteoclastic resorption *(55)*. In rare cases FD may be more aggressive, resulting in exophytic protuberances *(58)* or invasion into surrounding soft tissue *(59)*. These lesions are benign and do not metastasize. FD can undergo malignant degeneration, usually to osteosarcoma and less commonly to chondrosarcoma, fibrsarcoma, or malignant fibrohistiosarcoma *(14,15)*.

Pathogenesis of FD and MAS

It was noted that the cutaneous hyperpigmentation in MAS often follows the developmental lines of Blaschko. Happle proposed that MAS is caused by a dominant somatic mutation occurring early in development which would result in a mosaic with the widespead distribution of genetically abnormal cells *(23)*. This model predicts that the specific constellation of abnormalities within a given patient is determined by the distribution of mutant-bearing cells. The next important step in defining the pathogenesis of MAS was the demonstration that the abnormal endocrine glands in MAS patients were functioning autonomously *(6,26,28,60–62)*. cAMP is known to stimulate growth and hormonal secretion in many endocrine glands (including the thyroid, adrenal cortex, gonads, and somatotrophs) and the production of melanin pigment in melanocytes *(6,61,63,64)*. Therefore, a widespread defect leading to excess intracellular cAMP could explain many of the clinical manifestations of MAS.

The heterotrimeric G proteins are a family of proteins that couple a large number of receptors for extracellular ligands to intracellular enzymes and ion channels. Each G protein is a heterotrimer composed of a specific α, β, and γ subunit *(65)*. The α-subunit binds guanine nucleotide and interacts with specific receptors and effectors. In the inactive state, the guanosine diphosphate (GDP)-bound α-subunit is associated with a noncovalently bound βγ dimer. When a receptor is activated by binding of a specific ligand (e.g., hormone), it interacts with and activates specific G protein heterotrimers, leading to the exchange of guanosine triphosphate (GTP) for GDP on the α-subunit and dissociation of the α-subunit from βγ. GTP-bound α-subunits regulate the activity of specific effectors. The α-subunit of G_s ($G_s\alpha$) stimulates the activity of adenylyl cyclases, a family of enzymes that catalyze cAMP synthesis. Each α-subunit has an intrinsic GTPase activity which "turns off" the G protein by hydrolyzing bound GTP to GDP *(66)*. Modifications which disrupt the GTPase activity will result in constitutive activation. Constitutive activation of G_s leads to overproduction of cAMP. Mutations which encode substitutions of amino acid residues Arg^{201} or Gln^{227} in $G_s\alpha$ have been found in human thyroid and growth hormone-secreting pituitary tumors and shown to result in constitutive activation due to decreased GTPase activity *(67–71)*. Since both thyroid tumors and acromegaly are present in MAS patients, it seemed likely that activating $G_s\alpha$ mutations might be present in a more widespread distribution in MAS.

Activating $G_s\alpha$ mutations encoding Arg^{201} substitutions (but not Gln^{227} substitutions) have been found in tissues from many MAS patients *(19,20,72)*. Subsequently, elevated cAMP levels have been demonstrated in liver tissue and urine from MAS patients *(33,73)*. One specific mutation (Arg^{201} to His or Cys) is detected within multiple tissues of each patient. The mutation is present in variable abundance in different tissues, consistent with a widespread distribution of a population of cells harboring a dominant somatic mutation. These mutations are present in virtually all hyperplastic or adenomatous endocrine tissues examined and in a café-au-lait lesion from one MAS patient *(74)*. Mutations are also found in many nonendocrine tissues, some of which are abnormal (e.g., liver, heart, thymus) *(19,20)*. The role of G_s activation in the pathogenesis of these nonendocrine manifestations is not well established. It is of interest that in Albright hereditary osteodystrophy (AHO), $G_s\alpha$ loss-of-function mutations are associated with ectopic bone formation and resistance to multiple hormones which stimulate cAMP production *(75,76)*.

Activating $G_s\alpha$ mutations are also present in bone lesions from MAS patients *(72,77)* and in cells cultured from two MOFD lesions *(78)*. MOFD appears to result from the same somatic mutation as in MAS, but in a limited tissue distribution. An Arg^{201} to Ser was identified in abnormal bone from one severely affected patient *(79)*. In most bone lesions the mutant and wild-type alleles are present in roughly equal amounts, suggesting that the vast majority of the cells within these lesions are abnormal. This is consistent with the notion that FD results from excessive proliferation and abnormal differentiation of a mesenchymal osteoprogenitor cell *(1,72)*. In cultured cells, parathyroid hormone and forskolin (both stimulators of cAMP production) inhibit *(80,81)* whereas $G_s\alpha$ antisense oligonucleotides promote osteoblast differentiation *(82)*. Cells within FD lesions have increased basal intracellular cAMP levels *(57,83)* and an increased proliferation rate *(83)* but appear poorly differentiated morphologically and express proteins associated with early but not late stages of osteoblast differentiation *(55,83,84)*. cAMP has also been shown to alter the morphology of cultured osteoblasts, resulting in a retracted, stellate appearance similar to cells present in FD *(55)*.

Upon binding of cAMP to the regulatory subunits of cAMP-dependent protein kinase (PKA), these subunits dissociate from the catalytic subunits, allowing the catalytic subunits to translocate to the nucleus and phosphorylate cAMP-responsive transcription factors such as CREB and CREM (Fig. 2). Phosphorylated CREB can then activate cAMP-responsive genes, such as c-*fos* *(85)*. Fos, the product of c-*fos*, binds with Jun to form the heterodimer AP-1, which binds to the promoters of many genes and regulates their expression. AP-1 is highly expressed during the early proliferative phase of osteoblast development and its expression markedly decreases upon the onset of differentiation *(86)*. The gene for osteocalcin, a late marker of osteoblast differentiation, has AP-1 binding sites within two activating regions of its promoter (a vitamin D responsive element and the osteocalcin box). Binding of AP-1 to these regions suppresses both basal and vitamin D-induced expression of osteocalcin

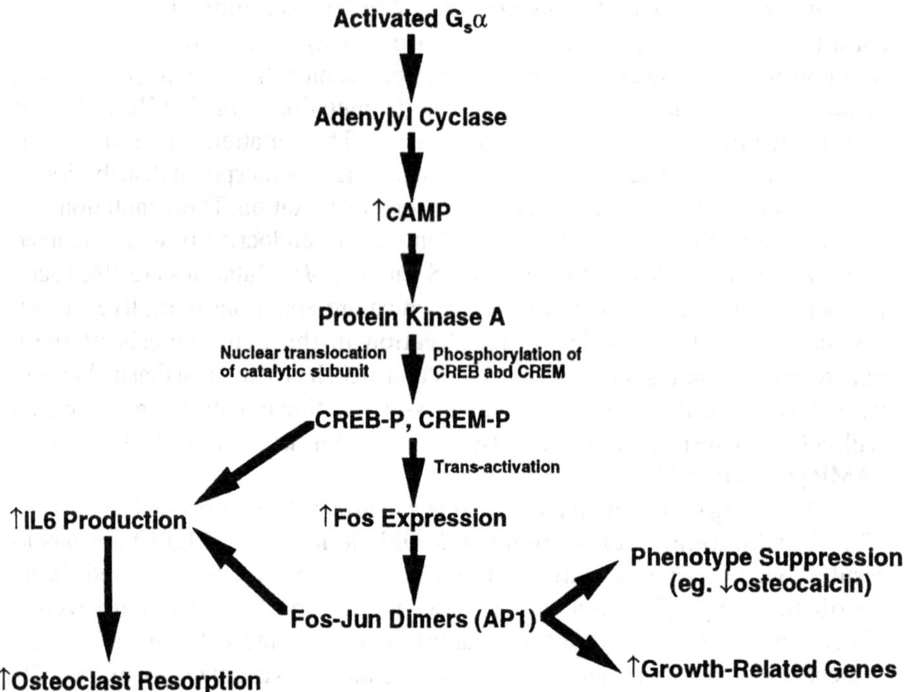

Fig. 2. Possible mechanisms by which activated G_s in osteogenic cells may lead to FD. G_s activation increases the activity of the effector adenylyl cyclase, leading to increased intracellular cAMP levels. Binding of cAMP to the regulatory subunits of cAMP-dependent protein kinase (PKA) allows release of its catalytic subunits, which translocate to the nucleus and phosphorylate proteins such as CREB and CREM. Phosphorylated CREB binds to promoters of cAMP-responsive immediate-early genes (e.g., c-*fos*) and increases their expression. Fos , the product of c-*fos*, binds with Jun to form AP-1. AP-1 is a transcription factor which increases the expression of growth-related genes and decreases the expression of osteoblast-specific genes, such as osteocalcin (phenotype suppression). CREB-P and AP-1 may both stimulate the transcription of the IL-6 gene. IL-6 may be important in recruiting osteoclasts and stimulating osteoclastic bone resorption.

(86). Therefore AP-1 expression during the proliferative stage of osteoblast development can suppress the expression of genes associated with osteoblast differentiation (phenotype suppression).

Several lines of evidence suggest that Fos overexpression in osteogenic precursors plays an important role in the pathogenesis of FD. Activated G_s has been shown to chronically increase the expression of c-*fos (87)* and Fos has been shown to be overexpressed in FD lesions *(88)*. The abnormal expression of Fos was localized to the stellate cells presumed to be immature osteoblastic precursors.

Fos overexpression in transgenic mice leads to abnormal bone remodeling and bone lesions which are similar to FD *(89)*. Fos is overexpressed in many human osteosarcomas *(90)* and mice which overexpress Fos eventually develop osteosarcomas *(91)*. Therefore Fos may play a role in the development of malignant bone lesions in patients with FD. In summary, the primary defect in FD is likely to be excess proliferation and abnormal differentiation of osteoblast precursors resulting from excess intracellular cAMP and abnormal expression of downstream transcription factors such as Fos.

Another characteristic feature of FD is increased osteoclastic bone resorption, which allows the abnormal medullary cells to expand into normal cortical bone. Cells isolated from FD lesions from two MAS patients had increased IL-6 (as well as IL-11) production which could not be stimulated further by added cAMP but could be decreased by the cAMP antagonist Rp-8Br-cAMP *(57)*. It is therefore likely that increased IL-6 production is the direct result of increased intracellular cAMP, especially since the IL-6 promoter has both cAMP response element and AP-1 sites. IL-6 overproduction is known to lead to increased numbers of osteoclasts and osteoclastic bone resorption, and it seems likely that IL-6 overproduction by osteogenic cells in FD leads to increased bone resorption. The platelet-derived growth factor β chain (PDGF-B) is expressed at abnormally high levels in FD and other fibrous bone lesions *(92)*. PDGF-B may stimulate fibroblast proliferation and osteoclast activation. Increased levels of sex steroid receptors in cells from FD lesions *(84,93)* and the ability of sex steroids to increase PDGF-B expression *(92)* may explain why FD sometimes progresses in puberty or pregnancy *(11)*.

Management of FD

In many cases no specific therapy is warranted since FD is often asymptomatic and nonprogressive. Fractures usually heal well with conservative management *(4)*. Surgery is required for nonhealing fractures, severe pain or deformity, or nerve compression *(2,4,94,95)*. Surgery usually involves excision or curretage and bone grafting. Radiotherapy is generally ineffective and may increase the risk of sarcomatous degeneration *(13–15)*. The important role of osteoclastic resorption in the expansion of FD lesions *(57)* suggests that osteoclastic resorption inhibitors might be effective therapeutic agents. Case reports have suggested that calcitonin, etidronate, and clodronate provide little benefit *(50,96,97)*. Short- and long-term use of intravenous pamidronate resulted in significantly decreased bone pain in all patients and radiological improvement in some but not all patients *(98–100)*. Biochemical markers of bone resorption were also decreased after pamidronate. It should be noted that no blinded, controlled prospective studies with pamidronate have been performed *(101)*. Reversible growth-plate widening was observed in a 13-yr-old patient *(98,99)*. Therefore younger patients on pamidronate need to be followed closely and all patients should be given calcium and vitamin D supplements to prevent hypocalcemia and elevated PTH.

References

1. Lichtenstein, L. and Jaffe, H. L. (1942) Fibrous dysplasia of bone: a condition affecting one, several or many bones, the graver cases of which may present abnormal pigmentation of skin, premature sexual development, hyperthyroidism or still other extraskeletal abnormalities. *Arch. Pathol.* **33,** 777–816.
2. Nager, G. T., Kennedy, D. W., and Kopstein, E. (1982) Fibrous dysplasia: a review of the disease and its manifestations in the temporal bone. *Ann. Otol. Rhinol. Laryngol. Suppl.* **92,** 1–52.
3. Schlumberger, H. G. (1946) Fibrous dysplasia of single bones (monostotic fibrous dysplasia). *Mil. Surg.* **99,** 504–527.
4. Harris, W. H., Dudley, H. R. Jr., and Barry, R. J. (1962) The natural history of fibrous dysplasia. *J. Bone Joint Surg.* **44–A,** 207–233.
5. Albright, F., Butler, A. M., Hampton, A. O., and Smith, P. (1937) Syndrome characterized by osteitis fibrosa disseminata, areas of pigmentation and endocrine dysfunction, with precocious puberty in females. *N. Engl. J. Med.* **216,** 727–746.
6. Mauras, N. and Blizzard, R. M. (1986) The McCune–Albright syndrome. *Acta Endocrinol. (Copenh)* **279 (Supp.),** 207–217.
7. Lucas, E., Sundaram, M., and Boccini, T. (1995) Radiological case study: polyostotic fibrous dysplasia. *Orthopedics* **18,** 311–313.
8. Danon, M. and Crawford, J. D. (1987) The McCune–Albright Syndrome. *Ergeb. Inn. Med. Kinderheilkd.* **55,** 81–115.
9. Fischer, J. A., Bollinger, A., Lichtlen, P., and Wellauer, J. (1970) Fibrous dysplasia of the bone and high cardiac output. *Am. J. Med.* **49,** 140–146.
10. Benedict, P. H. (1962) Endocrine features in Albright's syndrome (fibrous dysplasia of bone). *Metabolism* **11,** 30–45.
11. Stevens–Simon, C., Stewart, J., Nakashima, I. I., and White, M. (1991) Exacerbation of fibrous dysplasia associated with an adolescent pregnancy. *J. Adolesc. Health* **12,** 403–405.
12. Singer, F. R. (1997) Fibrous dysplasia of bone: the bone lesion unmasked. *Am. J. Pathol.* **151,** 1511–1515.
13. Tanner, H. C.,Jr., Dahlin, D. C., and Childs, D. S.,Jr. (1961) Sarcoma complicating fibrous dysplasia: probable role of radiation therapy. *Oral Surg. Oral Med. Oral Pathol.* **14,** 837–846.
14. Yabut, S. M., Kenan, S., Sissons, H. A., and Lewis, M. M. (1988) Malignant transformation of fibrous dysplasia: a case report and review of the literature. *Clin. Orthop.* **228,** 281–289.
15. Ruggieri, P., Sim, F. H., Bond, J. R., and Unni, K. K. (1994) Malignancies in fibrous dysplasia. *Cancer* **73,** 1411–1424.
16. Aoki, T., Kouho, H., Hisaoka, M., Hashimoto, H., Nakata, H., and Sakai, A. (1995) Intramuscular myxoma with fibrous dysplasia: a report of two cases with a review of the literature. *Pathol. Int.* **45,** 165–171.
17. McCune, D. J. (1936) Osteitis fibrosa cystica; the case of a nine year old girl who also exhibits precocious puberty, multiple pigmentation of the skin and hyperthyroidism. *Am. J. Dis. Child.* **52,** 743–744.
18. Schwindinger, W. F. and Levine, M. A. (1993) McCune–Albright syndrome. *Trends Endocrinol. Metab.* **4,** 238–242.

19. Weinstein, L. S., Shenker, A., Gejman, P. V., Merino, M. J., Friedman, E., and Spiegel, A. M. (1991) Activating mutations of the stimulatory G protein in the McCune–Albright syndrome. *N. Engl. J. Med.* **325,** 1688–1695.
20. Shenker, A., Weinstein, L. S., Moran, A., et al. (1993) Severe endocrine and nonendocrine manifestations of the McCune–Albright syndrome associated with activating mutations of stimulatory G protein G_s. *J. Pediatr.* **123,** 509–518.
21. Grant, D. B. and Martinez, L. (1983) The McCune–Albright syndrome without typical skin pigmentation. *Acta Paediatr. Scand.* **72,** 477–478.
22. Rieth, K. G., Comite, F., Shawker, T. H. and Cutler, G. B. (1984) Pituitary and ovarian abnormalities demonstrated by CT and ultrasound in children with features of the McCune–Albright syndrome. *Radiology* **153,** 389–393.
23. Happle, R. (1986) The McCune–Albright syndrome: a lethal gene surviving by mosaicism. *Clin. Genet.* **29,** 321–324.
24. Feuillan, P. P. (1993) Treatment of sexual precocity in girls with the McCune–Albright syndrome, in *Sexual Precocity: Etiology, Diagnosis and Management* (Grave, G. D. and Cutler, G. B., eds.), Raven Press, New York, pp. 243–251.
25. Comite, F., Shawker, T. H., Pescovitz, O. H., Loriaux, D. L., and Cutler, G. B. (1984) Cyclical ovarian function resistant to treatment with an analogue of luteinizing hormone releasing hormone in McCune–Albright syndrome. *N. Engl. J. Med.* **311,** 1032–1036.
26. Foster, C. M., Ross, J. L., Shawker, T., Pescovitz, O. H., Loriaux, D. L., and Cutler, G. B., Jr. (1984) Absence of pubertal gonadotropin secretion in girls with McCune–Albright syndrome. *J. Clin. Endocrinol. Metab.* **5,** 1161–1165.
27. Mastorakos, G., Koutras, D. A., Doufas, A. G., and Mitsiades, N. S. (1997) Hyperthyroidism in McCune–Albright syndrome with a review of thyroid abnormalities sixty years after the first report. *Thyroid* **7,** 433–439.
28. Feuillan, P. P., Shawker, T., Rose, S. R., Jones, J., Jeevanram, R. K., and Nisula, B. C. (1990) Thyroid abnormalities in the McCune–Albright syndrome: ultrasonography and hormone studies. *J. Clin. Endocrinol. Metab.* **71,** 1596–1601.
29. Benjamin, D. R. and McRoberts, J. W. (1973) Polyostotic fibrous dysplasia associated with Cushing syndrome. *Arch. Pathol.* **96,** 175–178.
30. Ryan, W. G., Nibbe, A. F., Schwartz, T. B., and Ray, R. D. (1968) Fibrous dysplasia of bone with vitamin D resistant rickets: a case study. *Metabolism* **17,** 988–998.
31. McArthur, R. G., Hayles, A. B., and Lambert, P. W. (1979) Albright's syndrome with rickets. *Mayo Clin. Proc.* **54,** 313–320.
32. Hahn, S. B., Lee, S. B., and Kim, D. H. (1991) Albright's syndrome with hypophosphatemic rickets and hyperthyroidism: a case report. *Yonsei Med. J.* **32,** 179–183.
33. Zung, A., Chalew, S. A., Schwindinger, W. F., et al. (1995) Urinary cyclic adenosine 3',5'-monophosphate response in McCune–Albright syndrome: clinical evidence for altered renal adenylate cyclase activity. *J. Clin. Endocrinol. Metab.* **80,** 3576–3581.
34. Dent, C. E. and Gertner, J. M. (1976) Hypophosphataemic osteomalacia in fibrous dysplasia. *Q. J. Med.* **45,** 411–420.
35. Tanaka, T. and Suwa, S. (1977) A case of McCune–Albright syndrome with hyperthyroidism and vitamin D-resistant rickets. *Helv. Paediat. Acta* **32,** 263–273.
36. Lever, E. G. and Pettingale, K. W. (1983) Albright's syndrome associated with a soft-tissue myxoma and hypophosphatemic osteomalacia: report of a case and review of the literature. *J. Bone Joint Surg.* **65–B,** 621–626.
37. Firat, D. and Stutzman, L. (1968) Fibrous dysplasia of the bone: a review of twenty-four cases. *Am. J. Med.* **44,** 421–429.

38. Ehrig, U. and Wilson, D. R. (1972) Fibrous dysplasia of bone and primary hyperparathyroidism. *Ann. Intern. Med.* **77,** 234–238.
39. Hammami, M. M., Hussain, S. S., Vencer, L. J., Butt, A., and al-Zahrani, A. (1997) Primary hyperparathyroidism-associated polyostotic fibrous dysplasia: absence of McCune–Albright syndrome mutations. *J. Endocrinol. Invest.* **20,** 552–558.
40. Jackson, C. E., Norum, R. A., Boyd, S. B., et al. (1990) Hereditary hyperparathyroidism and multiple ossifying jaw fibromas: a clinically and genetically distinct syndrome. *Surgery* **108,** 1006–1012.
41. Szabo, J., Heath, B., Hill, V. M., et al. (1995) Hereditary hyperparathyroidism-jaw tumor syndrome: the endocrine tumor gene HRPT2 maps to chromosome 1q21–q31. *Am. J. Hum. Genet.* **56,** 944–950.
42. Reitzik, M. and Lownie, J. F. (1975) Familial polyostotic fibrous dysplasia. *Oral Surg.* **40,** 769–774.
43. Hibbs, R. E. and Rush, H. P. (1952) Albright's syndrome. *Ann. Intern. Med.* **37,** 587–593.
44. Sarkar, A. K., Ghosh, A. K., Chowdhury, S. N., Biswas, S. K., and Bag, S. K. (1993) Fibrous dysplasia in two siblings. *Indian J. Pediatr.* **60,** 301–305.
45. Pfeffer, S., Molina, E., Feullian, P., and Simon, T. R. (1990) McCune–Albright syndrome: the patterns of scintigraphic abnormalities. *J. Nucl. Med.* **31,** 1474–1478.
46. Kapadia, K., Heyman, S., and Florio, F. (1996) Ga–67 uptake in fibrous dysplasia. *Clin. Nucl. Med.* **21,** 797–798.
47. Ohta, H., Okamoto, S., Komibuchi, T., Shintaku, M., and Hojo, M. (1997) Tc-99m HMDP and Ga–67 imaging along with CT and MRI in fibrous dysplasia of the temporal bone. *Clin. Nucl. Med.* **22,** 328–330.
48. Jimenez, C. E., Carpenter, A. L., Pacheco, E. J., and Moreno, A. J. (1996) SPECT imaging in a patient with monostotic rib fibrous dysplasia. *Clin. Nucl. Med.* **21,** 491–493.
49. Ishida, T. and Dorfman, H. D. (1993) Massive chondroid differentiation in fibrous dysplasia of bone (fibrocartilagenous dysplasia). *Am. J. Surg. Pathol.* **17,** 924–930.
50. Cole, D. E. C., Fraser, F. C., Glorieux, F. H., et al. (1983) Panostotic fibrous dysplasia: a congenital disorder of bone with unusual facial appearance, bone fragility, hyperphosphatasemia, and hypophosphatemia. *Am. J. Hum. Genet.* **14,** 725–735.
51. Inamo, Y., Hanawa, Y., Kin, H., and Okuni, M. (1993) Findings on magnetic resonance imaging of the spine and femur in a case of McCune–Albright syndrome. *Pediatr. Radiol.* **23,** 15–18.
52. Gober, G. A. and Nicholas, R. W. (1993) Case report 800. *Skeletal Radiol.* **22,** 452–455.
53. Jee, W. H., Shinn, K. S., Park, J. M., Choe, B. Y., and Choi, K. H. (1996) Fibrous dysplasia: MR imaging characteristics with radiopathologic correlation. *Am. J. Roentgenol.* **167,** 1523–1527.
54. Greco, M. A. and Steiner, G. C. (1986) Ultrastructure of fibrous dysplasia of bone: a study of its fibrous, osseous, and cartilaginous components. *Ultrastruct. Pathol.* **10,** 55–66.
55. Riminucci, M., Fisher, L. W., Shenker, A., Spiegel, A. M., Bianco, P., and Robey, P. G. (1997) Fibrous dysplasia of bone in the McCune–Albright syndrome: abnormalities in bone formation. *Am. J. Pathol.* **151,** 1587–1600.
56. Voytek, T. M., Ro, J. Y., Edeiken, J., and Ayala, A. G. (1995) Fibrous dysplasia and cemento-ossifying fibroma: a histologic spectrum. *Am. J. Surg. Pathol.* **19,** 775–781.
57. Yamamoto, T., Okada, S., Kishimoto, T., et al. (1996) Increased IL–6–production by cells isolated from the fibrous bone dysplasia tissues in patients with McCune–Albright syndrome. *J. Clin. Invest.* **98,** 30–35.

58. Dorfman, H. D., Ishida, T., and Tsuneyoshi, M. (1994) Exophytic variant of fibrous dysplasia (fibrous dysplasia protuberans). *Hum. Pathol.* **25,** 1234–1237.
59. Latham, P. D., Athanasou, N. A., and Woods, C. G. (1992) Fibrous dysplasia with locally aggressive malignant change. *Arch. Orthop. Trauma Surg.* **111,** 183–186.
60. Danon, M., Robboy, S. J., Kim, S., Scully, R., and Crawford, J. D. (1975) Cushing syndrome, sexual precocity, and polyostotic fibrous dysplasia (Albright syndrome) in infancy. *J. Pediatr.* **87,** 917–921.
61. Scully, R. E. and McNeely, B. U. (1975) Case records of the Massachusetts General Hospital: case 4-1975. *N. Engl. J. Med.* **292,** 199–203.
62. D'Armiento, M., Reda, G., Camagna, A., and Tardella, L. (1983) McCune–Albright syndrome: evidence for autonomous multiendocrine hyperfunction. *J. Pediatr.* **102,** 584–586.
63. Lee, P. A., Van Dop, C., and Migeon, C. J. (1986) McCune–Albright syndrome: Long term followup. *JAMA* **256,** 2980–2984.
64. Dumont, J. E., Jauniaux, J.-C., and Roger, P. P. (1989) The cyclic AMP-mediated stimulation of cell proliferation. *Trends Biochem. Sci.* **14,** 67–71.
65. Spiegel, A. M., Shenker, A., and Weinstein, L. S. (1992) Receptor-effector coupling by G proteins: implications for normal and abnormal signal transduction. *Endocr. Rev.* **13,** 536–565.
66. Bourne, H. R., Sanders, D. A., and McCormick, F. (1990) The GTPase superfamily: a conserved switch for diverse cell functions. *Nature* **348,** 125–132.
67. Landis, C. A., Masters, S. B., Spada, A., Pace, A. M., Bourne, H. R., and Vallar, L. (1989) GTPase inhibiting mutations activate the a chain of G_s and stimulate adenylyl cyclase in human pituitary tumours. *Nature* **340,** 692–696.
68. Masters, S. B., Miller, R. T., Chi, M.-H., et al. (1989) Mutations in the GTP-binding site of $G_s\alpha$ alter stimulation of adenylyl cyclase. *J. Biol. Chem.* **264,** 15,467–15,474.
69. Graziano, M. P. and Gilman, A. G. (1989) Synthesis in *Escherichia coli* of GTPase-deficient mutants of $G_s\alpha$. *J. Biol. Chem.* **264,** 15,475–15,482.
70. Lyons, J., Landis, C. A., Harsh, G., et al. (1990) Two G protein oncogenes in human endocrine tumors. *Science* **249,** 655–659.
71. Suarez, H. G., du Villard, J. A., Caillou, B., Schlumberger, M., Parmentier, C., and Monier, R. (1991) *gsp* mutations in human thyroid tumours. *Oncogene* **6,** 677–679.
72. Shenker, A., Weinstein, L. S., Sweet, D. E., and Spiegel, A. M. (1994) An activating $G_s\alpha$ mutation is present in fibrous dysplasia of bone in the McCune–Albright syndrome. *J. Clin. Endocrinol. Metab.* **79,** 750–755.
73. Schwindinger, W. F., Yang, S. Q., Miskovsky, E. P., Diehl, A. M., and Levine, M. A. (1993) An activating $G_s\alpha$ mutation in McCune–Albright syndrome increases hepatic adenylyl cyclase activity. *Program and Abstracts, The Endocrine Society 75th Annual Meeting,* p. 517 (Abstract).
74. Schwindinger, W. F., Francomano, C. A., and Levine, M. A. (1992) Identification of a mutation in the gene encoding the a subunit of the stimulatory G protein of adenylyl cyclase in McCune–Albright syndrome. *Proc. Natl. Acad. Sci. USA* **89,** 5152–5156.
75. Patten, J. L., Johns, D. R., Valle, D., et al. (1990) Mutation in the gene encoding the stimulatory G protein of adenylate cyclase in Albright's hereditary osteodystrophy. *N. Engl. J. Med.* **322,** 1412–1419.
76. Weinstein, L. S., Gejman, P. V., Friedman, E., et al. (1990) Mutations of the $G_s\alpha$-subunit gene in Albright hereditary osteodystrophy detected by denaturing gradient gel electrophoresis. *Proc. Natl. Acad. Sci. USA* **87,** 8287–8290.

77. Malchoff, C. D., Reardon, G., MacGillivray, D. C., Yamase, H., Rogol, A. D., and Malchoff, D. M. (1994) An unusual presentation of McCune–Albright Syndrome confirmed by an activating mutation of the $G_s\alpha$-subunit from a bone lesion. *J. Clin. Endocrinol. Metab.* **78,** 803–806.
78. Shenker, A., Chanson, P., Weinstein, L. S., et al. (1995) Osteoblastic cells derived from isolated lesions of fibrous dysplasia contain activating somatic mutations of the $G_s\alpha$ gene. *Hum. Mol. Genet.* **4,** 1675–1676.
79. Candeliere, G. A., Glorieux, F. H., and Roughley, P. J. (1997) Polymerase chain reaction-based technique for the selective enrichment and analysis of mosaic arg201 mutations in $G_s\alpha$ from patients with fibrous dysplasia of bone. *Bone* **21,** 201–206.
80. Bellows, C. G., Ishida, H., Aubin, J. E., and Heersche, J. N. M. (1990) Parathyroid hormone reversibly suppresses the differentiation of osteoprogenitor cells into functional osteoblasts. *Endocrinology* **127,** 3111–3116.
81. Turksen, K., Grigoriadis, A. E., Heersche, J. N. M., and Aubin, J. E. (1990) Forskolin has biphasic effects on osteoprogenitor cell differentiation in vitro. *J. Cell. Physiol.* **142,** 61–69.
82. Nanes, M. S., Boden, S., and Weinstein, L. S. (1995) Oligonucleotides antisense to $G_s\alpha$ promote osteoblast differentiation. *Endocrine Society 77th Annual Meeting Program and Abstracts* 62. (Abstract)
83. Marie, P. J., Lomri, A., Chanson, P., and de Pollak, C. (1997) Increased proliferation of osteoblastic cells expressing the activating $G_s\alpha$ mutation in monostotic and polyostotic fibrous dysplasia. *Am. J. Pathol.* **150,** 1059–1069.
84. Pensler, J. M., Langman, C. B., Radosevich, J. A., et al. (1990) Sex steroid hormone receptors in normal and dysplastic bone disorders in children. *J. Bone Miner. Res.* **5,** 493–498.
85. Sassone-Corsi, P. (1995) Signaling pathways and c-*fos* transcriptional response-links to inherited diseases. *N. Engl. J. Med.* **332,** 1576–1577.
86. Stein, G. S. and Lian, J. B. (1993) Molecular mechanisms mediating proliferation/differentiation interrelationships during progressive development of the osteoblast phenotype. *Endocr. Rev.* **14,** 424–442.
87. Gaiddon, C., Boutillier, A.-L., Monnier, D., Mercken, L. and Loeffler, J.-P. (1994) Genomic effects of the putative oncogene $G\alpha s$: chronic transcriptional activation of the c-*fos* proto-oncogene in endocrine cells. *J. Biol. Chem.* **269,** 22,663–22,671.
88. Candeliere, G. A., Glorieux, F. H., Prud'homme, J., and St.-Arnaud, R. (1995) Increased expression of the c-*fos* proto-oncogene in bone from patients with fibrous dysplasia. *N. Engl. J. Med.* **332,** 1546–1551.
89. Rüther, U., Garber, C., Komitowski, D., Müller, R., and Wagner, E. F. (1987) Deregulated c-*fos* expression interferes with normal bone development in transgenic mice. *Nature* **325,** 412–416.
90. Wu, J.-X., Carpenter, P. M., Gresens, C., et al. (1990) The proto-oncogene c-*fos* is overexpressed in the majority of human osteosarcomas. *Oncogene* **5,** 989–1000.
91. Grigoriadis, A. E., Schellander, K., Wang, Z.-Q., and Wagner, E. F. (1993) Osteoblasts are target cells for transformation in c-*fos* transgenic mice. *J. Cell Biol.* **122,** 685–701.
92. Alman, B. A., Naber, S. P., Terek, R. M., Jiranek, W. A., Goldberg, M. J., and Wolfe, H. J. (1995) Platelet derived growth factor in fibrous musculoskeletal disorders: a study of pathologic tissue sections and *in vitro* primary cell cultures. *J. Orthop. Res.* **13,** 67–77.
93. Kaplan, F. S., Fallon, M. D., Boden, S. D., Schmidt, R., Senior, M., and Haddad, J. G. (1988) Estrogen receptors in bone in a patient with polyostotic fibrous dysplasia (McCune–Albright syndrome). *N. Engl. J. Med.* **319,** 421–425.

94. Grabias, S. L. and Campbell, C. J. (1977) Fibrous dysplasia. *Orthop. Clin. North Am.* **8,** 771–783.
95. Edgerton, M. T., Persing, J. A., and Jane, J. A. (1985) The surgical treatment of fibrous dysplasia: with emphasis on recent contributions from cranio-maxillo-facial surgery. *Ann. Surg.* **202,** 459–479.
96. Hjelmstedt, A. and Ljunghall, S. (1979) A case of Albright syndrome treated with calcitonin. *Acta Orthop. Scand.* **50,** 251–253.
97. Grant, D. B., Savage, M. O., and Russell, R. G. G. (1982) McCune–Albright syndrome with severe progressive polyostotic fibrous dysplasia: failure of experimental treatment with salmon calcitonin and dichlorodiphosphonate. *Pediatr. Res.* **16,** 899.
98. Liens, D., Delmas, P. D., and Meunier, P. J. (1994) Long-term effects of intravenous pamidronate in fibrous dysplasia of bone. *Lancet* **343,** 953–954.
99. Chapurlat, R. D., Meunier, P. J., Liens, D., and Delmas, P. D. (1997) Long-term effects of intravenous pamidronate in fibrous dysplasia of bone. *J. Bone Miner. Res.* **12,** 1746–1752.
100. Weinstein, R. S. (1997) Long-term aminobisphosphonate treatment of fibrous dysplasia: spectacular increase in bone density. *J. Bone Miner. Res.* **12,** 1314–1315.
101. Czerwiec, F. S., Shenker, A., Feuillan, P., and Collins, M. (1997) Further study of the therapy for fibrous dysplasia is necessary [letter]. *J. Bone Miner. Res.* **12,** 128–130.

CHAPTER 11

The Molecular Basis for Parathyroid Hormone Resistance in Pseudohypoparathyroidism

Michael A. Levine

Introduction

The term "pseudohypoparathyroidism" (PHP) describes a collection of disorders that share in common biochemical hypoparathyroidism (i.e., hypocalcemia and hyperphosphatemia), increased secretion of parathyroid hormone (PTH), and target tissue unresponsiveness to the biological actions of PTH. Thus the pathophysiology of PHP differs fundamentally from true hypoparathyroidism, in which PTH secretion rather than PTH responsiveness is defective. In their original report of PHP, Fuller Albright and his associates described the failure of patients with this syndrome to show a phosphaturic response to injected parathyroid extract *(1)*. These observations led to the prescient speculation that biochemical hypoparathyroidism in PHP was due to an inability of the target organs, bone and kidney, to respond to PTH. During the more than fifty years since Albright's original description of PHP we have learned much about PTH signaling through extensive clinical and biochemical studies of these unusual patients.

In addition to functional hypoparathyroidism, the patients described by Albright exhibited a distinctive constellation of developmental and skeletal defects, subsequently referred to as Albright's hereditary osteodystrophy (AHO), that include a round face, short, stocky physique, brachydactyly, heterotopic ossification, and mental retardation (Fig. 1). The relationship between the biochemical abnormalities (hypocalcemia and hyperphosphatemia) and AHO could not be explained by Albright, and yet remains unclarified. Indeed, in certain families some affected members may show both AHO and PTH resistance whereas other family members may have AHO without evidence of any endocrine dysfunction, a disorder Albright termed "pseudo-pseudohypoparathyroidism"

The Genetics of Osteoporosis and Metabolic Bone Disease
Ed.: M. J. Econs © Humana Press Inc., Totowa, NJ

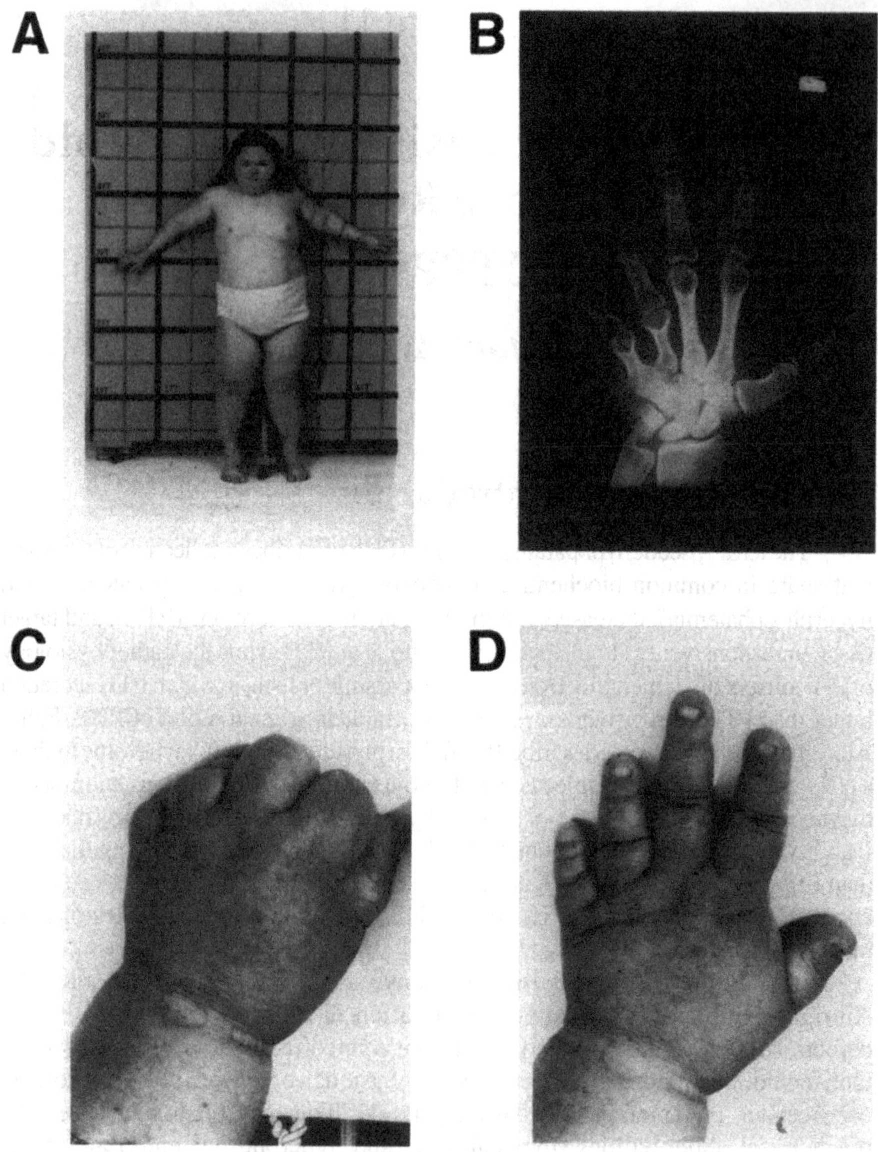

Fig. 1. Typical features of Albright hereditary osteodystrophy. **(A)** A young woman with characteristic features of AHO; note the short stature, disproportionate shortening of the limbs, obesity, and round face. **(B)** Radiograph of patient's showing marked shortening of 4th and 5th metacarpals. **(C)** Archibald sign, the replacement of "knuckles" with "dimples" due to the marked shortening of the metacarpal bones. **(D)** Brachydactyly of the hand, note thumb sign ("Murderer's thumb" or "potter's thumb") and shortening of the 4th and 5th digits.

(pseudoPHP) to emphasize the physical similarities but biochemical differences between these patients and patients with PHP *(2)*.

The diagnostic classification of PHP is further extended by the existence of additional variants in which patients manifest PTH resistance and biochemical hypoparathyroidism but lack any of the features of AHO *(3,4)*. A classification of the many different forms of PHP is presented in Table 1.

General Pathophysiology

Characterization of the molecular basis for PHP commenced with the observations by Chase and Aurbach that cAMP mediates many of the actions of PTH on kidney and bone, and that administration of biologically active PTH to normal subjects leads to a significant increase in the urinary excretion of nephrogenous cAMP and phosphate *(5)*. The PTH infusion test remains the most reliable test available for the diagnosis of PHP, and enables distinction between several variants of the syndrome (Fig. 2). Patients with PHP type I fail to show an appropriate increase in urinary excretion of both nephrogenous cAMP and phosphate *(5)*, suggesting that an abnormality in the renal PTH receptor adenylyl cyclase complex that produces cAMP is the basis for impaired PTH responsiveness. Subsequent studies by Bell et al., in which administration of dibutyryl cAMP to patients with PHP type I produced a phosphaturic response, provided additional support for this theory, and demonstrated that the renal response mechanism to cAMP was intact *(6)*. These studies have led to the conclusion that proximal renal tubule cells are unresponsive to PTH. By contrast, cells in other regions of the kidney appear responsive to PTH. For example, renal handling of calcium (and sodium) in response to exogenous PTH appears to be normal in patients with PHP type I *(7)*. In addition, urinary calcium excretion is markedly lower in patients with PHP type I than in patients with hypoparathyroidism *(8,9)*. These observations imply that calcium reabsorption in the distal tubule is responsive to circulating PTH in subjects with PHP type I, and suggest that PTH is capable to generating sufficient amounts of cAMP, or other second messengers (e.g. cytosolic calcium or diacylglycerol), in these cells to evoke a physiological response (Fig. 3).

Administration of PTH to subjects with PHP type II, a far less common form of the disorder, elicits a normal increase in nephrogenous cAMP that is not accompanied by an appropriate phosphaturic response *(4)*. These results are consistent with a biochemical defect that is distal to PTH-stimulated generation of cAMP.

The defective renal response to PTH in PHP type I has led to the general assumption that all PTH target cells, including bone cells, are resistant to PTH. This hypothesis remains unproved, however. The notion that bone cells are unresponsive to PTH has been drawn from observations that patients with PHP type I are hypocalcemic and that administration of PTH does not increase the plasma calcium level. However, patients with PHP type I frequently develop signs of hyperparathyroid bone disease *(10,11)*, and clinical, roentgenographic, or

Table 1
Classification and Characteristic Features of the Various Forms of Pseudohypoparathyroidism

	PHP type Ia	PseudoPHP	PHP type Ib	PHP type Ic	PHP type II
Physical appearance	Albright hereditary osteodystrophy, may be subtle or (rarely) absent		Normal hereditary	Albright osteodystrophy	Normal
Response to PTH					
Urine cAMP	Defective	Normal	Defective	Defective	Normal
Urine phosphorous	Defective	Normal	Defective	Defective	Defective
Serum calcium level	Low or (rarely) Normal	Normal	Low	Low	Low
Hormone resistance	Generalized	Absent	Limited to PTH target tissues	Generalized	Limited to PTH target tissues
$G_s\alpha$ activity	Reduced	Reduced	Normal	Normal	Normal
Inheritance	Autosomal dominant		Autosomal dominant (most cases)	Unknown	Unknown
Molecular defect	Heterozygous mutations in the GNAS1 gene		Unknown (*see text*)	Unknown	Unknown

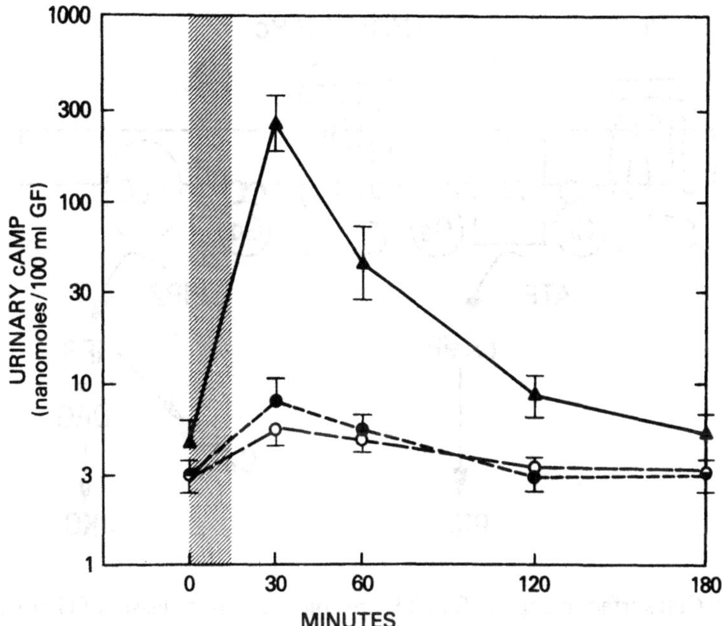

Fig. 2. Urinary cAMP excretion in response to an infusion of bovine parathyroid extract (300 USP units). The peak response in normal subjects (Δ) as well as those with pseudoPHP (not shown) is 50- to 100-fold times basal. Subjects with PHP type Ia (open circles) or PHP type Ib (closed circles) show only a two- to five-fold increase. Urinary cAMP is expressed as nanomoles per 100 mL of GF, U_{cAMP} (nanomoles per 100 mL GF) = U_{cAMP} (nanomoles/dL) X S_{Cre} (mg/dL) / U_{Cre} (mg/dL). (Reprinted by permission from Levine et al. 1986.)

histologic evidence of increased bone turnover and demineralization are not uncommon, particularly in subjects with PHP type Ib (Fig 4). These clinical indicators of PTH action are consistent with the in vitro demonstration of normal adenylyl cyclase responsiveness to PTH of cultured bone cells from one patient with PHP type Ib and osteitis fibrosa cystica *(12)*.

Patients with PHP may develop additional abnormalities in bone metabolism, including osteomalacia *(10)*, rickets *(13)* and osteopenia *(14)*, which may result from excessive PTH or deficient $1,25(OH)_2D_3$.

This unusual pattern of skeletal responsiveness to PTH may reflect the existence of two distinct signaling pathways in bone cells: the remodeling system and the mineral mobilization or homeostatic system. The bone remodeling system appears to be more responsive to PTH in patients with PHP type I than the homeostatic system, an observation that may reflect the lesser dependence of the remodeling system upon normal serum levels of $1,25(OH)_2D$. Circulating levels of $1,25(OH)_2D$ are typically low in patients with PHP type I *(15)*, and lead to the development of

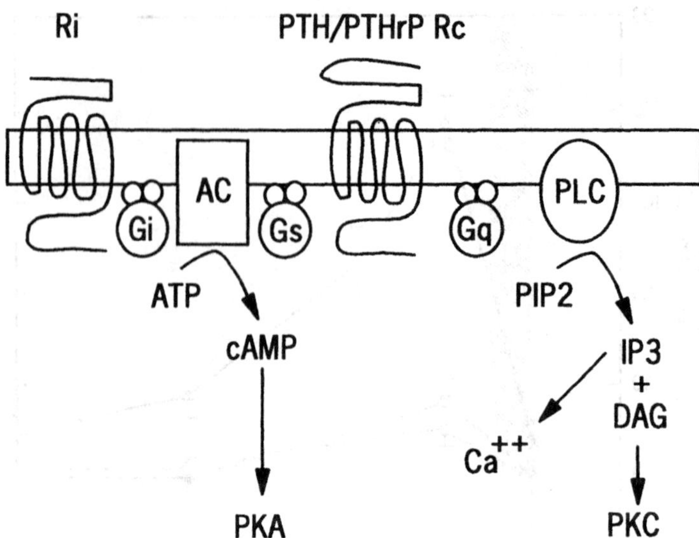

Fig. 3. Cell surface receptors for PTH are coupled to two classes of G proteins. G_s mediates stimulation of adenylyl cyclase (AC) and the production of cAMP, which in turn activates protein kinase A (PKA). G_q stimulates phospholipase C (PLC) to form the second messengers inositol-(1,4,5)-trisphosphate (IP_3) and diacylglycerol (DAG) from membrane bound phosphatidylinositol-(4,5)-bisphosphate. IP_3 increases intracellular calcium (Ca^{2+}) and DAG stimulates protein kinase C (PKC) activity. Each G protein consists of a unique α chain and a βγ dimer.

hypocalcemia and secondary hyperparathyroidism in these patients. As in chronic renal failure, elevated levels of serum PTH eventually overcome the $1,25(OH)_2D$ dependency for skeletal remodeling but not for calcium mobilization.

A role for $1,25(OH)_2D$ in modulating skeletal responsiveness to PTH in PHP type I is suggested by several observations. First, normalization of the serum calcium level in patients with PHP type I by administration of $1,25(OH)_2D$ (or pharmacological amounts of vitamin D) restores the calcemic response of the skeleton to PTH *(16)*. Second, patients with PHP type I who have normal serum levels of calcium and $1,25(OH)_2D_3$ without vitamin D treatment (so called "normocalcemic" PHP) show a normal calcemic response to administered PTH *(16)*. These findings suggest that $1,25(OH)_2D$ deficiency is the basis for the lack of a calcemic response to PTH in hypocalcemic patients with PHP type I, and contradict the premise that bone cells are intrinsically resistant to the actions of PTH.

Serum levels of phosphorous are elevated in PHP type I because of the inability of PTH to decrease the renal tubular reabsorption of phosphorous. Hypocalcemia *per se* may also contribute to the development of hyperphosphatemia, as renal phosphate clearance is impaired by very low levels of intracellular calcium

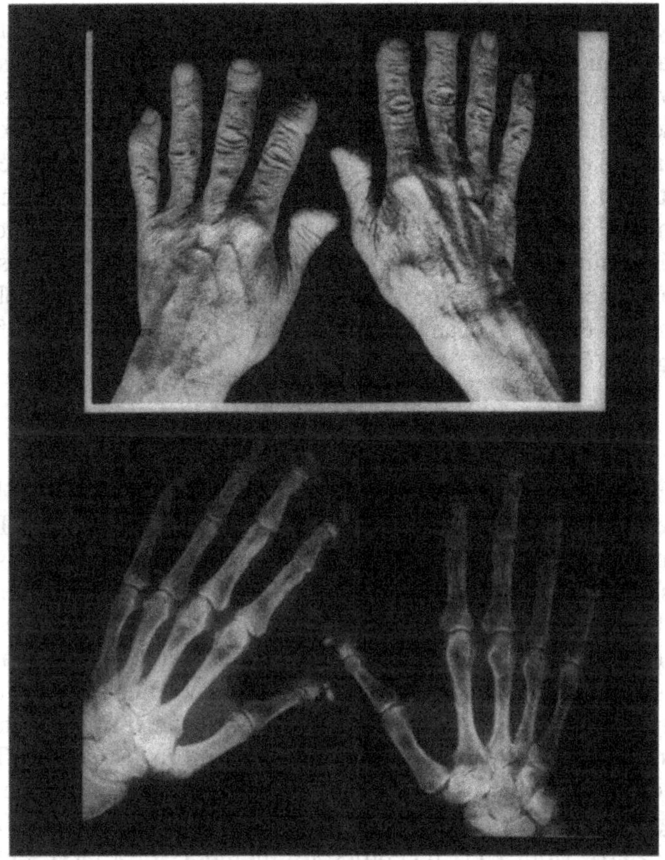

Fig. 4. Photograph and radiograph of hands of a patient with marked hyperparathyroid bone disease. Marked periosteal bone erosion in terminal phalanges has resulted in "pseudoclubbing." From ref. *149*.

(17). Accordingly, normalization of serum calcium levels by chronic treatment with calcium and/or vitamin D can reduce elevated levels of serum phosphorous. Similar therapy has been shown to reverse the defective phosphaturic response to administered PTH in certain patients with PHP type I, although the nephrogenous cAMP response remains markedly deficient *(18)*. Therefore, persistence of a blunted nephrogenous cAMP response to PTH in PHP type I patients in whom chronic vitamin D therapy has led to normalization of plasma calcium levels and restoration of a phosphaturic response need not imply, as has been at least suggested *(18)*, that there is no relationship between cAMP production and phosphate clearance.

The overall evidence suggests that the disturbances in calcium, phosphorous, and vitamin D metabolism in most patients with PHP type I result directly or indirectly from reduced responsiveness of both bone and kidney to PTH. Hypocalcemia results from impaired mobilization of calcium from bone, reduced intestinal absorption of calcium (via deficient generation of 1,25$(OH)_2$D), and urinary calcium loss. Of these defects, the diminished movement of calcium out of bone stores into the extracellular fluid probably has the greatest role in producing hypocalcemia. Intensive treatment with calcitriol (1,25$(OH)_2$D) or other vitamin D analogs improves intestinal calcium absorption and bone calcium mobilization, restores plasma calcium to normal, and reduces circulating PTH levels. Thus, although PTH resistance appears to be the proximate biochemical defect, the major abnormalities in mineral metabolism found in patients with PHP type I can be largely explained on the basis of deficiency of circulating 1,25$(OH)_2$D.

Molecular Basis for PTH Action

PTH regulates mineral metabolism and skeletal homeostasis by modulating the activity of specialized cells in bone and kidney. PTH binds to specific receptors located on the plasma membrane of target cells (Fig. 3). The classical PTH receptor that is expressed in bone and kidney is an approx 75-kDa glycoprotein that is often referred to as the PTH/PTHrP or type I PTH receptor (type I PTH-r). The type I PTH-r binds both PTH and parathyroid hormone-related protein (PTHrP), a factor made by diverse tumors that cause humorally mediated hypercalcemia, with equivalent affinity, which accounts for the similar activities of both hormones. By contrast, a second PTH receptor, termed the type II receptor protein, is not expressed in conventional PTH target tissues (i.e., bone and kidney), and interacts with PTH but not PTHrP *(19,20)*. Both PTH receptors are members of a large family of G protein coupled receptors that can bind hormones, neurotransmitters, cytokines, light photons, taste and odor molecules. These receptors consist of a single polypeptide chain that is predicted by hydrophobicity plots to span the plasma membrane seven times (i.e., heptahelical), forming three extracellular and three or four intracellular loops and a cytoplasmic carboxyl-terminal tail. The heptahelical receptors are coupled by heterotrimeric ($\alpha\beta\gamma$) G proteins *(21)* to signal effector molecules localized to the inner surface of the plasma membrane (Fig. 3). Highly specific associations among at least 20 α, six β, and 12 γ chains generate a diversity of heterotrimeric G proteins that have the ability to discriminate among a multitude of receptor and effector molecules. Hormone-binding to a receptor facilitates activation of the G protein, a process in which the α chain exchanges bound GDP for GTP and dissociates from the $\beta\gamma$ dimer and the receptor. The free, GTP-bound form of the α chain is the primary modulator of relevant effector molecules, although $\beta\gamma$ dimers can also influence activity of many effectors (e.g. some forms of adenylyl cyclase and phospholipase C). An intrinsic GTPase associated with the α chain acts as a molecular timing mechanism, and after a predetermined interval GTP is hydrolyzed to GDP. The inactive GDP-bound α chain reassociates with a βγ dimer, and the heterotrimeric G protein is ready for another cycle of hormone activation.

Interaction of PTH with its receptor activates intracellular signal effector systems that generate the second messengers cAMP *(22,23)*, inositol 1,4,5-trisphosphate and diacylglycerol *(24,25)*, and cytosolic calcium *(26–29)* . The best-characterized mediator of PTH action is cAMP, which rapidly activates protein kinase A *(30)*. The relevant target proteins that are phosphorylated by protein kinase A and the precise mode(s) of action of these proteins remain uncharacterized, though proteins that activate genes responsive to cAMP and ion channel proteins are strong candidates. In contrast to the well-recognized biologic effects of cAMP in PTH target tissues, the physiological importance of metabolites of phosphotidylinositol hydrolysis and intracellular calcium as PTH-induced second messengers has not yet been established. Studies of the expressed type I PTH-r have revealed that ligand activation of these diverse second messengers derives from the ability of the receptor to interact with several different G proteins. The agonist-bound type I PTH-r can activate members of the Gq/11 family, and thereby stimulate phospholipase C, and can activate Gs to stimulate adenylyl cyclase *(31,32)* (Fig. 3). These studies have revealed that the number of PTH-r's expressed, as well as the concentration of G protein and PTH, cooperate to determine the precise signal response.

Circulating Inhibitors of PTH Action

Hormone action may be divided conceptually into prereceptor, receptor, and postreceptor events; defects in each of these steps have been proposed as the basis of hormone resistance in PHP (Fig. 3). A circulating inhibitor of PTH action has been proposed as a cause of PTH resistance on the basis of studies showing an apparent dissociation between plasma levels of endogenous immunoreactive and bioactive PTH in subjects with PHP type I. Despite high circulating levels of immunoreactive PTH, the levels of bioactive PTH in many patients with PHP type I have been found to be within the normal range when measured with highly sensitive renal *(33)* and metatarsal *(34)* cytochemical bioassay systems. Furthermore, plasma from many of these patients has been shown to diminish the biological activity of exogenous PTH in these in vitro bioassays *(35)*. Currently, the nature of this putative inhibitor or antagonist remains unknown. The observation that chronic hypercalcemia can diminish or eliminate the inhibitory activity in the plasma of patients with PHP has suggested that the parathyroid gland may be the source of the inhibitor. This notion is supported by analyses of circulating PTH immunoactivity after fractionation of patient plasma by reversed-phase high-performance liquid chromatography (RP-HPLC), which has disclosed the presence of aberrant forms of immunoreactive PTH in many of these patients *(36)*. Although it is conceivable that a PTH inhibitor may cause PTH resistance in some patients with PHP, it is more likely that circulating antagonists of PTH action arise as a consequence of the sustained secondary hyperparathyroidism that results from the primary biochemical defect.

Pseudohypoparathyroidism Type Ia and Pseudopseudohypoparathyroidism

Cell membranes from most patients with AHO have an approx 50% reduction in expression or activity of $G_s\alpha$ protein *(37)* (Fig. 5). This form of PHP is termed PHP type Ia. The generalized deficiency of $G_s\alpha$ may impair the ability of PTH, as well as many other hormones and neurotransmitters (see below), to activate adenylyl cyclase and thereby may account for multihormone resistance.

Early studies of PHP type Ia led to the identification of families in which some individuals had signs of AHO but lacked apparent hormone resistance (i.e., pseudoPHP). The observation that PHP type Ia and pseudoPHP can occur in the same family first suggested that these two disorders might reflect variability in expression of a single genetic lesion. Further support for this view derives from recent studies which indicate that within a given kindred, subjects with either pseudoPHP or PHP type Ia have identical gene defects and similar deficiency of $G_s\alpha$ in accessible cells (Fig. 5) *(37,38)*. Moreover, a transition from hormone responsiveness to hormone resistance may occur in some patients *(39)*. It therefore seems reasonable to use the term AHO to simplify description of these two variants of the same syndrome, and to acknowledge the common clinical and biochemical characteristics that patients with PHP type Ia and pseudoPHP share.

Molecular Defect

The recent discovery that $G_s\alpha$ deficiency results from inactivating mutations in the GNAS1 gene resolved the controversy surrounding the pattern of inheritance of AHO. X-linked *(40)*, autosomal dominant *(41)*, and autosomal recessive *(42)* inheritance of AHO had been proposed. However, the observation of father to son transmission of AHO with $G_s($ deficiency excluded an X-linked mode of inheritance *(43)*, and the mapping of the GNAS1 gene to chromosome 20q13.2→13.3 *(44)* provided final confirmation that AHO, including both PHP type Ia and pseudoPHP, is inherited in an autosomal dominant fashion. *GNAS1* is a complex gene *(45)* comprised of at least 17 exons, including 3 alternative first exons *(46,47)*. Alternative splicing of nascent transcripts derived from exons 1–13 generates four mRNA's that encode $G_s\alpha$. Deletion of exon 3 results in the loss of 15 codons from the mRNA, while use of an alternative splice site in exon 4 results in the insertion of a single additional codon into the mRNA. This produces two $G_s\alpha$ proteins with apparent molecular weights of 45 kDa and two isoforms of apparent molecular weights of 52 kDa *(45)* that exhibit specific patterns of tissue expression *(48)*. Both long and short forms of $G_s\alpha$ can stimulate adenylyl cyclase and open calcium channels *(49)*, but biochemical characterization of these isoforms has revealed subtle differences in the binding constant for GDP, the rate at which the forms are activated by agonist binding, efficiency of adenylyl cyclase stimulation, and the rate of GTP hydrolysis. The significance of these differences remains unknown *(49–51)*, but these distinctions imply the existence of as yet unknown roles for these G proteins *(52)*.

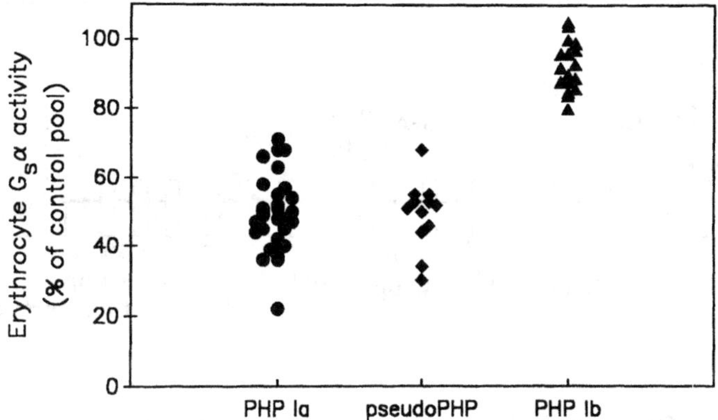

Fig. 5. $G_s\alpha$ activity of erythrocyte membranes. $G_s\alpha$ is quantified in complementation assays with S49 cyc⁻ membranes, which genetically lack G_s(but retain all other components necessary for hormone-response adenylyl cyclase activity. Activity is reduced approx 50% in patients with AHO subjects with either PHP type Ia or pseudoPHP, but is normal in patients with PHP type Ib.

Additional complexity in the processing of the GNAS1 gene derives from the use of alternative first exons that generate novel transcripts. Because these alternative forms of $G_s\alpha$ lack amino acid sequences encoded by exon 1, which are required for interaction with Gβγ and attachment to the plasma membrane, it is unlikely that these proteins can function as transmembrane signal transducers. In one case, a $G_s\alpha$ transcript is produced with an alternative first exon that lacks an initiator ATG; thus, a truncated, nonfunctional $G_s\alpha$ protein is translated from an inframe ATG in exon 2 *(53)*. The role of this $G_s\alpha$ chain is unknown. In two other instances unique transcripts are generated using additional coding exons that are present upstream of the exon 1 used to generate $G_s\alpha$. The more 5' of these exons encodes the neuroendocrine secretory protein NESP55, a chromogranin-like protein that contains sequences derived from exon 2 of GNAS1 in the 3' uncoded region *(54,55)*. The more downstream alternative exon encodes a 51-kDa protein, and when spliced to exons 2 – 13 results in a transcript that encodes a larger $G_s\alpha$ isoform ($XL\alpha_s$) *(56)*. Both of these alternative exons splice onto exon 2 of GNAS1, yet the encoded proteins share no amino acid sequences. Despite their structural unrelatedness, both NESP55 and XLαs have been implicated in regulated secretion in neuroendocrine tissues.

Molecular studies of DNA from subjects with AHO have disclosed inactivating mutations in the GNAS1 gene *(57–70)* that account for a 50% reduction in expression or function of $G_s\alpha$ protein (Fig. 6). All patients are heterozygous, and have one normal GNAS1 allele and one defective allele. A large variety of mutations in the GNAS1 gene have been identified, including missense mutations *(60,62,64,69)*, point mutations in sequences required for efficient splicing *(61)*, and small

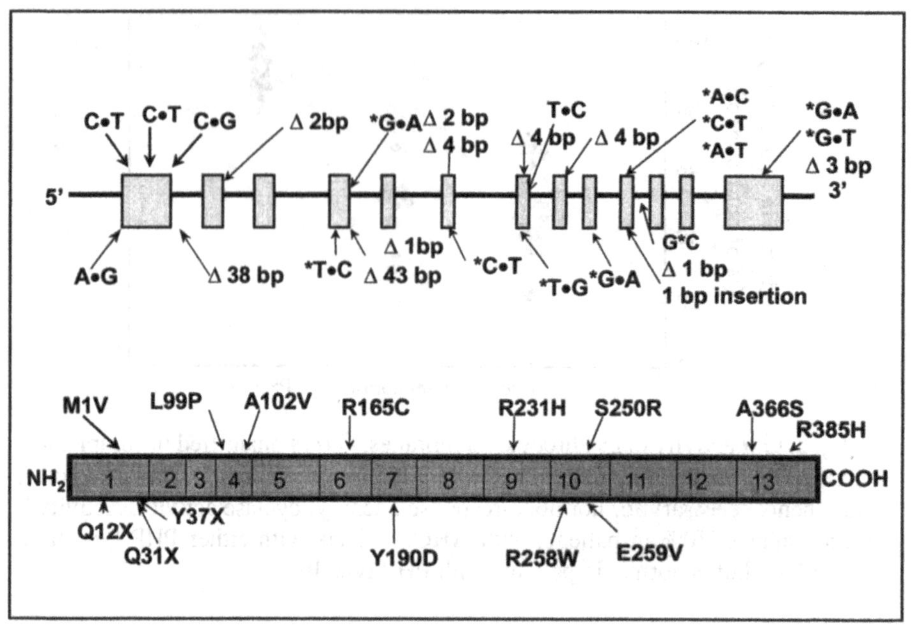

Fig. 6. Mutations in the GNAS1 gene. The upper panel (**A**) depicts the human GNAS1 gene, which spans over 20-kilobase pairs and contains at least 13 exons and 12 introns. Unique mutations that result in *loss of Gs function* are depicted; missense mutations are denoted by the symbol*. The lower panel (**B**) indicates the position of missense mutations above the protein structure. Two polymorphisms are denoted by the symbol +, and the position of the unchanged amino acid is denoted beneath the predicted G_s(protein (panel B). The site of two missense mutations that result in *gain of function* in patients with McCune–Albright syndrome (replacement of Arg^{201}) *(93,94156–158)* or in sporadic tumors (replacement of either Arg^{201} or Gln^{227}) *(159,160)* are depicted in italics. The mutation in exon 1 eliminates the initiator methionine codon and prevents synthesis of a normal $G_s\alpha$ protein *(60)*. The 4 base-pair deletions in exon 7 *(71,72)* and exon 8 *(62)*, and the 1 base-pair deletion and insertion in exon 10 all shift the normal reading frame and prevent normal mRNA and/or protein synthesis. Mutations in intron 3 and at the donor splice junction between exon 10 and intron 10 cause splicing abnormalities that prevent normal mRNA synthesis *(61)*. The mutations indicated with an asterisk represent missense mutations *(58,62,63)*; the resultant amino acid substitutions are indicated in the schematic diagram of the $G_s\alpha$ protein at the bottom of the figure. Some of these mutations may prevent normal protein synthesis by altering protein secondary structure; the R231H substitution in exon 9 prevents normal interaction of the (chain with the βγ dimer *(64)*; the R385H substitution in exon 13 appears to encode an altered protein that cannot couple normally to receptors *(63)* and the A366S mutation encodes an activated $G_s\alpha$ protein that is unstable at 37°C *(58)*.

deletions *(61,62,65,71)*. Although novel mutations have been found in nearly all of the kindreds studied, a 4-base deletion in exon 7 has been detected in multiple families *(70–72)* and an unusual missense mutation in exon 13 (A366S; *see* below) has been identified in two unrelated young boys *(58)*, suggesting that these two regions may be genetic "hot spots."

Most gene mutations lead to reduced expression of $G_s\alpha$ mRNA *(38,73)*, but in some subjects the mutant allele produces normal levels of G_s(mRNA *(38,73,74)* that encode dysfunctional $G_s\alpha$ proteins *(58,63,64,69)*. The replacement of arginine by histidine at codon 385 in the carboxyl terminal tail of $G_s\alpha$ selectively "uncouples" Gs from receptors and prevents receptor activation *(63)*. Substitution of histidine by arginine at position 231 also prevents receptor activation of Gs, but by an entirely different mechanism *(69)*. The replacement of histidine[231] hinders binding of GTP to the α chain, and thereby inhibits receptor-induced dissociation of Gsα from Gβγ.

Multiple Hormone Resistance

Although biochemical hypoparathyroidism is the most commonly recognized endocrine deficiency in PHP type Ia, early clinical studies described additional hormonal abnormalities, such as hypothyroidism *(75,76)* and hypogonadism *(77)*. Because available evidence suggests that $G_s\alpha$ is present in all tissues, generalized deficiency of this protein could be the basis for not only PTH resistance, the hallmark of PHP type Ia, but could also explain the decreased responsiveness of diverse tissues (e.g., kidney, thyroid gland, gonads, and liver) to hormones that act via activation of adenylyl cyclase (e.g., PTH, TSH, gonadotropins, and glucagon) *(9,78,79)*. Primary hypothyroidism occurs in most patients with PHP type Ia *(78)*. Typically, patients lack a goiter or anti-thyroid antibodies and have an elevated serum TSH with an exaggerated response to TRH. Serum levels of T_4 may be low or low normal. Hypothyroidism may occur early in life prior to the development of hypocalcemia, and elevated serum levels of TSH are not uncommonly detected during neonatal screening *(80–82)*. Unfortunately, early institution of thyroid hormone replacement does not seem to prevent the development of mental retardation *(81)*.

Hypogonadism is common in subjects with PHP type Ia. Women may have delayed puberty, oligomenorrhea, and infertility *(78)*. Plasma gonadotropins may be elevated, but are more commonly normal. Some patients show an exaggerated serum gonadotropin response to GnRH *(77,83)*. Features of hypogonadism may be less obvious in men. Serum testosterone may be normal or reduced. Testes may show evidence of a maturation arrest or may fail to descend normally. Fertility appears to be decreased in men with PHP type Ia.

Quite surprisingly, responsiveness to many other hormones that depend upon generation of cAMP appears unaffected in patients with PHP type Ia. For example, diabetes insipidus is not a feature of AHO, and urine is concentrated normally in response to vasopressin in patients with PHP type Ia *(84)*. Although there is a report of adrenal insufficiency in a single individual with PHP type Ia

(85), hypoadrenalism is not a typical feature of PHP type Ia and adrenocortical responsiveness to ACTH is normal *(78)*. One possible interpretation of variable hormonal responsiveness is that haploinsufficiency of Gsα is tissue-specific; that is, in some tissues a 50% reduction in $G_s\alpha$ is still sufficient to facilitate normal signal transduction. However, this explanation leaves unanswered the even more intriguing paradox of why some subjects with $G_s\alpha$ deficiency have hormone resistance (PHP type Ia) whereas others lack hormone resistance (pseudoPHP). Analysis of published pedigrees has indicated that in most cases maternal transmission of G_s(deficiency leads to PHP type Ia whereas paternal transmission of the defect leads to pseudoPHP *(37,68,86,87)*, findings which have implicated genomic imprinting of the GNAS1 gene as a possible regulatory mechanism *(87)*. Recent studies have indeed confirmed that the GNAS1 gene is imprinted, but in a far more complex manner than had been anticipated. Two upstream promoters, each associated with a large coding exon, lie 35 kb upstream of GNAS1 exon 1. These promoters are only 11 kb apart, yet show opposite patterns of allele-specific methylation and monoallelic transcription. The more 5' of these exons encodes NESP55, which is expressed exclusively from the maternal allele. By contrast, the XLαs exon is paternally expressed *(46,47)*. Despite the simultaneous imprinting in both the paternal and maternal directions of the GNAS1 gene, expression of $G_s\alpha$ appears to be biallelic in all human tissues examined *(46,47,90)*. The lack of access to relevant tissues in patients with PHP type Ia has hindered studies of $G_s\alpha$ expression and stimulated attempts to develop suitable animal models. Recently two groups have succeeded in developing mice in which one *Gnas* gene is disrupted, thereby generating murine models of PHP type Ia *(89,90)*. Although these mice have reduced levels of $G_s\alpha$ protein, they lack many of the features of the human disorder. Biochemical analyses of these heterozygous *Gnas* knockout mice suggest that Gsα expression may derive from only the maternal allele in some tissues (e.g., renal cortex) and from both alleles in other tissues (e.g., renal medulla). Accordingly, mice that inherit the defective *Gnas* gene maternally express only that allele in imprinted tissues, such as the PTH-sensitive renal proximal tubule, in which there is no functional $G_s\alpha$ protein. By contrast, the 50% reduction in $G_s\alpha$ expression that occurs in nonimprinted tissues, which express both *Gnas* alleles, may account for more variable and moderate hormone resistance in these sites (e.g., the thyroid). Confirmation of this proposed mechanism in patients with AHO will require demonstration that the human $G_s\alpha$ transcript is paternally imprinted in the renal cortex.

In AHO, inherited GNAS1 gene mutations reduce expression or function of $G_s\alpha$ protein. By contrast, in the McCune–Albright syndrome, post-zygotic somatic mutations in the GNAS1 gene (Fig. 6) enhance activity of the protein *(91,92)*. These mutations lead to constitutive activation of adenylyl cyclase, and result in proliferation and autonomous hyperfunction of hormonally responsive cells. The clinical significance of $G_s\alpha$ activity as a determinant of hormone action is emphasized by the recent description by Iiri et al. *(58)* of two males with both precocious puberty and PHP type Ia. These two unrelated boys had identical *GNAS1* gene mutations in exon 13 (A366S, Fig. 6) that resulted in a temperature-sensitive form of $G_s\alpha$. This $G_s\alpha$ is constitutively active in the cooler environment of the testis, while being rapidly degraded in other tissues at normal body temperature. Thus, different tissues in these two individuals could show hormone resistance (to PTH and TSH), hormone responsiveness (to ACTH), or hormone independent activation (to LH).

Albright Hereditary Osteodystrophy

Subjects with PHP type Ia or pseudoPHP typically manifest a characteristic constellation of developmental defects, termed Albright hereditary osteodystrophy, that includes short stature, obesity, a round face, shortening of the digits (brachydactyly), subcutaneous ossification, and dental hypoplasia (Fig. 1) *(1,2)*. Considerable variability occurs in the clinical expression of these features even among affected members of a single family, and all of these features may not be present in every case *(93)* . On rare occasion, it may be impossible to detect any features of AHO in an individual with $G_s\alpha$ deficiency*(61,62)*. The presence of AHO in patients with PHP type Ia and pseudoPHP suggests that the phenotype results from defective signaling function in cells in which GNAS1 is not imprinted, and in which a 50% reduction of $G_s\alpha$ can hinder activation of adenylyl cyclase.

Although patients with AHO may be of normal height and weight, approx 66% of children and 80% of adults are below the 10th percentile for height. This reflects a disproportionate shortening of the limbs, as arm span is less than height in the majority of patients. Obesity is a common feature of AHO and about one-third of all patients with AHO are above the 90th percentile of weight for their age, despite their short stature *(94)* (Fig. 1A). Patients with AHO typically have a round face, a short neck, and a flattened bridge of the nose. Numerous other abnormalities of the head and neck have also been noted. Ocular findings include hypertelorism, strabismus, nystagmus, unequal pupils, diplopia, microphthalmia, and a variety of abnormal findings on funduscopic exam that range from irregular pigmentation to optic atrophy and macular degeneration. Head circumference is above the 90th percentile in a significant minority of children *(94)*. Dental abnormalities are common in subjects with PHP type Ia and include dentin and enamel hypoplasia, short and blunted roots, and delayed or absent tooth eruption *(95)*.

Brachydactyly is the most reliable sign for the diagnosis of AHO, and may be symmetrical or asymmetrical and involve one or both hands or feet (Fig. 1). Shortening of the distal phalanx of the thumb is the most common abnormality; this is apparent on physical exam as a thumb in which the ratio of the width of the nail to its length is increased (so called "murderer's thumb" or "potter's thumb", Fig. 1D). Shortening of the metacarpals causes shortening of the digits, particularly the 4th and 5th. Shortening of the metacarpals may also be recognized on physical exam as dimpling over the knuckles of a clenched fist (Archibald sign, Fig. 1C). Often a definitive diagnosis requires careful examination of radiographs of the hands and feet (Fig. 1B). A specific pattern of shortening of the bones in the hand has been identified, in which the distal phalanx of the thumb and third through fifth metacarpals are the most severely shortened *(96,97)*. This may be useful in distinguishing AHO from other unrelated syndromes in which brachydactyly occurs, such as familial brachydactyly, Turner syndrome, and Klinefelter syndrome *(96)*.

In addition to brachydactyly, several other skeletal abnormalities are present in AHO. Numerous deformities of the long bones have been reported, including a short ulna, bowed radius, deformed elbow or cubitus valgus, coxa vara, coxa valga, genu varum, and genu valgus deformities *(94)*. The most common abnormalities of the skull are hyperostosis frontalis interna and a thickened calvarium. The skeletal abnormalities of AHO may not be apparent until a child is 5 yr old *(98)* . Bone age is advanced 2–3 yr in the majority of patients *(94)*. Spinal cord compression has been reported in several patients with AHO *(99)*.

Patients with AHO develop heterotopic ossifications of the soft tissues or skin (osteoma cutis). Although frequently confused with subcutaneous calcifications, these lesions are in fact ectopic islands of true bone, and their development and growth appear unrelated to abnormalities in serum calcium or phosphorous levels. Osteoma cutis is present in 25 to 50% of cases of AHO, and is usually first noted in infancy or early childhood. Ossification of the skin and subcutaneous tissues may be the presenting cardinal feature of AHO in infancy or childhood in the absence of hypocalcemia or other features of AHO *(100,101)*. Blue-tinged, stony hard papular or nodular lesions that range in size from pinpoint up to 5 cm in diameter often occur at sites of minor trauma and may appear to be migratory on repeated exams *(100)*. Biopsy of these lesions reveals heterotopic ossification with spicules of mineralizing osteoid and calcified cartilage.

The presence of these developmental and skeletal abnormalities does not necessarily indicate that the patient has AHO and $G_s\alpha$ deficiency. Features of AHO, particularly shortened metacarpals or metatarsals, may occur in normal subjects, as well as in patients with hormone deficient hypoparathyroidism *(101,102)*, renal hypercalciuria *(103)*, and primary hyperparathyroidism *(104)*. Moreover, several features of AHO, for example, obesity, round face, brachydactyly, and mental retardation, are common to other disorders (e.g., Prader–Willi syndrome, acrodysostosis, Ullrich-Turner syndrome, Gardener's syndrome), many of which are associated with chromosomal defects. In some instances overlapping clinical features between AHO and other syndromes may lead to confusion. For example, AHO in a mother and her daughter has been associated with a proximal 15q chromosomal deletion resembling that found in Prader–Willi syndrome *(105)*. A growing number of reports have described small terminal deletions of chromosome 2q in patients with variable AHO-like phenotypes. Terminal deletion of 2q37 [del(2)(q37.3)] is the first consistent karyotypic abnormality that has been documented in patients with an AHO-like syndrome *(106,107)*. These patients have normal endocrine function and normal $G_s\alpha$ activity, however *(107)*. Thus, high-resolution chromosome analysis, biochemical/molecular analysis, and careful physical and radiological examination are essential in discriminating between these phenocopies and AHO.

Pseudohypoparathyroidism Type Ib

Subjects with PHP type I who lack features of AHO typically manifest hormone resistance that is limited to PTH target organs and have normal $G_s\alpha$ activity (Fig. 5) *(78)*. This variant is termed PHP type Ib *(108)*. Although patients with PHP type Ib fail to show a nephrogenous cAMP response to PTH, they often manifest skeletal lesions similar to those that occur in patients with hyperparathyroidism (Fig. 4) *(109)*. These observations have suggested that at least one intracellular signaling pathway coupled to the PTH receptor may be intact in patients with PHP type Ib.

Specific resistance of target tissues to PTH, and normal activity of $G_s\alpha$, had implicated decreased expression or function of the PTH/PTHrP receptor as the cause for hormone resistance. In addition, cultured fibroblasts from some, but not all, PHP type Ib patients were shown to accumulate reduced levels of cAMP in response to PTH *(110)* and contain decreased levels of mRNA encoding the PTH/PTHrP receptor *(111)*. Several lines of evidence suggest that the primary defect in PHP type Ib is not in the gene encoding the PTH/PTHrP receptor, however. First, pretreatment of cultured fibroblasts from subjects with PHP type 1b with dexamethsone was found to normalize the PTH-induced cAMP response and to increase expression of PTH/PTHrP receptor mRNA *(111)*. Second, molecular studies have failed to disclose mutations in the coding exons *(112)* and promoter regions *(113)* of the PTH/PTHrP receptor gene or its mRNA *(114)*. Third, mice *(115)* and humans *(116)* that are heterozygous for inactivation of the gene encoding the PTH/PTHrP receptor do not manifest PTH resistance or hypocalcemia. And finally, inheritance of two defective type PTH/PTHrP receptor genes results in Blomstrand chondrodysplasia, a lethal genetic disorder characterized by advanced endochondral bone maturation (*see* Chapter 20). Thus, it is likely that the molecular defect in PHP type Ib resides in other gene(s) that regulate expression or activity of the PTH/PTHrP receptor.

Although most cases of PHP type Ib appear to be sporadic, familial cases have been described in which transmission of the defect is most consistent with an autosomal dominant pattern *(3,117)*. Recent studies have used gene mapping to identify the molecular defect in PHP type Ib *(118)*. In one study the unknown gene was mapped to a small region of chromosome 20q13.3 near the GNAS1 gene, thus raising the possibility that some patients with PHP type Ib have inherited a defective promoter or enhancer that regulates expression of $G_s\alpha$ in the kidney *(118)*.

Pseudohypoparathyroidism Type Ic

Resistance to multiple hormones has been described in several patients with AHO who do not have a demonstrable defect in G_s or G_i *(78,101,119)*.This disorder is termed PHP type Ic. The nature of the lesion in such patients is unclear, but it could be related to some other general component of the receptor-adenylyl cyclase system, such as the catalytic unit *(120)*. Alternatively, these patients could have functional defects of G_s (or G_i) that do not become apparent in the assays presently available *(121)*.

Pseudohypoparathyroidism Type II

PHP type II is the least common form of PHP. This variant is typically sporadic, although one case of familial PHP type II has been reported *(122)*. Patients do not have features of AHO. Renal resistance to PTH in PHP type II patients is manifested by a reduced phosphaturic response to administration of PTH, despite a normal increase in urinary excretion of nephrogenous cAMP*(4)*. These observations suggest that the PTH receptor-adenylyl cyclase complex functions normally to increase cAMP in response to PTH, and are consistent with a model in which PTH resistance arises from an inability of intracellular cAMP to initiate the chain of metabolic events that result in the ultimate expression of PTH action. Although supportive data are not yet available, a defect in cAMP-dependent protein kinase A has been proposed as the basis for this disorder *(4)*.

An alternative interpretation of these observations is that the defect in PHP type II is not an inability to generate a physiological response to intracellular cAMP: a defect in another PTH-sensitive signal transduction pathway may explain the lack of a phosphaturic response. One candidate is the PTH-sensitive phospholipase C pathway that leads to increased concentrations of the intracellular second messengers inositol 1,4,5-trisphosphate and diacylglycerol *(24,25)* and cytosolic calcium *(26–29)* (Fig. 3).

In some patients with PHP type II the phosphaturic response to PTH has been restored to normal after serum levels of calcium have been normalized by treatment with calcium infusion or vitamin D *(123)*. These results point to the importance of Ca^{2+} as an intracellular second messenger. Finally, a similar dissociation between the effects of PTH on generation of cAMP and tubular reabsorption of phosphate has been observed in patients with profound hypocalcemia due to vitamin D deficiency *(17)*, suggesting that some cases of PHP type II may in fact represent vitamin D deficiency.

Diagnosis

The diagnosis of PHP should be strongly suspected in any patient with hypocalcemia, hyperphosphatemia, and an elevated serum concentration of PTH. Occasionally serum levels of PTH are "inappropriately" normal in subjects with PHP owing to confounding hypomagnesemia *(117)* or other factors *(124)*. Although hypocalcemia is present in most patients with PHP by the end of the first decade of life, this biochemical finding may go undetected for many years. The circulating level of PTH generally increases prior to the development of hypocalcemia or hyperphosphatemia, and is an early marker of decreased renal responsiveness to the hormone. However, mild hypercalcemia has been found in several young patients with PHP type I who had markedly elevated circulating levels of PTH.

Cataracts and intracranial calcification, particularly of the basal ganglion, occur commonly in patients with all forms of chronic hypoparathyroidism. Thus, the presence of these ectopic or metastatic calcifications does not help to discriminate among the various causes of hypocalcemia and hyperphosphatemia *(125)*. Intracranial calcifications are readily detected when CT scanning is employed *(126,127)*, and may occasionally be associated with symptoms such as Parkinson's disease *(128)*. Unusual presenting manifestations of PHP include neonatal hypothyroidism *(80,81)*, unexplained cardiac failure *(129)*, Parkinson's disease *(136)*, and spinal cord compression *(130)*.

Corroboration of the diagnosis of PHP requires demonstration of normal renal function and normal serum levels of magnesium and 25-(OH)-vitamin D. The presence of AHO and/or multi-hormone resistance, such as hypothyroidism or hypogonadism, favors a diagnosis of PHP type Ia *(78)*. When most or all of these features are present, more sophisticated tests may not be necessary to confirm the clinical diagnosis. Serum calcium levels can fluctuate in patients with PHP, and may spontaneously change from low to normal and vice versa, thus contributing to the confusion regarding the distinction between PHP and pseudoPHP *(16,131)*. However, the abnormal cAMP response to administered PTH (below) does not become normal in PHP patients who become normocalcemic with or without treatment. Thus, the PTH infusion remains the most reliable test to distinguish between these two variants (Fig. 2).

Specialized Tests

The biochemical hallmark of PHP is the failure of the target organs, bone and kidney, to respond normally to PTH. Additional tests have been developed to identify subjects with PHP type Ia; these research tests, which are based on analysis of $G_s\alpha$ protein or the GNAS1 gene, are only rarely indicated under typical clinical circumstances. The classical tests of Ellsworth and Howard, and of Chase, Melson, and Aurbach involved the intravenous infusion of 200–300 USP units of bovine parathyroid extract (parathyroid injection, USP; Lilly) and subsequent measurement of urinary excretion of nephrogenous (or total) cAMP (Fig. 2) and phosphate. This relatively crude PTH preparation is no longer available, and has been replaced by synthetic peptides corresponding to the amino terminal region of human PTH (hPTH 1-34). After infusion of synthetic hPTH(1-34), normal subjects and patients with hormonopenic hypoparathyroidism usually display a 10- to 20-fold increase in plasma *(132)* or urinary *(133,134)* cAMP excretion, whereas patients with PHP type I (type Ia and type Ib) show a markedly blunted response regardless of their serum calcium concentration *(135)*. The urinary cAMP response to infusion of synthetic hPTH fragments in patients with PHP type I is unrelated to serum calcium levels, but may be related to endogenous serum PTH levels. The maximal urinary cAMP response to PTH increases after suppression of endogenous PTH in patients with PHP type I, but nevertheless does not reach that of the normal range . Thus, this test can distinguish patients with so-called "normocalcemic" PHP (i.e., patients with PTH resistance who are able to maintain normal serum calcium levels without treatment) from subjects with pseudoPHP (who will have a normal urinary cAMP response to PTH *[5,37]*)(Fig. 2). Calculation of the phosphaturic response to PTH as the percent decrease in tubular maximum for phosphate reabsorption [i.e., TmP/GFR, *(136)*] during the first hour after PTH infusion yields the best separation between normal subjects and patients with PHP or hypoparathyroidism *(133)*. However, distinction between groups is also possible when the results are expressed as the fall in percent tubular reabsorption of phosphorus (decrease in % TRP). Patients with hormone deficient hypoparathyroidism have a steep fall in TmP/GF during the first hour after beginning the infusion of PTH. This fall does not occur in patients with PHP [for further details see references by Mallette et al. *(133,134)*]. Although a normal phosphate response may occur in PHP type I patients with serum calcium or PTH levels in the normal range *(7)*, in patients with PHP type II the phosphaturic response to PTH is not changed despite at least a 10-fold increase in cAMP excretion.

The plasma cAMP response to PTH can also be used to differentiate patients with PHP type I from normal subjects and from patients with hypoparathyroidism *(132,135,137)*. Patients with PHP type II can be expected to have normal responsiveness, however. This test offers few advantages over protocols that assess the urinary excretion of cAMP, as changes in plasma cAMP in normal subjects and patients with hypoparathyroidism are much less dramatic than changes in urinary cAMP, and urine must still be collected if one wishes to assess the phosphaturic response to PTH. One reasonable indication for measuring the plasma cAMP response to PTH is the evaluation of patients in whom proper collection of urine is not possible, such as young children *(132)*.

The plasma $1,25(OH)_2D_3$ response to PTH has been used to differentiate between hormone deficient and hormone resistant hypoparathyroidism *(138,139)*. In contrast to normal subjects and patients with hypoparathyroidism, patients with PHP had no significant increase in circulating levels of $1,25(OH)_2D_3$. This proposed test readily demonstrates the difference in the pathophysiology between hypoparathyroidism and PHP. Its clinical relevance is probably limited to distinguishing type I from type II PHP where the expected increase in the latter form of PHP might be a more reliable parameter than the phosphaturic response to PTH.

Treatment

Urgent treatment of acute or severe symptomatic hypocalcemia in patients with hypoparathyroidism is best accomplished by the intravenous infusion of calcium. Vitamin D is not required. The long term treatment of hypocalcemia in patients with PHP involves the administration of oral calcium and vitamin D or analogs. Patients with PHP may require less intensive therapy than patients with PTH deficiency.

The goals of therapy are to maintain serum ionized calcium levels in the normal range, to avoid hypercalciuria, and to suppress PTH levels. Patients with PHP have significantly lower urinary calcium excretion than patients with hypoparathyroidism in relation to serum calcium *(140,141)* and can tolerate serum calcium levels that are within the normal range without developing hypercalciuria *(8)*.

Patients with PHP require lower doses of vitamin D than patients with hypoparathyroidism *(142)*, an observation that reflects the response of bone and renal distal tubular cells to endogenous PTH *(143)*. Treatment with calcium and vitamin D usually decreases the elevated serum phosphate to a high normal level because of a favorable balance between increased urinary phosphate excretion and decreased intestinal phosphate absorption. In general, phosphate binding gels such as aluminum hydroxide are not necessary.

Patients with AHO may require specific treatment for unusual problems related to their developmental and skeletal abnormalities. Patients with PHP type Ia should be treated for their associated hypogonadism and hypothyroidism. Ectopic ossification occurs in about 30% of patients with AHO *(94)*, but rarely causes a problem. However, at times large extraskeletal osteomas may occur *(100)*. These may require surgical removal to relieve pressure symptoms.

Patients with pseudohypoparathyroidism can develop intracranial calcifications and the extent of the calcification appears to be related to both the degree and the duration of functional hypoparathyroidism. Accordingly, correction of hypocalcemia and hyperphosphatemia can theoretically prevent development or progression of intracranial calcification, although no controlled studies are available to confirm this hypothesis.

Conclusion

The identification, and molecular characterization of the signal transduction pathways that regulate PTH secretion and action have facilitated development of new approaches to the investigation of PHP. Advanced immunoassays now make possible the accurate and precise measurement of circulating concentrations of biologically active PTH, and innovative genetic techniques now offer the promise of future molecular diagnosis of these disorders. Ultimately, the insights gained from studies of these unusual patients will provide new information concerning the physiological regulation of PTH responsiveness in classical target tissues, such as bone and kidney, as well as in nonclassical targets.

As with many other human disorders for which the disease gene has been identified, it is predicted that ability to diagnose these disorders on a molecular level will extend the clinical spectrum of disease. This prediction has already been fulfilled through our understanding of defects in genes encoding $G_s\alpha$. Future work will be directed toward identification of the molecular basis for other forms of PHP so that all disorders of PTH action can be described on the basis of their pathophysiology.

Acknowledgments

This work has been supported in part by grants from the National Institutes of Health (DK-34281 and DK-46720).

References

1. Albright, F., Burnett, C. H., and Smith, P. H. (1942) Pseudohypoparathyroidism, an example of "Seabright–Bantam syndrome". *Endocrinology* **30,** 922–932.
2. Albright, F., Forbes, A. P., and Henneman, P. H. (1952) Pseudopseudohypoparathyroidism. *Trans. Assoc. Am. Physicians* **65,** 337–350.
3. Winter, J. S. D. and Hughes, I. A. (1980) Familial pseudohypoparathyroidism without somatic anomalies. *Can. Med. Assoc. J.* **123,** 26–31.
4. Drezner, M. K., Neelon, F. A., and Lebovitz, H. E. (1973) Pseudohypoparathyroidism type II, a possible defect in the reception of the cyclic AMP signal. *N. Engl. J. Med.* **280,** 1056–1060.
5. Chase, L. R., Melson, G. L., and Aurbach, G. D. (1969) Pseudohypoparathyroidism, defective excretion of 3',5'-AMP in response to parathyroid hormone. *J. Clin. Invest.* **48,** 1832–1844.
6. Bell, N. H., Avery, S., Sinha, T. et al. (1972) Effects of dibutyryl cyclic adenosine 3',5'–monophosphate and parathyroid extract on calciuma nd phosphorous metabolism in hypoparathyroidisma and pseudohypoparathyroidism. *J. Clin. Invest.* **51,** 816–816.
7. Stone, M. D., Hosking, D. J., Garcia-Himmelstine, C., White, D. A., Rosenblum, D., and G. Worth, H. (1993) The renal response to exogenous parathyroid hormone in treated pseudohypoparathyroidism. *Bone* **14,** 727–735.
8. Mizunashi, K., Furukawa, Y., Sohn, H. E., Miura, R., Yumita, S., and Yoshinaga, K. (1990) Heterogeneity of pseudohypoparathyroidism type I from the aspect of urinary excretion of calcium and serum levels of parathyroid hormone. *Calcif. Tissue Int.* **46,** 227–232.
9. Shima, M., Nose, O., Shimizu, K., Seino,Y., Yabuuchi, H., and Saito, T. (1988) Multiple associated endocrine abnormalities in a patient with pseudohypoparathyroidism type 1a. *Eur. J. Pediatr.* **147,** 536–538.
10. Burnstein, M. I., Kottamasu, S. R., Pettifor, J. M., Sochett, E., Ellis, B. I., and Frame, B. (1985) Metabolic bone disease in pseudohypoparathyroidism, radiologic features. *Radiology* **155,** 351–356.
11. Eubanks, P. J. and Stabile, B. E. (1998) Osteitis fibrosa cystica with renal parathyroid hormone resistance, a review of pseudohypoparathyroidism with insight into calcium homeostasis. *Arch. Surg.* **133,** 673–676.
12. Murray, T. M., Rao, L. G., Wong, M. M., Waddell, J. P., McBroom, R., Tam, C. S., Rosen, F., and Levine, M. A. (1993) Pseudohypoparathyroidism with osteitis fibrosa cystica, direct demonstration of skeletal responsiveness to parathyroid hormone in cells cultured from bone. *J. Bone Miner. Res.* **8,** 83–91.
13. Dabbaugh, S., Chesney, R. W., Langer, L. O., DeLuca, H. F., Gilbert, E. F., and DeWeerd, J. H. Jr. (1984) Renal-non-responsive, bone–responsive pseudohypoparathyroidism. A case with normal vitamin D metabolite levels and clinical features of rickets. *Am. J. Dis. Child* **138,** 1030–1033.
14. Breslau, N. A., Moses, A. M., and Pak, C. Y. C. (1983) Evidence for bone remodeling but lack of calcium mobilization response to parathyroid hormone in pseudohypoparathyroidism. *J. Clin. Endocrinol. Metab.* **57,** 638–644.
15. Drezner, M. K., Neelon, F. A., Haussler, M. McPherson, H. T., and Lebovitz, H. E. (1976) 1,25-Dihydroxycholecalciferol deficiency, the probable cause of hypocalcemia and metabolic bone disease in pseudohypoparathyroidism. *J. Clin. Endocrinol. Metab.* **42,** 621–628.

16. Drezner, M. K. and Haussler,M. R. (1979) Normocalcemic pseudohypoparathyroidism. *Am. J. Med.* **66,** 503–508.
17. Rao, D. S., Parfitt, A. M., Kleerekoper, M., Pumo, B. S., and Frame,B. (1985) Dissociation between the effects of endogenous parathyroid hormone on adenosine 3',5'-monophosphate generation and phosphate reabsorption in hypocalcemia due to vitamin D depletion, An acquired disorder resembling pseudohypoparathyroidism type II. *J. Clin. Endocrinol. Metab.* **61,** 285–290.
18. Stogmann, W. and Fischer, J. A. (1975) Pseudohypoparathyroidism. Disappearance of the resistance to parathyroid extract during treatment with vitamin D. *Am. J. Med.* **59,** 140–144.
19. Behar, V., Pines, M., Nakamoto, C., Greenberg, Z., Bisello, A., Stueckle, S. M. et al. (1996) The human PTH2 receptor, binding and signal transduction properties of the stably expressed recombinant receptor. *Endocrinology* **137,** 2748–2757.
20. Usdin, T. B., Gruber, C., and Bonner, T. I. (1995) Identification and functional expression of a receptor selectively recognizing parathyroid hormone, the PTH2. *J. Biol. Chem.* **270,** 15,455–15,458.
21. Neer, E. J. (1995) Heterotrimeric G Proteins: Organizers of transmembrane Signals. *Cell* **80,** 249–257.
22. Melson, G. L., Chase, L. R., and Aurbach, G. D. (1970) Parathyroid hormone-sensitive adenyl cyclase in isolated renal tubules. *Endocrinology* **86,** 511–518.
23. Chase, L. R., Fedak, S. A., and Aurbach, G. D. (1969) Activation of skeletal adenyl cyclase by parathyroid hormone in vitro. *Endocrinology* **84,** 761–768.
24. Civitelli, R., Reid, I. R., Westbrook, S., Avioli, L. V., and Hruska, K. A. (1988) PTH elevates inositol polyphosphates and diacylglycerol in a rat osteoblast-like cell line. *Am. J. Physiol.* **255,** E660–E667.
25. Dunlay, R. and Hruska, K. (1990) PTH receptor coupling to phospholipase C is an alternate pathway of signal transduction in bone and kidney. *Am. J. Physiol.* **258,** F223–F231.
26. Gupta, A., Martin, K. J., Miyauchi, A., and Hruska, K. A. (1991) Regulation of cytosolic calcium by parathyroid hormone and oscillations of cytosolic calcium in fibroblasts from normal and pseudohypoparathyroid patients. *Endocrinology* **128,** 2825–2836.
27. Civitelli, R., Martin, T. J., Fausto, A., Gunsten, S. L., Hruska, K. A., and Avioli, L. V. (1989) Parathyroid hormone-related peptide transiently increases cytosolic calcium in osteoblast-like cells, comparison with parathyroid hormone. *Endocrinology* **125,** 1204–1210.
28. Reid, I. R., Civitelli, R., Halstead, L. R., Avioli, L. V., and Hruska, K. A. (1987) Parathyroid hormone acutely elevates intracellular calcium in osteoblastlike cells. *Am. J. Physiol.* **253,** E45–E51.
29. Yamaguchi, D. T., Hahn, T. J., Iida-Klein, A., Kleeman, C. R., and Muallem, S. (1987) Parathyroid hormone-activated calcium channels in an osteoblast-like clonal osteosarcoma cell line. *J. Biol. Chem.* **262,** 7711–7718.
30. Bringhurst, F. R., Zajac, J. D., Daggett, A. S., Skurat, R. N., and Kronenberg, H. M. (1989) Inhibition of parathyroid hormone responsiveness in clonal osteoblastic cells expressing a mutant form of 3',5'-cyclic adenosine monophosphate-dependent protein kinase. *Mol. Endocrinol.* **3,** 60–67.
31. Schwindinger, W. F., Fredericks, J., Watkins, L., Robinson, H., Bathon, J. M., Pines, M. Suva, L. J., and Levine, M. A. (1998) Coupling of the PTH/PTHrP receptor to multiple G-proteins. Direct demonstration of receptor activation of Gs, Gq/11, and

Gi(1) by [alpha-32P]GTP-gamma-azidoanilide photoaffinity labeling. *Endocrine* **8,** 201–209.
32. Offermanns, S., A. Iida-Klein, G. V. Segre, and M. I. Simon. (1996) G alpha q family members couple parathyroid hormone (PTH)/PTH–related peptide and calcitonin receptors to phospholipase C in COS-7 cells. *Mol. Endocrinol.* **10,** 566–574.
33. de Deuxchaisnes, C. N., Fischer, J. A., Dambacher, M. A., Devogelaer, J. P. et al. (1981) Dissociation of parathyroid hormone bioactivity and immunoreactivity in pseudohypoparathyroidism type I. *J. Clin. Endocrinol. Metab.* **53,** 1105–1109.
34. Bradbeer, J. N., Dunham, J., Fischer, J. A., Nagant de Deuxchaisnes, C., and Loveridge, N. (1988) The metatarsal cytochemical bioassay of parathyroid hormone, validation, specificity, and application to the study of pseudohypoparathyroidism type I. *J. Clin. Endocrinol. Metab.* **67,** 1237–1243.
35. Loveridge, N., Fischer, J. A., Nagant de Deuxchaisnes, C., Dambacher, M. A., Tschopp, F., Werder, E., et al. (1982) Inhibition of cytochemical bioactivity of parathyroid hormone by plasma in pseudohypoparathyroidism type I. *J. Clin. Endocrinol. Metab.* **54,** 1274–1275.
36. Mitchell, J. and Goltzman, D. (1985) Examination of circulating parathyroid hormone in pseudohypoparathyroidism. *J. Clin. Endocrinol. Metab.* **61,** 328–334.
37. Levine, M. A., Jap, T. S., Mauseth, R. S., Downs, R. W., and Spiegel, A. M. (1986) Activity of the stimulatory guanine nucleotide-binding protein is reduced in erythrocytes from patients with pseudohypoparathyroidism and pseudopseudohypoparathyroidism, biochemical, endocrine, and genetic analysis of Albright's hereditary osteodystrophy in six kindreds. *J. Clin. Endocrinol. Metab.* **62,** 497–502.
38. Levine, M. A., Ahn, T. G., Klupt, S. F., Kaufman, K. D., Smallwood, P. M., Bourne, H. R., Sullivan, K. A., and Van Dop, C. (1988) Genetic deficiency of the alpha subunit of the guanine nucleotide-binding protein Gs as the molecular basis for Albright hereditary osteodystrophy. *Proc. Natl. Acad. Sci. USA* **85,** 617–621.
39. Barr, D. G., Stirling, H. F., and Darling, J. A. (1994) Evolution of pseudohypoparathyroidism, an informative family study. *Arch. Dis. Child.* **70,** 337–338.
40. Mann, J. B., Alterman, S., and Hills, A. G. (1962) Albright's hereditary osteodystrophy comprising pseudohypoparathyroidism and pseudo-pseudohypoparathyroidism with a report of two cases representing the complete syndrome occuring in successive generations. *Ann. Intern. Med.* **56,** 315–342.
41. Weinberg, A. G. and Stone, R. T. (1971) Autosomal dominant inheritence in Albright's hereditary osteodystrophy. *J. Pediatr.* **79,** 996–999.
42. Cedarbaum, S. D. and Lippe, B. M. (1973) Probable autosomal recessive inheritance in a family with Albright's hereditary osteodystrophy and an evaluation of the genetics of the disorder. *Am. J. Hum. Genet.* **25,** 638–645.
43. Van Dop, C., Bourne, H. R., and Neer, R. M. (1984) Father to son transmission of decreased Ns activity in pseudohypoparathyroidism type Ia. *J. Clin. Endocrinol. Metab.* **59,** 825–828.
44. Levine, M. A., Modi, W. S., and OBrien, S. J. (1991) Mapping of the gene encoding the alpha subunit of the stimulatory G protein of adenylyl cyclase (GNAS1) to 20q13. 2--q13. 3 in human by in situ hybridization. *Genomics* **11,** 478–479.
45. Kozasa, T., Itoh, H., Tsukamoto, T., and Kaziro, Y. (1988) Isolation and characterization of the human Gs alpha gene. *Proc. Natl. Acad. Sci. USA* **85,** 2081–2085.
46. Hayward, B. E., Moran, V., Strain, L., and Bonthron, D. T. (1998) Bidirectional imprinting of a single gene, GNAS1 encodes maternally, paternally, and biallelically derived proteins. *Proc. Natl. Acad. Sci. USA* **95,** 15,475–15,480.

47. Hayward, B. E., Kamiya, M., Strain, L. Moran, V., Campbell, R., Hayashizaki, Y., and Bonthron, D. T. (1998) The human GNAS1 gene is imprinted and encodes distinct paternally and biallelically expressed G proteins. *Proc. Natl. Acad. Sci. USA* **95,** 10,038–10,043.
48. Bhatt, B., Burns, J., Flanner, D., and McGee, J. (1988) Direct visualization of single copy genes on banded metaphase chromosomes by nonisotopic *in situ* hybridization. *Nucleic Acids Res.* **16,** 3951–3961.
49. Mattera, R., Graziano, M. P., Yatani, A., Zhou, Z., Graf, R., Codina, J., Birnbaumer, L., Gilman, A. G., and Brown, A. M. (1989) Splice variants of the alpha subunit of the G protein Gs activate both adenylyl cyclase and calcium channels. *Science* **243,** 804–807.
50. Jones, D. T., Masters, S. B., Bourne, H. R., and Reed, R. R. (1990) Biochemical characterization of three stimulatory GTP-binding proteins. *J. Biol. Chem.* **265,** 2671–2676.
51. Graziano, M. P., Freissmuth, M., and Gilman, A. G. (1989) Expression of Gs alpha in Escherichia coli. Purification and properties of two forms of the protein. *J. Biol. Chem.* **264,** 409–418.
52. Novotny, J. and Svoboda, P. (1998) The long (Gs(alpha)-L) and short (Gs(alpha)-S) variants of the stimulatory guanine nucleotide-binding protein. Do they behave in an identical way? *J. Mol. Endocrinol.* **20,** 163–173.
53. Ishikawa, Y., Bianchi, C., Nadal-Ginard, B., and Homcy, C. J. (1990) Alternative promoter and 5' exon generate a novel G_s alpha mRNA. *J. Biol. Chem.* **265,** 8458–8462.
54. Leitner, B., Lovisetti-Scamihorn, P., Heilmann, J., Striessnig, J., Blakely, R. D., Eiden, L. E., and Winkler, H. (1999) Subcellular localization of chromogranins, calcium channels, amine carriers, and proteins of the exocytotic machinery in bovine splenic nerve. *J. Neurochem.* **72,** 1110–1116.
55. Ischia, R., Lovisetti-Scamihorn, P., Hogue-Angeletti, R., Wolkersdorfer, M., Winkler, H., and Fischer-Colbrie, R. (1997) Molecular cloning and characterization of NESP55, a novel chromogranin-like precursor of a peptide with 5-HT1B receptor antagonist activity. *J. Biol. Chem.* **272,** 11,657–11,662.
56. Kehlenbach, R. H., Matthey, J., and Huttner, W. B. (1994) XLαs is a new type of G protein. *Nature* **372,** 804–808.
57. Lin, C. K., Hakakha, M. J., Nakamoto, J. M., Englund, A. T., Brickman, A. S., Scott, M. L., and Van Dop, C. (1992) Prevalence of three mutations in the Gs alpha gene among 24 families with pseudohypoparathyroidism type Ia. *Biochem. Biophys. Res. Commun.* **189,** 343–349.
58. Iiri, T., Herzmark, P., Nakamoto, J. M., Van Dop, C., and Bourne, H. R. (1994) Rapid GDP release from Gsα in patients with gain and loss of function. *Nature* **371,** 164–168.
59. Luttikhuis, M. E., Wilson, L. C., Leonard, J. V., and Trembath, R. C. (1994) Characterization of a de novo 43-bp deletion of the Gs alpha gene (GNAS1) in Albright hereditary osteodystrophy. *Genomics* **21,** 455–457.
60. Patten, J. L., Johns, D. R., Valle, D., Eil, C., Gruppuso, P. A., Steele, G., Smallwood, P. M., and Levine, M. A. (1990) Mutation in the gene encoding the stimulatory G protein of adenylate cyclase in Albright's hereditary osteodystrophy. *N. Engl. J. Med.* **322,** 1412–1419.
61. Weinstein, L. S., Gejman, P. V., Friedman, E., Kadowaki, T., Collins, R. M., Gershon, E. S., and Spiegel, A. M. (1990) Mutations of the Gs alpha-subunit gene in Albright hereditary osteodystrophy detected by denaturing gradient gel electrophoresis. *Proc. Natl. Acad. Sci. USA* **87,** 8287–8290.

62. Miric, A., Vechio, J. D., and Levine, M. A. (1993) Heterogeneous mutations in the gene encoding the alpha subunit of the stimulatory G protein of adenylyl cyclase in Albright hereditary osteodystrophy. *J. Clin. Endocrinol. Metab.* **76,** 1560–1568.
63. Schwindinger, W. F., Miric, A., Zimmerman, D., and Levine, M. A. (1994) A novel Gsα mutant in a patient with Albright hereditary osteodystrophy uncouples cell surface receptors from adenylyl cyclase. *J. Biol. Chem.* **269,** 25,387–25,391.
64. Farfel, Z., Iiri, T., Shapira, H., Roitman, A., Mouallem, M., and Bourne, H. R. (1996) Pseudohypoparathyroidism, a novel mutation in the betagamma-contact region of Gsalpha impairs receptor stimulation. *J. Biol Chem.* **271,** 19,653–19,655.
65. Shapira, H., Mouallem, M., Shapiro, M. S., Weisman, Y., and Farfel, Z. (1996) Pseudohypoparathyroidism type Ia, two new heterozygous frameshift mutations in exons 5 and 10 of the Gs alpha gene. *Hum. Genet.* **97,** 73–75.
66. Fischer, J. A., Egert, F., Werder, E., and Born, W. (1998) An inherited mutation associated with functional deficiency of the alpha-subunit of the guanine nucleotide-binding protein Gs in pseudo- and pseudopseudohypoparathyroidism. *J. Clin. Endocrinol. Metab.* **83,** 935–938.
67. Jan de Beur, S. M., Deng, Z., Ding, C. L., and Levine, M. A. (1998) Amplification of the GC-rich exon 1 of GNAS1 and identification of three novel nonsense mutations in Albright's hereditary osteodystrophy. *Endocr. Soc.* (Abstr.), 62.
68. Nakamoto, J. M., Sandstrom, A. T., Brickman, A. S., Christenson, R. A., and Van Dop, C. (1998) Pseudohypoparathyroidism type Ia from maternal but not paternal transmission of a Gsalpha gene mutation. *Am. J. Med. Genet.* **77,** 261–267.
69. Warner, D. R., Weng, G., Yu, S., Matalon, R., and Weinstein, L. S. (1998) A novel mutation in the switch 3 region of Gsalpha in a patient with Albright hereditary osteodystrophy impairs GDP binding and receptor activation. *J. Biol. Chem.* **273,** 23,976–23,983.
70. Ahmed, S. F., Dixon, P. H., Bonthron, D. T., Stirling, H. F., Barr, D. G., Kelnar, C. J., and Thakker, R. V. (1998) GNAS1 mutational analysis in pseudohypoparathyroidism. *Clin. Endocrinol. (Oxford)* **49,** 525–531.
71. Weinstein, L. S., Gejman, P. V., de Mazancourt, P., American, N., and Spiegel, A. M. (1992) A heterozygous 4-bp deletion mutation in the $G_s\alpha$ gene (GNAS1) in a patient with Albright hereditary osteodystrophy. *Genomics* **13,** 1319–1321.
72. Yu, S., Yu, D., Hainline, B. E., Brener, J. L., Wilson, K. A., Wilson, L. C., Oude-Luttikhuis, M. E., Trembath, R. C., and Weinstein, L. S. (1995) A deletion hot-spot in exon 7 of the Gs alpha gene (GNAS1) in patients with Albright hereditary osteodystrophy. *Hum. Mol. Genet.* **4,** 2001–2002.
73. Carter, A., Bardin, C., Collins, R., Simons, C., Bray, P., and Spiegel, A. (1987) Reduced expression of multiple forms of the alpha subunit of the stimulatory GTP-binding protein in pseudohypoparathyroidism type Ia. *Proc. Natl. Acad. Sci. USA* **84,** 7266–7269.
74. Mallet, E., Carayon, P., Amr, S., Brunelle, P., Ducastelle, T., Basuyau, J. P., and de Menibus, C. H. (1982) Coupling defect of thyrotropin receptor and adenylate cyclase in a pseudohypoparathyroid patient. *J. Clin. Endocrinol Metab.* **54,** 1028–1032.
75. Marx, S. J., Hershman, J. M., and Aurbach, G. D. (1971) Thyroid dysfunction in pseudohypoparathyroidism. *J. Clin. Endocrinol. Metab.* **33,** 822–828.
76. Werder, E. A., Illig, R., Bernasconi, S., Kind, H., and Prader, A. (1975) Excessive thyrotropin-releasing hormone in pseudohypoparathyroidism. *Pediatr. Res.* **9,** 12–16.

77. Wolfsdorf, J. I., Rosenfield, R. L., Fang, V. S. and et al. (1978) Partial gonadotrophin-resistance in pseudohypoparathyroidism. *Acta Endocrinol.* **88,** 321–328.
78. Levine, M. A., Downs, R. W. Jr., Moses, A. M., Breslau, N. A., Marx, S. J., Lasker, R. D., Rizzoli, R. E., Aurbach, G. D., and Spiegel, A. M. (1983) Resistance to multiple hormones in patients with pseudohypoparathyroidism. Association with deficient activity of guanine nucleotide regulatory protein. *Am. J. Med.* **74,** 545–556.
79. Tsai, K. S., Chang, C. C., Wu, D. J., Huang, T. S.. Tsai, I. H., and Chen, F. W. (1989) Deficient erythrocyte membrane Gs alpha activity and resistance to trophic hormones of multiple endocrine organs in two cases of pseudohypoparathyroidism. *Taiwan. I. Hsueh. Hui. Tsa. Chih.* **88,** 450–455.
80. Levine, M. A., Jap, T. S., and Hung, W. (1985) Infantile hypothyroidism in two sibs, an unusual presentation of pseudohypoparathyroidism type Ia. *J. Pediatr.* **107,** 919–922.
81. Weisman, Y., Golander, A., Spirer, Z., and Farfel, Z. (1985) Pseudohypoparathyroidism type Ia presenting as congenital hypothyroidism. *J. Pediatr.* **107,** 413–415.
82. Yokoro, S., Matsuo, M., Ohtsuka, T., and Ohzeki, T. (1990) Hyperthyrotropinemia in a neonate with normal thyroid hormone levels, the earliest diagnostic clue for pseudohypoparathyroidism. *Biol. Neonate* **58,** 69–72.
83. Downs, R. W., Jr., Levine, M. A., Drezner, M. K., Burch, W. M., Jr., and Spiegel, A. M. (1983) Deficient adenylate cyclase regulatory protein in renal membranes from a patient with pseudohypoparathyroidism. *J. Clin. Invest.* **71,** 231–235.
84. Moses, A. M., Weinstock, R. S., Levine, M. A., and Breslau, N. A. (1986) Evidence for normal antidiuretic responses to endogenous and exogenous arginine vasopressin in patients with guanine nucleotide-binding stimulatory protein-deficient pseudohypoparathyroidism. *J. Clin. Endocrinol. Metab.* **62,** 221–224.
85. Ridderskamp, P. and Schlaghecke, R. (1990) Pseudohyoparathyroidism and adreanal cortex insufficiency. A case of multiple endocrinopathy due to peripheral hormone resistance. *Klin. Wochenschr.* **68,** 927–931.
86. Wilson, L. C., Oude Luttikhuis, M. E., Clayton, P. T., Fraser, W. D., and Trembath, R. C. (1994) Parental origin of Gs alpha gene mutations in Albright's hereditary osteodystrophy. *J. Med. Genet.* **31,** 835–839.
87. Davies, S. J. and Hughes, H. E. (1993) Imprinting in Albright's hereditary osteodystrophy. *J. Med. Genet.* **30,** 101–103.
88. Campbell, R., Gosden, C. M., and Bonthron, D. T. (1994) Parental origin of transcription from the human GNAS1 gene. *J. Med.Genet.* **31,** 607–614.
89. Yu, S., Yu, D., Lee, E., Eckhaus, M., Lee, R., Corria, Z., Accili, D., Westphal, H., and Weinstein, L. S. (1998) Variable and tissue-specific hormone resistance in heterotrimeric Gs protein alpha-subunit (Gs alpha) knockout mice is due to tissue-specific imprinting of the gsalpha gene. *Proc. Natl. Acad. Sci. USA* **95,** 8715–8720.
90. Schwindinger, W. F., Lawler, A. M., Gearhart, J. D., and Levine, M. A. (1998) A murine model of Albright hereditary osteodystrophy. *Endocr. Soc.* (Abstr.)
91. Schwindinger, W. F., Francomano, C. A., and Levine, M. A. (1992) Identification of a mutation in the gene encoding the alpha subunit of the stimulatory G protein of adenylyl cyclase in McCune–Albright syndrome. *Proc. Natl. Acad. Sci. USA* **89,** 5152–5156.
92. Weinstein, L. S., Shenker, A., Gejman, P. V., Merino, M. J., Friedman, E., and Spiegel, A. M. (1991) Activating mutations of the stimulatory G protein in the McCune–Albright syndrome. *N. Engl. J. Med.* **325,** 1688–1695.

93. Faull, C. M., Welbury, R. R., Paul, B., and Kendall Taylor, P. (1991) Pseudohypoparathyroidism, its phenotypic variability and associated disorders in a large family. *Q. J. Med.* **78,** 251–264.
94. Fitch, N. (1982) Albright's hereditary osteodystrophy, a review. *Am. J. Med. Genet.* **11,** 11–29.
95. Croft, L. K., Witkop, C. J., and Glas, J.-E. (1965) Pseudohypoparathyroidism. *Oral Surg. Oral Med. Oral Pathol.* **20,** 758–770.
96. Poznanski, A. K., Werder, E. A., and Giedion, A. (1977) The pattern of shortening of the bones of the hand in PHP and PPHP: a comparison with brachydactyly E, Turner syndrome, and acrodysostosis. *Radiology* **123,** 707–718.
97. Graudal, N., Galloe, A., Christensen, H., and Olesen, K. (1988) The pattern of shortened hand and foot bones in D- and E-brachydactyly and pseudohypoparathyroidism/pseudopseudohypoparathyroidism. *ROFO. Fortschr. Geb. Rontgenstr. Nuklearmed.* **148,** 460–462.
98. Steinbach, H. L., Rudhe, U., Jonsson, M., et al. (1965) Evolution of skeletal lesions in pseudohypoparathyroidism. *Radiology* **85,** 670–676.
99. Alam, S. M. and Kelly, W. (1990) Spinal cord compression associated with pseudohypoparathyroidism. *J. R. Soc. Med.* **83,** 50–51.
100. Prendiville, J. S., Lucky, A. W., Mallory, S. B., Mughal, Z., Mimouni, F., and Langman, C. B. (1992) Osteoma cutis as a presenting sign of pseudohypoparathyroidism. *Pediatr. Dermatol.* **9,** 11–18.
101. Izraeli, S., Metzker, A., Horev, G., Karmi, D., Merlob, P., and Farfel, Z. (1992) Albright hereditary osteodystrophy with hypothyroidism, normocalcemia, and normal Gs protein activity. *Am. J. Med.* **43,** 764–767.
102. Le Roith, D., Burshell, A. C., Ilia, R., and Glick, S. M. (1979) Short metacarpal in a patient with idiopathic hypoparathyroidism. *Isr. J. Med. Sci.* **15,** 460–461.
103. Moses, A. M. and Notman, D. D. (1979) Albright's osteodystrophy in a patient with renal hypercalciuria. *J. Clin. Endocrinol. Metab.* **49,** 794–797.
104. Sasaki, H., Tsutsu, N., Asano, T., Yamamoto, T., Kikuchi, M., and Okumura, M. (1985) Co-existing primary hyperparathyroidism and Albright's hereditary osteodystrophy—an unusual association. *Postgrad. Med. J.* **61,** 153–155.
105. Hedeland, H., Berntorp, K., Arheden, K., and Kristoffersson, U. (1992) Pseudohypoparathyroidism type I and Albright's hereditary osteodystrophy with a proximal 15q chromosomal deletion in mother and daughter. *Clin. Genet.* **42,** 129–134.
106. Wilson, L. C., Leverton, K., Oude Luttikhuis, M. E., Oley, C. A., Flint, J., Wolstenholme, J., Duckett, D. P., Barrow, M. A., Leonard, J. V., Read, A. P. and et al. (1995) Brachydactyly and mental retardation, an Albright hereditary osteodystrophy-like syndrome localized to 2q37. *Am. J. Hum. Genet.* **56,** 400–407.
107. Phelan, M. C., Rogers, R. C., Clarkson, K. B., Bowyer, F. P., Levine, M. A., Estabrooks, L. L., Severson, M. C., and Dobyns, W. B. (1995) Albright hereditary osteodystrophy and del(2)(q37. 3) in four unrelated individuals. *Am. J. Med. Genet.* **58,** 1–7.
108. Silve, C., Santora, A., Breslau, N., Moses, A., and Spiegel, A. (1986) Selective resistance to parathyroid hormone in cultured skin fibroblasts from patients with pseudohypoparathyroidism type Ib. *J. Clin. Endocrinol. Metab.* **62,** 640–644.
109. Kidd, G. S., Schaaf, M., Adler, R. A., Lassman, M. N., and Wray, H. L. (1980) Skeletal responsiveness in pseudohypoparathyroidism: a spectrum of clinical disease. *Am. J. Med.* **68,** 772–781.

110. Silve, C., Suarez, F., el Hessni, A., Loiseau, A., Graulet, A. M., and Gueris, J. (1990) The resistance to parathyroid hormone of fibroblasts from some patients with type Ib pseudohypoparathyroidism is reversible with dexamethasone. *J. Clin. Endocrinol. Metab.* **71,** 631–638.
111. Suarez, F., Lebrun, J. J., Lecossier, D., Escoubet, B., Coureau, C., and Silve, C. (1995) Expression and modulation of the parathyroid hormone (PTH)/PTH-related peptide receptor messenger ribonucleic acid in skin fibroblasts from patients with type Ib pseudohypoparathyroidism. *J. Clin. Endocrinol. Metab.* **80,** 965–970.
112. Schipani, E., Weinstein, L. S., Bergwitz, C., Iida-Klein, A., Kong, X. F., Stuhrmann, M., Kruse, K., Whyte, M. P., Murray, T., Schmidtke, J. et al. (1995) Pseudohypoparathyroidism type Ib is not caused by mutations in the coding exons of the human parathyroid hormone (PTH)/PTH-related peptide receptor gene. *J. Clin. Endocrinol. Metab.* **80,** 1611–1621.
113. Bettoun, J. D., Minagawa, M., Kwan, M. Y., Lee, H. S., Yasuda, T., Hendy, G. N., Goltzman, D., and White, J. H. (1997) Cloning and characterization of the promoter regions of the human parathyroid hormone (PTH)/PTH-related peptide receptor gene, Analysis of deoxyribonucleic acid from normal subjects and patients with pseudohypoparathyroidism type 1b. *J. Clin. Endocrinol. Metab.* **82,** 1031–1040.
114. Fukumoto, S., Suzawa, M., Takeuchi, Y., Kodama, Y., Nakayama, K., Ogata, E., Matsumoto, T., and Fujita, T. (1996) Absence of mutations in parathyroid hormone (PTH)/PTH-related protein receptor complementary deoxyribonucleic acid in patients with pseudohypoparathyroidism type Ib. *J. Clin. Endocrinol. Metab.* **81,** 2554–2558.
115. Lanske, B., Karaplis, A. C., Lee, K., Luz, A., Vortkamp, A., Pirro, A., Karperien, M., Defize, L. K., Ho, C., Mulligan, R. C., Abou-Samra, A. B., Juppner, H., Segre, G. V., and Kronenberg, H. M. (1996) PTH/PTHrP receptor in early development and Indian hedgehog-regulated bone growth. *Science* **273,** 663–666.
116. Jobert, A. S., Zhang, P., Couvineau, A., Bonaventure, J., Roume, J., Le Merrer, M., and Silve, C. (1998) Absence of functional receptors for parathyroid hormone and parathyroid hormone-related peptide in Blomstrand chondrodysplasia. *J. Clin. Invest.* **102,** 34–40.
117. Allen, D. B., Friedman, A. L., Greer, F. R., and Chesney, R. W. (1988) Hypomagnesemia masking the appearance of elevated parathyroid hormone concentrations in familial pseudohypoparathyroidism. *Am. J. Med. Genet.* **31,**153–158.
118. Juppner, H., Schipani, E., Bastepe, M., Cole, D. E., Lawson, M. L., Mannstadt, M. et al. (1998) The gene responsible for pseudohypoparathyroidism type Ib is paternally imprinted and maps in four unrelated kindreds to chromosome 20q13. 3. *Proc. Natl. Acad. Sci. USA* **95,** 11,798–11,803.
119. Farfel, Z., Brothers, V. M., Brickman, A. S., Conte, F., Neer, R., and Bourne, H. R. (1981) Pseudohypoparathyroidism, inheritance of deficient receptor-cyclase coupling activity. *Proc. Natl. Acad. Sci. USA* **78,** 3098–3102.
120. Barrett, D., Breslau, N. A., Wax, M. B., Molinoff, P. B., and Downs, R. W., Jr. (1989) New form of pseudohypoparathyroidism with abnormal catalytic adenylate cyclase. *Am. J. Physiol.* **257,** E277–E283
121. Farfel, Z., Bourne, H. R., and Iiri, T. (1999) The expanding spectrum of G protein diseases. *N. Engl. J Med.* **340,** 1012–1020.
122. Van Dop, C. (1989) Pseudohypoparathyroidism, clinical and molecular aspects. *Semin. Nephrol.* **9,** 168–178.

123. Kruse, K., Kracht, U., Wohlfart, K., and Kruse, U. (1989) Biochemical markers of bone turnover, intact serum parathyroid horn and renal calcium excretion in patients with pseudohypoparathyroidism and hypoparathyroidism before and during vitamin D treatment. *Eur. J. Pediatr.* **148,** 535–539.
124. Attanasio, R., Curcio, T., Giusti, M., Monachesi, M., Nalin, R., and Giordano, G. (1986) Pseudohypoparathyroidism. A case report with low immunoreactive parathyroid hormone and multiple endocrine dysfunctions. *Minerva. Endocrinol.* **11,** 267–273.
125. Litvin, Y.,Rosler, A., and Bloom. R. A. (1981) Extensive cerebral calcification in hypoparathyroidism. *Neuroradiology* **21,** 271–271.
126. Sachs, C., Sjoberg, H. E., and Ericson, K. (1982) Basal ganglia calcifications on CT, Relation to hypoparathyroidism. *Neurology* **32,** 779–782.
127. Korn-Lubetzki, I., Rubinger, D., and Siew, F. (1980) Visualization of basal ganglion calcification by cranial computed tomography in a patient with pseudohypoparathyroidism. *Isr. J. Med. Sci.* **16,** 40–41.
128. Pearson, D. W. M., Durward, W. F., Fogelman, I., Boyle, I. T., and Beastall, G. (1981) Pseudohypoparathyroidism presenting as severe Parkinsonism. *Postgrad. Med. J.* **57,** 445–447.
129. Miano, A., Casadel, G., and Biasini, G. (1981) Cardiac failure in pseudohypoparathyroidism. *Helv. Paediat. Acta* **36,** 191–192.
130. Cavallo, A., Meyer, W. J., III, Bodensteiner, J. B., and Chesson, A. L. (1980) Spinal cord compression, An unusual manifestation of pseudohypoparathyroidism. *Am. J. Dis. Child* **134,** 706–707.
131. Breslau, N. A., Notman, D., Canterbury, J. M., and Moses, A. M. (1980) Studies on the attainment of normocalcemia in patients with pseudohypoparathyroidism. *Am. J. Med.* **68,** 856–860.
132. Stirling, H. F., Darling, J. A., and Barr, D. G. (1991) Plasma cyclic AMP response to intravenous parathyroid hormone in pseudohypoparathyroidism. *Acta Paediatr. Scand.* **80,** 333–338.
133. Mallette, L. E., Kirkland, J. L., Gagel, R. F., Law, W. M., Jr. and Heath, H. III. (1988) Synthetic human parathyroid hormone-(1–34) for the study of pseudohypoparathyroidism. *J. Clin. Endocrinol. Metab.* **67,** 964–972.
134. Mallette, L. E. (1988) Synthetic human parathyroid hormone 1–34 fragment for diagnostic testing. *Ann. Intern. Med.* **109,** 800–804.
135. Furlong, T. J., Seshadri, M. S., Wilkinson, M. R., Cornish, C. J., Luttrell, B., and Posen, S. (1986) Clinical experiences with human parathyroid hormone 1–34. *Aust. N. Z. J. Med.* **16,** 794–798.
136. Walton, R. J. and Bijvoet, O. L. M. (1975) Nomogram for derivation of renal threshold phosphate concentration. *Lancet* **309**, 310.
137. Sohn, H.E., Furukawa, Y., Yumita, S., Miura, R., Unakami, H., and Yoshinaga, K. (1984) Effect of synthetic 1–34 fragment of human parathyroid hormone on plasma adenosine 3', 5'–monophosphate (cAMP) concentrations and the diagnostic criteria based on the plasma cAMP response in Ellsworth–Howard test. *Endocrinol. Jpn.* **31,** 33–40.
138. Miura, R., Yumita, S., Yoshinaga, K., and Furukawa, Y. (1990) Response of plasma 1,25-dihydroxyvitamin D in the human PTH(1–34) infusion test, an improved index for the diagnosis of idiopathic hypoparathyroidism and pseudohypoparathyroidism. *Calcif. Tissue Int.* **46,** 309–313.

139. McElduff, A., Lissner, D., Wilkinson, M., Cornish, C., and Posen, S. (1987) A 6-hour human parathyroid hormone (1–34) infusion protocol, studies in normal and hypoparathyroid subjects. *Calcif. Tissue Int.* **41,** 267–273.
140. Litvak, J., Moldawer, M. P., Forbes, A. P., and Henneman, P. H. (1958) Hypocalcemic hypercalciuria during vitamin D and dihydrotachysterol therpay of hypoparathyroidism. *J. Clin. Endocrinol. Metab.* **18,** 246–252.
141. Yamamoto, M., Takuwa, Y., Masuko, S., and Ogata, E. (1988) Effects of endogenous and exogenous parathyroid hormone on tubular reabsorption of calcium in pseudohypoparathyroidism. *J. Clin. Endocrinol. Metab.* **66,** 618–625.
142. Okano, K., Furukawa, Y., Morii, H., and Fujita, T. (1982) Comparative efficacy of various vitamin D metabolites in the treatment of various types of hypoparathyroidism. *J. Clin. Endocrinol. Metab.* **55,** 238–243.
143. Breslau, N. A. (1989) Pseudohypoparathyroidism, current concepts. *Am. J. Med. Sci.* **298,** 130–140.
144. Shenker, A., Weinstein, L. S., Sweet, D. E., and Spiegel, A. M. (1994) An activating Gsa mutation is present in fibrous dysplasia of bone in McCune–Albright syndrome. *J. Clin. Endocrinol. Metab.* **79,** 750–755.
145. Shenker, A., Weinstein, L. S., Moran, A., Pescovitz, O. H., Charest, N. J., Boney, C. M., Van Wyk, J. J., Merino, M. J., Feuillan, P. P., and Spiegel, A. M. (1993) Severe endocrine and nonendocrine manifestations of the McCune– Albright syndrome associated with activating mutations of stimulatory G protein GS. *J. Pediatr.* **123,** 509–518.
146. Levine, M. A., Schwindinger, W. F., Downs, R. W. Jr., and Moses, A. M. (1994) Pseudohypoparathyroidism: clinical, biochemical, and molecular features, in *The Parathyroids, Basic and Clinical Concepts.* (Bilezikian, J. P., Marcus, R., and Levine, M. A., eds.)Raven Press, New York, pp. 781–800.
147. Landis, C. A., Masters, S. B., Spada, A., Pace, A. M., Bourne, H. R., and Vallar, L. (1989) GTPase inhibiting mutations activate the alpha chain of Gs and stimulate adenylyl cyclase in human pituitary tumours. *Nature* **340,** 692–696.
148. Lyons, J., Landis, C. A., Griffith, H., Vallar, L., Grunewald, K., Feichtinger, H., Yuh, Q. Y., Clark, O. H., Kawasaki, E., Bourne, H. R., and McCormick, F. (1990) Two G protein oncogenes in human endocrine tumors. *Science* **249,** 655–659.
149. Levine, M. A., Parfrey, N. A., and Feinstein, R. S. (1982) Pseudohypoparathyroidism. *Johns Hopkins Med. J.* **151,** 137–146.

Chapter 12

Fibrodysplasia Ossificans Progressiva

Eileen M. Shore, John G. Rogers, Roger Smith, Francis H. Gannon, Martin Delatycki, J. Andoni Urtizberea, James Triffitt, Martine Le Merrer, and Frederick S. Kaplan

Introduction

Fibrodysplasia ossificans progressiva (FOP) is a rare genetic disorder of connective tissue characterized by congenital malformation of the great toes and by progressive heterotopic osteogenesis that occurs in predictable anatomic patterns. The rate of disease progression is variable *(1)*; however, onset of heterotopic bone formation typically occurs before age 10. Cumulative episodes of heterotopic ossification commonly result in ankylosis of all major joints of the axial and appendicular skeleton, preventing movement of affected joints. Most patients are confined to a wheelchair by the third decade of life and require lifelong assistance in performing activities of daily living. Surgical trauma associated with attempts to remove heterotopic bone typically leads to increased local ossification. There is currently no effective treatment.

Neither the genetic defect nor pathophysiology of fibrodysplasia ossificans progressiva are known. A candidate gene approach to identify the cause of this disorder is being pursued since no karyotype abnormalities have been detected in patients with FOP, and gene identification through linkage analysis is difficult, as few families with inheritance of fibrodysplasia ossificans progressiva have been identified worldwide *(1–6)*. The bone morphogenetic protein (BMP) genes and other genes in the BMP pathway have been implicated as plausible candidate genes *(7–10)*.

Phenotypic Features of FOP

The three major diagnostic criteria for FOP are congenital malformations of the great toes *(11)*, progressive heterotopic endochondral ossification *(12)*, and disease progression in well-defined anatomic patterns *(13,14)*.

The Genetics of Osteoporosis and Metabolic Bone Disease
Ed.: M. J. Econs © Humana Press Inc., Totowa, NJ

Congenital Skeletal Malformations

The skeleton that develops during embryogenesis in people who have FOP is grossly normal, with the most characteristic skeletal malformation being the shortening and deviation of the big toes (hallux valgus), due to malformations in the cartilaginous anlage of the first metatarsal and proximal phalanx *(11,15)*. In some cases, the thumbs may also be strikingly short and malformed *(11,16,17)*. Additional sporadic exceptions to normal skeletal formation include segmentation defects in the cervical spine (hypoplasia of the vertebral bodies of the cervical spine and synostosis of the posterior elements) *(6,18)*, broad short femoral necks *(19,20)*, osteochondromas of the proximal tibias *(12)* and rarely enchondromas *(21)*. An association with synovial chondromatosis also has been reported *(22)*.

Congenital malformation of the great toes is the earliest recognizable phenotypic feature of FOP and is present in nearly all affected individuals *(15,23)* (Fig. 1), occurring in greater than 95% of cases of FOP, and should be considered a hallmark of the disease *(15)*. Eventual fusion of the proximal and distal phalanges of the great toe is typical. Fibrodysplasia ossificans progressiva can be suspected at birth, before soft-tissue lesions occur, if the characteristic congenital skeletal malformations are recognized *(12)*. Usually, FOP is diagnosed only when soft-tissue swellings and radiologic evidence of heterotopic ossification are noted in the presence of congenital malformations of the toes.

Heterotopic Ossification

Impending heterotopic ossification is signaled by the appearance of large, often painful, lesions of highly vascular fibroproliferative tissue *(12,24)* involving skeletal muscle, tendons, and ligaments (Fig. 2). It is not yet known whether these lesions are monoclonal fibroproliferative tumors or polyclonal reactive lesions. These soft-tissue lesions generally appear spontaneously, but also may be precipitated by minor trauma such as intramuscular childhood immunizations *(25)* or falls *(26)*. Lesion-associated swelling develops rapidly over the course of several days *(27)*. Fever may occur during this development, mistakenly suggesting an infectious process or tumor. Aponeuroses, fascia, tendons, ligaments, and connective tissue of voluntary muscles may be affected *(15,23,28)*. Typically, lesions occur in paraspinal muscles in the back or in the limb girdles and may evolve over months. While many early swellings may regress spontaneously, others form heterotopic bone *(27)*. Factors responsible for the regression of some lesions and the progression of others are not known. Regardless of the cause, the lesions in FOP mature through an endochondral pathway to form normal lamellar bone that bridges and immobilizes the joints of the axial and appendicular skeleton *(12)* (Fig. 3). The episodes of FOP lesion formation occur at unpredictable frequencies *(17,20)*, and some patients enter periods of disease quiescence.

Once ossification develops, it is permanent, although bone remodeling may occur at heterotopic sites, and the shape and size of the lesion may change over time. Radiographic evidence indicates normal modeling and remodeling of the heterotopic skeleton *(29,30)*, including:

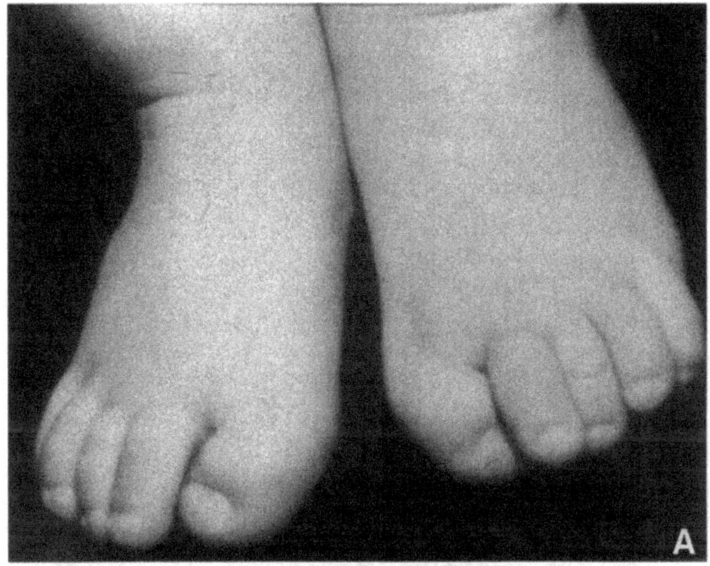

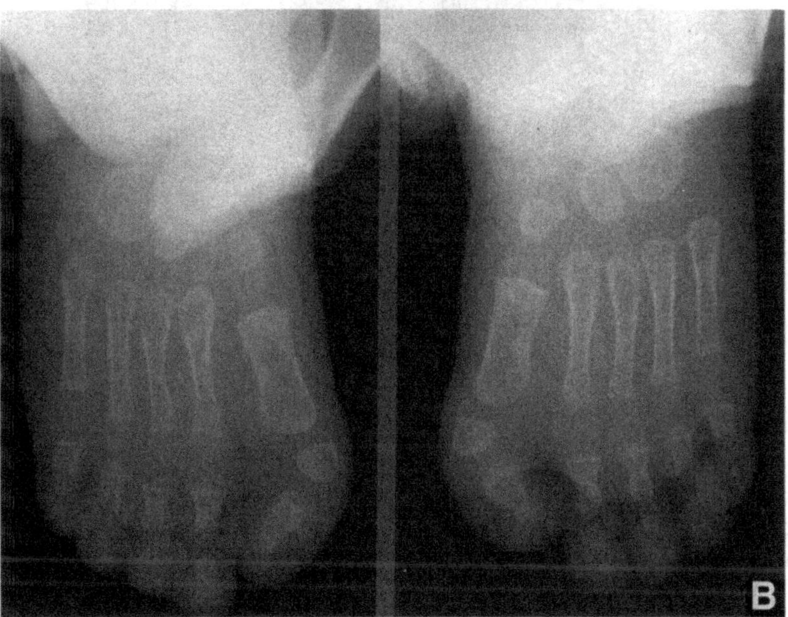

Fig. 1. Toe malformation in FOP. (**A**) Clinical photograph of the feet of a 13-mo-old child with FOP. Note the short malformed great toes with valgus deviation at the metatarsophalangeal joints. (**B**) Anteroposterior radiographs reveal an anteroposterior patterning defect with malformed first metatarsals, delta-shaped proximal phalanges, and valgus deviation at the metatarsophalangeal joints.

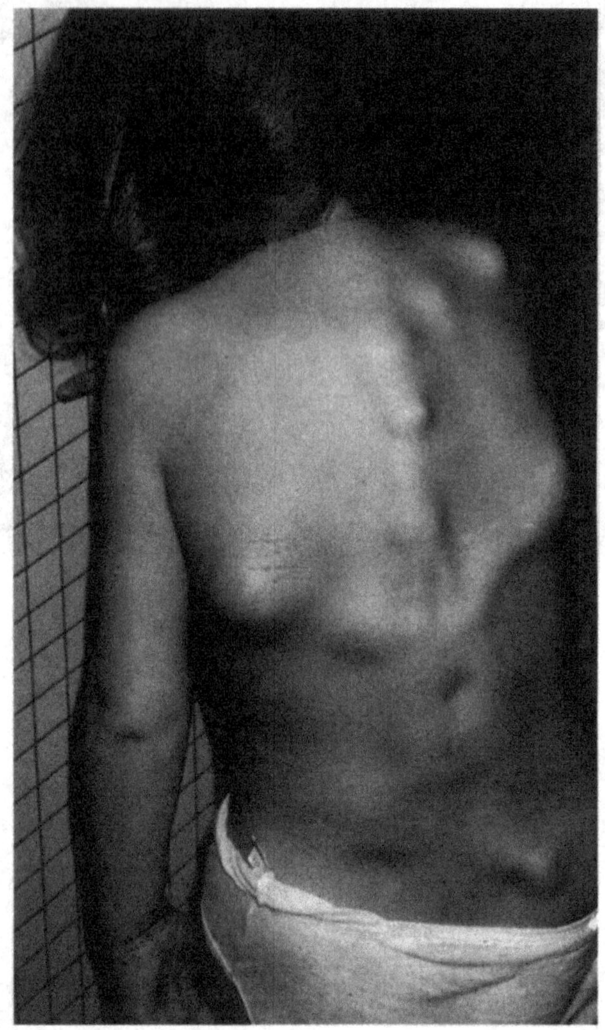

Fig. 2. Clinical photograph of the back of a 4-yr-old child with FOP. Note the appearance of multiple pre-osseous soft tissue lesions along with areas of more mature heterotopic bone during the time of an acute flareup of the condition.

1. Tubular and flat bones with mature cortical and trabecular organization;
2. Well-defined cortical-endosteal borders enclosing medullary canals;
3. Metaphyseal funnelization in isolated ossicles or at sites of synostoses;
4. Osteosclerosis from use (weight bearing) and osteopenia from disuse; and
5. Absence of pathologic fractures or stress fractures from fatigue failure.

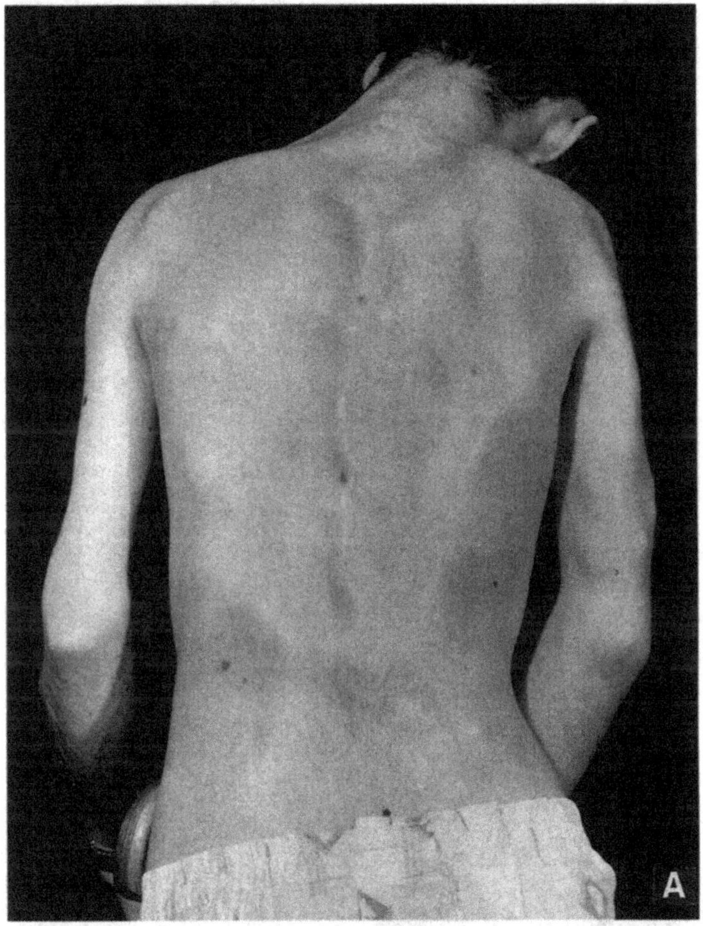

Fig. 3. Clinical photograph and skeleton of a 25-yr-old man with FOP. The rigid posture noted in this man with FOP is due to ankylosis of the spine,shoulders, and elbows. Plates and ribbons of ectopic bone contour the skin over the back and arms **(A)**, and can be visualized directly on the skeleton **(B)** (following death from pneumonia at age 40 yr). (Courtesy of the Mutter Museum, College of Physicians of Philadelphia. Reprinted with permission from ref. *10*.)

Isotope bone scans also suggest that remodeling of mature heterotopic bone is normal. Fracture healing in the heterotopic and normotopic bone is similar, although healing of heterotopic bone may be accelerated *(30,31)*.

Isotope bone scans show abnormalities before ossification can be detected by conventional radiographs *(32)*. Computerized tomography and magnetic resonance imaging of early lesions have been described *(33,34)*. In early ectopic

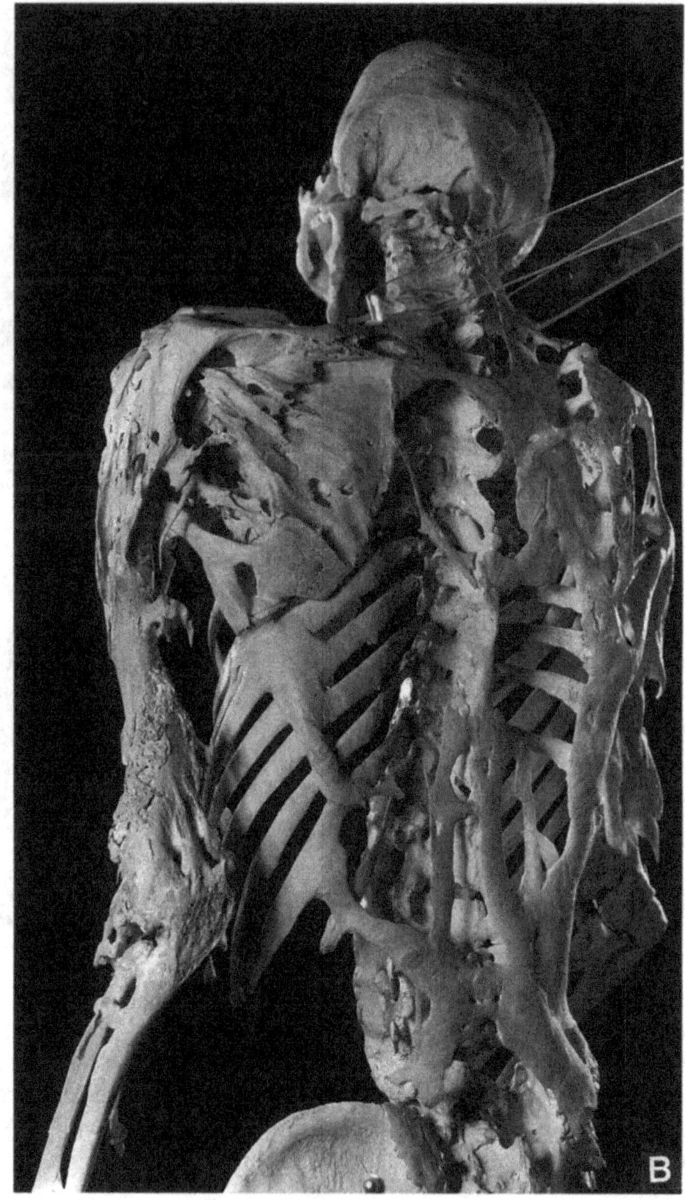

Fig. 3B

ossification, the isotope uptake is considerably increased and the CT scan detects calcification earlier than on plain films. Ultrasound and angiography have also been used to examine lesions.

Patterns of Disease Progression

The anatomic progression of heterotopic bone formation in FOP occurs in specific patterns (or gradients) over time, beginning early in post-natal life and proceeding in predictable temporal and spatial patterns, with the first involvement typically occurring in muscles along the upper back and neck *(13,14)*. Involvement is typically seen earliest in dorsal, axial, cranial, and proximal regions of the body and later in ventral, appendicular, caudal, and distal regions *(13)*. This sequence of events is similar to the developmental pattern of embryonic skeletal formation, although the exact cause of this pattern of progression is unknown.

The presentation and course of FOP was described in a recent clinical series *(20)* of 28 patients studied for up to 24 yr. Painful swelling of muscles (myositis) leading to ossification began at a mean age of 4.6 yr (range: 0–16 yr), initially in the neck and upper spine (in 25 subjects) and later around the hips and jaw.

The recognized temporal and spatial sequence of myositis leading to ossification in fibrodysplasia ossificans progressiva can vary among individuals *(20)*, with injury, surgical procedures, or immunization injections as potential determinants of the first site. This variation makes individual prognosis very difficult. Nevertheless a statistical analysis of 44 patients suggested that new joint involvement could be predicted in individuals *(14)*.

Typically, episodes of soft-tissue swelling begin during the first decade of life, although occasionally, the onset is as late as early adulthood *(1)*. The severity of FOP may differ dramatically among patients *(1)*, although most affected individuals become completely immobilized and confined to a wheelchair by the third decade *(14)*. The rate and extent of disability was unrelated to the time of onset of postnatal complications *(20)*.

Other Phenotypic Features

Over time, heterotopic bone causes joint immobilization. Ossification around the hips, typically formed by the third decade of life, commonly prevents ambulation. Limb swelling is a frequently reported complication of the acute myositis *(27)*. The intense angiogenesis and edema seen on histopathologic evaluation of pre-osseous fibroproliferative lesions may play a role in the acute limb swelling, but the pathogenesis of this complication is complex and may involve numerous factors including lymphedema and rarely thrombophlebitis *(27)*.

Ankylosis of the spine and rib cage also restrict patient mobility and may impair cardiopulmonary function. Scoliosis is a common finding and is associated with asymmetric bars of heterotopic bone connecting the rib cage to the pelvis *(35)*. A decrease in the normal thoracic kyphosis results from early ossification of the paravertebral musculature. Restrictive lung disease and predisposition to pneumonia may follow. While cor pulmonale might be an expected long-term result, no evidence of clinically significant right ventricular dysfunction has been reported, although many patients have electrocardiographic evidence of right ventricular dysfunction *(36)*.

Involvement of the muscles of mastication (often due to injury by injection of local anesthetic or stretching of the jaw during dental procedures) can cause ankylosis of the temporomandibular joint, leading to severe nutritional impairment *(37)*. Submandibular swelling can be a life-threatening complication with massive anterior neck swelling and difficulty swallowing. Special measures to decrease swelling, including a course of glucocorticoids, may be warranted *(38)*.

The heart, diaphragm, extraocular muscles, smooth muscles, and tongue are characteristically spared, and the intrinsic muscles of the hands are involved late in the course of the disease or not at all. Although secondary amenorrhea may develop, successful reproduction has been reported (*see* Inheritance section). Breast development in females is often impaired, and exacerbation of FOP at puberty has been reported anecdotally. Hearing impairment (beginning in late childhood or adolescence) has been reported but definitive studies to determine the nature of the hearing loss have not been undertaken *(15)*. Alopecia also has been reported frequently *(20)*.

Despite the unique clinical features of this disorder, the initial diagnosis of fibrodysplasia ossificans progressiva has often been incorrect and usually considerably delayed from the onset of symptoms. Mistaken histological diagnoses such as soft tissue sarcoma or fibromatosis has led to inappropriate treatment.

Histopathology of FOP

Adequate histopathology of FOP lesion formation has been hampered by the lack of specimens for study. Biopsy specimens of developing FOP lesions are exceedingly rare, since surgical trauma to tissues of FOP patients often leads to additional heterotopic ossification at the operative site, and occasionally at sites remote from the operative trauma *(6,12)*. Occasional tissue samples are available from nonelective surgical procedures or from biopsies taken prior to the diagnosis of FOP.

Early and Late Stage Lesions

Histological examination of early FOP lesions reveals an intense perivascular lymphocytic aggregate followed by lymphocytic invasion into the surrounding muscle with subsequent myocyte death. The lesion then progresses to a fibroproliferative tissue with extensive neovascularity *(39)*. A role for hematopoietic cells in heterotopic osteogenesis has been suggested *(40)*. Immunohistochemical evaluation of lymphocyte markers revealed a predominance of perivascular B-lymphocytes and a mixed population of B-lymphocytes and T-lymphocytes weakly positive for bone morphogenetic protein-4 (BMP-4) invading the skeletal muscle *(39)*. Whether the early lymphocytic infiltrate is a causative or reactive event, or both, cannot be determined from the observations in the small sample of patients examined. In addition, levels of basic fibroblast growth factor (bFGF), an extremely potent angiogenic peptide, are markedly elevated in the urine of patients with FOP during times of disease flare-up *(41)*, correlating with the appearance of a vascular fibroproliferative lesion.

Intermediate-stage FOP lesions cannot be distinguished histologically from aggressive juvenile fibromatosis, a condition which does not progress to form bone *(24)*, but immunohistochemistry can be useful *(12,20)*. BMP-4 expression has been detected in cultured fibroproliferative cells and in intact tissue specimens from pre-osseous FOP lesions, but not in aggressive juvenile fibromatosis lesions *(10,24)*. Later-stage FOP lesions show characteristic features of endochondral ossification including chondrocyte hypertrophy, calcification of cartilage, and formation of lamellar bone with marrow elements, almost identical to the pattern seen in a normally developing growth plate.

Animal Models for FOP

A fibrodysplasia ossificans progressiva-like condition has been recognized in cats, and six cases have been reported *(42–45)*. The disease occurs in both males and females, and affected breeds were the domestic short hair and domestic long hair cat. Affected cats ranged from ten months to six years of age at diagnosis. Unlike the disease in man, affected cats do not have congenital malformations of the distal limbs. Affected cats developed progressive joint stiffness with enlargement of proximal limb musculature. Radiography revealed multiple foci of heterotopic ossification within affected musculature. Pathologic examination revealed intense perivascular lymphocytic infiltration at the advancing edge of fibroproliferative lesions nearly identical to that seen in human FOP lesions. Marked proliferation of connective tissue followed by cartilage and bone formation within epimysium, tendons, and fasciae was observed. The clinical course of the feline disease is rapid, with the development of severe disability within weeks to months. The disease in the cat closely mimics FOP in humans, and may serve as an animal model for this disorder. Unfortunately, all evaluations performed to date have been post-mortem studies on pet cats, and no live animals are currently available for examination.

In another animal model, murine embryonic overexpression of the *c-fos* proto-oncogene leads to postnatal heterotopic chondrogenesis and osteogenesis with phenotypic features similar to those seen in children who have fibrodysplasia ossificans progressiva *(46)*. The overexpression of Fos protein in embryonic stem cell chimeras leads to heterotopic endochondral osteogenesis mediated at least in part through a BMP-4 signal transduction pathway. In contrast, early FOP lesions express abundant BMP-4 without overexpression of *c-Fos*, suggesting that the primary molecular defect in FOP may be independent of sustained Fos effects on chondrogenesis and osteogenesis *(46)*. The *c-fos* embryonic stem cell chimera may be relevant to the study of FOP *(47)*.

Inheritance

Prevalence and Distribution

FOP was first described in 1692 *(48,49)* and more than 700 cases have since been reported. The disorder is among the rarest of human afflictions, with an estimated incidence of one per two million live births in Great Britain *(50)*, the United States, and France. Currently, the authors know of fewer than 200 individuals with FOP worldwide. Although caucasian patients have been described most often, the disorder has been reported in all ethnic groups *(5,28)* including African *(51,52)*, Japanese *(53)*, Indian *(54)*, West Indian *(55)*, and native American *(4)* populations. The excess of cases reported from Europe and North America is likely due to circumstances influencing ascertainment and survival rather than a result of significantly different mutation rates in these populations *(56)*. FOP appears to affect both sexes equally *(15,56)*.

Reproductive Fitness

Reproductive fitness in this severe condition is low. Two explanations for this low reproductive fitness in FOP have been suggested *(3)*. First, the severe deformity in FOP may lead to difficulty with sexual intercourse, gestation, and delivery. Second, there may be decreased fertility in patients with FOP. Connor and Evans *(15)* found that one of 17 females studied did not develop normal secondary sexual characteristics and that many of their female patients had premature menopause. Two female patients in their twenties with "sexual infantilism" were described *(57)*, and another amenorrheic patient has been reported *(58,59)*. Two viable pregnancies in females with FOP are documented *(60,61)*. Both authors comment on the potential complications of pregnancy in such patients, including worsening of restrictive pulmonary disease *(62)* with uterine enlargement and a potential risk of exacerbation of the ectopic ossification, although this latter complication was not found in the two patients reported.

Genetic Transmission

Most described cases of FOP result from new mutations, with the mutation rate estimated to be 1.8 (SE $\pm$ 1.04) $\times 10^{-6}$ mutations per gene per generation *(50)*. The rarity of FOP suggests the likelihood of a single mutated locus causing the disorder in all or most individuals, but the possibility of genetic heterogeneity cannot be excluded.

Due to low reproductive fitness, only a few examples of inheritance of FOP within a family have been documented, and previous major reviews of FOP reported no clear examples of dominant transmission *(15,63)*. The autosomal dominant inheritance of FOP was first documented in 1886 in a 7-yr-old boy with characteristic features of FOP whose father had the same congenital deformity of the great toes but had no other features of this disorder *(64)*. A similar occurrence was reported soon after *(65)*, as was father to son transmission of classic FOP *(66)*. Further reports indicating dominant inheritance described the condition in a grandfather, a father and his three sons *(67)*, and a father and daughter with this disease *(68)*.

Kaplan et al. *(3)* reported a father, two daughters, and a son all affected by FOP. This family showed little variability in the phenotype between affected individuals. Connor et al. *(2)* reported a three-generation family with FOP with a wide range of phenotypic severity ranging from disabling ectopic bone formation and premature death to an asymptomatic adult whose only manifestation was a malformation of the big toes.

Two case reports of FOP in identical twins *(69,70)* whose parents had no sign of the condition have been noted. The first suggestion of gonadal mosaicism in FOP was reported in two half-sisters with the same unaffected mother and different unaffected fathers *(4)*, raising the possibility that the mother had a mutant gene for FOP in multiple ova but that the mutant gene was present in few or no somatic cells. Gonadal mosaicism is a proven cause of recurrence in sibs of autosomal dominant disorders *(71)*.

Although there is variable expressivity of the FOP phenotype, there is little evidence that the condition is nonpenetrant *(50)*. However, a report of one family with affected cousins does suggest the possibility of nonpenetrance *(58,59)*.

Risk of Inheritance

An autosomal dominant mode of inheritance predicts a 50% chance that any child of a person with FOP will themselves have the condition. There is no documentation of successful prenatal diagnosis of FOP. Theoretically ultrasound may be able to identify skeletal changes, but it is unknown whether these are apparent early enough in the pregnancy when termination is generally considered acceptable. An increased paternal age as an associated risk factor for occurence of FOP has been suggested *(50,72,73)*.

Counseling a family who has one child with FOP requires that both parents be thoroughly examined. Examples of a parent with mild features, such as short laterally deviated great toes, with a child showing the complete FOP phenotype have been observed *(2,64,65)*. If both parents are phenotypically normal then a low recurrence risk can be given. The possibility of gonadal mosaicism *(4)* means that the parents cannot be absolutely reassured, but can be given a very low recurrence risk.

Molecular Genetics of FOP

Candidate Gene Approach

A common approach to identifying the genetic basis of a disease, genetic linkage analysis, and positional cloning, presently is difficult for FOP due the small number of affected individuals and lack of multigenerational families showing inheritance of the disease. The candidate gene approach has been pursued as an alternative indirect method in an attempt to identify the mutated gene. In selecting a candidate gene for FOP, the main diagnostic criteria (congenital malformations of the great toes, heterotopic endochondral ossification, temporal and spatial patterns of ectopic bone formation) must be considered. The candidate gene for FOP must be functional during normal embryonic development (to account for the malformations of the great toe), as well as being active postnatally to induce heterotopic ossification in tendon, ligament, fascia, and skeletal muscle.

Bone Morphogenetic Protein (BMP) Genes

The genes that best fit the criteria of an FOP candidate gene are those that encode the bone morphogenetic protein (BMP) genes and other components in the BMP signal transduction pathways *(8,74–80)*. The term "bone morphogenetic protein" (BMP) was first used to describe a demineralized bone extract with the ability to induce ectopic bone formation in animal assay systems *(81)*. When BMP is implanted subcutaneously, the complete pathway of endochondral bone and bone marrow formation is induced at the implant site *(74,75)*. Individual components of the demineralized extract with bone-inducing activity were identified and four human cDNAs encoding these bone-inducing proteins were cloned and named the BMP genes *(74)*. Several additional members of what has become a large family of structurally related BMP genes have subsequently been identified and cloned *(77,79)*.

Mutations in the genes of two members of the BMP family which cause skeletal abnormalities during embryogenesis have been identified in the mouse. Homozygous deletions of the BMP-5 gene lead to malformations of the axial skeleton and result in abnormal fracture repair *(82)*. Homozygous mutations of Gdf-5 (growth-differentation factor-5) preferentially affect the appendicular skeleton *(83)*. A mutation in the human homologue of the Gdf-5 gene, CDMP-1 (cartilage-derived morphogenetic protein 1), has been correlated with a recessive human chondrodysplasia, acromesomelic chondrodysplasia, Hunter–Thompson type *(84)*. These mutations provide evidence for a direct role of at least some of the BMPs in embryonic and postnatal bone formation *(77,79)*.

The BMP genes, members of the larger transforming growth factor beta (TGF-β) superfamily of peptides, have been highly conserved throughout evolution *(8)*, and genes with a high degree of homology to members of the mammalian BMP family have been found in the fruit fly, *Drosophila melanogaster (8,77,79)*. The BMP-2 and BMP-4 genes, which produce proteins that are about 90% similar to each other, are homologous to the *Drosophilia* decapentaplegic (dpp) gene. The DPP protein shows approx 75% amino acid identity to BMP-2 and BMP-4 in the mature carboxyl-terminal region which is the mature functional protein domain of these proteins.

In *Drosophila*, the dpp gene is an essential gene for early embryonic development as well as later in development when it provides necessary information for limb formation *(8)*. The pattern of dpp expression is analogous to the expression of BMP-2 and BMP-4 in vertebrate development *(8,77,79)*. These BMPs play critical roles both in early embryogenesis and in skeletal formation, important criteria for FOP candidate genes. BMP-4 and DPP both appear to function by directing cell fate *(8,85)*. The absence of BMP-4 in a transgenic knockout mouse is lethal in early embryogenesis, showing little or no mesodermal differentiation, and no hematopoiesis *(78,86)*. BMP-4 has also been implicated in patterning of the developing mouse limb. Overexpression of BMP-4 in the chick embryonic limb bud is associated with ectopic osteogenesis and polarizing defects in limb formation *(87)*.

The significance of the conservation of the *Drosophila* dpp and human BMP-2 and BMP-4 gene structures is reflected in the functional similarities of their protein products. Experiments have demonstrated that the BMP-4 gene can rescue embryonic dorsal-ventral lethal pattern mutations of dpp-deficient flies *(88)*. Furthermore, when implanted into an animal assay system used to evaluate bone induction by BMPs, DPP protein can induce bone formation *(89)*. These data support the idea that the dpp and BMP-2/4 genes provide the same signaling information that is interpreted by cells in widely-varying developmental and phylogenetic contexts according to the type of cell, the cell environment, and/or the concentration of the BMP/DPP signal.

BMP Expression in FOP

Drosophila genetics and developmental biology have provided us with several clues to understand BMP function and to select the BMPs as plausible candidate genes for FOP *(8)*. Recent studies have examined the expression of many of the BMPs in cells from FOP patients *(10,24)*.

Although early FOP lesions are histologically identical to those of aggressive juvenile fibromatosis, these two disorders can be distinguished by immunohistochemistry with BMP-2/4 antibodies *(24)*. Tissue from aggressive juvenile fibromatosis lesions (which do not progress to form bone) shows no binding of the BMP2/4 antibody, while FOP lesional tissue binds the antibody, indicating the presence of the BMP proteins within early stage lesions that will progress to endochondral ossification. The antibody used for these experiments cannot distinguish between BMP-2 and BMP-4, however the activity of these two BMP genes can be distinguished by examining specific mRNA expression *(24)*.

Cells derived from a pre-osseous FOP lesion and from immortalized lymphoblastoid cell lines established from FOP patients showed increased expression (by Northern analysis and ribonuclease protection assays) of BMP-4 but not BMP-2 compared to controls. In addition, correlation of BMP-4 expression with FOP was observed in a family showing inheritance of FOP: the affected father and three affected children expressed BMP-4, while the unaffected mother did not *(10)*. Further studies have verified that BMP-4 protein is synthesized in cells from patients who have FOP *(90,91)*.

Steady-state levels of mRNA expression for BMP-4 and the BMP receptors were evaluated using semiquantitative reverse transcription polymerase chain reaction (RT-PCR) and documented the presence of Type I and Type II BMP-4 receptor mRNAs in FOP lesional tissue as well as in unaffected muscle tissue *(91)*. In lymphoblastoid cell lines of affected individuals in a family that exhibited autosomal dominant inheritance of FOP, the previous finding of elevated steady-state levels of BMP-4 mRNA was confirmed *(91)*, but no differences in the steady-state levels of mRNA for either the Type I or Type II BMP-4 receptors were observed between affected and unaffected individuals in the same family.

Given the evidence of BMP-4 overexpression associated with heterotopic ossification in FOP, several directions to understand the exact involvement of BMP-4 in the pathophysiology of FOP are being examined. Recent results have indicated that the increased levels of BMP-4 mRNA in FOP cells result from an increased rate of transcription of the BMP-4 gene *(90)*. The increased activation of BMP-4 in FOP cells may be due to a mutation within the BMP-4 gene itself or to a mutation in another genetic locus that causes overexpression of BMP-4 in the cells of FOP patients. The structure and function of the human BMP-4 gene is being examined in order to understand how the BMP-4 gene is regulated *(92)*. An examination of the exon-coding sequences of the BMP-4 genes of patients with FOP have identified no mutations in these transcribed regions *(93)*.

Linkage analysis of two small families with autosomal dominant transmission of FOP has been performed using a highly polymorphic microsatellite marker near the BMP-4 gene locus *(94)* in order to determine whether the BMP-4 gene is consistent with or excluded from linkage with FOP in these two families. In one family *(3)*, which showed the classic phenotypic features of FOP (as described previously), the results were consistent with linkage to BMP-4 and the lymphoblastoid cells of affected members expressed high levels of BMP-4 mRNA. In the second family *(2)*, in which affected members showed mild phenotypic features of FOP, linkage of FOP and BMP-4 was excluded; interestingly, BMP-4 expression levels were not elevated in affected members of this family *(94a)*.

The appearance of large aggregates of B-cell and T-cell lymphocytes in the intramuscular perivascular space of the earliest detectable lesions of FOP supports the possibility of involvement of lymphocytes and perivascular cells in the induction of osteogenesis *(39)*. These observations suggest a mechanism to explain the pathophysiology of heterotopic bone formation in this disorder. One hypothesis is that lymphocytes capable of expressing BMP-4 circulate in the peripheral blood of patients with FOP, and are recruited to connective tissue sites after soft-tissue injury *(10)*. Alternatively, an event at a soft-tissue site may cause an immune-like response and recruitment of lymphocytes, with cells within the soft tissue induced to produce BMP-4. Type IV collagen, a primary constituent of the basement membrane of endothelial cells, muscle cells, and myoblast-like satellite cells, binds BMP-4, and this binding could result in increased local concentrations of BMP-4 *(75)*. At high concentrations, BMP-4 acts as a morphogen that up-regulates its own mesenchymal expression *(76)* followed by the development of pre-osseous lesions around muscle satellite cells, muscle fibroblasts or pericytes *(95)* capable of transducing the BMP signal. To test the hypothesis that BMP-4 expression and delivery by lymphocytes to a soft-tissue site can result in FOP-like bone forming lesions, transgenic animal models are being developed to over-express BMP-4 in B-lymphocytes and T-lymphocytes. The expression of BMPs and BMP receptors in hematopoietic stem cells is also being investigated.

The stringent temporal and spatial patterns of postnatal heterotopic ossification in patients with FOP are reminiscent of the patterns of mesenchymal cell condensation during skeletal embryogenesis and suggest a common molecular basis for prenatal and postnatal osteogenesis. Postnatal osteogenesis in humans most commonly occurs during fracture healing. Fracture callus and heterotopic bone formation in FOP form by endochondral pathways and both involve increased BMP-4 expression *(96,97)*. BMP-4 overexpression at connective tissue sites leads to focal osteogenesis at those sites *(98,99)*.

A direct link of FOP to the BMP-4 gene has not yet been proven and remains circumstantial. Genetic mutations in FOP could reside anywhere in the BMP-4 signaling pathway, or in other molecular pathways that affect the level of BMP-4 expression (Fig. 4). Additional information about the cellular and molecular events that occur during progression of FOP lesion formation as well as a better understanding of the events that induce bone formation during normal embryonic development and fracture healing will both expand the list of candidate genes and focus on the most likely causes of this disorder.

Other Candidate Genes

Homeotic genes, sonic hedgehog, Indian hedgehog, patched, smoothened, gli, jun, PTHrp, scleraxis, and the newly described osteogenic transcription factor Osf2/Cbfa1 are involved in upstream and downstream BMP-4 signaling *(100–110)*. In addition, Type I and Type II BMP receptors as well as the intracellular signaling molecules SMADs 1, 4, 5, 6, and 7 are involved in the regulation of pathways involved in endochondral osteogenesis *(111–113)*. These genes, as well as those that encode inhibitors Noggin and Chordin are all plausible candidate genes for FOP *(103,114–118)*. The presence of multiple osteochondromas in some FOP patients raises the intriguing possibility that the exostoses genes (EXT1, 2, 3, and EXT-L) may be involved in this family. EXT1, EXT2, and EXT-L have been cloned and all four genes have been mapped to the human chromosomes *(119,120)*. Linkage exclusion analyses with markers for these and other promising candidate genes may be revealing.

Prevention Regimens in FOP

Preventive measures are directed at decreasing or avoiding episodes of trauma that might stimulate the induction of a new lesion. Early diagnosis of FOP is critical in preventing unnecessary biopsies which are likely to provoke disease flare-ups.

Once FOP is diagnosed, all intramuscular injections and all dental blocks using local anesthetic must be avoided *(25,37)*. Assiduous attention should be directed to dental hygiene in order to decrease the necessity for therapeutic dental intervention *(37,121)*.

Falls are a common cause of severe morbidity in patients with FOP *(26)*. Trauma to the head has been found to be a common site of injury in FOP, and the injury profile included traumatic brain injuries, intracranial hemorrhage, and death. Deficiencies in coordinate gait and protective function likely accounted for the severity of head injuries in the FOP population. Precautions are recommended

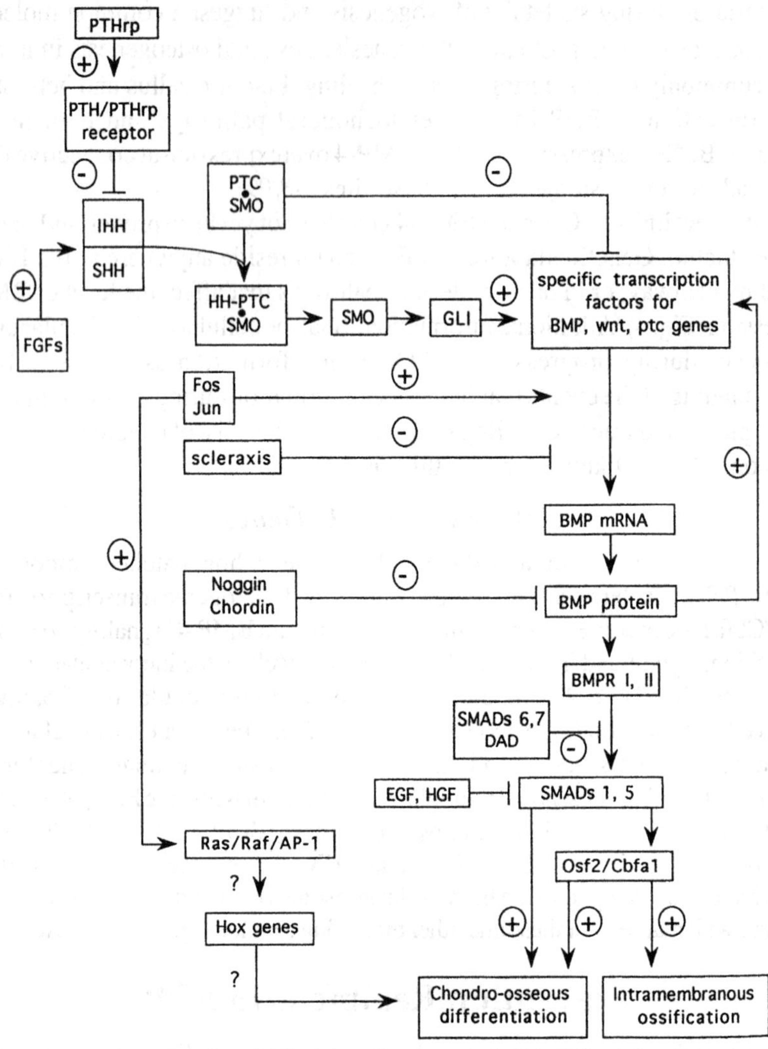

Fig. 4. Putative BMP signaling pathways. This composite schematic diagram depicts experimentally determined features of BMP signaling that have been identified in numerous in vitro and in vivo model systems including *Drosophila*, *Xenopus*, chicken, mouse, and humans. Each component of this pathway may not be active in every model system or in every cell type within a model system. + indicates an activating pathway; – indicates an inhibitory pathway. PTHrp, parathyroid hormone-related protein; PTH, parathyroid hormone; FGF, fibroblast growth factor; IHH, Indian hedgehog; SHH, sonic hedgehog; PTC, ptc, patched; SMO, smoothened; GLI, glioblastoma-derived oncogene family; BMP, bone morphogenetic protein; wnt, vertebrate wingless family; BMPR, receptors for BMPs*; Hox, vertebrate homeobox family; Fos and Jun, members of the AP1

which are intended to minimize the risk of injury without compromising a patient's functional level or independence. These include limitation of high risk activities, the use of protective head gear, and institution of safety improvements in living environments.

Treatment of FOP

There is no established medical treatment for FOP *(56,122,123)*. See Table 1 for treatment possibilities. The rarity of the disorder, its variable severity, and the fluctuating clinical course are substantial difficulties for evaluating potential therapies.

Physical therapy used in an attempt to maintain joint mobility may be harmful if pursued aggressively provoking or exacerbating lesions *(50)*. Surgical release of joint contractures is generally unsuccessful and risks new, trauma-induced heterotopic ossification *(50)*. Osteotomy of ectopic bone to mobilize a joint is usually counterproductive because of robust heterotopic ossification at the operative site. Spinal bracing is ineffective and surgical intervention is associated with numerous complications *(35)*. Dental therapy should preclude routine injection of local anesthetics and stretching of the jaw *(37,38)*. Newer dental techniques for focused administration of anesthetic are available. Guidelines for general anesthesia have been reported *(124)*. All intramuscular injections should be avoided *(25)*.

Adrenocorticotrophic hormone, corticosteroids, binders of dietary calcium, intravenous infusion of ethylenediaminetetraacetic acid (EDTA), nonsteroidal anti-inflammatory agents, radiotherapy, oral disodium etidronate, and warfarin (to inhibit gamma-carboxylation of osteocalcin) are ineffective *(125,126)*. Two recent studies suggest possible limited benefits from a course of intravenous etidronate *(127)* or prophylactic use of 13 cis-retinoic acid *(127,128)*. Accordingly, medical intervention is currently supportive.

Creative use of BMP technology will likely have important applications in the inhibition of heterotopic ossification in diseases such as FOP. Soluble BMP receptors, dominant negative receptors, as well as pharmacologic use of recombinant BMP antagonists may be promising in binding and physiologically inactivating BMP where it is not needed or wanted *(129)*. The hope for an effective treatment for FOP has been increased by the recent discovery of BMP-4 overexpression in the condition *(6,9,10)*. "With so much being discovered about how the BMPs act," says Brigid Hogan, a developmental geneticist at Vanderbilt University in Nashville, TN, "it might be possible to develop drugs that would block some part of the BMP-

---

Fig. 4. *(continued)* family of transcription factors; SMADs, members of the mothers-against-decapentaplegic family of signaling molecules; DAD, daughters against decapentaplegic; EGF, epidermal growth factor; HGF, hepatocyte growth factor; Osf2/Cbfa1, osteogenic induction transcription factor.

*BMP signaling is mediated through a complex of Type I and Type II BMPRs; BMPR-IA is specific for cartilage differentiation and BMPR-IB is specific for apoptosis and cartilage formation in the embryo *(111)*.

Table 1
FOP: Laboratory Observations and Treatment Possibilities

Observation	Ref.	Type of analysis	Proposed pharmacologic class	Rationale for treatment
Severe lesional swelling and edema	*(27,38)*	Clinical	Glucocorticoids	Decrease edema
Perivascular lymphocytic infiltrate	*(39)*	Histologic	Glucocorticoids	Decrease early lymphocytic infiltration
Intense angiogenesis in early fibroproliferative lesions	*(12,41)*	Histologic	Anti-angiogenic agents	Inhibit angiogenesis
Elevated urinary bFGF during disease flareups	*(41)*	Biochemical, in vivo	Interferon, thalidomide	Down-regulate expression and/or action of bFGF
Increased serum prostaglandin E_2-like molecules	*(131)*	Biochemical, in vitro	Prostaglandin inhibitors	Decrease production of prostaglandin
Increased BMP-4 expression in FOP tissue	*(10)*	Molecular	BMP inhibitors	Decrease production or inhibit activity of BMP-4

4 pathway—and therefore prevent the progression of what is a horrible nightmare disease" *(130)*.

Acknowledgments

The authors are indebted to Drs. Judah Folkman, William Gelbart, Victor McKusick, Maximilian Muenke, Vicki Rosen, Marshall Urist, Beth Valentine, Michael Whyte, John Wozney, and Michael Zasloff for their enduring intellectual contributions to this field and to the evolution of the work presented here.

The authors dedicate this work to Jeannie Peeper (President of The International Fibrodysplasia Ossificans Progressiva Association) and to all of the patients worldwide affected with FOP in appreciation for their continuous inspiration and in admiration of their steadfast courage. This work was supported in part by grants from the Medical Research Council (UK), International Fibrodysplasia Ossificans Progressiva Association, The Orthopaedic Research and Education Foundation, The Ian Cali Fellowship, The Gund Foundation, The European Neuromuscular Center, The Isaac & Rose Nassau Professorship of Orthopaedic Molecular Medicine, and the National Institutes of Health (R01-AR-41916).

References

1. Janoff, H. B., Tabas, J. A., Shore, E. M., Muenke, M., Dalinka, M. K., Schlesinger, S., Zasloff, M. A., and Kaplan, F. S. (1995) Mild expression of fibrodysplasia ossificans progressiva: a report of 3 cases. *J. Rheumatol.* **22,** 976–978.
2. Connor, J. M., Skirton, H., and Lunt, P. W. (1993) A three generation family with fibrodysplasia ossificans progressiva. *J. Med. Genet.* **30,** 687–689.
3. Kaplan, F. S., McCluskey, W., Hahn, G., Tabas, J. A., Muenke, M., and Zasloff, M. A. (1993) Genetic transmission of fibrodysplasia ossificans progressiva. Report of a family. *J. Bone Joint Surg. (Am).* **75,** 1214–1220.
4. Janoff, H. B., Muenke, M., Johnson, L. O., Rosenberg, A., Shore, E. M., Okereke, E., Zasloff, M., and Kaplan, F. S. (1996) Fibrodysplasia ossificans progressiva in two half–sisters: evidence for maternal mosaicism. *Am. J. Med. Genet.* **61,** 320–324.
5. Delatycki, M. and Rogers, J. G. (1998) The genetics of fibrodysplasia ossificans progressiva. *Clin. Orthop.* **346,** 15–18.
6. Kaplan, F. S., Shore, E. M., and Zasloff, M. A. (1996) Fibrodysplasia ossificans progressiva: searching for the skeleton key. *Calcif. Tissue Int.* **59,** 75–78.
7. Smith, R. and Triffitt, J. T. (1986) Bones in muscles: the problems of soft tissue ossification. *Q. J. Med.* **61,** 985–990.
8. Kaplan, F. S., Tabas, J. A., and Zasloff, M. A. (1990) Fibrodysplasia ossificans progressiva: a clue from the fly? *Calcif. Tissue Int.* **47,** 117–125.
9. Connor, J. M. (1996) Fibrodysplasia ossificans progressiva—lessons from rare maladies. *N. Engl. J. Med.* **335,** 591–593.
10. Shafritz, A. B., Shore, E. M., Gannon, F. H., Zasloff, M. A., Taub, R., Muenke, M., and Kaplan, F. S. (1996) Overexpression of an osteogenic morphogen in fibrodysplasia ossificans progressiva. *N. Engl. J. Med.* **335,** 555–561.
11. Schroeder, H. W., Jr. and Zasloff, M. (1980) The hand and foot malformations in fibrodysplasia ossificans progressiva. *Johns Hopkins Med. J.* **147,** 73–78.

12. Kaplan, F. S., Tabas, J. A., Gannon, F. H., Finkel, G., Hahn, G. V., and Zasloff, M. A. (1993) The histopathology of fibrodysplasia ossificans progressiva. An endochondral process. *J. Bone Joint Surg. (Am).* **75,** 220–230.
13. Cohen, R. B., Hahn, G. V., Tabas, J. A., Peeper, J., Levitz, C. L., Sando, et al. (1993) The natural history of heterotopic ossification in patients who have fibrodysplasia ossificans progressiva. A study of forty-four patients. *J. Bone Joint Surg. (Am).* **75,** 215–219.
14. Rocke, D. M., Zasloff, M., Peeper, J., Cohen, R. B., and Kaplan, F. S. (1994) Age- and joint-specific risk of initial heterotopic ossification in patients who have fibrodysplasia ossificans progressiva. *Clin. Orthop.* **301,** 243–248.
15. Connor, J. M. and Evans, D. A. (1982) Fibrodysplasia ossificans progressiva. The clinical features and natural history of 34 patients. *J. Bone Joint Surg. (Br).* **64,** 76–83.
16. Smith, R., Russell, R. G., and Woods, C. G. (1976) Myositis ossificans progressiva. Clinical features of eight patients and their response to treatment. *J. Bone Joint Surg. (Br).* **58,** 48–57.
17. Smith, R. (1998) Fibrodysplasia (myositis) ossificans progressiva: clinical lessons from a rare disease. *Clin. Orthop.* **346,** 7–14.
18. Connor, J. M. and Smith, R. (1982) The cervical spine in fibrodysplasia ossificans progressiva. *Br. J. Radiol.* **55,** 492–496.
19. O'Reilly, M. and Renton, P. (1993) Metaphyseal abnormalities in fibrodysplasia ossificans progressiva. *Br. J. Radiol.* **66,** 112–116.
20. Smith, R., Athanasou, N. A., and Vipond, S. E. (1996) Fibrodysplasia (myositis) ossificans progressiva: clinicopathological features and natural history. *Q. J. Med.* **89,** 445–446.
21. Tabas, J. A., Zasloff, M., Fallon, M. D., Gannon, F. H., Cohen, R. B., and Kaplan, F. S. (1993) Enchondroma in a patient with fibrodysplasia ossificans progressiva. *Clin. Orthop.* **294,** 277–280.
22. Kalifa, G., Adamsbaum, C., Job-Deslande, C., and Dubousset, J. (1993) Fibrodysplasia ossificans progressiva and synovial chondromatosis. *Pediatr. Radiol.* **23,** 91–93.
23. Kaplan, F. S., Hahn, G. V., and Zasloff, M. A. (1994) Heterotopic ossification: Two rare forms and what they can teach us. *J. Am. Acad. Orthop. Surg.* **2,** 288–296.
24. Gannon, F. H., Kaplan, F. S., Olmsted, E., Finkel, G. C., Zasloff, M., and Shore, E. (1997) Bone morphogenetic protein (BMP) 2/4 in early fibromatous lesions of fibrodysplasia ossificans progressiva. *Hum. Pathol.* **28,** 339–343.
25. Lanchoney, T. F., Cohen, R. B., Rocke, D. M., Zasloff, M. A., and Kaplan, F. S. (1995) Permanent heterotopic ossification at the injection site after diphtheria–tetanus-pertussis immunizations in children who have fibrodysplasia ossificans progressiva. *J. Pediatr.* **126,** 762–764.
26. Glaser, D. L., Rocke, D. M., and Kaplan, F. S. (1998) Catastrophic falls in patients who have fibrodysplasia ossificans progressiva. *Clin. Orthop.* **346,** 110–116.
27. Moriatis, J. M., Gannon, F. H., Shore, E. M., Bilker, W., Zasloff, M. A., and Kaplan, F. S. (1997) Limb swelling in patients who have fibrodysplasia ossificans progressiva. *Clin. Orthop.* **336,** 247–253.
28. Bridges, A. J., Hsu, K. C., Singh, A., Churchill, R., and Miles, J. (1994) Fibrodysplasia (myositis) ossificans progressiva. *Semin. Arthritis Rheum.* **24,** 155–164.

29. Cremin, B., Connor, J. M., and Beighton, P. (1982) The radiological spectrum of fibrodysplasia ossificans progressiva. *Clin. Radiol.* **33,** 499–508.
30. Kaplan, F. S., Strear, C. M., and Zasloff, M. A. (1994) Radiographic and scintigraphic features of modeling and remodeling in the heterotopic skeleton of patients who have fibrodysplasia ossificans progressiva. *Clin. Orthop.* **304,** 238–247.
31. Einhorn, T. A. and Kaplan, F. S. (1994) Traumatic fractures of heterotopic bone in patients who have fibrodysplasia ossificans progressiva. A report of 2 cases. *Clin. Orthop.* **308,** 173–177.
32. Fang, M. A., Reinig, J. W., Hill, S. C., Marini, J., and Zasloff, M. A. (1986) Technetium-99m MDP demonstration of heterotopic ossification in fibrodysplasia ossificans progressiva. *Clin. Nucl. Med.* **11,** 8–9.
33. Reinig, J. W., Hill, S. C., Fang, M., Marini, J., and Zasloff, M. A. (1986) Fibrodysplasia ossificans progressiva: CT appearance. *Radiology* **159,** 153–157.
34. Shirkhoda, A., Armin, A. R., Bis, K. G., Makris, J., Irwin, R. B., and Shetty, A. N. (1995) MR imaging of myositis ossificans: variable patterns at different stages. *J. Magn. Res. Imag.* **5,** 287–292.
35. Shah, P. B., Zasloff, M. A., Drummond, D., and Kaplan, F. S. (1994) Spinal deformity in patients who have fibrodysplasia ossificans progressiva. *J. Bone Joint Surg. (Am).* **76,** 1442–1450.
36. Kussmaul, W. G., Esmail, A. N., Sagir, Y., Ross, J., Gregory, S., and Kaplan, F. S. (1998) Pulmonary and cardiac function in advanced fibrodysplasia ossificans progressiva. *Clin. Orthop.* **346,** 104–109.
37. Luchetti, W., Cohen, R. B., Hahn, G. V., Rocke, D. M., Helpin, M., Zasloff, M., and Kaplan, F. S. (1996) Severe restriction in jaw movement after routine injection of local anesthetic in patients who have fibrodysplasia ossificans progressiva. *Oral Surg. Oral Med. Oral Pathol. Oral Radiol. Endod.* **81,** 21–25.
38. Janoff, H. B., Zasloff, M. A., and Kaplan, F. S. (1996) Submandibular swelling in patients with fibrodysplasia ossificans progressiva. *Otolaryngol. Head Neck Surg.* **114,** 599–604.
39. Gannon, F. H., Valentine, B. A., Shore, E. M., Zasloff, M. A., and Kaplan, F. S. (1998) Acute lymphocytic infiltration in extremely early lesions of fibrodysplasia ossificans progressiva. *Clin. Orthop.* **346,** 19–25.
40. Buring, K. (1975) On the origin of cells in heterotopic bone formation. *Clin. Orthop.* **110,** 293–302.
41. Kaplan, F. S., Sawyer, J., Connors, S., Keough, K., Shore, E. M., Gannon, F., Glaser, D., Rocke, D., Zasloff, M., and Folkman, J. (1998) Urinary basic fibroblast growth factor: a biochemical marker for pre-osseous fibroproliferative lesions in patients who have fibrodysplasia ossificans progressiva. *Clin. Orthop.* **346,** 59–65.
42. Warren, H. B. and Carpenter, J. L. (1984) Fibrodysplasia ossificans in three cats. *Vet. Pathol.* **21,** 495–499.
43. Waldron, D., Pettigrew, V., Turk, M., Turk, J., and Gibson, R. (1985) Progressive ossifying myositis in a cat. *J. Am. Vet. Med. Assoc.* **187,** 64–65.
44. Valentine, B. A., George, C., Randolph, J. F., Center, S. A., Fuhrer, L., and Beck, K. A. (1992) Fibrodysplasia ossificans progressiva in the cat. A case report. *J. Vet. Intern. Med.* **6,** 335–340.
45. Valentine, B. A. and Kaplan, F. S. (1996) Fibrodysplasia ossificans progressiva in cats: a potentially important animal model of the human disease. *Feline Pract.* **24,** 6.
46. Olmsted, E. A., Gannon, F. H., Wang, Z.-Q., Grigoriadis, A. E., Wagner, E. F., Zasloff, M. A., Shore, E. M., and Kaplan, F. S. (1998) Embryonic over-expression

of the c-fos proto-oncogene: a murine stem cell chimera applicable to the study of fibrodysplasia ossificans progressiva in humans. *Clin. Orthop.* **346,** 81–94.
47. Wang, Z. Q., Grigoriadis, A. E., Mohle–Steinlein, U., and Wagner, E. F. (1991) A novel target cell for c-fos-induced oncogenesis: development of chondrogenic tumours in embryonic stem cell chimeras. *EMBO J.* **10,** 2437–2450.
48. Rang, M. (1966) *Anthology of Orthopaedics*. Churchill Livingstone, New York.
49. Buyse, G., Silberstein, J., Goemans, N., and Casaer, P. (1995) Fibrodysplasia ossificans progressiva: still turning into wood after 300 years? *Eur. J. Pediatr.* **154,** 694–699.
50. Connor, J. M. and Evans, D. A. (1982) Genetic aspects of fibrodysplasia ossificans progressiva. *J. Med. Genet.* **19,** 35–39.
51. Connor, J. M. and Beighton, P. (1982) Fibrodysplasia ossificans progressiva in South Africa. Case reports. *S. Afr. Med. J.* **61,** 404–406.
52. Ebrahim, G. J., Grech, P., and Slavin, G. (1966) Myositis ossificans progressiva in an African child. *Br. J. Radiol.* **39,** 952–953.
53. Suzuki, T., Ishikawa, S., Akanuma, N., and Tsunoda, H. (1976) Myositis ossificans progressiva with parathyroid hyperplasia and polycystic ovary. *Acta Pathol. Jpn.* **26,** 251–262.
54. Chopra, K., Saha, M. M., and Saluja, S. (1987) Fibrodysplasia ossificans progressiva. *Indian Pediatr.* **24,** 677–680.
55. Cooles, P., Favot, I., and Madhavan, R. (1989) Fibrodysplasia (myositis) ossificans progressiva in Dominica. *West Indian Med. J.* **38,** 48–50.
56. Beighton, P. (1993) Fibrodysplasia ossificans progressiva, in *McKusick's Heritable Disorders of Connective Tissue* (Beighton, P., ed.), C.V. Mosby, St. Louis, pp. 501–518.
57. Lutwak, L. (1964) Myositis ossificans progressiva. Mineral, metabolic and radioactive calcium studies of the effects of hormones. *Am. J. Med.* **37,** 269–293.
58. McKusick, V. A. (1972) *Heritable Disorders of Connective Tissue*, 4th ed., C.V. Mosby, St. Louis, MO.
59. Koontz, A. R. (1927) Myositis ossificans progressiva. *Am. J. Med. Sci.* **174,** 406–412.
60. Fox, S., Khoury, A., Mootabar, H., and Greenwald, E. F. (1987) Myositis ossificans progressiva and pregnancy. *Obstet. Gynecol.* **69,** 453–455.
61. Thornton, Y. S., Birnbaum, S. J., and Lebowitz, N. (1987) A viable pregnancy in a patient with myositis ossificans progressiva. *Amer. J. Obstet. Gynecol.* **156,** 577–578.
62. Connor, J. M., Evans, C. C., and Evans, D. A. (1981) Cardiopulmonary function in fibrodysplasia ossificans progressiva. *Thorax* **36,** 419–423.
63. Rogers, J. G. and Geho, W. B. (1979) Fibrodysplasia ossificans progressiva. A survey of forty–two cases. *J. Bone Joint Surg. (Am).* **61,** 909–914.
64. Sympson, T. (1886) Case of myositis ossificans. *BMJ* **2,** 1026.
65. Stonham, C. (1892) Myositis ossificans. *Lancet* **2,** 1485–1491.
66. Burton-Fanning, F. W. and Vaughan, A. L. (1901) A case of myositis ossificans. *Lancet* **ii,** 849–850.
67. Gaster, A. (1905) A case of myositis ossificans. *West London Med. J.* **10,** 37.
68. Harris, N. H. (1961) Myositis ossificans progressiva. *Proc. Roy. Soc. Med.* **54,** 70–71.
69. Eaton, W. L., Conkling, W. S., and Daeschner, C. W. (1957) Early myositis ossificans progressiva occurring in homozygotic twins. *J. Pediatr.* **50,** 591–598.
70. Vastine, J. H., Vastine, M. F., and Orango, O. (1948) Myositis ossificans progressiva in homozygotic twins. *Am. J. Roentgenol.* **59,** 204–212.

71. Bernards, A. and Gusella, J. F. (1994) The importance of genetic mosaicism in human disease. *N. Engl. J. Med.* **331,** 1447–1449.
72. Tunte, W., Becker, P. E., and Knorre, G. V. (1967) On the genetics of myositis ossificans progressiva. *Humangenetik* **4,** 320–351.
73. Rogers, J. G. and Chase, G. A. (1979) Paternal age effect in fibrodysplasia ossificans progressiva. *J. Med. Genet.* **16,** 147–148.
74. Wozney, J. M., Rosen, V., Celeste, A. J., Mitsock, L. M., Whitters, M. J., Kriz, R. W., Hewick, R. M., and Wang, E. A. (1988) Novel regulators of bone formation: molecular clones and activities. *Science* **242,** 1528–1534.
75. Reddi, A. H. and Cunningham, N. S. (1993) Initiation and promotion of bone differentiation by bone morphogenetic proteins. *J. Bone Miner. Res.* **8(Suppl 2),** S499–502.
76. Vainio, S., Karavanova, I., Jowett, A., and Thesleff, I. (1993) Identification of BMP-4 as a signal mediating secondary induction between epithelial and mesenchymal tissues during early tooth development. *Cell* **75,** 45–58.
77. Kingsley, D. M. (1994) The TGF-beta superfamily: new members, new receptors, and new genetic tests of function in different organisms. *Genes Dev.* **8,** 133–146.
78. Winnier, G., Blessing, M., Labosky, P. A., and Hogan, B. L. (1995) Bone morphogenetic protein-4 is required for mesoderm formation and patterning in the mouse. *Genes Dev.* **9,** 2105–2116.
79. Hogan, B. L. (1996) Bone morphogenetic proteins: multifunctional regulators of vertebrate development. *Genes Dev.* **10,** 1580–1594.
80. Urist, M. R. (1997) Bone morphogenetic protein: the molecularization of skeletal system development. *J. Bone Miner. Res.* **12,** 343–346.
81. Urist, M. R. (1965) Bone formation by autoinduction. *Science* **150,** 893–899.
82. Kingsley, D. M., Bland, A. E., Grubber, J. M., Marker, P. C., Russell, L. B., Copeland, N. G., and Jenkins, N. A. (1992) The mouse short ear skeletal morphogenesis locus is associated with defects in a bone morphogenetic member of the TGF beta superfamily. *Cell* **71,** 399–410.
83. Storm, E. E., Huynh, T. V., Copeland, N. G., Jenkins, N. A., Kingsley, D. M., and Lee, S. J. (1994) Limb alterations in brachypodism mice due to mutations in a new member of the TGF beta-superfamily. *Nature* **368,** 639–643.
84. Thomas, J. T., Lin, K., Nandedkar, M., Camargo, M., Cervenka, J., and Luyten, F. P. (1996) A human chondrodysplasia due to a mutation in a TGF-beta superfamily member. *Nat. Genet.* **12,** 315–317.
85. Jones, C. M., Lyons, K. M., and Hogan, B. L. (1991) Involvement of bone morphogenetic protein-4 (BMP-4) and Vgr-1 in morphogenesis and neurogenesis in the mouse. *Development* **111,** 531–542.
86. Johansson, B. M. and Wiles, M. V. (1995) Evidence for involvement of activin A and bone morphogenetic protein 4 in mammalian mesoderm and hematopoietic development. *Mol. Cell. Biol.* **15,** 141–151.
87. Francis-West, P. H., Richardson, M. K., Bell, E., Chen, P., Luyten, F., Brickell, P., L., W., and Archer, C. W. (1996) The effect of overexpression of BMP-4 and GDF-5 on the development of limb skeletal elements. *Trans. Orthop. Res. Soc.* **21,** 62–11.
88. Padgett, R. W., Wozney, J. M., and Gelbart, W. M. (1993) Human BMP sequences can confer normal dorsal-ventral patterning in the Drosophila embryo. *Proc. Natl. Acad. Sci. USA* **90,** 2905–2909.

89. Sampath, T. K., Rashka, K. E., Doctor, J. S., Tucker, R. F., and Hoffmann, F. M. (1993) *Drosophila* transforming growth factor beta superfamily proteins induce endochondral bone formation in mammals. *Proc. Natl. Acad. Sci. USA* **90,** 6004–6008.
90. Olmsted, E. A., Liu, C., Haddad, J. G., Shore, E. M., and Kaplan, F. S. (1996) Characterization of mechanisms controlling bone morphogenetic protein-4 message expression in fibrodysplasia ossificans progressiva. *J. Bone Miner. Res.* **11,** S164.
91. Lanchoney, T. F., Olmsted, E. A., Shore, E. M., Gannon, F. H., Zasloff, M. A., Rosen, V., and Kaplan, F. S. (1998) Characterization of bone morphogenetic protein-4 receptors in fibrodysplasia ossificans progressiva. *Clin. Orthop.* **346,** 38–45.
92. Shore, E. M., Xu, M., Shah, P. B., Janoff, H. B., Hahn, G. V., Deardorff, M. A., Sovinsky, L., et al.(1998) The human bone morphogenetic protein 4 (BMP-4) gene: Molecular structure and transcriptional regulation. *Calcif. Tissue Int.* **63,** 221–229.
93. Xu, M. and Shore, E. M. (1998) Mutational screening of the bone morphogenetic protein 4 gene in a family with fibrodysplasia ossificans progressiva. *Clin. Orthop.* **346,** 53–58.
93a. Virdi, A. S., Shore, E. M., Oreffo, R. O. C., Li, M., Connor, J. M., Smith, R., Kaplan, F. S., and Triffitt, J. T., (1999) Phenotypic and molecular heterogeneity in fibrodyplasia ossificans progressiva. *Calif. Tissue Int.* **65,** 250–255.
94. Shore, E. M., Li, M., Calvert, G., Xu, M., Zasloff, M., and Kaplan, F. S. (1997) Identification of polymorphic markers for the human BMP-2 and BMP-4 genes. *J. Bone Miner. Res.* **12,** S309.
95. Brighton, C. T., Lorich, D. G., Kupcha, R., Reilly, T. M., Jones, A. R., and Woodbury, R. A. (1992) The pericyte as a possible osteoblast progenitor cell. *Clin. Orthop.* **275,** 287–299.
96. Nakase, T., Nomura, S., Yoshikawa, H., Hashimoto, J., Hirota, S., Kitamura, Y., et al. (1994) Transient and localized expression of bone morphogenetic protein 4 messenger RNA during fracture healing. *J. Bone Miner. Res.* **9,** 651–659.
97. Bostrom, M. P., Lane, J. M., Berberian, W. S., Missri, A. A., Tomin, E., Weiland, A., et al. (1995) Immunolocalization and expression of bone morphogenetic proteins 2 and 4 in fracture healing. *J. Orthop. Res.* **13,** 357–367.
98. Shimizu, K., Yoshikawa, H., Matsui, M., Masuhara, K., and Takaoka, K. (1994) Periosteal and intratumorous bone formation in athymic nude mice by Chinese hamster ovary tumors expressing murine bone morphogenetic protein-4. *Clin. Orthop.* **300,** 274–280.
99. Takaoka, K., Yoshikawa, H., Hashimoto, J., Ono, K., Matsui, M., and Nakazato, H. (1994) Transfilter bone induction by Chinese hamster ovary (CHO) cells transfected by DNA encoding bone morphogenetic protein-4. *Clin. Orthop.* **300,** 269–273.
100. Jabs, E. W., Muller, U., Li, X., Ma, L., Luo, W., Haworth, I. S., et al. (1993) A mutation in the homeodomain of the human MSX2 gene in a family affected with autosomal dominant craniosynostosis. *Cell* **75,** 443–450.
101. Chen, Y. and Struhl, G. (1996) Dual roles for patched in sequestering and transducing Hedgehog. *Cell* **87,** 553–563.
102. Vortkamp, A., Lee, K., Lanske, B., Segre, G. V., Kronenberg, H. M., and Tabin, C. J. (1996) Regulation of rate of cartilage differentiation by Indian hedgehog and PTH–related protein. *Science* **273,** 613–622.
103. Holley, S. A., Neul, J. L., Attisano, L., Wrana, J. L., Sasai, Y., O'Connor, M. B., De Robertis, E. M., and Ferguson, E. L. (1996) The *Xenopus* dorsalizing factor

noggin ventralizes *Drosophila* embryos by preventing DPP from activating its receptor. *Cell* **86,** 607–617.
104. Scott, M. P. (1997) Hox genes, arms and the man. *Nat. Genet.* **15,** 117–118.
105. Ducy, P., Zhang, R., Geoffroy, V., Ridall, A. L., and Karsensky, G. (1997) Osf2/Cbfa1: a transcriptional activator of osteoblast differentiation. *Cell* **89,** 747–754.
106. Cserjesi, P., Brown, D., Ligon, K. L., Lyons, G. E., Copeland, N. G., Gilbert, D. J., Jenkins, N. A., and Olson, E. N. (1995) Scleraxis: a basic helix–loop–helix protein that prefigures skeletal formation during mouse embryogenesis. *Development* **121,** 1099–1110.
107. Liu, Y., Cserjesi, P., Nifuji, A., Olson, E. N., and Noda, M. (1996) Sclerotome–related helix-loop-helix type transcription factor (scleraxis) mRNA is expressed in osteoblasts and its level is enhanced by type-beta transforming growth factor. *J. Endocrinol.* **151,** 491–499.
108. Ruiz i Altaba, A. (1997) Catching a glimpse of hedgehog. *Cell* **90,** 193–196.
109. Marigo, V., Davey, R. A., Zuo, Y., Cunningham, J. M., and Tabin, C. J. (1996) Biochemical evidence that patched is the hedgehog receptor. *Nature* **384,** 176–179.
110. Stone, D. M., Hynes, M., Armanini, M., Swanson, T. A., Gu, Q., Johnson, R. L., et al. (1996) The tumour-suppressor gene patched encodes a candidate receptor for Sonic hedgehog. *Nature* **384,** 129–134.
111. Zou, H., Wieser, R., Massague, J., and Niswander, L. (1997) Distinct roles of type I bone morphogenetic protein receptors in the formation and differentiation of cartilage. *Genes Dev.* **11,** 2191–2203.
112. Whitman, M. (1997) Feedback from inhibitory SMADs. *Nature* **389,** 549–551.
113. Massague, J., Hata, A., and Liu, F. (1997) TGF-β signaling through the Smad pathway. *Trends Cell Biol.* **7,** 187–192.
114. Lamb, T. M. and Harland, R. M. (1995) Fibroblast growth factor is a direct neural inducer, which combined with noggin generates anterior-posterior neural pattern. *Development* **121,** 3627–3636.
115. Piccolo, S., Sasai, Y., Lu, B., and De Robertis, E. M. (1996) Dorsoventral patterning in *Xenopus:* inhibition of ventral signals by direct binding of chordin to BMP-4. *Cell* **86,** 589–598.
116. Re'em-Kalma, Y., Lamb, T., and Frank, D. (1995) Competition between noggin and bone morphogenetic protein 4 activities may regulate dorsalization during *Xenopus* development. *Proc. Natl. Acad. Sci. USA* **92,** 12,141–12,145.
117. Sasai, Y., Lu, B., Steinbeisser, H., Geissert, D., Gont, L. K., and De Robertis, E. M. (1994) *Xenopus* chordin: a novel dorsalizing factor activated by organizer-specific homeobox genes. *Cell* **79,** 779–790.
118. Zimmerman, L. B., De Jesus–Escobar, J. M., and Harland, R. M. (1996) The Spemann organizer signal noggin binds and inactivates bone morphogenetic protein 4. *Cell* **86,** 599–606.
119. Wise, C. A., Clines, G. A., Massa, H., Trask, B. J., and Lovett, M. (1997) Identification and localization of the gene for EXTL, a third member of the multiple exostoses gene family. *Genome Res.* **7,** 10–16.
120. Stickens, D., Clines, G., Burbee, D., Ramos, P., Thomas, S., Hogue, D., et al. (1996) The EXT2 multiple exostoses gene defines a family of putative tumour suppressor genes. *Nat. Genet.* **14,** 25–32.
121. Nussbaum, B. L., O'Hara, I., and Kaplan, F. S. (1996) Fibrodysplasia ossificans progressiva: report of a case with guidelines for pediatric dental and anesthetic management. *ASDC J. Dent. Child.* **63,** 448–450.

122. Connor, J. M. (1993) Fibrodysplasia ossificans progressiva, in *Connective Tissue and Its Heritable Disorders* (Royce, P. M. and Steinmann, B., eds.), Wiley-Liss, New York, pp. 603–611.
123. Whyte, M. P., Kaplan, F. S., and Shore, E. M. (1996) Fibrodysplasia ossificans progressiva, in *Primer on the Metabolic Bone Diseases and Disorders of Mineral Metabolism*, (Favus, M. J., ed.), Lipincott-Raven, Philadelphia, pp. 428–430.
124. Lininger, T. E., Brown, E. M., and Brown, M. (1989) General anesthesia and fibrodysplasia ossificans progressiva. *Anesth. Analg.* **68,** 175–176.
125. Bar Oz, B. and Boneh, A. (1994) Myositis ossificans progressiva: a 10-year follow-up on a patient treated with etidronate disodium. *Acta Paediatr.* **83,** 1332–1334.
126. Pazzaglia, U. E., Beluffi, G., Ravelli, A., Zatti, G., and Martini, A. (1993) Chronic intoxication by ethane-1-hydroxy-1, 1–diphosphonate (EHDP) in a child with myositis ossificans progressiva. *Pediatr. Radiol.* **23,** 459–462.
127. Brantus, J.-F. and Meunier, P. J. (1998) Effects of intravenous etidronate in acute episodes of fibrodysplasia ossificans progressiva. An open study. *Clin. Orthop.* **346,** 117–120.
128. Zasloff, M. A., Rocke, D., Crofford, L. J., Hahn, G. V., and Kaplan, F. S. (1998) Treatment of patients who have fibrodysplasia ossificans progressiva with 13-cis-retinoic acid (isotretinoin). *Clin. Orthop.* **346,** 121–129.
129. Graff, J. M. (1997) Embryonic patterning: to BMP or not to BMP, that is the question. *Cell* **89,** 171–174.
130. Roush, W. (1996) Protein builds second skeleton. *Science* **273,** 1170.
131. Levitz, C. L., Cohen, R. B., Zasloff, M. A., and Kaplan, F. S. (1992) The role of prostaglandins in the pathogenesis of fibrodysplasia ossificans progressiva. *Calcif. Tissue Int.* **50,** 378.

CHAPTER 13

Disorders Resulting from Inactivating or Activating Mutations in the Ca^{2+}_o-Sensing Receptor

Edward M. Brown

Introduction

The cloning of the Ca^{2+}_o-sensing receptor (CaR), which is a G protein-coupled receptor (GPCR) that responds to changes in the extracellular calcium concentration (Ca^{2+}_o), has enabled identification of several inherited disorders of Ca^{2+}_o homeostasis that result from either activating or inactivating mutations of this recently recognized receptor. Inactivating mutations produce hypercalcemic syndromes, while activating mutations produce a form of hypocalcemia resembling hypoparathyroidism. In addition to elucidating the molecular pathogenesis of these disorders exhibiting "resistance" or "oversensitivity" to actions of Ca^{2+}_o that are mediated by the CaR, the identification of inherited diseases of this receptor has afforded "experiments-in-nature" that have clarified substantially the CaR's normal physiological roles in parathyroid and kidney. This chapter will briefly describe the discovery of the CaR and its roles in normal physiology, delineate in more detail the principal clinical and biochemical features of these inherited diseases of the receptor and illustrate how these disorders have clarified further the CaR's physiological roles. More detailed descriptions of the molecular biology, regulation and other properties of this novel receptor and its role in regulating diverse tissues, both those involved and those uninvolved in systemic mineral ion homeostasis, may be found in recent reviews *(1,2)*.

Roles of the Ca^{2+}_o-Sensing Receptor (CaR) in Normal Calcium Homeostasis

Virtually all physiological processes utilize intra- and/or extracellular calcium (Ca^{2+}) ions in some fashion *(3,4)*. Cytosolic free calcium ions (Ca^{2+}_i) play

The Genetics of Osteoporosis and Metabolic Bone Disease
Ed.: M. J. Econs © Humana Press Inc., Totowa, NJ

key roles as an intracellular second messenger and as an enzymic cofactor, coordinating and controlling cellular functions as diverse as hormonal secretion, muscular contraction, glycogen metabolism, cellular differentiation, proliferation and motility *(3)*. The basal level of Ca^{2+}_i, generally in the range of 100 n*M*, is about four orders of magnitude lower than the extracellular ionized calcium concentration (Ca^{2+}_o) (~1 m*M*). Ca^{2+}_i undergoes large, rapid increases upon cellular activation due to release of Ca^{2+} from various intracellular stores and/or uptake of calcium ions through Ca^{2+}-permeable channels in the plasma membrane. In contrast, the level of Ca^{2+}_o measured in the blood remains almost invariant under normal circumstances, fluctuating from its mean value by only a few percent *(4–6)*. Ca^{2+}_o also serves diverse essential functions, being crucial for clotting of the blood, maintaining skeletal integrity, and regulating neuromuscular excitability and other processes.

The homeostatic system maintaining near constancy of Ca^{2+}_o includes two principal elements (Fig. 1) *(3a,4–6)*. The first are several types of cells that recognize Ca^{2+}_o as their major physiological, "first" messenger, which controls the secretion of calciotropic hormones from parathyroid cells, thyroidal C-cells, and renal proximal tubular cells. These Ca^{2+}_o-induced changes in the secretion of parathyroid hormone (PTH), calcitonin (CT), and 1,25-dihydroxyvitamin D (1,25$(OH)_2$D), respectively, modulate the second element of the homeostatic system, namely the effector tissues, bone, intestine, and kidney (*see* Fig. 1), that normalize Ca^{2+}_o by altering their transport of calcium and/or phosphate ions into or out of the extracellular fluid. Although it was for many years clear that the capacity of parathyroid and other cells to sense Ca^{2+}_o was crucial for the maintenance of mineral ion homeostasis, the mechanism(s) underlying the Ca^{2+}_o-sensing ability of these cells remained obscure until recently.

Cloning and Characterization of a G Protein-Coupled CaR

Expression cloning in *Xenopus laevis* has provided a useful vehicle for isolating the cDNAs encoding phosphoinositide (PI)-coupled receptors for which there are no molecular probes available. *X. laevis* oocytes are injected with RNA extracted from a tissue expressing such a receptor. The oocytes then synthesize the receptor protein, which, in turn, couples to the oocyte's endogenous G protein(s) and phospholipase C (PLC), resulting in an IP_3- and Ca^{2+}_i-mediated stimulation of Ca^{2+}-activated chloride channels following exposure of the oocytes to that receptor's agonists. Parathyroid cells were known to respond to elevated levels of Ca^{2+}_o with activation of PLC *(7,8)*, transient and then sustained rises in Ca^{2+}_i *(9)* and inhibition of adenylate cyclase that is sensitive to pertussis toxin *(10)*, suggesting that the putative CaR was a GPCR that was linked to stimulation and inhibition, respectively, of PLC and adenylate cyclase *(4)*. Furthermore, injection of *X. laevis* oocytes with parathyroid mRNA isolated from bovine parathyroid glands rendered them responsive to Ca^{2+}_o *(11,12)*. Brown et al. *(13)* subsequently used the oocyte system to screen a cDNA library constructed from a highly active

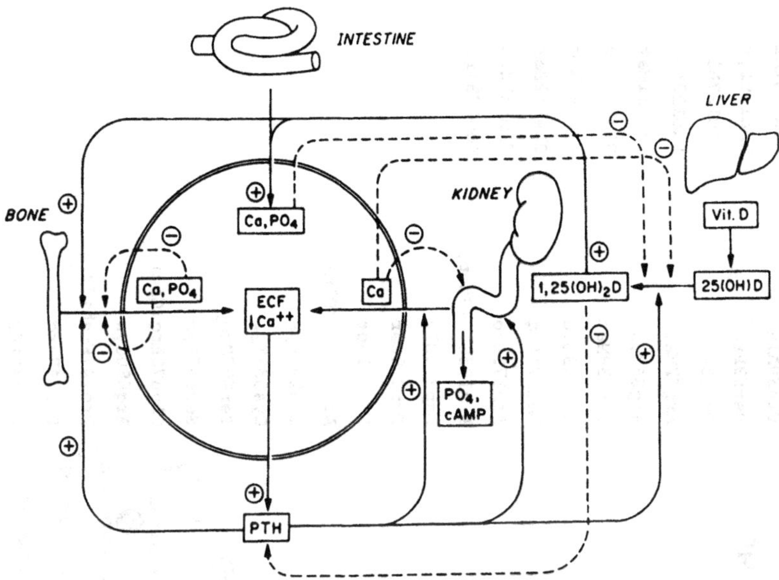

Fig. 1. Schematic diagram illustrating the regulatory system maintaining Ca^{2+}_o homeostasis. The solid arrows and lines show the effects of PTH and $1,25(OH)_2D_3$; the dotted arrows and lines demonstrate examples of how Ca^{2+} or phosphate ions exert direct actions on target tissues. Abbreviations are the following: Ca^{2+}, calcium; $P0_4$, phosphate; ECF, extracellular fluid; PTH, parathyroid hormone; $1,25(OH)_2D$, 1,25-dihydroxyvitamin D; 25(OH)D, 25-hydroxyvitamin D; minus signs show inhibitory actions while plus signs illustrate positive effects. (Reproduced with permission from ref. *3a*.)

fraction of this mRNA to isolate a full length, functionally active CaR clone. The use of hybridization-based screening techniques subsequently permitted cloning of additional, highly homologous CaRs from human *(14)* (Fig. 2; *14a*) and chicken parathyroid *(15)*, human *(16)*, rat *(17)*, and rabbit kidney *(18)*, rat C-cell *(19,20)*, and rat brain *(21)*. All of these CaRs are activated not only by elevated levels of Ca^{2+}_o but also by Mg^{2+}_o as well as a variety of inorganic (e.g., the trivalent cation, gadolinium [Gd^{3+}]) and organic polycations (i.e., spermine and neomycin). Of these various polycations, both Mg^{2+}_o *(22)* and spermine *(23)* are present in vivo at levels that might permit them to act as physiological agonists of the CaR.

All of these CaRs represent species and tissue homologs of the same ancestral gene and share three principal structural domains on the basis of their deduced amino acid sequences. The first is a largely hydrophilic, amino-terminal extracellular domain (ECD) comprising more than 600 amino acids. A second, predominantly hydrophobic region follows, which contains about 250 amino acids, including those encoding seven transmembrane (TM) segments that are characteristic of the superfamily of G protein-coupled receptors (GPCR). The third

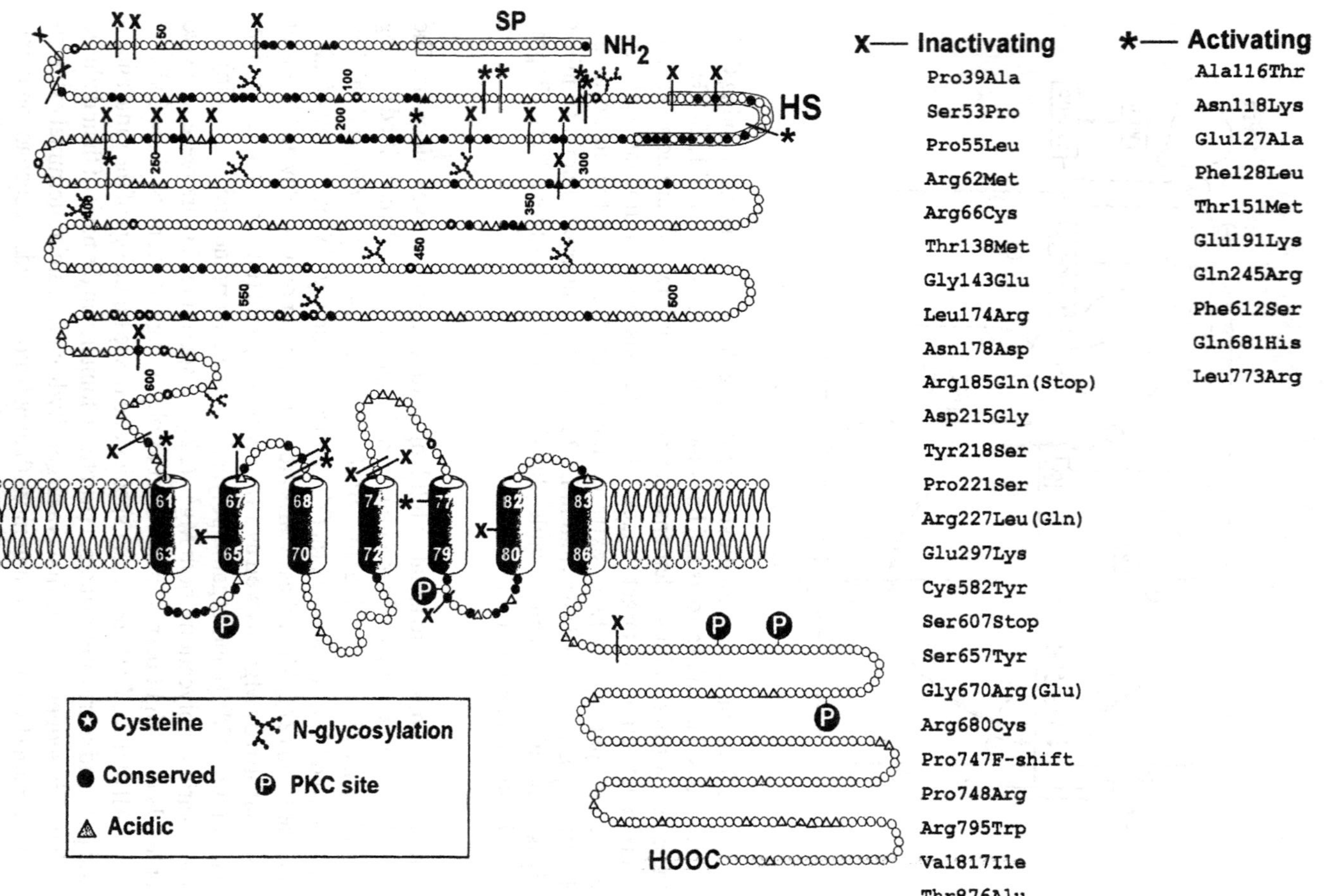
SP
NH2
HS
HOOC
X— Inactivating
Pro39Ala
Ser53Pro
Pro55Leu
Arg62Met
Arg66Cys
Thr138Met
Gly143Glu
Leu174Arg
Asn178Asp
Arg185Gln(Stop)
Asp215Gly
Tyr218Ser
Pro221Ser
Arg227Leu(Gln)
Glu297Lys
Cys582Tyr
Ser607Stop
Ser657Tyr
Gly670Arg(Glu)
Arg680Cys
Pro747F-shift
Pro748Arg
Arg795Trp
Val817Ile
Thr876Alu
*— Activating
Ala116Thr
Asn118Lys
Glu127Ala
Phe128Leu
Thr151Met
Glu191Lys
Gln245Arg
Phe612Ser
Gln681His
Leu773Arg
Cysteine
Conserved
Acidic
N-glycosylation
PKC site

domain is a cytoplasmic, carboxyl (C)-terminal tail of slightly more than 200 amino acids. The sensing of polycationic CaR agonists is thought to take place within the ECD based on studies using chimeric receptors created from the CaR and the structurally related, metabotropic glutamate receptors (mGluRs). For example, a chimeric receptor containing the CaR's ECD fused to the TMs and C-terminal tail of one of the mGluRs responds to agonists of the CaR but not to those of the mGluRs *(24)*. Conversely, a chimeric receptor with an mGluR's ECD and the CaR's TMs and C-terminal tail recognizes mGluR agonists but not Ca^{2+}_o.

Additional members of a growing family of the GPCRs to which the CaR and the mGluRs belong, the so-called family C GPCRs, are the recently-cloned $GABA_B$ receptors *(25)* and a substantial subfamily of putative pheromone receptors cloned from the rat vomeronasal organ *(26,27)*. The latter respond to environmental clues thought to be involved in regulating instinctual behavior. All of the family C GPCRs have large ECDs that likely evolved from the bacterial periplasmic binding proteins (PBPs) *(25,28,29)*. The latter bind a variety of extracellular ligands involved in chemotaxis or destined for cellular uptake by associated bacterial transport systems *(30,31)*.

The CaR is thought to bind through its intracellular domains (i.e., intracellular loops and carboxyl-terminal tail) to the G proteins linking it to modulation of various intracellular effector systems (most likely $G_{q/11}$ for activation of PLC *[32]* and G_i for inhibition of adenylate cyclase *[10,32,33]*), although the cloned receptor has not yet been definitively proven to couple directly to adenylate cyclase. The CaR also activates phospholipase A_2 (PLA_2) *(34,35)* and phospholipase D (PLD) *(34)*, most likely indirectly through a protein kinase C (PKC)-mediated mechanism *(34)*. The receptor has also recently been shown to activate the mitogen-activated protein kinase (MAP kinase) pathway in rat-1 fibroblasts, probably via tyrosine phosphorylation of a member of the c-SRC tyrosine kinase family *(36)*. Only a single isoform of the CaR apparently activates all of these diverse signal transduction pathways. In contrast, there are multiple mGluR isoforms, each of which is linked to one principal effector system (i.e., mGluRs 1 and 5, for instance, couple to PLC) *(37)*. The existence of additional isoforms of the CaR (or for that matter GPCRs activated by other ions), however, has by no means been excluded.

Fig. 2. Schematic illustration of the predicted structure of the Ca^{2+}_o-sensing receptor protein, showing activating and inactivating mutations. Symbols are given in key. Additional abbreviations include the following: SP, predicted signal peptide; HS, hydrophobic segment. Also shown are the positions of missense and nonsense mutations that cause either familial hypocalciuric hypercalcemia (FHH) or autosomal dominant hypocalcemia; mutations are indicated with the three letter amino acid code. The normal amino acid is indicated prior to and the mutant amino acid after the number of the relevant codon. (Reproduced with permission from ref. *14a*.)

Tissue Distribution and Physiological Roles of the CaR

Transcripts for the CaR are present in a wide variety of tissues, many of which play no obvious roles in mineral ion metabolism. These tissues and cell types include the parathyroid glands, C-cells, kidney, stomach *(38)* and intestines *(39)*, lung, and various regions of the brain *(1,21,40)*, as well as lens epithelial cells *(41)*, fibroblasts *(36)*, and diverse cells within the bone marrow *(42)*. The use of *in situ* hybridization with CaR-specific probes combined with immunohistochemistry using anti-CaR antibodies has permitted more detailed localization of the CaR in these tissues, including two key tissues involved in Ca^{2+}_o homeostasis, parathyroid and kidney *(21,40,43,44)*, where the CaR's putative roles are delineated in more detail shortly.

In bovine parathyroid cells, the CaR stimulates PLC, PLA_2 and PLD *(34)* and likely also inhibits adenylate cyclase *(4,10)*, as noted above. Which, if any, of these intracellular signaling pathways, however, is/are the major one(s) through which the CaR produces its atypical inhibition, as opposed to stimulation, of PTH secretion remains a key unsolved problem. In any event, the marked impairment of high Ca^{2+}_o-induced inhibition of PTH secretion in patients with neonatal severe hyperparathyroidism (NSHPT) *(45,46)* as a result of their harboring homozygous inactivating CaR mutations *(1,2,4)* or in mice homozygous for targeted disruption of the CaR gene *(47)* (*see* below) provides strong support for the crucial, nonredundant role of the CaR in Ca^{2+}_o-regulated PTH release. In addition, the use of "calcimimetic" CaR agonists has shown that the CaR is probably also responsible for the high Ca^{2+}_o-mediated reduction in preproPTH mRNA levels *(48)*.

Finally, the pronounced chief cell hyperplasia in both NSHPT *(49,50)* and mice that are homozygous for "knockout" of the CaR *(47)* provides indirect evidence for an important role of this receptor in tonically suppressing parathyroid cellular proliferation. Interestingly, in the C-cell the CaR couples to stimulation, rather than inhibition, of secretion *(19,20,51)*, as it does in the ACTH-secreting AtT-20 cell line *(52)*. Thus depending upon the cellular context in which it is expressed, the CaR can either stimulate or inhibit hormonal secretion.

Transcripts for the CaR are expressed along much of the nephron, based on the use of reverse transcription-based polymerase chain reaction (RT-PCR). In one study CaR transcripts were present in the glomerulus, proximal convoluted and straight tubule, MTAL and cortical thick ascending limb (CTAL), distal convoluted tubule (DCT) and cortical (CCD), outer medullary (OMCD) and inner medullary collecting duct (IMCD) *(43)*. In another study, transcripts were identified in MTAL, CTAL, DCT, and CCD *(44)*. Additional studies using specific anti-CaR antisera have helped to resolve the differences between the results of these two studies *(53)*. In CTAL, where CaR transcripts and protein are present at the highest levels, the CaR is located mainly on the basolateral plasma membrane where it likely senses systemic (e.g., blood) levels of Ca^{2+}_o. The CaR in CTAL and perhaps also in DCT regulates the tubular handling of Ca^{2+} and Mg^{2+}, enhancing their reabsorption if Ca^{2+}_o is low and reducing it when Ca^{2+}_o is high *(54)*. The CaR and PTH receptors are both expressed in CTAL and DCT, which may permit mutually antagonistic interactions between the actions of these two receptors on the reabsorption of Ca^{2+} in the distal nephron *(55,56)*. In the IMCD, the CaR is situated largely on the apical (e.g., luminal) cell surface, thereby permitting monitoring of the level of Ca^{2+}_o within the final urine *(57)*. This apical CaR likely mediates the reduction in vasopressin-stimulated reabsorption of water that is observed when isolated tubules from the rat IMCD are perfused with high Ca^{2+}_o, an action that could potentially diminish the risk of renal stone formation when renal Ca^{2+} excretion is increased *(57)*. Moreover, through inhibition of NaCl reabsorption in the MTAL *(2)*, the CaR may further diminish maximal urinary concentrating capacity by decreasing the medullary hypertonicity that drives vasopressin-mediated, transepithelial water flow in the renal collecting duct *(58)*.

Inherited Disorders Exhibiting Extracellular Calcium Resistance

Familial Hypocalciuric Hypercalcemia (FHH)

Clinical and Biochemical Features of FHH

In 1972, Foley et al. described the unusually benign clinical features of a form of hypercalcemia that they termed familial benign hypercalcemia (FBH) *(59)*. Although several forms of familial hypercalcemia had previously been described, this report was the first to outline clearly the characteristic clinical features of this syndrome. Later studies confirmed and extended the initial desciption of FBH by Foley et al. *(59)*. Marx and coworkers called this syndrome of mild and largely asymptomatic hypercalcemia, familial hypocalciuric hypercalcemia (FHH), because of the characteristic alteration in renal handling of Ca^{2+} exhibited by affected family members *(60,61)*. Both the terms FHH and FBH are still used to describe this syndrome, but I shall use the former of these two names in this chapter.

FHH is an uncommon genetic syndrome, occurring with a frequency that is probably about 1% of that of primary hyperparathyroidism. It is inherited in an autosomal dominant fashion, being characterized by lifelong, usually asymptomatic hypercalcemia that is mild to moderate in its severity (usually <12 mg/dL) *(60–62)*. There is some variability in the degree of severity from family to family that appears to result from the particular functional properties of a given family's defective gene. A few families exhibit serum calcium concentrations that are minimally elevated or even consistently within the upper part of the normal range *(63)*, and occasional kindreds have serum calcium concentrations averaging greater than 12 or even 13 mg/dL *(50,64,65)*.

Despite being hypercalcemic, affected patients commonly have little, if any, in the way of the symptomatology and complications characteristic of other hypercalcemic disorders. These symptoms most commonly include gastrointestinal abnormalities, especially anorexia, nausea, and constipation, mental disturbances and renal complications (i.e., nephrolithiasis or nephrocalcinosis, impaired renal function and defective urinary concentrating ability) *(66,67)*. Even in FHH families with higher than average concentrations of serum calcium, however, affected members are generally remarkably asymptomatic. Nonspecific manifestations present in other forms of hypercalcemia, i.e., fatigue, were reported in some early clinical descriptions of FHH *(61)* but were not confirmed subsequently *(62,68)*. It is possible that ascertainment bias attributed symptoms to the disorder in probands of FHH families that were not, in fact, found to be present more commonly in affected than in unaffected family members when those kindreds were subjected to closer scrutiny.

Affected individuals in some FHH kindreds have had pancreatitis or chondrocalcinosis (calcification of the cartilage that covers the joint surfaces) *(61)*, perhaps because these conditions represented true complications of this syndrome. Subsequent studies, however, have revealed that pancreatitis is no more prevalent in affected than in unaffected members of FHH kindreds or, for that matter, in the general population *(68)*. In addition, most patients with FHH who have developed pancreatitis had other coexistent factors that might have predisposed to this condition, such as alcoholism or gallstones *(68)*. Further studies have also not confirmed that chondrocalcinosis is more common in FHH than in the population as a whole *(62,68)*. Although one study *(62)* described an apparently increased incidence of gallstones in FHH, most large series of FHH kindreds have not reported this to be a complication of the disorder.

The degree of elevation in the serum calcium concentration in FHH is similar to that encountered in patients with primary hyperparathyroidism of mild to moderate severity, and there are equivalent increases in both the serum total and ionized calcium concentrations in both conditions *(61,62)*. Persons with FHH often have some degree of reduction in serum phosphate concentration, although the latter parameter generally remains within the lower half of the normal range, and the degree of reduction in serum phosphate concentration is less than that found in primary hyperparathyroidism. Serum magnesium concentrations in FHH can be in the upper half of the normal range or in some cases frankly, albeit mildly elevated. Unlike primary hyperparathyroidism, there is a positive correlation between the serum calcium and magnesium concentrations in FHH, so that hypermagnesemia may be more common in kindreds with more severe hypercalcemia *(61)*.

A very characteristic biochemical finding in FHH is an inappropriately "normal" PTH level in the face of concomitant hypercalcemia *(68)*, particularly when assays for intact PTH are employed *(69,70)*. Occasionally PTH levels are in the lower portion of the normal range or are frankly elevated *(71)*. It is in patients with FHH who exhibit overtly elevated PTH levels that differentiating them from patients with mild primary hyperparathyroidism on the basis of their PTH levels alone may be difficult *(71)*. This is especially true in the 5–10% of cases of primary hyperparathyroidism whose intact PTH levels are in the upper part of the normal range.

Studies utilizing induced changes in serum calcium concentration have confirmed that patients with FHH exhibit dysregulation of Ca^{2+}_o-regulated PTH secretion, documenting an increase in "set-point" (the level of Ca^{2+}_o half-maximally suppressing circulating PTH levels) *(72,73)*. Therefore, there is mild to moderate resistance of the parathyroid glands to the inhibitory effects of Ca^{2+}_o on PTH secretion in FHH. A similar, but somewhat more severe increase in set-point is exhibited by most patients with primary hyperparathyroidism *(74)*; in the latter condition, pathological parathyroid glands have additional defects in secretory control, including increases in the maximal and minimal secretory rates observed at low and high Ca^{2+}_o, respectively *(73,74)*. In view of their generally normal circulating PTH levels, it is not surprising that there is often normal histology of the parathyroid glands in FHH; or, at most, such glands exhibit mild chief cell hyperplasia *(75,76)*.

A number of patients with FHH have undergone partial or total parathyroidectomy because they were thought to have primary hyperparathyroidism. Such patients have exhibited a distinctly atypical course following surgical intervention that has afforded additional indirect evidence that this disorder differs in some fundamental way from primary hyperparathyroidism. In 27 patients with FHH, each of whom had undergone from one to four neck explorations, recurrence of hypercalcemia took place within a few days or weeks in the majority (21 patients); only two of these individuals remained permanently normocalcemic without any additional therapy *(68)*. More commonly, long term remission of hypercalcemia in patients with FHH required that they be rendered aparathyroid and then be treated with vitamin D (5 of the 27 patients). Recurrent hypercalcemia following resection of a parathyroid adenoma, in contrast, occurs in less than 10% of cases, and, although recurrence of hypercalcemia occurs more commonly in the various forms of primary parathyroid hyperplasia, it generally only occurs after several years *(66,67)*.

Serum 25(OH)D and $1,25(OH)_2D$ levels in patients with FHH are most commonly within the normal range *(77–79)*, and their intestinal absorption of calcium is normal or modestly reduced. Some individuals with FHH exhibit a blunted homeostatic response to a decrease in dietary intake of calcium, showing smaller than expected increases in their gastrointestinal absorption of Ca^{2+} and their $1,25(OH)_2D$ levels *(79)*. Patients with primary hyperparathyroidism, in contrast, frequently show elevated levels of the latter two parameters *(67)*. Although markers of bone turnover, such as urinary hydroxyproline excretion, can be mildly increased *(80,81)*, bone mineral density is usually within the normal range in FHH *(62,80,82)*, and there is no increase in fracture risk. Several members of a recently reported FHH kindred from Oklahoma manifested osteomalacia, but this form of bone disease has not been encountered in other FHH kindreds *(83)*. In addition, this Oklahoman kindred has a form of FHH that is a genetically distinct from that present in the majority of families with this condition (*see* below).

Another characteristic biochemical feature of patients with FHH is their excessively avid renal tubular reabsorption of Ca^{2+} and Mg^{2+}, particularly given their concomitant hypercalcemia *(60,71)*. The parameter of renal Ca^{2+} handling that is employed most commonly to demonstrate this abnormality is the ratio of the renal clearance of calcium to that for creatinine. The calcium to creatinine clearance ratio is less than 0.01 in about 80% of individuals with FHH, while it is higher than this value in the great majority of patients with primary hyperparathyroidism and is markedly greater in other hypercalcemic conditions, since the accompanying inhibition of PTH secretion in the latter circumstance further reduces renal tubular Ca^{2+} reabsorption. Therefore, the combination of a low urinary calcium to creatinine clearance ratio and a normal PTH level in the setting of an autosomal dominant pattern of inheritance of mild, asymptomatic hypercalcemia usually makes the diagnosis of FHH straightforward. Causes of relative hypocalciuria that can be a source of diagnostic confusion in patients with what otherwise appears to be typical primary hyperparathyroidism include concomitant vitamin D deficiency, very low intake of calcium, use of thiazides or lithium, and hypothyroidism.

Occasional kindreds with FHH have been encountered in which there is hypercalciuria and even overt renal stone disease in some family members *(84)*. It is not known at present whether these families have a variant of FHH or two separate disease genes—one conferring the FHH trait and the other promoting increased urinary calcium excretion, thereby outweighing the hypocalciuric effect of the FHH gene(s). It is of interest that the excessively avid renal tubular Ca^{2+} reabsorption in patients with FHH persists even after total parathyroidectomy *(77,85)*. Therefore, the characteristic abnormality in renal handling of calcium in this disorder is not dependent upon PTH but is an independent derangement in renal sensing/handling of Ca^{2+}_o.

Several additional parameters of renal function that have been examined in patients with FHH have suggested altered responsiveness of the kidney to Ca^{2+}_o. Renal blood flow and glomerular filtration rate are both normal in FHH, despite the fact that both of these parameters are reduced in a sizable proportion of patients with other causes of hypercalcemia *(61)*. Moreover, persons with FHH are able to concentrate their urine normally *(86)*, despite the fact that hypercalcemia of other causes may diminish urinary concentrating ability and can sometimes cause overt nephrogenic diabetes insipidus *(58)*.

Therefore, both the clinical and biochemical features of patients with FHH have afforded compelling evidence that this disorder represents an inherited abnormality in the sensing and/or handling of Ca^{2+}_o by parathyroid, kidney, and perhaps other tissues (for instance, there is an apparent absence of the other gastrointestinal or mental symptoms encountered in the more usual forms of hypercalcemia). Because of the benign clinical course of patients with FHH and because it is so difficult to achieve a biochemical "cure" (which would be of dubious value in an otherwise asymptomatic individual), a consensus has evolved that surgical intervention should be avoided in FHH *(68)*. Differentiating FHH from primary hyperparathyroidism, therefore, is very important to avoid unnecessary and inadvisable exploration of the neck in patients with FHH.

Genetics of FHH

FHH is an autosomal dominantly inherited trait with a penetrance approaching 100% *(61,62,68)*. Its biochemical abnormalities have been detected immediately postnatally in affected infants. The disease gene was initially mapped to chromosome 3 (band q21–24) utilizing linkage analysis by Chou et al. in four large FHH kindreds *(70)*. Furthermore, formal genetic analysis proved that persons with FHH are heterozygous for the FHH gene *(70,87)*. Subsequent studies revealed that 90% or more of kindreds sufficiently large for genetic analysis exhibited linkage of the FHH gene to the locus on chromosome 3 *(88,89)*. One family, however, had linkage of a disorder phenotypically indistinguishable from FHH to the short arm of chromosome 19, band 19p13.3 *(88)*, documenting that this condition is genetically heterogeneous. Furthermore, the Oklahoma kindred described previously that exhibits atypical clinical features (e.g., osteomalacia in a few affected family members and a tendency toward progressive elevation in serum PTH with increasing age) showed linkage to neither the chromosome 3 nor the chromosome 19 loci *(83,90)*. This variant of FHH has recently been mapped to the long arm of chromosome 19, band 19q13 *(89a)*. A severe form of hyperparathyroidism in newborn infants (neonatal severe hyperparathyroidism [NSHPT]) is sometimes found in FHH families; in some cases it represents the homozygous form of FHH that is linked to chromosome 3 *(87,91)*. The clinical, biochemical, and genetic features of NSHPT will be delineated in detail later (*see* below).

Identification and Functional Expression of CaR Mutations in FHH

Because there was abnormal Ca^{2+}_o-sensing in FHH by kidney, parathyroid, and probably other tissues, the newly cloned CaR was clearly a good candidate for the disease gene in this condition. Pollak et al. *(92)* first demonstrated that the location of the CaR gene was on the long arm of chromosome 3, where the FHH gene was known to be localized *(70)*. They then utilized a ribonuclease A (RNAse A) protection assay to search for mutations in the CaR gene in three unrelated FHH families that had already been shown to be linked to the chromosome 3 locus *(92)*. These workers identified a different missense mutation in the coding region of the CaR gene in each of these three families (i.e., an alteration in a single nucleotide base substituting a new amino acid for the one normally encoded), arg185gln, glu297lys, and arg795trp. (Note that the arg 185 gln mutation was inadvertently described as arg186glu in the original publication and that the numbering of the amino acid residues in the bovine CaR *(92)* is numerically one higher than that for the human receptor *(89)* because an extra amino acid is present in the ECD of the former.) Furthermore, these mutations were not present in the genomic DNA of 50 normocalcemic control subjects (Fig. 2) *(92)*. Further studies have subsequently identified between two and three dozen additional mutations in the CaR of families with the form of FHH that is linked to chromosome 3 *(63,89,93–96)*. Each family most commonly has its own unique mutation, although occasional, apparently unrelated families share the same mutation. Most are missense mutations that are present within several distinct portions of the predicted CaR protein (Fig. 2):

1. The first half of the ECD;
2. A region of the ECD that immediately precedes TM1; and
3. The TMs, intra- and/or extracellular loops. Heath and coworkers have also identified several seemingly benign polymorphisms within the CaR's C-terminal tail that are present in a substantial fraction of the population (e.g., from about 10 – 30%) *(94)*. Whether these polymorphisms predispose to disorders of Ca^{2+}_o homeostasis or other diseases involving CaR-expressing tissues remains to be determined.

In addition to missense mutations, several other types of mutations have been described in affected members of FHH families. There is a nonsense mutation present in the CaR of one family that is just proximal to TM1 (i.e., ser607stop—substitution of a stop codon for the serine that is normally encoded by this codon) *(89)*. The resultant mutant CaR would almost certainly be inactive as a result of being truncated, since it would be predicted to lack all of its transmembrane domains and might well be secreted. Another mutation includes both a deletion of a single nucleotide and transversion of an adjacent nucleotide (e.g., substitution of one nucleotide for another) within codon 747. This mutation would alter the downstream reading frame of its encoded mutant CaR, thereby resulting in premature termination of the protein after residue 776 within the TMs *(89)*. Finally, a family living in Nova Scotia harbors the insertion at codon 876 of a 383-base pair Alu repetitive sequence *(95)*. The Alu element is present in an orientation opposite to that of the CaR gene and contains a very long poly A tract. Stop signals within all three reading frames of the Alu sequence would generate a truncated CaR protein that contains a long stretch of repeated phenylalanines within its C-terminus (resulting from the AAA codons encoded by the poly A tract). Interestingly, the length of the Alu repetitive element has approximately doubled in size in a subsequent generation of this family *(97)*. Although the vast majority of families with FHH have their disease gene linked to the locus on chromosome 3, only about two-thirds of these families have identifiable mutations in the CaR's coding sequence. In the remainder, it is probable that mutations reside within the receptor's introns or its upstream or downstream regulatory elements and interfere with the normal level of expression of a CaR gene that has a normal coding sequence.

Recent studies have utilized transient transfection in human embryonic kidney (HEK293) cells to express mutant CaRs engineered to include several of the mutations defined to date in FHH kindreds *(64,65,98,99)*. Figure 3 illustrates the impact of several point mutations on high Ca^{2+}_o-evoked increases in Ca^{2+}_i when expressed in HEK293 cells. Some of the mutations, including arg185gln and arg795trp, substantially diminish the apparent affinity and/or maximal activity of the mutated CaRs. Others (e.g., thr138met or arg62met) only modestly reduce apparent affinity and produce no obvious changes in the receptor's maximal response *(64)*. In many cases, the mutant CaRs showing the most marked decreases in biological activity exhibit substantial reductions in the expression of the putatively mature, glycosylated form of the receptor as determined by Western analysis of cellular proteins. Of interest, the degree of elevation in serum calcium concentration in families harboring these mutations is, in general, relatively mild (e.g., ≤1 mg/dL). Indeed, the family in which the nonsense mutation is present at codon 607 shows serum calcium concentrations that are only at or slightly above the upper limit of the normal range *(98)*. Furthermore, as described in greater detail later, mice with targeted disruption (e.g., "knockout") of one allele of the CaR gene likewise exhibit very mild hypercalcemia *(47)*.

Transient transfection in HEK cells has also been performed with two mutant CaRs containing the deletion and transversion mutation in codon 747 *(98)* or the insertion of the Alu repetitive element at codon 876 *(99)*. In both cases, truncated proteins were produced on Western analysis that were of the sizes predicted from the presence of the predicted premature stop codons introduced by these two mutations, but there was essentially no biological activity present in the transfected cells.

Mutations markedly reducing the CaR's biological activity despite their having an apparently normal expression pattern on Western analysis, in contrast, tend to be those producing the greatest degree of elevation is serum calcium concentration. The arg795trp or arg185gln mutations *(64,65)*, for example, produce serum calcium concentrations in affected family members that are about 2 mg/dL and 3 mg/dL higher, respectively, than the levels in unaffected members. These mutant receptors appear to exert a so-called dominant negative effect on the wild-type (i.e., normal) receptor when the two CaRs are cotransfected. Indeed, while coexpressing normal and mutant receptors (to mimic the heterozygous state that is present in vivo in FHH patients) has little or no effect on the function of the normal receptor in cases where the mature form of the mutant CaR is expressed in reduced amounts, both the arg795trp and arg185gln mutations right-shift the EC_{50} (the effective concentration of agonist evoking half of the maximal response) of cells cotransfected with the wild-type receptor (Fig. 4). This dominant negative action of the latter two mutant receptors probably results from some interference by the mutant receptor with the wild-type CaR's expression or action. Such interference could take place in several possible ways:

1. A reduction in the quantity of the normal CaR that reaches the cell surface;
2. A decrease in the effective concentration of the G protein(s) that are available to the wild-type CaR as a result of the formation of an inactive complex of G protein(s) with the mutant receptor; and/or
3. The presence of inactive complexes of the normal and mutant CaRs on the cell surface.

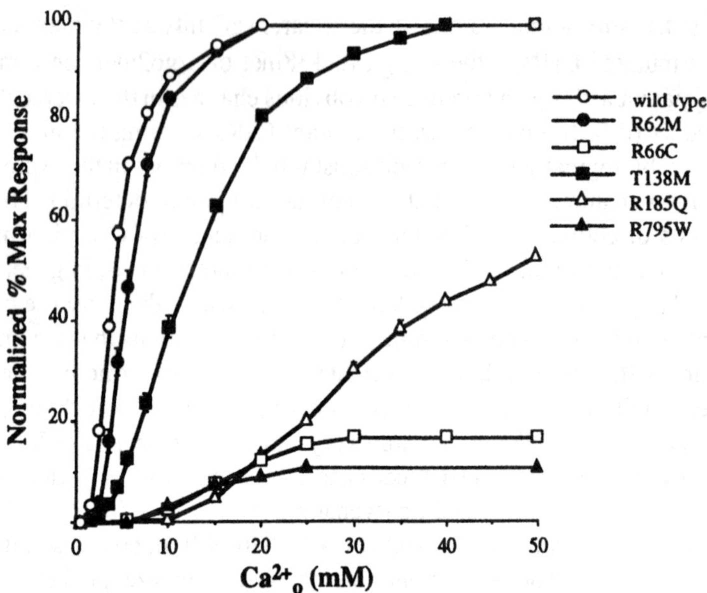

Fig. 3. Expression of CaRs with FHH mutations in HEK293 cells. The results show the effects of varying levels of Ca^{2+}_o on Ca^{2+}_i in HEK293 cells transiently transfected with the wild-type CaR or the indicated mutant CaRs. Results are normalized to indicate the percent of the maximal response of the wild type CaR. (Reproduced with permission from ref. *64*.) Note that R62M = arg62met; R66C = arg66cys; T138M = thr138met; R185Q = arg185gln; and R795W = arg795trp.

Available data do not permit differentiation among these possibilities at present, although we have recently found that the CaR resides on the surface of parathyroid and HEK cells largely in the form of a dimer, indicating that the third of the possible mechanisms just listed may contribute to the apparently dominant negative action of some CaRs harboring inactivating mutations on the wild-type receptor. Many FHH families have levels of serum calcium that are higher than those in mice heterozygous for CaR knockout or in FHH kindreds harboring what are effectively null mutations (e.g., there is essentially no receptor protein produced from the abnormal allele, as in the ser607stop mutation). Therefore, it is quite possible that some degree of dominant negative interaction of mutant and wild-type receptors is the rule rather than the exception in FHH.

Several tentative conclusions can be made concerning the structure-function relationships for the calcium-sensing receptor on the basis of the work just outlined. Some missense mutations present within the receptor's ECD produce a spectrum of changes in the CaR's apparent affinity for Ca^{2+}_o (as well as for Gd^{3+}_o) without altering the apparent level of expression of the mature receptor protein, at least as assessed by Western analysis *(64)*. Thus the mutated amino acid may

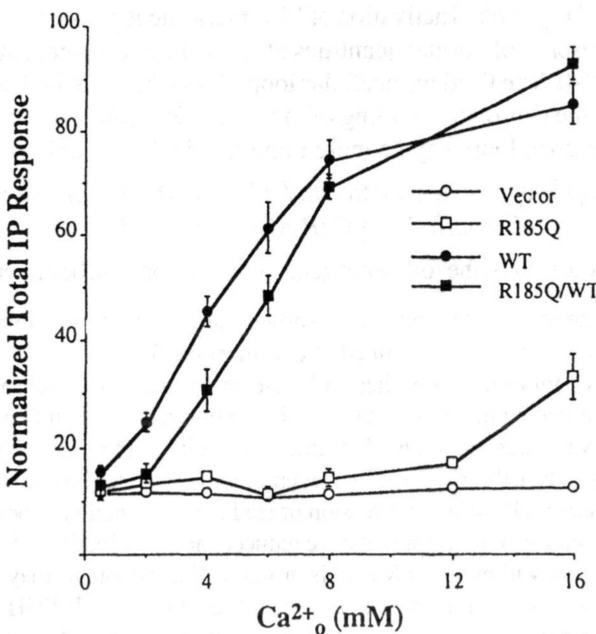

Fig. 4. Coexpression of a mutant CaR bearing an inactivating CaR mutation (arg185gln) and the wild-type CaR in HEK293 cells. The results illustrate the high Ca^{2+}_o-elicited increases in total cellular inositol phosphates in HEK 293 cells transiently transfected with empty vector (e.g., not containing cDNA), wild-type CaR, a mutant CaR bearing the inactivating CaR mutation, arg185gln, or both the mutant and wild-type CaRs. Note the "dominant negative" effect of the CaR bearing arg185gln when it is co-transfected with the wild-type CaR, thereby right-shifting the high Ca^{2+}_o-induced activation of the wild-type receptor and likely contributing to the more severe hypercalcemia found in the neonate with *de novo* heterozygous FHH resulting from this mutation. (Reproduced with permission from ref. *65*.) Note that R185Q = arg185gln.

directly or indirectly alter the CaR's affinity for its polycationic ligands. The eventual solution of the three dimensional structure of the CaR's ECD by X-ray crystallography will be essential for elucidating how this protein interacts with its polycationic ligands. The Hill coefficient for the stimulation of the CaR by Ca^{2+}_o in transiently transfected HEK cells is about three, suggesting that there are three (or possibly more) interacting binding sites for Ca^{2+}_o *(64)*.

Mutations within the CaR's TMs probably interfere with activation of the receptor by its agonists by reducing its cell surface expression and/or disrupting the conformational changes in the TMs and/or ICLs that occur with agonist binding and are required for activation of G protein(s). As noted previously, the single FHH mutation described to date that is present in an ICL (e.g., arg795trp), severely reduces high Ca^{2+}_o-evoked activation of PLC in transiently transfected HEK cells despite the presence of normal quantities of the mature receptor protein on Western analysis *(64)*. The third intracellular loop plays a key role in determining the specificity of the G protein coupling of many GPCRs *(100,101)*, although in the mGluRs the second loop may be more important in this regard *(102)*.

Physiologic, Diagnostic, and Therapeutic Implications of Inactivating CaR Mutations in FHH

From these results, the following general conclusions can be drawn about FHH:

1. It is a genetically heterogeneous disorder, but 90% or more of families have the form of the condition linked to chromosome 3.
2. About two-thirds of all families with FHH due to the locus on chromosome 3 have inactivating mutations in the CaR's coding region. Each family usually has its own unique mutation. Most mutations reside within the CaR's ECD and probably reduce the affinity of the receptor for Ca^{2+}_o, interfere with its biosynthesis and/or cell surface expression or lead to the formation of heterodimers with the wild-type receptor that have reduced biological activity. Some mutations present within the CaR's TMs or intracellular domains may impair the processes required for productive signal transduction. All FHH mutations appear to render patients with FHH mildly to moderately "resistant" to the normal actions of extracellular Ca^{2+}_o that are mediated by the CaR.
3. The remaining persons with the form of FHH that is linked to chromosome 3 who do not have detectable mutations in the receptor's coding region may have mutations in promoter or enhancer sequences of the CaR gene that eliminate or reduce the expression of the otherwise normal receptor encoded by the mutated gene.
4. The altered parathyroid dynamics in individuals with FHH confirm that the CaR is a central player in Ca^{2+}_o-regulated PTH secretion. Moreover, the PTH-independent alterations in the regulation of renal Ca^{2+}, Mg^{2+} and water handling by Ca^{2+}_o (i.e., excessive renal tubular reabsorption of these two divalent cations despite hypercalcemia and the absence of the normally inhibitory action of high Ca^{2+}_o on urinary concentration) provide in vivo evidence supporting a central role for the CaR in regulating several aspects of renal function.
5. In occasional families with conditions phenotypically nearly indistinguishable from FHH, the disease gene maps to other, as yet undefined genetic loci on chromosome 19p or 19q13. Identifying these genes may enable isolation of additional Ca^{2+}_o-sensing receptors or other molecular elements required for the CaR's normal biological activities.
6. Since the disorder is genetically heterogeneous and a substantial fraction of patients with FHH linked to chromosome 3 do not have mutations that can be identified within the CaR's coding region, the diagnosis of FHH will likely continue to require documenting the presence of mild, PTH-dependent hypercalcemia in combination with relative hypocalciuria (a calcium to creatinine clearance ratio < 0.01) that exhibits an autosomal dominant pattern of inheritance. Direct mutational analysis may be of utility in specific clinical settings, such as in the differentiation of FHH from primary hyperparathyroid-

ism in persons who do not have relatives available for biochemical and genetic screening or in patients with apparently de novo CaR mutations.

7. Finally, because persons with FHH usually have a benign clinical course, parathyroidectomy should only be carried in very unusual clinical circumstances, i.e., in cases where patients are suffering adverse consequences of their hypercalcemia.

Neonatal Severe Primary Hyperparathyroidism (NSHPT)

Clinical and Biochemical Features of NSHPT

Neonatal primary hyperparathyroidism often presents dramatically as severe, symptomatic hypercalcemia that is associated with hyperparathyroid bone disease before the age of six months—the clinical syndrome of neonatal severe hyperparathyroidism (NSHPT) *(68)*. NSHPT was described well before FHH *(103)*. A recent review of 49 cases of NSHPT showed that most present clinically at birth or shortly thereafter, often during the first week of life *(68)*. Common symptoms include anorexia, constipation, failure to thrive, hypotonia, and respiratory distress. Additional clinical features that may be encountered include chest wall deformity and, occasionally, dysmorphic facies, craniotabes, and anovaginal or rectovaginal fistula *(50,104–107)*. Respiratory complications may supervene as a result of thoracic deformity, sometimes leading to a flail chest syndrome owing to multiple rib fractures, which can cause substantial morbidity *(103,104)*.

The hypercalcemia in NSHPT is most commonly severe, on the order of 14 to 20 mg/dL, and levels as high as 30.8 mg/dL have been recorded *(105)*. In spite of this marked hypercalcemia, some cases have exhibited relative hypocalciuria, even in the absence of a family history of FHH *(108)*. Serum magnesium concentrations, when available, have sometimes been elevated well above the normal range *(63)*. Serum PTH levels have been markedly elevated in most cases, often being 5-10-fold elevated, although the degree of the increase can be more modest on occasion *(45,109)*. Skeletal X-rays often show profound reductions in bony mineralization, accompanied by fractures of the long bones and ribs, widening of the metaphyses, subperiosteal erosion, and, occasionally, rickets *(104,110)*. Skeletal histology usually reveals the typical osteitis fibrosa cystica that is seen in severe hyperparathyroidism *(106)*. At the time of parathyroidectomy, all four parathyroid glands are usually enlarged, and their combined mass may be many times that of the parathyroid glands of normal children of this age, exhibiting chief cell or water-clear cell hyperplasia. Occasionally, when the parathyroid enlargement is less marked, the low content of fat that is normally present in the parathyroid glands of children can complicate interpretation of the parathyroid histology *(68,106,111)*. There have been no cases reported of NSHPT caused by a parathyroid adenoma.

In some cases, the hypercalcemia encountered in neonatal hyperparathyroidism is less severe, in the range of 11–12 mg/dL; and occasional cases have run a self-limited course, reverting to a milder form of hypercalcemia at the age of 6 – 7 mo following only conservative medical therapy *(104)*. It is likely that the recent discovery that inactivating CaR mutations cause NSHPT will widen further the spectrum of this disease as milder cases are uncovered. A particularly interesting case was identified recently—a homozygous 32-yr-old female who was the offspring of a consanguineous union between two individuals with unrecognized FHH and the same FHH mutation. Both of the parents' serum calcium concentrations were in the upper range of normal *(63)*. This homozygous individual did not initially present as NSHPT and was only diagnosed as an adult, when her hypercalcemia and her homozygous CaR mutations were identified serendipitously and by mutational analysis, respectively. In spite of serum calcium concentrations between 15 and 17 mg/dL, this patient was felt to be asymptomatic, although she was characterized as mildly retarded. Her serum magnesium concentration was also elevated to a substantial degree (about 50% above the upper limit of normal), and her serum intact PTH level was just at the upper limit of the normal range. Despite her marked hypercalcemia, renal function was apparently entirely normal.

Before 1982 *(68)*, NSHPT often had a fatal outcome unless there was prompt and aggressive combined medical and surgical treatment. This has been less true in more recent clinical experience, however, and wider recognition of the broadening clinical spectrum of the disease combined with improvements in the medical treatment of severe hypercalcemia have resulted in successful medical management in a number of cases during the past 15 yr *(68)*. In symptomatic cases, initial management includes vigorous hydration, the use of inhibitors of bone resorption and respiratory support. If the infant's condition is very severe or deteriorates during medical therapy, total parathyroidectomy with autotransplantation of part of one of the glands is generally recommended within the first month of life *(46,68,109)*. Some authors recommend total parathyroidectomy followed by lifelong management of the resultant hypoparathyroidism with oral calcium and vitamin D therapy (generally with 1,25-dihydroxyvitamin D) as needed to prevent symptomatic hypocalcemia *(45,106)*. There is generally rapid and dramatic clinical improvement after parathyroidectomy, with rapid healing of the skeletal lesions, even though the hypercalcemia generally recurs rapidly with less than a total parathyroidectomy or following autotransplantation *(68,106)*. Similar clinical improvement has been observed more recently in infants with NSHPT managed medically *(68)*, indicating that biochemical improvement in the degree of hyperparathyroidism can be part of the natural history of NSHPT, a point that will be returned to later.

Genetics of NSHPT

Early descriptions of FHH showed that infants with NSHPT could occur in kindreds with this condition *(61,91,106,112)*. In 15 kindreds with FHH, Marx et al. identified three patients with FHH in two of the families *(61,106)*, providing strong indirect evidence that NSHPT, in some cases, can be the homozygous form of FHH. In another family with two children exhibiting NSHPT, the parents, who were related, showed mild increases in their levels of serum ionized calcium (despite having levels of total calcium that were normal) and relative hypocalciuria *(91)*, again suggesting that NSHPT could represent homozygous FHH. Pollak and co-workers subsequently showed in an additional 11 FHH families in whom the disease gene mapped to chromosome 3 *(87)* that consanguineous unions of affected individuals in four families produced NSHPT in some offspring. The inheritance of specific genetic markers, closely linked to the FHH gene, provided very strong evidence that NSHPT in these families was the homozygous form of FHH. Later studies of FHH documented to arise from CaR mutations confirmed that inheritance of two abnormal copies of the mutant gene can cause NSHPT *(92,93,95)*. Because such infants have no normal CaR genes, they exhibit much more severe clinical and biochemical manifestations than observed in the heterozygous state (FHH), principally as a result of having a greater degree of resistance of the parathyroid glands to Ca^{2+}_{o}.

NSHPT Caused by Homozygous, Compound Heterozygous or Heterozygous CaR Mutations

Not all cases of NSHPT, however, represent homozygous FHH. Kobayashi et al. recently described an infant with the clinical picture of NSHPT, each of whose parents had a separate mutation in the coding region of the CaR gene—arg185stop in the father and gly670glu in the mother *(96)*. Although the mother was normocalcemic, her serum calcium concentration averaged 10.4 mg/dL (with an upper limit of 10.5 mg/dL), suggesting the presence of a very mild FHH phenotype. Therefore, co-expression in the infant's CaR-expressing tissues of the mother's mutant CaR with the father's CaR nonsense mutation (which produced clear-cut, albeit mild paternal hypercalcemia [averaging 10.6 mg/dL]) caused the NSHPT phenotype, with a serum calcium concentration of 26.5 mg/dL. At the time of parathyroidectomy, four hyperplastic parathyroid glands were identified.

In a number of other cases of NSHPT, however, it appears this condition was associated with a single abnormal CaR allele in the affected neonate(s), although this has been formally proven in only a minority of cases. In most instances, NSHPT has occurred sporadically or in FHH kindreds in which there was only one affected parent *(50,113,114)*. What was the basis for the occurrence of NSHPT in these cases? Such children could also potentially have been compound heterozygotes, harboring two distinct different mutant CaR alleles—as in the case of Kobayashi et al. *(96)*—the first producing clear-cut hypercalcemia in one parent, but the second being so mild as to be biochemically silent in the other parent. Alternatively, there could conceivably be a mutation in one CaR allele combined with a separate mutation in one allele of another gene causing an FHH-like clinical picture (e.g., the one on chromosome 19p *[88]*)or that linked to neither chromosome 19q13 *(89a)* that was inherited from the other parent. No such cases, however, have been documented to date.

Another possible contributory factor for the development of NSHPT that occurs in a child with a single mutant CaR allele arising from a father with FHH but with an unaffected mother is the impact of normal maternal calcium homeostasis on the fetus' abnormal Ca^{2+}_o-sensing *in utero (91)*. Calcium is transported actively across the placenta from the maternal to the fetal circulation, engendering a higher level of the fetal than of the maternal calcium concentration *(91)*. Therefore, a normal mother would expose the fetal parathyroid glands to a level of Ca^{2+}_o that would be sensed as relatively hypocalcemic owing to the presence of the FHH mutation in one allele of the CaR expressed in those glands. The latter would lead to "overstimulation" of the fetal parathyroids, causing an additional degree of "secondary" fetal/neonatal hyperparathyroidism that would be superimposed on the abnormal Ca^{2+}_o-sensing already present in those parathyroid glands as a result of the FHH mutation by itself. Support for this explanation has been provided by the occurrence of cases of NSHPT with an autosomal dominant pattern of inheritance in cases where the father had FHH and the mother was thought to be normal *(68,71,106)*. In the postnatal period, the "secondary" hyperparathyroidism would gradually resolve over a period of several months, eventually returning to the clinical and biochemical characteristics of FHH. It is clear, however, that in most cases children with FHH born to normal mothers do not have any greater severity of their hypercalcemia than those born to affected mothers. In addition, there are no apparent differences between the mice heterozygous for targeted disruption of the CaR gene that are born to normal mothers compared to mothers that are heterozygous for CaR knockout *(47)*. Recent evidence suggests that some families may be more susceptible to the development of NSHPT in heterozygous infants because their CaR mutations exert a dominant negative action on the normal CaR, presumably as a result of the defect in Ca^{2+}_o-sensing being more severe than that observed in FHH families with mild hypercalcemia or in the CaR knockout mice *(64)*.

Recent studies have demonstrated that neonatal hyperparathyroidism can likewise occur in the setting of heterozygous *de novo* CaR mutations *(89)* (i.e., with a spontaneous, apparently germline CaR mutation occurring *de novo* in the child of normal parents). Two such infants exhibited hyperparathyroid bone disease but had less severe hypercalcemia than is generally observed in NSHPT resulting from homozygous FHH *(89)*. We recently identified another case of *de novo* heterozygous NSHPT occurring in a child who harbored the same Arg185Gln mutation that has previously been associated with a greater degree of elevation in serum calcium concentration than seen in most FHH kindreds *(65,92,106)*. As in the cases of NSHPT described in the families with this mutation, the relatively large disparity between the set-points of the maternal and fetal parathyroid glands in this *de novo* case of FHH may have caused more severe prenatal hyperparathyroidism and, in turn, hyperparathyroid bone disease in the newborn infant.

Therefore, the clinical and biochemical features of NSHPT, which in homozygous cases is equivalent to "knockout" of the human CaR gene, support the following additional conclusions about the receptor's function in humans: (1) They further point out its importance in fetal and neonatal calcium metabolism.

(2) They indicate that, beyond its role in Ca^{2+}_o-regulated PTH release, which is markedly deranged in NSHPT particularly that resulting from homozygous FHH, the CaR likely serves to inhibit parathyroid cellular proliferation tonically, because there is often florid parathyroid hyperplasia in NSHPT.

Mouse Models of FHH and NSHPT

Recently, Ho et al. have utilized targeted disruption of the CaR gene to create mice that are either heterozygous or homozygous for inactivation of the CaR gene. These mice provide animal models of FHH and NSHPT, respectively. Introduction of DNA encoding the neomycin resistance gene by homologous recombination into the CaR gene's third exon resulted in essentially a complete absence of CaR protein in the parathyroid glands and kidneys of homozygous mice, although there were approx 50% reductions in the levels of the CaR protein in the heterozygotes *(47)*. Phenotypically, the heterozygous mice appeared normal, were fertile and had a normal life span. The level of their serum calcium concentration was 10.4 mg/dL, a value about 10% higher than that of their normal littermates. The heterozygous mice also had mild, but significant ~10% elevations in their serum magnesium concentrations. Serum PTH levels were ~50% higher in the heterozygous mice than in normal mice of the same age; despite the hypercalcemia, the calcium concentration in bladder urine was slightly lower than that in the normal mice. Skeletal X-rays in the wild-type and heterozygous mice were essentially indistinguishable. Therefore, mice that are heterozygous for "knock-out" of the CaR gene appear to share many of the phenotypic and biochemical features of individuals with FHH.

Interestingly, the heterozygous mice showed little, if any, apparent up-regulation in their production of CaR protein expression in parathyroid and kidney by the remaining normal CaR allele, since the levels of expression of the CaR protein in kidney and parathyroid were approximately one-half of those in the wild-type animals *(47)*. This approx 50% reduction in the level of expression of the CaR protein in the parathyroid led to a mild (approx 10%) elevation in the apparent set-point of Ca^{2+}_o-regulated PTH release. The latter abnormality was not dissimilar from that encountered in FHH families that harbor mutations expected to produce a totally inactive CaR (e.g., ser607stop). Therefore, the results observed in the heterozygous mice further supported the notion that the abnormal CaR allele in FHH can act as a null mutation (e.g., it produces no gene product or one that is totally inactive), thereby producing an abnormality in parathyroid function that is simply the result of a reduction in the density of normally functioning CaRs on the parathyroid cell surface *(61,62,68)*. This pathophysiology is not unlike that which we and others have recently shown to occur in parathyroid adenomas. Although such adenomas do not appear to harbor mutations in the CaR gene *(115)* they show an average approx 60% reduction in CaR expression as assessed by *in situ* hybridization and/or immunohistochemistry *(116,117)*. Parathyroid adenomas usually exhibit a somewhat greater increase in set-point in vitro and in vivo than is observed in FHH *(72,74)*, perhaps as a result of the greater reduction in cell surface CaRs in the former. It is also apparent, however, as noted previously, that in occasional FHH families the serum calcium concentration of affected members is higher than in most other FHH families, probably as a result of an additional, "dominant negative" interaction of the mutant with the wild-type CaR protein *(64,65)*.

Mice homozygous for inactivation of the CaR, in contrast, while nearly normal in size at birth, subsequently grew much more slowly than their normal or heterozygous littermates *(47)*. This poor growth may have resulted, in part, from their inability to compete successfully with their more vigorous normal and heterozygous littermates for their mothers' milk. The homozygous mice exhibited severe hypercalcemia, with serum calcium levels averaging 14.8 mg/dL. Their serum magnesium levels, in contrast, were only slightly and not significantly higher than those in the heterozygous mice. Serum PTH levels were almost 10-fold greater than those observed in normal mice, an increase that was comparable to what is seen in infants with NSHPT. Despite their severe hypercalcemia, the calcium concentration in the bladder urine of the homozygous mice was lower than that in normal mice *(47)*. Skeletal X-rays showed striking abnormalities, with appreciable reductions in mineral density, bowing of the long bones, and kyphoscoliosis. The majority of the homozygous mice died within the first two postnatal weeks, and only occasional homozygotes survived for up to 3 or 4 wk. Therefore, the biochemical and clinical characteristics of mice homozygous for "knock-out" of the CaR gene exhibited numerous similarities to the those of the human disorder, NSHPT. Much remains to be learned, however, from the use of this animal model to investigate alterations in Ca^{2+}_o-sensing in a variety of tissues that express the CaR, both those involved in and those not thought to be play any role in systemic calcium homeostasis, such as the brain.

Syndrome of Overresponsiveness to Ca^{2+}_o Owing to Activating CaR Mutations

Clinical and Biochemical Features Resulting from Activating CaR Mutations

Familial isolated hypoparathyroidism is a rare disorder that occurs in several forms—autosomal recessive, autosomal dominant, and X-linked *(118)*. The molecular pathogenesis of the autosomal recessive and X-linked forms have yet to be discovered. In a study of eight families with autosomal dominant hypoparathyroidism, there was linkage of the disorder to the PTH gene in two of them *(119)*. One of these two families was subsequently shown to harbor a mutation within the region of the preproPTH gene encoding the signal peptide *(120)*. Another family has since been described with a mutation in a splice junction of the preproPTH gene *(121)*. The identification of inactivating mutations in the CaR gene as the cause of FHH, combined with the discovery of activating mutations in other G protein-coupled receptors *(122–125)*, suggested the possibility that activating mutations of the CaR might produce an autosomal dominant form of hypocalcemia (e.g., familial hypercalciuric hypocalcemia). This hypothesis, in fact, has turned out to be correct.

Autosomal dominant hypocalcemia, prior to its recognition as the clinical expression of activating mutations in the CaR, had been lumped together with other forms of hypoparathyroidism. Nevertheless, families subsequently shown to harbor CaR mutations exhibit certain clinical features that might have been predicted to be the result of "resetting" downward of the set-points of both parathyroid and kidney for Ca^{2+}_o *(98,126–131)*. In effect, this disorder represents the clinical expression of mild to moderate increases in the responsiveness of CaR-expressing tissues to Ca^{2+}_o (vs the resistance to Ca^{2+}_o that is present in FHH). Doubtless, the identification of further families with this disorder as a result of screening hypoparathyroid families for CaR mutations will provide a more detailed picture of its prevalence, presentation, and clinical course.

Individuals with autosomal dominant hypocalcemia exhibit mild to moderate hypocalcemia (~6-8 mg/dL) *(126,130–132)*, although occasional patients have more severe hypocalcemia (4–6 mg/dL) *(126)*. Some individuals with this disorder experience relatively little symptomatology despite their hypocalcemia *(131)*, while others share many of the signs and symptoms exhibited by patients with other hypocalcemic disorders, including seizures, paresthesias, muscle cramps, and laryngospasm *(126,130)*. The seizures appear to be more common within the first few weeks or months of life. In several cases seizures occurred during febrile episodes and in the majority of patients were not difficult to control *(130)*. Individuals with autosomal dominant hypocalcemia, similar to those with classical hypoparathyroidism, exhibit hyperphosphatemia, although in some kindreds the serum phosphate levels of affected individuals can be normal *(131)*, probably in those families with mild hypocalcemia and normal PTH levels. Serum magnesium levels are often in the lower half of the normal range and may be overtly low in the untreated state *(126,128,130,131)*. Intact PTH levels are generally in the lower part of the normal range *(131)*. In one case of autosomal dominant hypocalcemia, reducing serum calcium further caused a brisk rise in serum PTH, consistent with the presence of a leftward shift in the set-point for Ca^{2+}_o-regulated PTH release without frank parathyroid failure *(133)*. $1,25(OH)_2$ vitamin D levels have been measured in relatively few cases and were usually normal *(130)*. In two studies, the urinary excretion of calcium in the untreated state was approximately twice as high in patients with autosomal dominant hypocalcemia as in those with other causes of hypoparathyroidism, despite the fact that PTH levels are often higher in the former than in the latter *(126,130,132)*. As described in more detail later, this increased excretion of calcium is thought to reflect direct inhibition of renal tubular Ca^{2+} (and Mg^{2+}) reabsorption by mutant CaRs activated at inappropriately low levels of Ca^{2+}_o—the opposite of the effect of inactivating FHH mutations on renal handling of calcium by the same nephron segments.

Patients with autosomal dominant hypocalcemia appear to respond to treatment with vitamin D in a manner that differs in a characteristic way from that observed in patients with true hypoparathyroidism. The former are unusually susceptible to the development of marked hypercalciuria and other renal complications of overtreatment with vitamin D, even in the absence of frank hypercalcemia *(130)*. These deleterious effects of vitamin D therapy include renal stones, nephrocalcinosis, reversible (and, in some cases, irreversible) reductions in renal function as well as polydipsia and polyuria, probably as a result of poor urinary concentrating ability *(130)*.

Linkage to Chromosome 3 and Identification of Activating CaR Mutations

Finegold and colleagues first identified a family with a form of autosomal dominant hypocalcemia that was linked to a locus on chromosome 3 that was close to that of the CaR gene *(134)*. Shortly afterward, Pollak, et al. identified a heterozygous missense mutation in codon 127 of the CaR (glu127ala) *(131)* in another family with autosomal dominant hypocalcemia that had previously been postulated to have an inherited reduction in the set-point of the parathyroid glands to Ca^{2+}_o *(133)*. Subsequent studies have identified a total of approximately a dozen heterozygous missense, activating mutations in the CaR gene, which cause either autosomal dominant hypocalcemia or *de novo* sporadic cases of hypocalcemia *(98,126–131,135)* (Fig. 2). The majority are present within the CaR's ECD, providing further indirect evidence for the importance of this region of the receptor in the mechanisms underlying its activation by Ca^{2+}_o, while several families harbor mutations residing within the receptor's TMs *(126,127,129)*. To date, no cases of homozygous activating CaR mutations have been identified in sporadic cases of hypocalcemia or in kindreds with autosomal dominant hypocalcemia.

Expression of several of the known mutations causing autosomal dominant hypocalcemia in HEK293 cells showed a clear leftward shift in Ca^{2+}_o-evoked increases in Ca^{2+}_i (Fig. 5) *(64,98)* or in inositol phosphates *(127,129)*. In addition, in the studies characterizing the effects of such activating mutations on the accumulation of inositol phosphates, there was also an increase in the maximal activity of the mutant receptors at high Ca^{2+}_o. It is possible, however, that this apparent increase in maximal activity was related to greater labeling of the phosphoinositide pool during the preincubation of the cells with tritiated inositol as a consequence of a greater degree of activation of the mutant as opposed to the wild-type receptors at the calcium concentration present in the culture medium. In a case in which the mutant CaR has been co-expressed with the wild-type CaR to mimic the heterozygous state present in patients, the pattern of receptor activation was more similar to that of the mutant than of the wild-type receptor (Fig. 5). This observation may simply reflect the fact that the number of mutant receptors expressed in the

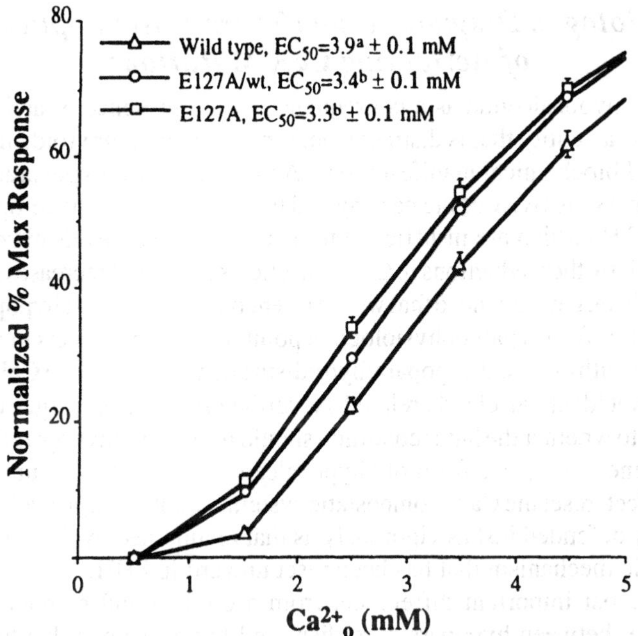

Fig. 5. Expression of an activating CaR mutation (glu127ala) in HEK293 cells. Results indicate the effects of the indicated levels of Ca^{2+}_o on Ca^{2+}_i in HEK293 cells transiently transfected with the wild-type CaR, a mutant CaR bearing the activating mutation, glu127ala, or cotransfected with both the wild-type and mutant receptors. (Reproduced with permission from ref. *64*.) Note that E127A = glu127ala.

cotransfected HEK cells is sufficient to give a pattern of activation by Ca^{2+}_o not dissimilar from that produced in HEK cells transfected with the mutant receptor alone. Alternatively, as noted previously, recent evidence suggests that the CaR is present on the cell surface of parathyroid and HEK cells largely in the form of a disulfide-linked dimer *(135a,135b)*. It is possible, therefore, that heterodimers of wild-type and activated CaRs more closely resemble the latter than the former in their functional properties, a possibility that has not yet been formally tested.

Activating mutations present in other GPCRs, such as the TSH or LH receptors, are most commonly found in the transmembrane domains, where they presumably facilitate the activation of signal transduction or mimic the receptor's active state if there is ligand-independent activation of the receptor *(123,136)*. Those mutations present in the transmembrane domains of the CaR may act in a similar manner. Mutations within the CaR's ECD, in contrast, may increase its affinity for Ca^{2+}_o, and/or favor the active conformation of the receptor, thereby promoting subsequent events in signal transduction at levels of Ca^{2+}_o too low to produce similar effects on the wild-type CaR.

Physiologic, Diagnostic, and Therapeutic Implications of Activating CaR Mutations.

Thus, hypocalcemia as a consequence of the presence of activating CaR mutations is an entity that is distinct from typical hypoparathyroidism in both its clinical and biochemical manifestations. As with classical hypoparathyroidism, the excessive sensitivity of the parathyroid to Ca^{2+}_o produces inappropriately low levels of PTH (which are insufficient to maintain normal levels of serum Ca^{2+}_o) even though further reductions in Ca^{2+}_o can elicit substantial increases in PTH that are probably larger than those that would be encountered in most hypoparathyroid subjects. Thus from a pathophysiological point of view the defects in parathyroid physiology with classical hypoparathyroidism and with activating CaR mutations are, while not identical, clearly related. Nevertheless, one could argue on a semantic basis as to whether the latter condition should be termed "hypoparathyroidism" or more generically, as a form of "hypocalcemia." Activating mutations of the CaR, in effect, reset the Ca^{2+}_o homeostatic system, maintaining a level of Ca^{2+}_o that is probably defended just as vigorously as that maintained by the Ca^{2+}_o-resistant homeostatic mechanism that has been reset upward in FHH.

The most important difference, from a clinical and pathophysiological perspective, between hypoparathyroidism and hypocalcemia due to activating mutations of the CaR is the result of the presence of "overresponsive" CaRs in the kidney, particularly in the distal tubule. The latter elevate the level of urinary calcium excretion substantially above that generally present in hypoparathyroidism, at least in the untreated state. Further increases in serum calcium as a result of well-intentioned treatment with vitamin D and calcium, elevate urinary calcium excretion even further, producing a substantial risk of nephrolithiasis and nephrocalcinosis. Furthermore, during such treatment these individuals not infrequently develop the same reductions in renal function at low-normal levels of Ca^{2+}_o that are only encountered in patients with classical hypoparathyroidism when they are rendered frankly hypercalcemic by treatment with calcium and vitamin D. The polyuria, enuresis, and polydipsia that can develop in these patients during such treatment also appear from the reports available to date to occur more commonly and at lower levels of Ca^{2+}_o than in patients being treated for classical hypoparathyroidism. It is likely, therefore, that the kidneys in patients with activating CaR mutations manifest a generalized increase in sensitivity to the usual "toxic" actions of calcium, although more detailed studies are needed in patients with this condition or in animal models that could potentially be developed in which the normal CaR gene is replaced with one harboring an activating mutation.

Further studies are also needed to determine the true prevalence of hypocalcemia due to CaR activating mutations among the hypocalcemic population previously thought to have hypoparathyroidism. It may well be that a larger number of families with autosomal dominant hypocalcemia or individual cases arising from *de novo* activating mutations in the CaR will be uncovered, which were previously identified as familial isolated or sporadic hypoparathyroidism. To date only about one-third as many activating as inactivating CaR mutations have been identified. Nevertheless, the recognition of the relatively benign, asymptomatic nature of FHH led to systematic family screening in hypercalcemic patients that uncovered a substantial number of kindreds whose DNA could be subjected to systematic mutational analysis after the cloning of the CaR and recognition of its gene as the disease gene in FHH. Perhaps, more vigorous family screening of hypocalcemic probands will identify a larger reservoir of both sporadic hypocalcemia and autosomal dominant forms of hypocalcemia resulting from activating CaR mutations.

This distinction of hypocalcemia due to activating CaR mutations from that due to classical isolated hypoparathyroidism is clinically important because of the reversible or even irreversible renal damage that can occur in the former following overly aggressive treatment of their hypocalcemia with calcitriol in an attempt to normalize their serum calcium concentrations *(130)*. Identifying individuals with activating CaR mutations requires a prepared mind and careful clinical, biochemical, and genetic evaluation. The most helpful diagnostic clues are the presence of hypocalcemia, which, in a familial setting, has an autosomal dominant pattern of transmission, and is accompanied by hypomagnesemia (in some cases), intact PTH levels in the lower half of the normal range and urinary calcium excretion that, on average, is greater than that observed in classical hypoparathyroidism. Nevertheless, differentiation from the usual case of hypoparathyroidism may not be straightforward, and in some cases the diagnosis has only been entertained subsequent to the development of severe hypercalciuria and/or renal impairment during therapy with vitamin D.

Summary

The cloning of a G protein-coupled CaR, coupled with the identification of naturally occurring syndromes of Ca^{2+}_o resistance and oversensitivity, has permitted direct documentation that a variety of cell types can sense small changes in Ca^{2+}_o via a receptor-mediated mechanism similar to that through which numerous cells respond to a wide variety of other extracellular messengers. Thus, Ca^{2+}_o can function in a hormone-like role as an extracellular first messenger in addition to carrying out its better recognized functions as an important intracellular second messenger. Of the numerous tissues that express the CaR, several represent important components of the mineral ion homeostatic system that have long been known to sense Ca^{2+}_o, such as parathyroid and C-cells. Furthermore, the CaR's presence on several types of renal cells strongly supports the notion that several of the long-recognized but poorly understood effects of Ca^{2+}_o on the function of the kidney may likewise be CaR-mediated. These effects include the enhanced excretion of calcium and magnesium that occur with hypercalcemia, probably as a result of direct actions of high Ca^{2+}_o on CaRs in the distal tubule, which complement the reduction in renal reabsorption of Ca^{2+} that results from the accompanying, high Ca^{2+}_o-induced inhibition of PTH secretion. The diminished urinary concentrating capacity exhibited by some hypercalcemic individuals is likely a manifestation of a functionally relevant integration of the homeostatic mechanisms controlling renal calcium and water handling.

The inherited human syndromes of Ca^{2+}_o "resistance" or "overresponsiveness" represented by FHH and autosomal dominant hypocalcemia offer interesting "experiments-in-nature." They are, in effect, syndromes in which the body's "calciostat" has been reset upward or downward, respectively, thereby producing predictable alterations in the regulation of parathyroid and kidney by Ca^{2+}_o. The lack of obvious symptoms of hypercalcemia in most patients with FHH supports the idea that not only the regulation of parathyroid and renal function by Ca^{2+}_o but also many of the other symptoms of hypercalcemia are mediated by the CaR. Conversely, it is clear that individuals with activating mutations can exhibit classical symptoms of hypocalcemia; therefore, neuromuscular manifestations, such as seizures and tetany, are presumably, at least in part, CaR-independent. Much more remains to be learned, however, about the CaR's role in the brain and in other parts of the body, where in many cases it likely responds to local rather than systemic changes in Ca^{2+}_o. Further studies of humans with mutations in the CaR as well as of mice with targeted disruption of the CaR and of tissues derived from these mice should provide additional insights into the range of cellular functions that are controlled by the CaR both in systemic and in local ionic homeostasis as well as in tissues where this receptor plays roles unrelated to fluid and electrolyte metabolism.

The development of therapeutic agents that stimulate or inhibit the CaR has substantial potential clinical utility for treating conditions in which the receptor is under- or overactive, respectively. For example, clinical trials are currently in progress on the efficacy of "calcimimetic" CaR agonists for the medical therapy of primary and secondary hyperparathyroidism *(137,138)*. Based on clinical clues provided by inherited disorders of Ca^{2+}_o-sensing, there are several settings where CaR antagonists, so-called "calcilytics," would be of clinical utility. If such agents increased the set-point of the parathyroid and kidney in a manner reciprocal to the decrease in set-point produced by the calcimimetics, calcilytics would represent an effective means of "resetting" the parathyroid and kidney in individuals with activating mutations. Thus it should be possible by this means to raise the level of Ca^{2+}_o in those individuals who experience complications of hypocalcemia (i.e., seizures) without, presumably, incurring undue hypercalciuria. Similarly, in view of the markedly enhanced renal tubular reabsorption of calcium in FHH, a calcilytic with specificity for the kidney as opposed to the parathyroid could represent an effective form of treatment for renal stones caused by hypercalciuria. Finally, there may well be further receptors for Ca^{2+}_o *(139–143)*, perhaps encoded by the additional genetic loci associated with the clinical and biochemical picture of FHH, or, for that matter, for other ions (indeed, the CaR likely acts as a physiologically relevant Mg^{2+}_o receptor).

Acknowledgments

The author gratefully acknowledges generous grant support provided by the following sources: the USPHS (DK41415, 44588, 46422, 48330 and 52005), the St. Giles Foundation and NPS Pharmaceuticals, Inc., Salt Lake City, UT.

References

1. Chattopadhyay, N. and Brown, E. M. (1997) Calcium-sensing receptor: roles in and beyond systemic calcium homeostasis. *Biol. Chem.* **378,** 759–768.
2. Hebert, S. C., Brown, E. M., and Harris, H. W. (1997) Role of the Ca^{2+}-sensing Receptor in divalent mineral ion homeostasis. *J. Exp. Biol.* **200,** 295–302.
3. Pietrobon, D., Di Virgilio, F., and Pozzan, T. (1990) Structural and functional aspects of calcium homeostasis in eukaryotic cells. *Eur. J. Biochem.* **120,** 599–622.
3a. Brown, E. M., Pollak, M., and Hebert, S. C. (1994) Cloning and characterization of extracellular Ca^{2+}-sensing receptors from parathyroid and kidney: molecular physiology and pathophysiology of Ca^{2+}-sensing. *Endocrinologist* **4,** 419-426.
4. Brown, E. M. (1991) Extracellular Ca^{2+} sensing, regulation of parathyroid cell function, and role of Ca^{2+} and other ions as extracellular (first) messengers. *Physiol. Rev.* **71,** 371–411.
5. Parfitt, A. M. (1987) Bone and plasma calcium homeostasis. *Bone* **8(Suppl. 1),** 1–8.
6. Kurokawa, K. (1994) The kidney and calcium homeostasis. *Kidney Int.* **45(Suppl. 44),** S97–S105.
7. Kifor, O., Kifor, I., and Brown, E. M. (1992) Effects of high extracellular calcium concentrations on phosphoinositide turnover and inositol phosphate metabolism in dispersed bovine parathyroid cells. *J. Bone Miner. Res.* **7,** 1327–1335.
8. Shoback, D., Membreno, L. A., and McGhee, J. (1988) High calcium and other divalent cations in increase inositol trisphosphate in bovine parathyroid cells. *Endocrinology* **123,** 382–389.
9. Nemeth, E., Wallace, J., and Scarpa, A. (1986) Stimulus–secretion coupling in bovine parathyroid cells. Dissociation between secretion and net changes in cytosolic Ca^{++}. *J. Biol. Chem.* **261,** 2668–2674.
10. Chen, C., Barnett, J., Congo, D., and Brown, E. (1989) Divalent cations suppress 3',5'-adenosine monophosphate accumulation by stimulating a pertussis toxin–sensitive guanine nucleotide-binding protein in cultured bovine parathyroid cells. *Endocrinology* **124,** 233–239.
11. Chen, T., Pratt, S., and Shoback, D. (1994) Injection of bovine parathyroid poly(A)$^+$ RNA into Xenopus oocytes confers sensitivity to high extracellular calcium. *J. Bone Miner. Res.* **9,** 293–300.
12. Racke, F., Hammerland, L., Dubyak, G., and Nemeth, E. (1993) Functional expression of the parathyroid cell calcium receptor in Xenopus oocytes. *FEBS Lett.* **333,** 132–136.
13. Brown, E., Gamba, G., Riccardi, D., Lombardi, D., Butters, R., Kifor, O., et al. (1993) Cloning and characterization of an extracellular Ca^{2+}-sensing receptor from bovine parathyroid. *Nature* **366,** 575–580.
14. Garrett, J. E., Capuano, I. V., Hammerland, L. G., Hung, B. C. P., Brown, E. M., Hebert, S. C., et al. (1995) Molecular cloning and functional expression of human parathyroid calcium receptor cDNAs. *J. Biol. Chem.* **270,** 12,919–12,925.

14a. Brown, E. M., Bai, M., and Pollak, M. (1997) Familial benign hypocalciuric hypercalcemia and other syndromes of altered responsiveness to extracellular calcium, in *Metabolic Bone Diseases*, 3rd ed. (Krane, S. M. and Avioli, L. V. eds.) Academic Press, San Diego, CA, pp. 479-499.
15. Diaz, R., Hurwitz, S., Chattopadhyay, N., Pines, M., Yang, Y., Kifor, O., et al. (1997) Cloning, expression and tissue localization of the calcium-sensing receptor in the chicken (Gallus domesticus). *Am. J. Physiol.* **273,** R1008–R1016.
16. Aida, K., Koishi, S., Tawata, M., and Onaya, T. (1995) Molecular cloning of a putative Ca^{2+}-sensing receptor cDNA from human kidney. *Biochem. Biophys. Res. Commun.* **214,** 524–529.
17. Riccardi, D., Park, J., Lee, W.-S., Gamba, G., Brown, E. M., and Hebert, S. C. (1995) Cloning and functional expression of a rat kidney extracellular calcium/polyvalent cation-sensing receptor. *Proc. Natl. Acad. Sci. USA* **92,** 131–135.
18. Butters, R. R. Jr.,Chattopadhyay, N., Nielsen, P., Smith, C. P., Mithal, A., Kifor, O., et al. (1997) Cloning and characterization of a calcium–sensing receptor from the hypercalcemic New Zealand white rabbit reveals unaltered responsiveness to extracellular calcium. *J. Bone Miner. Res.* **12,** 568–579.
19. Freichel, M., Zinc-Lorenz, A., Hollishi, A., Hafner, M., Flockerzi, V., and Raue, F. (1996) Expression of a calcium-sensing receptor in a human medullary thyroid carcinoma cell line and its contribution to calcitonin secretion. *Endocrinology* **137,** 3842–3848.
20. Garrett, J. E., Tamir, H., Kifor, O., Simin, R. T., Rogers, K. V., Mithal, A., Gagel, R. F., and Brown, E. M. (1995) Calcitonin-secreting cells of the thyroid express an extracellular calcium receptor gene. *Endocrinology* **136,** 5202–5211.
21. Ruat, M., Molliver, M. E., Snowman, A. M., and Snyder, S. H. (1995) Calcium sensing receptor: molecular cloning in rat and localization to nerve terminals. *Proc. Natl. Acad. Sci. USA* **92,** 3161–3165.
22. Strewler, G. J. (1994) Familial hypocalciuric hypercalcemia—from the clinic to the calcium sensor. *West. J. Med.* **160,** 579–580.
23. Quinn, S. J., Ye, C. P., Diaz, R., Kifor, O., Bai, M., Vassilev, P. and Brown, E. M. (1997) The calcium-sensing receptor: a target for polyamines. *Am. J. Physiol.* **273,** C1315–C1323.
24. Nemeth, E. F., (1996) Calcium receptors as novel drug targets, in *Principles of Bone Biology*, 1st ed. (Bilezikian, J. P., Raisz, L. G., and Rodan, G. A., eds.), Academic Press, San Diego, CA, pp. 1019–1035.
25. Kaupmann, K., Huggel, K., Heid, J., Flor, P. J., Bischoff, S., Kickel, S. J., et al. (1997) Expression cloning of GABAB receptors uncovers similarity to metabotropic glutamate receptor. *Nature* **386,** 239–246.
26. Ryba, N. J. P. and Trindell, R. (1997) A new multigene family of putative pheromone receptors. *Neuron* **19,** 371–379.
27. Matsunami, H. and Buck, L. B. (1997) A multigene family encoding a diverse array of putative pheromone receptors in mammals. *Cell* **90,** 775–784.
28. O'Hara, P., Sheppard, P., Thogersen, H., Venezia, D., et al. (1993) The ligand binding domain in metabotropic glutamate receptors is related to bacterial periplasmic binding proteins. *Neuron* **11,** 41–52.
29. Conklin, B. and Bourne, H. (1994) Marriage of the flytrap and the serpent. *Nature* **367,** 22.

30. Sharff, A. J., Rodseth, L. E., Spurlino, J. C., and Quiocho, F. A. (1992) Crystallographic evidence for a large ligand-induced hinge-twist motion between the two domains of the maltodextrin binding protein involved in active transport and chemotaxis. *Biochemistry* **31,** 10,657–10,663.
31. Tam, R. and Saier, M. H., Jr. (1993) Structural, functional, and evolutionary relationships among extracellular solute-binding receptors of bacteria. *Microbiol. Rev.* **57,** 320–346.
32. Varrault, A., Pena, M. S., Goldsmith, P. K., Mithal, A., Brown, E. M., and Spiegel, A. M. (1995) Expression of G protein alpha subunits in bovine parathyroid. *Endocrinology* **136,** 4390–4396.
33. Chang, W. Pratt, S., Chen, T. H., Nemeth, E., Huang, Z., and Shoback, D. M. (1998) Coupling of calcium receptors to inositol phosphate and cyclic AMP generation in mammalian cells and *Xenopus laevis* oocytes and immunidiction of receptor protein by region-specific anticipated antisera. *J. Bone Miner. Res.* **13,** 578–580.
34. Kifor, O., Diaz, R., Butters, R., and Brown, E. M. (1997) The Ca^{2+}-sensing receptor activates phospholipases C, A_2, and D by high extracellular Ca^{2+} in bovine parathyroid and CaR-transfected, human embryonic kidney (HEK293) cells. *J. Bone Miner. Res.* **12,** 715–725.
35. Ruat, M., Snowman, A. M., Hester, L. D., and Snyder, S. H. (1996) Cloned and expressed rat Ca^{2+}-sensing receptor. *J. Biol. Chem.* **271,** 5972–5976.
36. McNeill, S. E., Hobson, S. A., Nipper, K. D., and Rodland, K. D. (1998) Functional calcium-sensing receptors in rat fibroblasts are required for activation of SRC kinase and mitogen-activated protein kinase in response to extracellular calcium. *J. Biol. Chem.* **273,** 1114–1120.
37. Nakanishi, S. (1994) Metabotropic glutamate receptors: synaptic transmission, modulation and plasticity. *Neuron* **13,** 1031–1037.
38. Ray, J. M., Squires, P. E., Curtis, S. B., Meloche, M. R., and Buchan, A. M. J. (1997) Expression of the calcium-sensing receptor on human antral gastrin cells. *J. Clin. Invest.* **99,** 2328–2333.
39. Chattopadhyay, N., Cheng, I., Rogers, K., Riccardi, D., Hall, A., Diaz, R., Hebert, S. C., Soybel, D. I., and Brown, E. M. (1998) Identification and localization of extracellular Ca^{2+}-sensing receptor in rat intestine. *Am. J. Physiol.* **274,** G122–G130.
40. Rogers, K. V., Dunn, C. E., Brown, E. M., and Hebert, S. C. (1997) Localization of calcium receptor mRNA in the adult rat central nervous system by *in situ* hybridization. *Brain Res.* **744,** 47–56.
41. Chattopadhyay, N., Ye, C., Singh, D. P., Kifor, O., Vassilev, P. M., Sinohara, T., et al. (1997) Expression of extracellular calcium-sensing receptor by human lens epithelial cells. *Biochem. Biophys. Res. Commun.* **233,** 801–805.
42. House, M. G., Kohlmeier, L., Chattopadhyay, N., Kifor, O., LeBoff, M. S., Glowacki, J., and Brown, E. M. (1997) Expression of an extracellular calcium-sensing receptor in human and mouse bone marrow cells. *J. Bone Miner. Res.* **12,** 1959–1970.
43. Riccardi, D., Lee, W.-S., Lee, K., Segre, G. V., Brown, E. M., and Hebert, S. C. (1996) Localization of the extracellular Ca^{2+}-sensing receptor and PTH/PTHrP receptor in rat kidney. *Am. J. Physiol.* **271,** F951–F956.
44. Yang, T., Hassan, S., Huang, Y. G., Smart, A. M., Briggs, J. P., and Schnermann, J. B. (1997) Expression of PTHrP, PTH/PTHrP receptor, and Ca^{2+}-sensing receptor mRNAs along the rat nephron. *Am. J. Physiol.* **272,** F751–F758.

45. Marx, S., Lasker, R., Brown, E., Fitzpatrick, L., Sweezey, N., Goldbloom, R., et al. (1986) Secretory dysfunction in parathyroid cells from a neonate with severe primary hyperparathyroidism. *J. Clin. Endocrinol. Metab.* **62,** 445–449.
46. Cooper, L., Wertheimer, J., Levey, R., Brown, E., LeBoff, M., Wilkinson, R., and Anast, C. (1986) Severe primary hyperparathyroidism in a neonate with two hypercalcemic parents: management with parathyroidectomy and heterotopic autotransplantation. *Pediatrics* **78,** 263–268.
47. Ho, C., Conner, D. A., Pollak, M., Ladd, D. J., Kifor, O., Warren, H., et al. (1995) A mouse model for familial hypocalciuric hypercalcemia and neonatal severe hyperparathyroidism. *Nat. Genet.* **11,** 389–394.
48. Garrett, J. E., Steffey, M. E., and Nemeth, E. F. (1995) The calcium receptor agonist R–568 suppresses PTH mRNA in cultured bovine parathyroid cells. *J. Bone Miner. Res.* **10(Suppl 1),** 387(Abstract).
49. Randall, C. and Lauchlan, S. C. (1963) Parathyroid hyperplasia in an infant. *Am. J. Dis. Child.* **105,** 364–367.
50. Spiegel, A. M., Harrison, H. E., Marx, S. J., Brown, E. M., and Aurbach, G. D. (1977) Neonatal primary hyperparathyroidism with autosomal dominant inheritance. *J. Pediatr.* **90,** 269–272.
51. McGehee, D. S., Aldersberg, M., Liu, K.-P., Hsuing, S.-C., Heath, M. J. S., and Tamir, H. (1997) Mechanism of extracellular Ca^{2+} receptor–stimulated hormone release from sheep thyroid parafollicular cells. *J. Physiol.* **502,** 31–44.
52. Emanuel, R. L., Adler, G. K., Kifor, O., Quinn, S. Q., Fuller, F., Krapcho, K., and Brown, E. M. (1996) Ca^{2+}-sensing receptor expression and regulation by extracellular calcium in the AtT-20 pituitary cell line. *Mol. Endocrinol.* **10,** 555–565.
53. Riccardi, D., Hall, A. E., Chattopadhyay, N., Xu, J., Brown, E. M., and Hebert, S. C. (1998) Localization of the extracellular Ca^{2+}/(polyvalent cation)-sensing receptor protein in rat kidney. *Am. J. Physiol.* **274,** F611–F620.
54. Brown, E. and Hebert, S. (1995) A cloned Ca^{2+}-sensing receptor: A mediator of direct effects of extracellular Ca^{2+} on renal function? *J. Am. Soc. Nephrol.* **6,** 1530–1540.
55. Chabardes, D., Imbert, M., Clique, A., Montegut, M., and Morel, F. (1975) PTH-sensitive adenyl cyclase activity in different segments of the rabbit nephron. *Pflugers Arch.* **354,** 229–239.
56. Champignuelle, A., Siga, E., Vassent, G., and Imbert-Teboul, M. (1997) Relationship between extra- and intracellular calcium in distal segments of the renal tubule. Role of the Ca^{2+} receptor RaKCaR. *J. Membr. Biol.* **156,** 117–129.
57. Sands, J. M., Naruse, M., Baum, M., Jo, I., Hebert, S. C., Brown, E. M., and Harris, W. H. (1997) Apical extracellular calcium/polyvalent cation-sensing receptor regulates vasopressin-elicited water permeability in rat kidney inner medullary collecting duct. *J. Clin. Invest.* **99,** 1399–1405.
58. Suki, W. M., Eknoyan, G., Rector, F. C. Jr., and Seldin, D. W. (1969) The renal diluting and concentrating mechanism in hypercalcemia. *Nephron* **6,** 50–61.
59. Foley, T. Jr., Harrison, H., Arnaud, C., and Harrison, H. (1972) Familial benign hypercalcemia. *J. Pediatr.* **81,** 1060–1067.
60. Marx, S., Spiegel, A., Brown, E., Koehler, J., Gardner, D., Brennan, M., and Aurbach, G. (1978) Divalent cation metabolism. Familial hypocalciuric hypercalcemia versus typical primary hyperparathyroidism. *Am. J. Med.* **65,** 235–242.
61. Marx, S. J., Attie, M. F., Levine, M. A., Spiegel, A. M., Downs, R. W. Jr., and Lasker, R. D. (1981) The hypocalciuric or benign variant of familial hypercalce-

mia: clinical and biochemical features in fifteen kindreds. *Medicine (Baltimore)* **60,** 397–412.
62. Law, W. M. Jr. and Heath, H. III (1985) Familial benign hypercalcemia (hypocalciuric hypercalcemia). Clinical and pathogenetic studies in 21 families. *Ann. Int. Med.* **105,** 511–519.
63. Aida, K., Koishi, S., Inoue, M., Nakazato, M., Tawata, M., and Onaya, T. (1995) Familial hypocalciuric hypercalcemia associated with mutation in the human Ca^{2+}-sensing receptor gene. *J. Clin. Endocrinol. Metab.* **80,** 2594–2598.
64. Bai, M., Quinn, S., Trivedi, S., Kifor, O., Pearce, S. H. S., Pollak, M. R., Krapcho, K., et al. (1996) Expression and characterization of inactivating and activating mutations of the human Ca^{2+}_{o}-sensing receptor. *J. Biol. Chem.* **271,** 19,537–19,545.
65. Bai, M., Pearce, S. H. S., Kifor, O., Trivedi, S., Stauffer, U. G., Thakker, R. V., et al. (1997) In vivo and in vitro characterization of neonatal hyperparathyroidism resulting from a de novo, heterozygous mutation in the Ca^{2+}-sensing receptor gene: Normal maternal calcium homeostasis as a cause of secondary hyperparathyroidism in familial benign hypocalciuric hypercalcemia. *J. Clin. Invest.* **99,** 88–96.
66. Aurbach, G. D., Marx, S. J., and Spiegel, A. M. (1985) Parathyroid hormone, calcitonin, and the calciferols, in *Textbook of Endocrinology,* 7th ed. (Wilson, J. D., and Foster, D. W., eds.), Saunders, Philadelphia, PA, pp. 1137–1217.
67. Stewart, A. F. and Broadus, A. E. (1987) Mineral Metabolism, in *Endocrinology and Metabolism,* 2nd ed. (Felig, P., Baxter, J. D., Broadus, A. E., and Frohman, L. A., eds.), McGraw-Hill, New York, pp. 1317–1453.
68. Heath, D. A. (1994) Familial hypocalciuric hypercalcemia, in: *The Parathyroids,* (Bilezikian, J. P., Marcus, R., and Levine, M. A., eds), Raven Press, New York, NY. pp. 699–710.
69. Gunn, I. and Wallace, J. (1992) Urine calcium and serum ionized calcium, total calcium and parathyroid hormone concentrations in the diagnosis of primary hyperparathyroidism and familial benign hypercalcaemia. *Ann. Clin. Biochem.* **29,** 52–58.
70. Chou, Y.-H., Brown, E., Levi, T., Crowe, G., Atkinson, A., Arnqvist, H., Toss, G., Fuleihan, G., Seidman, J., and Seidman, C. (1992) The gene responsible for familial hypocalciuric hypercalcemia maps to chromosome 3q in four unrelated families. *Nature Genet.* **1,** 295–300.
71. Heath, D. (1989) Familial benign hypercalcemia. *Trends Endocrinol. Metab.* **1,** 6–9.
72. Auwerx, J., Demedts, M., and Bouillon, R. (1984) Altered parathyroid set point to calcium in familial hypocalciuric hypercalcaemia. *Acta Endocrinologica (Copenh.)* **106,** 215–218.
73. Khosla, S., Ebeling, P. R., Firek, A. F., Burritt, M. M., Kao, P. C., and Heath, H., III. (1993) Calcium infusion suggests a "set-point" abnormality of parathyroid gland function in familial benign hypercalcemia and more complex disturbances in primary hyperparathyroidism. *J. Clin. Endocrinol. Metab.* **76,** 715–720.
74. Brown, E. (1983) Four parameter model of the sigmoidal relationship between parathyroid hormone release and extracellular calcium concentration in normal and abnormal parathyroid tissue. *J. Clin. Endocrinol. Metab.* **56,** 572–581.
75. Law, W. M. Jr., Carney, J. A., and Heath, H., III. (1984) Parathyroid glands in familial benign hypercalcemia (familial hypocalciuric hypercalcemia). *Am. J. Med.* **76,** 1021–1026.

76. Thogeirsson, U., Costa, J., and Marx, S. J. (1981) The parathyroid glands in familial hypocalciuric hypercalcemia. *Hum. Pathol.* **12,** 229–237.
77. Davies, M., Adams, P. H., Lumb, G. A., Berry, J. L., and Loveridge, N. (1984) Familial hypocalciuric hypercalcemia: evidence for continued enhanced renal tubular reabsorption of calcium following total parathyroidectomy. *Acta Endocrinol.* **106,** 499–504.
78. Kristiansen, J. H., Rodbro, P., Christiansen, C., Brochner Mortensen, J., and Carl, J. (1985) Familial hypocalciuric hypercalcemia II: Intestinal calcium absorption and vitamin D metabolism. *Clin. Endocrinol.* **23,** 511–515.
79. Law, W. M. Jr., Bollman, S., Kumar, R., and Heath, H. III. (1984) Vitamin D metabolism in familial benign hypercalcemia (hypocalciuric hypercalcemia) differs from that in primary hyperparathyroidism. *J. Clin. Endocrinol. Metab.* **58,** 744–747.
80. Kristiansen, J. H., Rodbro, P., Christiansen, C., Johansen, J., and Jensen. J. T. (1987) Familial hypocalciuric hypercalcemia. III: Bone mineral metabolism. *Clin. Endocrinol. (Oxford)* **26,** 713–716.
81. Menko, F. H., Bijouvet, O. L. M., Fronen, J. L. H. H. et al. (1983) Familial benign hypercalcemia: study of a large family. *Q. J. Med.* **206,** 120–140.
82. Abugassa, S., Nordenstrom, J., and Jarhult, J. (1992) Bone mineral density in patients with familial hypocalciuric hypercalcemia (FHH). *Eur. J. Surg.* **158,** 397–402.
83. McMurtry, C., Schranck, F., Walkenhorst, D., Murphy, W., Kocher, D., Teitelbaum, S., Rupich, R., and Whyte, M. (1992) Significant developmental elevation in serum parathyroid hormone levels in a large kindred with familial benign (hypocalciuric) hypercalcemia. *Am. J. Med.* **93,** 247–258.
84. Pasieka, J. L., Andersen, M. A., and Hanley, D. A. (1990) Familial benign hypercalcemia: hypercalciuria and hypocalciuria in affected members of a small kindred. *Clin. Endocrinol.* **33,** 429–433.
85. Attie, M. F., Gill, J., Jr., Stock, J. L., Spiegel, A. M., Downs, R. W., Jr., Levine, M. A., and Marx, S. J. (1983) Urinary calcium excretion in familial hypocalciuric hypercalcemia. Persistence of relative hypocalciuria after induction of hypoparathyroidism. *J. Clin. Invest.* **72,** 667–676.
86. Marx, S. J., Attie, M. F., Stock, J. L., Spiegel, A. M., and Levine, M. A. (1981) Maximal urine-concentrating ability: familial hypocalciuric hypercalcemia versus typical primary hyperparathyroidism. *J. Clin. Endocrinol. Metab.* **52,** 736–740.
87. Pollak, M., Chou, Y. H., Marx, S. J., Steinmann, B., Cole, D. E. C., Brandi, M. L., et al. (1994) Familial hypocalciuric hypercalcemia and neonatal severe hyperparathyroidism. effects of mutant gene dosage on phenotype. *J. Clin. Invest.* **93,** 1108–1112.
88. Heath, H., Jackson, C., Otterud, B., and Leppert, M. (1993) Genetic linkage analysis of familial benign (hypocalciuric) hypercalcemia: evidence for locus heterogeneity. *Am. J. Hum. Genet.* **53,** 193–200.
89. Pearce, S., Trump, D., Wooding, C., Besser, G., Chew, S., Heath, D., Hughes, I., and Thakker, R. (1995) Calcium-sensing receptor mutations in familial benign hypercalcaemia and neonatal hyperparathyroidism. *J. Clin. Invest.* **96,** 2683–2692.
89a. Lloyd, S. E., Dannett, A. A., Dixon, P. H., Whyte, M. P., and Thakker, R. V. (1999) Localization of falmilial benign hypercalcemia, Oklahoma variant (FBHOK), to chromosome 19q13. *Am. J. Hum. Genet.* **64,** 189–195.
90. Trump, D., Whyte, M. P., Wooding, C., Pang, J. T., Pearce, S. H. S., Kocher, D. B., and Thakker, R. V. (1995) Linkage studies in a kindred from Oklahoma, with famil-

ial benign (hypocalciuric) hypercalcaemia (FBH) and developmental elevations in serum parathyroid hormone levels, indicate a third locus for FBH. *Hum. Genet.* **96,** 183–187.

91. Marx, S. J., Fraser, D., and Rapoport, A. (1985) Familial hypocalciuric hypercalcemia. Mild expression of the gene in heterozygotes and severe expression in homozygotes. *Am. J. Med.* **78,** 15–22.
92. Pollak, M., Brown, E. M., Chou, Y. H., Hebert, S. C., Marx, S. J., Steinmann, B., et al. (1993) Mutations in the human Ca^{2+}-sensing receptor gene cause familial hypocalciuric hypercalcemia and neonatal severe hyperparathyroidism. *Cell* **75,** 1297–1303.
93. Chou, Y.-H., Pollak, M., Brandi, M., Toss, G., Arnqvist, H., Atkinson, A., et al. (1995) Mutations in the human Ca^{2+}-sensing receptor gene that cause familial hypocalciuric hypercalcemia. *Am. J. Hum. Genet.* **56,** 1075–1079.
94. Heath, H. I., Odelberg, S., Jackson, C. E., Teh, B. T., Hayward, N., Larsson, C., et al. (1996) Clustered inactivating mutations and benign polymorphisms of the calcium receptor gene in familial benign hypocalciuric hypercalcemia suggest receptor functional domains. *J. Clin. Endocrinol. Metab.* **81,** 1312–1317.
95. Janicic, N., Pausova, Z., Cole, D. E. C., and Hendy, G. N. (1995) Insertion of an Alu sequence in the Ca^{2+}-sensing receptor gene in familial hypocalciuric hypercalcemia and neonatal severe hyperparathyroidism. *Am. J. Hum. Genet.* **56,** 880–886.
96. Kobayashi, M., Tanaka, H., Tsuzuki, K., Tsuyuki, M., Igaki, H., Ichinose, Y., et al. (1997) Two novel missense mutations in calcium-sensing receptor gene associated with neonatal severe hyperparathyroidism. *J. Clin. Endocrinol. Metab.* **82,** 2716–2719.
97. Janicic, N., Pausova, Z., Cole, D. E. C., and Hendy, G. N. (1995) De novo expansion of an Alu insertion mutation of the Ca^{2+}-sensing receptor gene in familial hypocalciuric hypercalcemia and neonatal severe hyperparathyroidism. *J. Bone Miner. Res.* **10(Suppl. 1),** S191.
98. Pearce, S. H. S., Bai, M., Quinn, S. J., Kifor, O., Brown, E. M., and Thakker, R. V. (1996) Functional characterization of calcium-sensing receptor mutations expressed in human embryonic kidney cells. *J. Clin. Invest.* **98,** 1860–1866.
99. Bai, M., Janicic, N., Trivedi, S., Quinn, S. J., Cole, D. E. C., Brown, E. M., and Hendy, G. N. (1997) Markedly reduced activity of mutant calcium–sensing receptor with an inserted Alu element from a kindred with familial hypocalciuric hypercalcemia and neonatal severe hyperparathyroidism. *J. Clin. Invest.* **99,** 1917–1925.
100. Bockaert, J. (1991) G proteins, G protein-coupled receptors: structure, function and interactions. *Curr. Opin. Neurobiol.* **1,** 32–42.
101. Jackson, T. (1991) Structure and function of G protein coupled receptors. *Pharmacol. Ther.* **50,** 425–442.
102. Pin, J.-P., Gomeza, T., Joly, C., and Bockaert, J. (1994) The metabotropic glutamate receptors: their second intracellular loop plays a critical role in the G-protein coupling specificity. *Biochem. Soc. Trans.* **23,** 910–996.
103. Landon, J. F. (1932) Parathyroidectomy in generalized osteitis fibrosa cystica. *J. Pediatr.* **1,** 544–560.
104. Eftekhari, F. and Yousefzadeh, D. (1982) Primary infantile hyperparathyroidism: clinical, laboratory, and radiographic features in 21 cases. *Skeletal Radiol.* **8,** 201–208.

105. Gaudelus, J., Dandine, M., Nathanson, M., Perelman, R., and Hassan, M. (1983) Rib cage deformity in neonatal hyperparathyroidism [letter]. *Am. J. Dis. Child.* **137,** 408–409.
106. Marx, S., Attie, M., Spiegel, A., Levine, M., Lasker, R., and Fox, M. (1982) An association between neonatal severe primary hyperparathyroidism and familial hypocalciuric hypercalcemia in three kindreds. *N Engl. J. Med.* **306,** 257–284.
107. Steinmann, B., Gnehm, H. E., Rao, V. H., Kind, H. P., and Prader, A. (1984) Neonatal severe primary hyperparathyroidism and alkaptonuria in a boy born to related parents with familial hypocalciuric hypercalcemia. *Helv. Paediatr. Acta* **39,** 171–186.
108. Mallette, L. A. (1994) The functional and pathologic spectrum of parathyroid abnormalities in hyperparathyroidism, in *The Parathyroids* (Bilezikian, J. P., Marcus, R., and Levine, M. A., eds.), Raven Press, New York, pp. 423–455.
109. Fujimoto, Y., Hazama, H., and Oku, K. (1990) Severe primary hyperparathyroidism in a neonate having a parent with hypercalcemia: treatment by total parathyroidectomy and simultaneous heterotopic autotransplantation. *Surgery* **108,** 933–938.
110. Grantmyre, E. (1973) Roentgenographic features of "primary" hyperparathyroidism in infancy. *J. Can. Assoc. Radiol.* **24,** 257–260.
111. Fujita, T., Watanabe, N., Fukase, M., Tsutsumi, M., Fukami, T., Imai, Y. et al. (1983) Familial hypocalciuric hypercalcemia involving four members of a kindred including a girl with severe neonatal primary hyperparathyroidism. *Miner. Electr. Metab.* **9,** 51–54.
112. Matsuo, M., Okita, K., Takemine, H., and Fujita, T. (1982) Neonatal primary hyperparathyroidism in familial hypocalciuric hypercalcemia. *Am. J. Dis. Child.* **136,** 728–731.
113. Page, L. and Haddow, J. (1987) Self–limited neonatal hyperparathyroidism in familial hypocalciuric hypercalcemia. *J. Pediatr.* **111,** 261–264.
114. Harris, S. S. and D'Ercole, A. J. (1989) Neonatal hyperparathyroidism: the natural course in the absence of surgical intervention. *Pediatrics* **83,** 53–56.
115. Hosokawa, Y., Pollak, M. R., Brown, E. M., and Arnold, A. (1995) Mutational analysis of the extracellular Ca^{2+}-sensing receptor gene in human parathyroid tumors. *J. Clin. Endocrinol. Metab.* **80,** 3107–3110.
116. Kifor, O., Moore, F. D. Jr. Wang, P., Goldstein, M., Vassilev, P., Kifor, I., Hebert, S. C., and Brown, E. M. (1996) Reduced Immunostaining for the Extracellular Ca^{2+}-Sensing Receptor in Primary and Uremic Secondary Hyperparathyroidism. *J. Clin. Endocrinol. Metab.* **81,** 1598–1606.
117. Gogusev, J., Duchambon, P., Hory, B., Giovannini, M., Goureau, Y., Sarfati, E., and Drueke, T. (1997) Depressed expression of calcium receptor in parathyroid gland tissue of patients with hyperparathyroidism. *Kidney Int.* **51,** 328–336.
118. Eastell, R. and Heath, H. III (1992) The hypocalcemic states: their differential diagnosis and management, in *Disorders of Bone Metabolism* (Coe, F. and Favus, M., eds.), Raven Press, New York, pp. 571–585.
119. Ahn, T. J., Antonarakis, S. E., Kronenberg, H. M., Igarashi, T., and Levine, M. A. (1986) Familial isolated hypoparathyroidism: a molecular genetic analysis of 8 families with 23 affected persons. *Medicine (Baltimore)* **65,** 573–81.
120. Arnold, A., Horst, S. A., Gardella, T. J., Baba, H., Levine, M. A., and Kronenberg, H. M. (1990) Mutation of the signal peptide-encoding region of the preproparathyroid hormone gene in familial isolated hypoparathyroidism. *J. Clin. Invest.* **86,** 1084–1087.

121. Parkinson, D. B. and Thakker, R. V. (1992) A donor splice site mutation in the parathyroid hormone gene is associated with autosomal recessive hypoparathyroidism. *Nat. Genet.* **1,** 149–153.
122. Spiegel, A. M. (1996) Mutations in G protein and G protein-coupled receptors in endocrine disease. *J. Clin. Endocrinol. Metab.* **81,** 2434–2442.
123. Parma, J., Van Sande, J., Swillens, S., Tonacchera, M., Dumont, J., and Vassart, G. (1995) Somatic mutations causing constitutive activity of the thyrotropin receptor are a major cause of hyperfunctioning thyroid adenomas: Identification of additional mutations activating both the cyclic adenosine 3',5'-monophosphate and inositol phosphate–Ca^{2+} cascades. *Mol. Endocrinol.* **9,** 725–733.
124. Lefkowitz, R. J. and Premont, R. T. (1993) Diseased G protein-coupled receptors. *J. Clin. Invest.* **92,** 2089.
125. Coughlin, S. (1994) Expanding horizons for receptors coupled to G proteins: diversity and disease. *Curr. Opin. Cell. Biol.* **6,** 191–197.
126. Baron, J., Winer, K. K., Yanovski, J. A., Cunningham, A. W., Laue, L., Zimmerman, D., and Cutler, G. B. Jr. (1996) Mutations in the Ca^{2+}-sensing receptor gene cause autosomal dominant and sporadic hypoparathyroidism. *Human Mol. Genet.* **5,** 601–606.
127. De Luca, F., Ray, K., Mancilla, E. E., Fan, G.-F., Winer, K. K., Gore, P., et al. (1997) Sporadic hypoparathyroidism caused by *de novo* gain-of-function mutations in the Ca^{2+}-sensing receptor. *J. Clin. Endocrinol. Metab.* **82,** 2710–2715.
128. Lovlie, R., Eiken, H. G., and Sorheim, H. (1996) The Ca^{2+}–sensing receptor gene (PCAR1) mutation T151M in isolated autosomal dominant hypoparathyroidism. *Hum. Genet.* **98,** 129–133.
129. Mancilla, E. E., De Luca, F., Ray, K., Winer, K. K., Fan, G.-F., and Baron, J. (1997) A Ca^{2+}-sensing receptor mutation causes hypoparathyroidism by increasing receptor sensitivity to Ca^{2+} and maximal signal transduction. *Pediatr. Res.* **42,** 443–447.
130. Pearce, S. H. S., Williamson, C., Kifor, O., Bai, M., Coulthard, M. G., Davies, M., et al. (1996) A familial syndrome of hypocalcemia with hypercalciuria due to mutations in the calcium-sensing receptor. *N. Engl. J. Med.* **335,** 1115–1122.
131. Pollak, M., Brown, E., Estep, H., McLaine, P., Kifor, O., Park, J., et al. (1994) Autosomal dominant hypocalcaemia caused by Ca^{2+}-sensing receptor gene mutation. *Nat. Genet.* **8,** 303–307.
132. Davies, M., Mughal, Z., Selby, P., Tymms, D., and Mawer, E. (1995) Familial benign hypocalcemia. *J. Bone Miner. Res.* **10(Suppl. 1),** S507.
133. Estep, H., Mistry, Z., and Burke, P. (1981) Familial idiopathic hypocalcemia, in *Proceedings and Abstracts of the 63rd Annual Meeting of the Endocrine Society,* Cincinnati, OH; 275 (Abstract).
134. Finegold, D. N., Armitage, M. M., Galiani, M., Matise, T. C., Pandian, M. R., Perry, Y. M., et al. (1994) Preliminary localization of a gene for autosomal dominant hypoparathyroidism to chromosome 3q13. *Pediatr. Res.* **36,** 414–417.
135. Perry, Y. M., Finegold, D. M., Armitage, M. M., and Ferrell, R. E. (1994) A missense mutation in the Ca-sensing receptor causes familial autosomal dominant hypoparathyroidism. *Am. J. Hum. Genet.* **55(Suppl.),** A17(Abstract).

135a. Ward, D. T., Brown, E. M., and Harris, H. W. (1998) The extracellular calcium-polyvalent cation-sensing receptor exists as a putative disulfide-linked dimer altered by divalent cations in vitro. *J. Biol. Chem.* **273,** 14,476–14,483.

135b. Bai, M., Trivedi, S., and Brown, E. M. (1998) Dimerization of extracellular calcium (CA^{2+}_o)-sensing receptor on the cell surface of CaR-transfected HEK293 cells. *J. Biol. Chem.* **273,** 23,605–23,610.
136. Shenker, A., Laue, L., Kosugi, S., Merendino, J. J. Jr., Mineyshi, T., and Cutler, G. B. Jr. (1993) A constitutively activating mutation of the luteinizing hormone receptor in familial male precocious puberty. *Nature* **65,** 652–654.
137. Nemeth, E. F. (1995) Ca^{2+} receptor-dependent regulation of cellular functions. *News Physiol. Sci.* **10,** 1–5.
138. Silverberg, S. J., Bone, H. G. III., Marriott, T. B., Locker, F. G., Thys-Jacobs, S., Dziem, G., et al. (1997) Short-term inhibition of parathyroid hormone secretion by a calcium-receptor agonist in patients with primary hyperparathyroidism. *N. Engl. J. Med.* **337,** 1506–1510.
139. Hinson, T. K., Damodaran, T. V., Chen, J., Zhang, X., Qumsiyeh, M. B., Seldin, M. F., and Quarles, L. D. (1997) Identification of putative transmembrane receptor sequences homologous to the calcium-sensing G-protein-coupled receptor. *Genomics* **45,** 279–289.
140. Hjalm, G., Murray, E., Crumley, G., Harazim, W., Lundgren, S., Onyango, I., et al. (1996) Cloning and sequencing of human gp330, a Ca^{2+}-binding receptor with potential intracellular signaling properties. *Eur. J. Biochem.* **239,** 132–137.
141. Saito, A., Pietromonaco, S., Loo, A. K., and Farquhar, M. G. (1994) Complete cloning and sequencing of rat gp330/"megalin," a distinctive member of the low density lipoprotein receptor gene family. *Proc. Natl. Acad. Sci. USA* **91,** 9725–9729.
142. Zaidi, M., Shankar, V. S., Tunwell, R., Adebanjo, O. A., Mackrill, J., Pazianis, M., et al. (1995) A ryanodine receptor-like molecule expressed in the osteoclast plasma membrane functions in extracellular Ca^{2+} sensing. *J. Clin. Invest.* **96,** 1582–1590.
143. Malgaroli, A., Meldolesi, J., Zambone-Zallone, A., and Teti, A. (1989) Control of cytosolic free calcium in rat and chicken osteoclasts. The role of extracellular calcium and calcitonin. *J. Biol. Chem.* **264,** 14,342–14,349.

CHAPTER 14

Multiple Endocrine Neoplasia Type 1 (MEN1)

Rajesh V. Thakker

Introduction

Multiple endocrine neoplasia *(1–3)* is characterized by the occurrence of tumors involving two or more endocrine glands within a single patient. The disorder has previously been referred to as multiple endocrine adenopathy (MEA) or the pluriglandular syndrome. However, glandular hyperplasia and malignancy may also occur in some patients and the term multiple endocrine neoplasia (MEN) is now preferred. There are two major forms of multiple endocrine neoplasia referred to as type 1 and type 2 and each form is characterized by the development of tumors within specific endocrine glands (*see* Table 1). Thus, the combined occurrence of tumors of the parathyroid glands, the pancreatic islet cells, and the anterior pituitary is characteristic of multiple endocrine neoplasia type 1 (MEN1), which is also referred to as Wermer's syndrome. In addition to these tumors, adrenal cortical, carcinoid, facial angiofibromas, collagenomas, and lipomatous tumors have also been described in patients with MEN1 *(3,4)*. However, in multiple endocrine neoplasia type 2 (MEN2), which is also called Sipple's syndrome, medullary thyroid carcinoma (MTC) occurs in association with phaeochromocytoma, and three clinical variants referred to as MEN2a, MEN2b and MTC-only are recognized *(1,5)*. In MEN2a, which is the most common variant, the development of MTC is associated with phaeochromocytoma and parathyroid tumors. However, in MEN2b parathyroid involvement is absent and the occurrence of MTC and phaeochromocytoma is found in association with a marfanoid habitus mucosal neuromas, medullated corneal fibers and intestinal autonomic ganglion dysfunction leading to a megacolon. In the variant of MTC only, medullary thyroid carcinoma appears to be the sole manifestation of the syndrome. Although MEN1 and MEN2 usually occur as distinct and separate syndromes as outlined above, some patients occasionally may develop tumors that are associated with both

The Genetics of Osteoporosis and Metabolic Bone Disease
Ed.: M. J. Econs © Humana Press Inc., Totowa, NJ

Table 1
The Multiple Endocrine Neoplasia (MEN) Syndromes: Their Characteristic Tumors and Associated Genetic Abnormalities[a]

Type (chromosomal location)	Tumors	Gene: most frequently (%) mutated codons
MEN1	Parathyroids	MEN1:
(11q13)	Pancreatic islets	83/84, 4bp del (≈10%)
	Gastrinoma	209–211, 4bp del (≈10%)
	Insulinoma	514–516, del or ins (≈5%)
	Glucagonoma	
	VIPoma	
	PPoma	
	Pituitary (anterior)	
	Prolactinoma	
	Somatotrophinoma	
	Corticotrophinoma	
	Nonfunctioning	
	Associated tumors	
	Adrenal cortical	
	Carcinoid	
	Lipoma	
	Angiofibromas	
	Collagenomas	
MEN2		
(10 cen-10q.11.2)		
MEN2a	Medullary thyroid carcinoma (MTC)	ret: 634, missense, e.g., Cys(Arg (≈85%)
	Phaeochromocytoma parathyroid	
MTC-only	Medullary thryoid carcinoma (MTC)	ret: 618, missense (>50%)
MEN2b	Medullary thyroid carcinoma (MTC)	ret: 918, Met (Thr (>95%)
	Phaeochromocytoma	
	Associated abnormalities	
	Mucosal neuromas	
	Marfanoid habitus	
	Medullated corneal nerve fibers	
	Megacolon	

[a]Autosomal dominant inheritance of the MEN syndromes has been established.
Abbreviations: del = deletion; ins = insert.

MEN1 and MEN2. For example, patients suffering from islet cell tumors of the pancreas and phaeochromocytomas, or from acromegaly and phaeochromocytoma have been described and these patients may represent an "overlap" syndrome. All these forms of MEN may either be inherited as autosomal dominant syndromes, or they may occur sporadically i.e., without a family history. However, this distinction between sporadic and familial cases may sometimes be difficult as in some sporadic cases the family history may be absent because the parent with the disease may have died before developing symptoms. In this chapter, the main clinical features and molecular genetics of MEN1 will be discussed. MEN2 is discussed in Chapter 15.

MEN1: Clinical Findings, Biochemical Abnormalities, and Treatment

The incidence of MEN1 has been estimated from randomly chosen post mortem studies to be 0.25%, and to be 18% amongst patients with primary hyperparathyroidism *(2,6)*. The disorder affects all age groups, with a reported age range of 5–81 yr, and 80% of patients have developed clinical manifestations of the disorder by the fifth decade *(2,4)*. The clinical manifestations of MEN1 are related to the sites of tumors and to their products of secretion. In addition to the triad of parathyroid, pancreatic, and pituitary tumors, which consistitute the major components of MEN1, adrenal cortical, carcinoid, facial angiofibromas, collagenomas, and lipomatous tumors have also been described *(3,4)*.

Parathyroid Tumors

Primary hyperparathyroidism is the most common feature of MEN1 and occurs in more than 95% of all MEN1 patients *(2,4)*. Patients may present with asymptomatic hypercalcaemia, or nephrolithiasis, or osteitis fibrosa cystica, or vague symptoms associated with hypercalcaemia, for example polyuria, polydipsia, constipation, malaise, or occasionally with peptic ulcers. Biochemical investigations reveal hypercalcaemia usually in association with raised circulating parathyroid hormone (PTH) concentrations. No effective medical treatment for primary hyperparathyroidism is generally available and surgical removal of the abnormally overactive parathyroids is the definitive treatment. However, all four parathyroid glands are usually affected with multiple adenomas or hyperplasia, although this histological distinction may be difficult, and total parathyroidectomy has been proposed as the definitive treatment for primary hyperparathyroidism in MEN1, with the resultant lifelong hypocalcaemia being treated with oral calcitriol (1,25 dihydroxy vitamin D_3) *(7)*. It is recommended that such total parathyroidectomy should be reserved for the symptomatic hypercalcaemic patient with MEN1, and that the asymptomatic hypercalcaemic MEN1 patient should not have parathyroid surgery but have regular assessments for the onset of symptoms and complications, when total parathyroidectomy should be undertaken.

Pancreatic Tumors

The incidence of pancreatic islet cell tumors in MEN1 patients varies from 30–80% in different series *(1,2,4)*. The majority of these tumors produce excessive amounts of hormone, for example gastrin, insulin, glucagon, or vasoactive intestinal polypeptide (VIP), and are associated with distinct clinical syndromes.

Gastrinomas

These gastrin-secreting tumors represent over 50% of all pancreatic islet cell tumors in MEN1, and are the major cause of morbidity and mortality in MEN1 patients. This is due to the recurrent severe multiple peptic ulcers which may perforate. This association of recurrent peptic ulceration, marked gastric acid production and non β-islet cell tumors of the pancreas is referred to as the Zollinger-Ellison syndrome. Additional prominent clinical features of this syndrome include diarrhoea and steatorrhoea. The diagnosis is established by demonstration of a raised fasting serum gastrin concentration in association with an increased basal gastric acid secretion *(8)*. Medical treatment of MEN1 patients with the Zollinger-Ellison syndrome is directed to reducing basal acid output to less than 10 mmol/L, and this may be achieved by the parietal cell H+-K+-ATPase inhibitor, omeprazole. The ideal treatment for a nonmetastastic gastrinoma is surgical excision of the gastrinoma. However, in patients with MEN1 the gastrinomas are frequently multiple or extrapancreatic and surgery has not been successful *(9,10)*. The treatment of disseminated gastrinomas is difficult and hormonal therapy with octreotide, which is a human somatostatin analog, chemotherapy with streptozotocin and 5-fluoroaracil, hepatic artery embolization, and removal of all resectable tumor have all occasionally been successful *(2)*.

Insulinoma

These β-islet cell tumors secreting insulin represent one-third of all pancreatic tumors in MEN1 patients *(2,4)*. Insulinomas also occur in association with gastrinomas in 10% of MEN1 patients, and the two tumors may arise at different times. Patients with an insulinoma present with hypoglycemic symptoms that develop after a fast or exertion and improve after glucose intake. Biochemical investigations reveal raised plasma insulin concentrations in association with hypoglycaemia. Circulating concentrations of C-peptide and proinsulin, which are also raised, may be useful in establishing the diagnosis, as may an insulin suppression test. Medical treatment, which consists of frequent carbohydrate feeds and diazoxide, is not always successful and surgery is often required. Most insulinomas are multiple and small, and preoperative localization with computed tomography scanning, coeliac axis angiography, and preperi operative percutaneous transhepatic portal venous sampling is difficult and success rates have varied. Surgical treatment, which ranges from enucleation of a single tumor to a distal pancreatectomy or partial pancreatectomy, has been curative in some patients. Chemotherapy, which consists of streptozotocin or octreotide, is used for metastatic disease.

Glucagonoma

These α-islet cell, glucagon-secreting pancreatic tumors, have been reported in a few MEN1 patients *(2–4)*. The characteristic clinical manifestations of a skin rash (necrolytic migratory erythyema), weight loss, anemia, and stomatitis may be absent and the presence of the tumor is indicated only by glucose intolerance and hyperglucagonemia. The tail of the pancreas is the most frequent site for glucagonomas and surgical removal of these is the treatment of choice. However, treatment may be difficult as 50% of patients have metastases at the time of diagnosis. Medical treatment of these with octreotide, or with streptozotocin has been successful in some patients.

VIPoma

Patients with VIPomas, which are vasoactive intestinal peptide (VIP) secreting pancreatic tumors, develop watery diarrhea, hypokalemia and achlorhydria (the WDHA syndrome). This clinical syndrome has also been referred to as the Verner-Morrison syndrome or the VIPoma syndrome. VIPomas have been reported in only a few MEN1 patients and the diagnosis is established by documenting a markedly raised plasma VIP concentration *(2)*. Surgical management of VIPomas, which are mostly located in the tail of the pancreas, has been curative. However, in patients with unresectable tumor, treatment with streptozotocin, octreotide, corticosteroids, indomethicin, metoclopramide, and lithium carbonate has proved beneficial.

PPoma

These tumors, which secrete pancreatic polypeptide (PP) are found in a large number of patients with MEN1 *(2)*. No pathological sequelae of excessive PP secretion are apparent and the clinical significance of PP is unknown, although the use of serum PP measurements has been suggested for the detection of pancreatic tumors in MEN1 patients.

Pituitary Tumors

The incidence of pituitary tumors in MEN1 patients varies from 15–90% in different series *(2,4)*. Approximately 60% of MEN1 associated pituitary tumors secrete prolactin, 25% secrete growth hormone (GH), 3% secrete adenocorticotrophin (ACTH) and the remainder appear to be nonfunctioning. The clinical manifestations depend upon the size of the pituitary tumor and its product of secretion. Enlarging pituitary tumors may compress adjacent structures such as the optic chiasm or normal pituitary tissue and cause bitemporal hemianopia or hypopituitarism, respectively. The tumor size and extension are radiologically assessed by computed tomography scanning and nuclear magnetic resonance imaging. Treatment of pituitary tumors in MEN1 patients is similar to that in non-MEN1 patients and consists of medical therapy or selective hypophysectomy by the transphenoidal approach if feasible, with radiotherapy being reserved for residual unresectable tumor.

Associated Tumors

Patients with MEN1 may have tumors involving glands other than the parathyroids, pancreas, and pituitary. Thus carcinoid, adrenal cortical, facial angiofibromas, collagenomas, thyroid, and lipomatous tumors have been described in association with MEN1 *(2–4)*.

Carcinoid tumors, which occur more frequently in patients with MEN1 may be inherited as an autosomal dominant trait in association with MEN1. The carcinoid tumor may be located in the bronchi, the gastrointestinal tract, the pancreas, or the thymus. Most patients are asymptomatic and do not suffer from the flushing attacks and dyspnoea associated with the carcinoid syndrome, which usually develops after the tumor has metastasized to the liver.

The incidence of asymptomatic *adrenal cortical tumors* in MEN1 patients has been reported to be as high as 40%. The majority of these tumors are nonfunctioning. However, functioning adrenal cortical tumors in MEN1 patients have been documented to cause hypercortisolaemia and Cushing's syndrome, and primary hyperaldosteronism, as in Conn's syndrome.

Thyroid tumors, consisting of adenomas, colloid goiters, and carcinomas have been reported to occur in over 25% of MEN1 patients. However, the prevalence of thyroid disorders in the general population is high and it has been suggested that the association of thyroid abnormalities in MEN1 patients may be incidental and not significant.

Multiple *facial angiofibromas*, which are identical to those observed in patients with tuberous sclerosis, have been observed in 88% of MEN1 patients *(3)*, and *collagenomas* have been reported in >70% of MEN1 patients *(3)*.

Molecular Genetics of MEN1

Models of Tumor Development

The development of tumors may be associated with mutations or inappropriate expression of specific normal cellular genes, which are referred to as *oncogenes* (reviewed in refs. *1*, *2*, and *11*). Two types of oncogenes referred to as "dominant" and "recessive" oncogenes have been described. An activation of "dominant" oncogenes leads to transformation of the cells containing them, and examples of this are the chromosomal translocations associated with the occurrence of chronic myeloid leukemia and Burkitt's lymphoma. In these conditions, the mutations that lead to activation of the oncogene are dominant at the cellular level, and therefore only one copy of the mutated gene is required for the phenotypic effect. Such dominantly acting oncogenes may be assayed in cell culture by first transferring them into recipient cells and then scoring the numbers of transformed colonies, and this is referred to as the "transfection assay." However, in some inherited neoplasms that may also arise sporadically, such as retinoblastoma, tumor development is associated with two recessive mutations that inactivate oncogenes, and these are referred to as "recessive oncogenes." In the inherited tumors, the first of the two recessive mutations is inherited via the germ cell line and is present in all the cells. This recessive mutation is not expressed until a second mutation, within a somatic cell, causes loss of the normal dominant allele. The mutations causing the inherited and sporadic tumors are similar but the cell types in which they occur are different. In the inherited tumors the first mutation occurs in the germ cell, whereas in the sporadic tumors both mutations occur in the somatic cell. Thus, the risk of tumor development in an individual who has not inherited the first germ-line mutation is much smaller, as both mutational events must coincide in the same somatic cell. In addition, the apparent paradox that the inherited cancer syndromes are due to recessive mutations but dominantly inherited at the level of the family is explained because, in individuals who have inherited the first recessive mutation, a loss of a single remaining wild-type allele is almost certain to occur in at least one of the large number of cells in the target tissue. This cell will be detected because it forms a tumor, and almost all individuals who have inherited the germ-line mutation will express the disease, even though they inherited a single copy of the recessive gene. This model involving two (or more) mutations in the development of tumors is known as the "two hit" or Knudson's hypothesis. The normal function of these recessive oncogenes appears to be in regulating cell growth and differentiation, and these genes have also been referred to as "anti-oncogenes" or "tumor suppressor genes." An important feature which has facilitated the investigation of these genetic abnormalities associated with tumor development is that the loss of the remaining allele (i.e., the "second hit"), which occurs in the somatic cell and gives rise to the tumor, often involves a large scale loss of chromosomal material. This "second hit" may be detected by a comparison of the DNA sequence polymorphisms (Fig. 1) in the leukocytes and tumor obtained from a patient, and observing a loss of heterozygosity (LOH) in the tumors (Fig. 2).

The MEN1 Gene

The gene causing MEN1 was localized to chromosome 11q13 by genetic mapping studies that investigated MEN1 associated tumors for loss of heterozygosity (LOH) (Fig. 2) and by segregation studies in MEN1 families (Fig. 3) *(12–14)*. The results of these studies, which were consistent with Knudson's model for tumor development, indicated that the MEN1 gene represented a putative tumor suppressor gene. Further genetic mapping studies defined a <300-kb region as the minimal critical segment that contained the MEN1 gene and characterization of genes from this region led to the identification of the MEN1 gene *(15,16)*, which consists of 10 exons with a 1830-bp coding region (Fig. 4) that encodes a novel 610 amino acid protein, referred to as "MENIN" *(15)*. Mutations of the MEN1 gene (Figs. 4 and 5) have been identified *(15–20)* and the total number of germ-line mutations of the MEN1 gene that have now been identified in MEN1 patients is over 150. Approximately 25% are nonsense mutations, ≈ 45% are deletions, ≈ 15% are insertions, <5% are donor-splice mutations and ≈ 10% are missense mutations. More than 10% of the MEN1

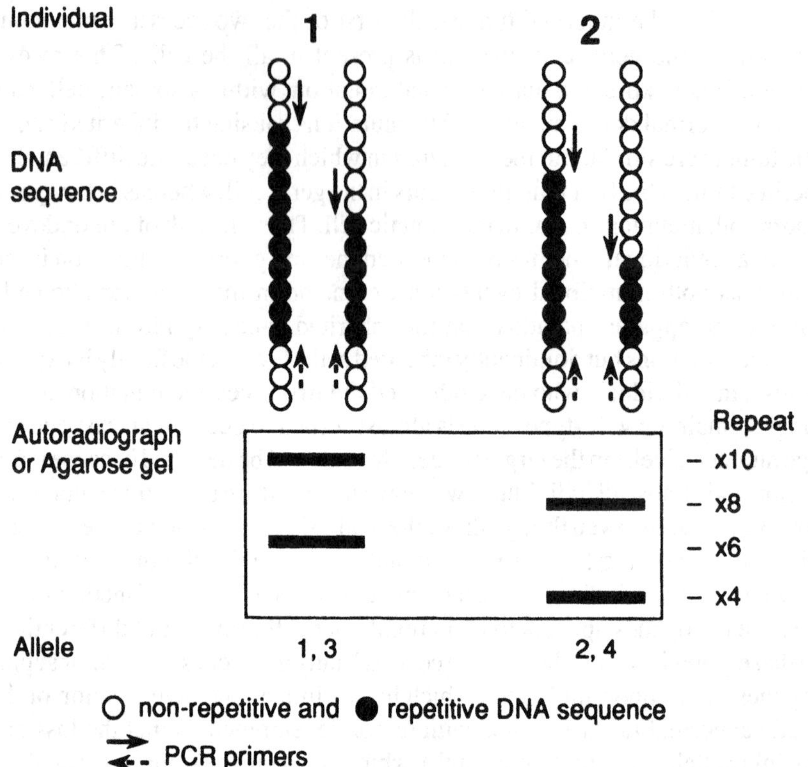

Fig. 1. Schematic representation of polymorphisms in microsatellite tandem repetitive DNA sequences, which may consist, for example, of the dinucleotide CA, or the trinucleotide ATT, or the tetranucleotide ATTT, or the hexanucleotide TATATG. Oligonucleotides primers (- - →) corresponding to the nonrepetitive sequences (O) on either side of the repetitive DNA sequence (●) are synthesised and the polymerase chain reaction (PCR) is utilised to amplify the repeat in genomic DNA obtained from different individuals. The resulting PCR products are separated either by polyacrylamide gel or agarose gel electrophoresis, and the polymorphisms are revealed by autoradiography or by viewing of an ethidium bromide-stained agarose gel under ultraviolet light. Thus, of the pair of chromosomes from individual (1), 1 has 10 repeats and the other has 6 repeats, whereas of the pair of chromosomes from individual (2), 1 has 8 repeats and the other has 4 repeats. Following PCR amplification and separation by gel electrophoresis, these variations in the length of the repeats will be revealed by the difference in the size of the bands, which have been designated alleles; for example, the larger band consisting of 10 repeats is designated allele 1, and those consisting of 8, 6, and 4 repeats are designated alleles 2, 3, and 4 respectively. These microsatellite tandem repetitive sequences, which are highly polymorphic, show Mendelian inheritance (*see* Fig. 3) and can be used as genetic markers in family studies or for the detection of abnormalities in tumors (Fig. 2). (Adapted with permission from ref. *11*.)

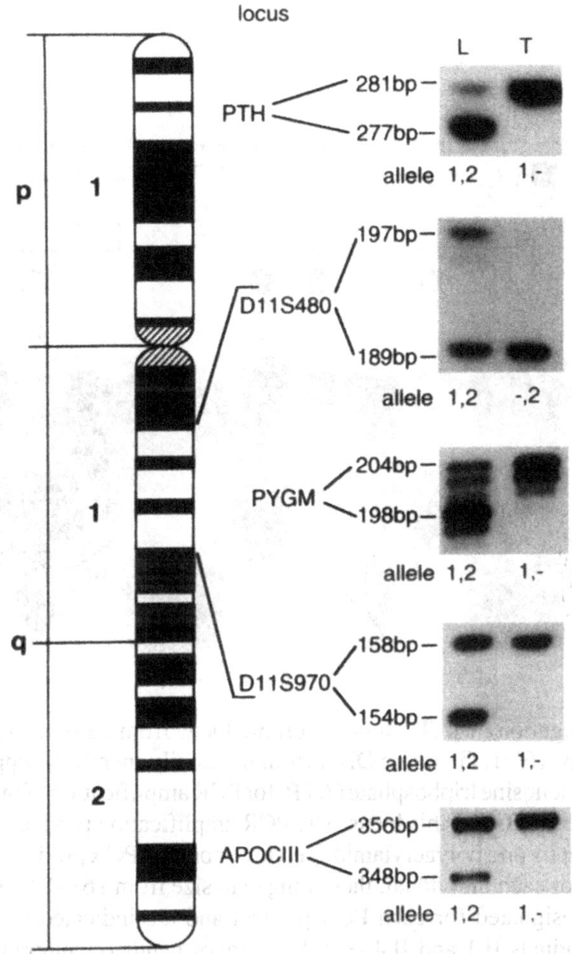

Fig. 2. Loss of heterozygosity (LOH) involving polymorphic loci from chromosome 11 in a parathyroid tumor from a patient with familial MEN1. The microsatellite polymorphisms obtained from the patient's leukocyte (L) and parathyroid tumor (T) DNA at the PTH, D11S480, PYGM, D11S970 and APOCIII loci are shown. These microsatellite polymorphisms have been identified using specific primers for each of the loci which have been localized to chromosome 11, and are shown juxtaposed to their region of origin on the short (p) and long (q) arms of chromosome 11. The microsatellite polymorphisms are assigned alleles (*see* Fig. 1). For example, D11S480 yielded a 197-bp product (allele 1) and a 189-bp product (allele 2) following PCR amplification of leukocyte DNA, but the tumor cells have lost the 197-bp product (allele 1) and are hemizygous (alleles -,2). Similar losses of alleles are detected using the other DNA markers, and an extensive loss of alleles involving the whole of chromosome 11 is observed in the parathyroid tumor of this patient with

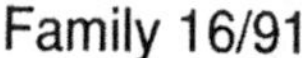

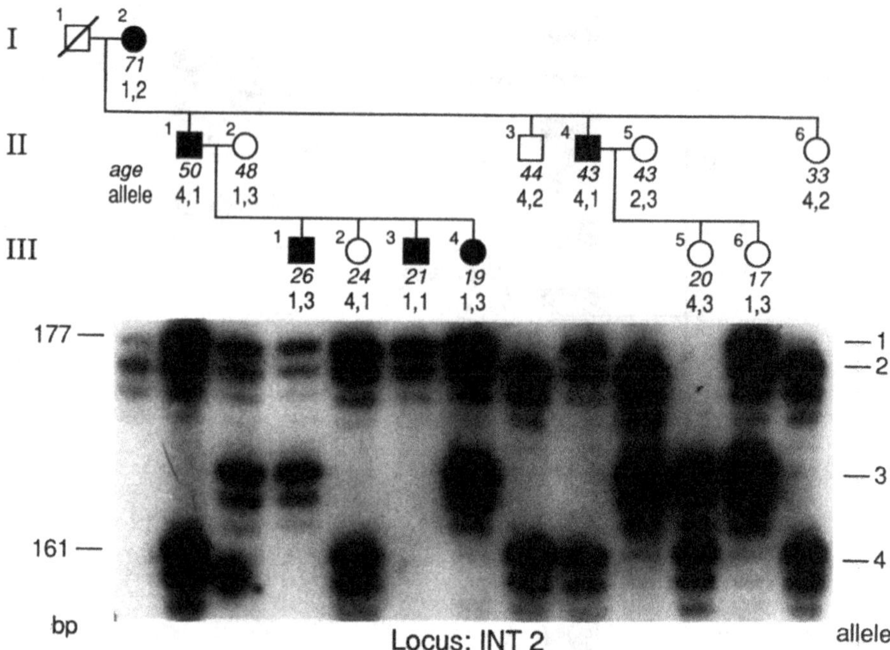

Fig. 3. Segregation of INT2, a polymorphic locus from chromosome 11q13, and MEN1 in family 16/91. Genomic DNA from the family members (upper panel) was used with γ^{32}P adenosine triphosphate (ATP) for PCR amplification of the polymorphic repetitive element $(TG)_n$ at this locus. The PCR amplification products were detected by autoradiography on a polyacrylamide gel (lower panel). PCR products were detected from the DNA of each individual; these ranged in size from 161–177 base pairs (bp). Alleles were designated for each PCR product and are indicated on the right. For example, individuals II.1 and II.4 reveal 2 pairs of bands on autoradiography. The upper pair of bands is designated allele 1 and the lower pair of bands is designated allele 4; and these 2 individuals are therefore heterozygous (alleles 1, 4). A pair of bands for each allele is frequently observed in the PCR detection of microsatellite repeats. The upper band in the pair is the "true" allele and the lower band in the pair is its associated "shadow," which results from slipped-strand mispairing during the PCR. The segregation of these bands and their respective alleles together with the disease can be studied in the family members whose alleles and ages are shown. In some individuals, the inheritance of paternal and maternal alleles can be ascertained; the paternal allele

---

Fig. 2. *(continued)* MEN1. In addition, the complete absence of bands suggests that this abnormality has occurred within all the tumor cell studies, and indicates a monoclonal origin for this MEN1 parathyroid tumor. (Adapted with permission from ref. *36*.)

mutations arise *de novo* and may be transmitted to subsequent generations *(17–19)*. It is also important to note that between 5–20% of MEN1 patients may not harbor mutations in the coding region of the MEN1 gene *(15–20)*, and that these individuals may have mutations in the promoter or untranslated regions (UTRs), which remain to be investigated.

The majority (>80%) of the MEN1 mutations are inactivating, and are consistent with those expected in a tumor suppressor gene. The mutations are not only diverse in their types but are also scattered (Fig. 4) throughout the 1830-bp coding region of the MEN1 gene with no evidence for clustering as observed in MEN2 (*see* Chapter 15). However, some of the mutations have been observed to occur several times in unrelated families (Table 1), and the 3 deletional and insertional mutations involving codons 83 and 84, 209–211, and codons 514–516, account for approx 25% of all the germ-line MEN1 mutations, and thus these may represent potential "hot" spots. Such deletional and insertional hot spots may be associated with DNA sequence repeats that may consist of long tracts of either single nucleotides or shorter elements, ranging from dinucleotides to octanucleotides. Indeed, the DNA sequence in the vicinity of codons 83 and 84 in exon 2, and codons 209 to 211 in exon 3, contains CT and CA dinucleotide repeats, respectively, flanking the 4-bp deletions (Table 1); these would be consistent with a replication-slippage model in which there is misalignment of

---

is shown on the left. Individuals are represented as unaffected male (□), affected male (■), unaffected female (O), and affected female (●). Individual II.1 is affected and heterozygous (alleles 4, 1) and an examination of his affected children (III.1, III.3 and III.4) and his mother (I.2) and sibling (II.4) reveals inheritance of allele 1 with the disease. The unaffected individuals II.3, II.6, III.2 and III.5 have not inherited this allele 1. However, the daughter (III.6) of individual II.4 has inherited allele 1, but remains unaffected at the age of 17 yr; this may either be a representation of age-related penetrance, or a recombination between the disease and INT2 loci. Thus, in this family, the disease and INT2 loci are co-segregating in 9 out of the 10 children, but in one individual (III.6), assuming a 100% penetrance (see below) in early childhood, recombination is observed. Thus, MEN1 and INT2 are cosegregating in 9/10 of the meioses and not segregating in 1/10 meioses, and the likelihood that the two loci are *linked* at $\theta = 0.10$, i.e., 10% recombination, is $(9/10)^9 \times (1/10)^1$. If the disease and the INT2 loci were not linked, then the disease would be associated with allele 1 in one half (1/2) of the children and with allele 2 in the remaining half (1/2) of the children, and the likelihood that the two loci are *not linked* is $(1/2)^{10}$. Thus, the odds ratio in favor of linkage between the MEN1 and INT2 loci at $\theta = 0.10$, i.e., 10% recombination in this family, is therefore $(9/10)^9 \times (1/10)^1 \div (1/2)^{10} = 39.67:1$, and the LOD score (i.e., $\log_{10}$ of the odds ratio favoring linkage) = 1.60 (i.e., $\log_{10}$ 39.67). A LOD score of +3, which indicates a probability in favor of linkage of 1000:1, establishes linkage (also *see* Chapter 20). LOD scores from individual families can also be summated, and such studies revealed that the peak LOD score between MEN1 and the INT2 locus was >+3, thereby establishing linkage between MEN1 and INT2 loci. (Adapted with permission from ref. *32*.)

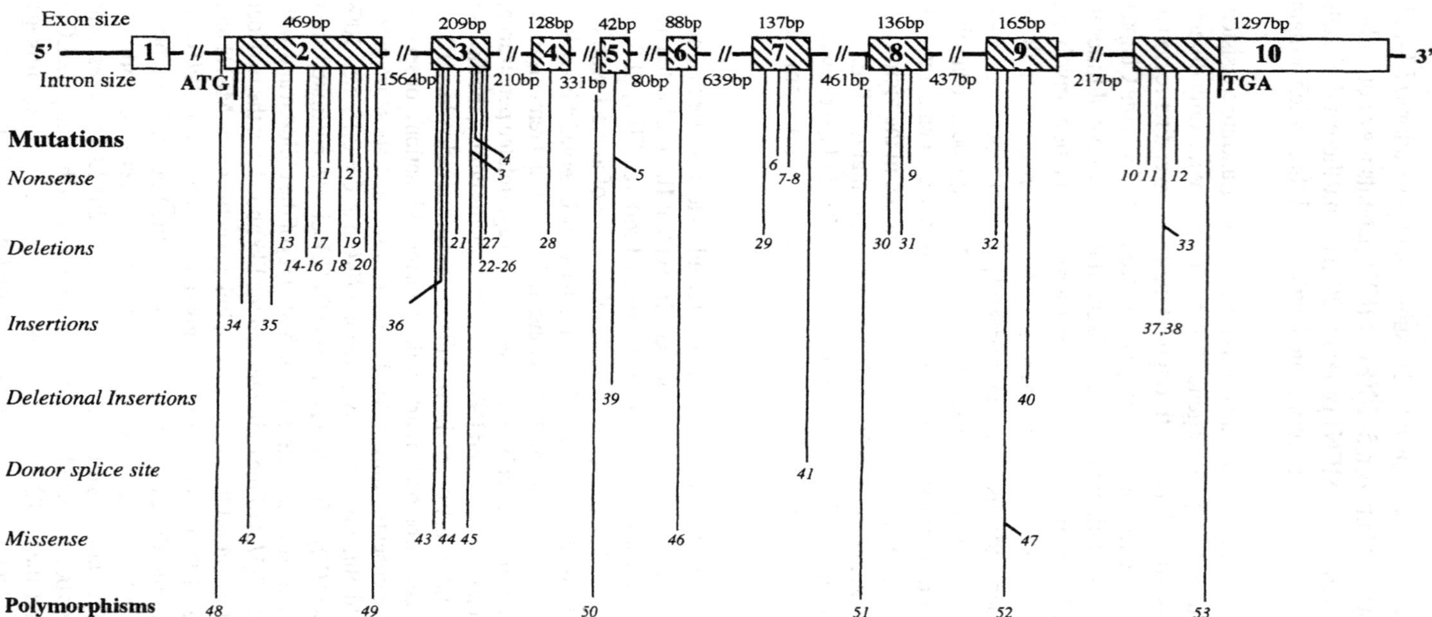

Fig. 4. Schematic representation of the genomic organization of the MEN1 gene. The human MEN1 gene consists of 10 exons that span >9 kb of genomic DNA and encodes a 610 amino acid protein (4,5). The 1.83-kb coding region is organized into 9 exons (exons 2–10, indicated by the hatched boxes) and 8 introns (indicated by a line but not to scale). The sizes of the exons (size range 88–1312bp) and introns (size range 41 to 1564 bp) are shown, and the start (ATG) and Stop (TGA) sites in exons 2 and 10, respectively, are indicated. Exon 1, the 5' part of exon 2 and 3' part of exon 10 are untranslated (indicated by the open boxes). The sites of 44 mutations (11 nonsense, 19 deletions, 3 duplications, 2 insertion, 2 insertional substitutions, 1 donor splice site, and 6 missense) and 6 different polymorphisms identified by one study (18) are shown below. (Adapted with permission from ref. *18*.)

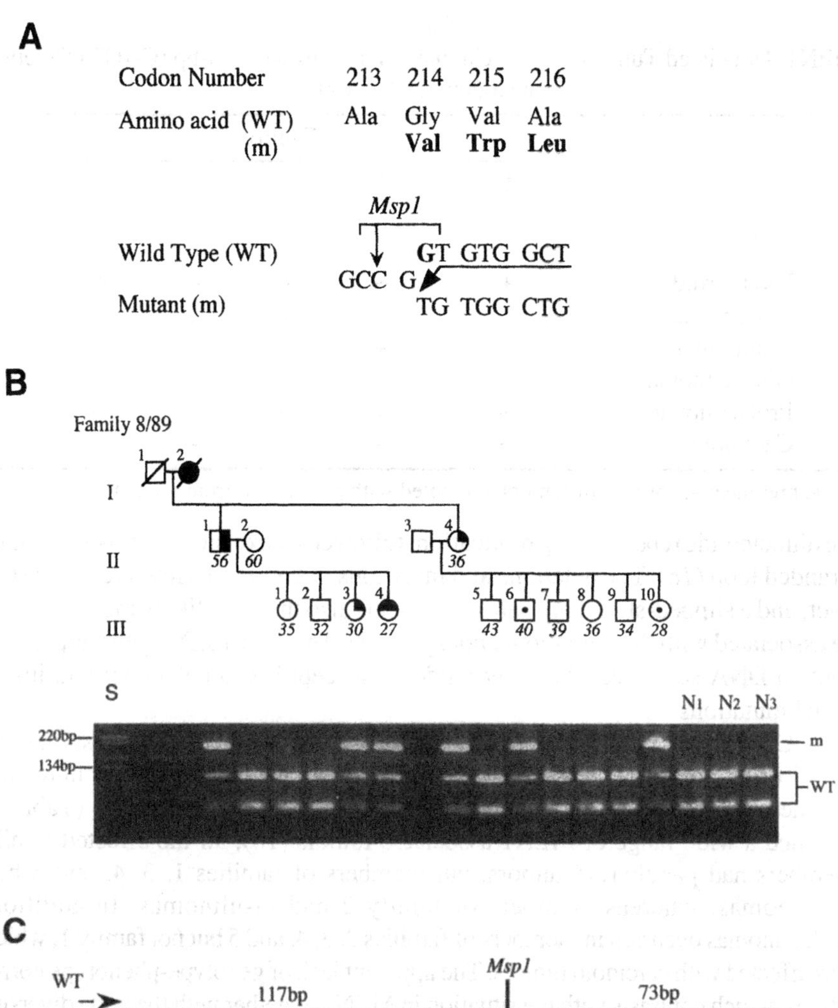

Fig. 5. Detection of mutation in exon 3 in family 8/89 by restriction enzyme analysis. DNA sequence analysis of individual II.1 revealed a 1-bp deletion at the second position (GGT) of codon 214 (**A**). The deletion has caused a frameshift that continues to codon 223 before a stop codon (TGA) is encountered in the new frame. The 1-bp deletion results in the loss of an *MspI* restriction enzyme site (C/CGG) from the normal (wild type, WT) sequence (**A**) and this has facilitated the detection of this mutation in the other affected members (II.4, III.3, and III.4) of this family (**B**). The mutant (*m*) PCR product is 190 bp, whereas the wild-type (WT) products are 117 and 73 bp (**C**). The affected individuals were heterozygous, and the unaffected members were homozygous for the wild-type sequence. Individuals III.6 and III.10, who are 40-and 28-yr-old, respectively, are mutant gene carriers who are clinically and biochemically normal and this is due to the age-related penetrance

Table 2
MEN1-Associated Tumors in Five Unrelated Families with a 4-bp (CAGT) Deletion at Codons 210 and 211

	Family				
	1	2	3	4	5
Tumors					
Parathyroid	+	+	+	+	+
Gastrinoma	+	–	+	+	+
Insulinoma	–	+	–	–	–
Glucagonoma	–	–	–	–	+
Prolactinoma	–	+	+	+	+
Carcinoid	+	–	–	–	–

+, presence; –, absence of tumors. (Adapted with permission from ref. *5*.)

the dinucleotide repeat during replication, followed by excision of the 4-bp single-stranded loop *(18)*. The deletions and insertions of codon 516 involve a poly$(C)_7$ tract, and a slipped-strand mispairing model is also the most likely mechanism to be associated with this mutational hot spot *(18)*. Thus, the MEN1 gene appears to contain DNA sequences that may render it susceptible to deletional and insertional mutations.

Correlations between the MEN1 mutations and the clinical manifestations of the disorder appear to be absent. For example, a detailed study of 5 unrelated families with the same 4-bp deletion (CAGT) in codons 210 and 211 (Table 2) revealed a wide range of MEN1-associated tumors *(18)*; all the affected family members had parathyroid tumors, but members of families 1, 3, 4, and 5 had gastrinomas, whereas members of family 2 had insulinomas. In addition, prolactinomas occurred in members of families 2, 3, 4, and 5 but not family 1, which was affected with carcinoid tumors. The apparent lack of genotype-phenotype correlations, which contrasts with the situation in MEN2, together with the wide diversity of mutations in the 1830-bp coding region of the MEN1 gene will make mutational analysis for diagnostic purposes in MEN1 time-consuming and expensive *(5)*.

Fig. 5. *(conintued)* of this disorder (Fig. 6). Individuals are represented as: male (square); female (circle); unaffected (open); affected with parathyroid tumors (filled upper right quadrant), with gastrinoma (filled lower right quadrant), with prolactinoma (filled upper left quadrant); and unaffected mutant gene carriers (dot in the middle of the open symbol). Individual I.2 who is deceased but was known to be affected (tumor details not known) is shown as a filled symbol. The age is indicated below for each individual at diagnosis or at the time of the last biochemical screening. The standard size marker (S) in the form of the 1-kb ladder is indicated. Cosegregation of this mutation with MEN1 in family 8/89 and its absence in 110 alleles from 55 unrelated normal individuals (N_{1-3} shown) indicates that it is not a common DNA sequence polymorphism. (Adapted with permission from ref. *18*.)

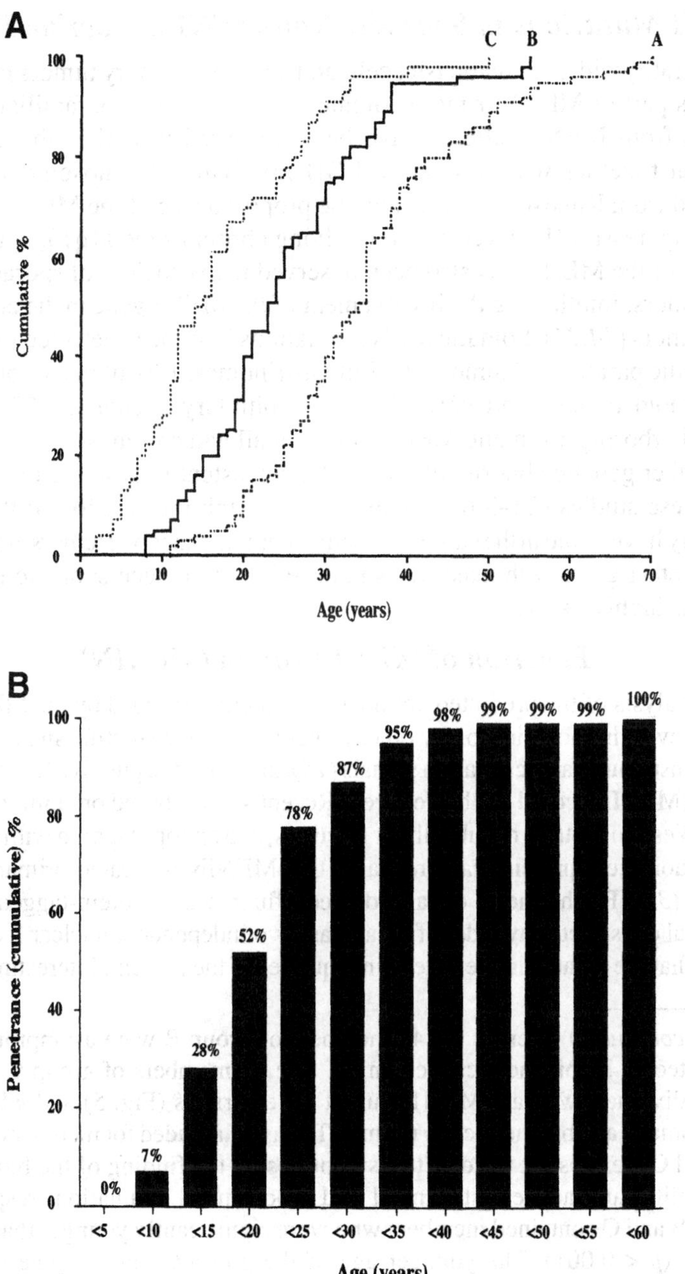

Fig. 6. The age distributions (**A**) and age-related penetrances (**B**) of MEN1 determined from an analysis of 174 mutant gene carriers. The age distributions were determined for 3 groups of MEN1 mutant gene carriers from 40 families in whom mutations were detected *(18)*. The 91 members of group A presented with symptoms,

MEN1 Mutations in Sporadic Non-MEN1 Endocrine Tumors

Parathyroid, pancreatic islet cell, and anterior pituitary tumors may occur either as part of MEN1 or more commonly as sporadic, nonfamilial, tumors. Tumors from MEN1 patients have been observed to harbor the germ-line mutation together with a somatic LOH involving chromosome 11q13, as expected from Knudson's model and the proposed role of the MEN1 gene as a tumor suppressor. However, LOH involving chromosome 11q13, which is the location of the MEN1, has also been observed in 5% to 50% of sporadic endocrine tumors, implicating the involvement of the MEN1 gene in the etiology of these tumors *(14,21)*. Somatic MEN1 mutations have been detected in 12–21% of sporadic parathyroid tumors, 33% of gastrinomas, 17% of insulinomas, 36% of carcinoid tumors, and <5% of anterior pituitary adenomas *(22–30)*. The tumors harboring a somatic MEN1 mutation all had chromosome 11q13 LOH as the other genetic abnormality, or "hit", consistent with Knudson's hypothesis. These studies (22–30) indicate that although inactivation of the MEN1 gene may have a role in the etiology of some sporadic endocrine tumors, the involvement of other genes with major roles in the etiology of such sporadic endocrine tumors is highly likely.

Function of MEN1 Protein (MENIN)

Analysis of the predicted amino acid sequence encoded by the MEN1 gene did not reveal homologies to any other proteins, sequence motifs, signal peptides, or consensus nuclear localization signals *(15)*, and thus, the putative function of the protein (MENIN) could not be deduced. Recent studies based on immunofluorescence, Western blotting of subcellular fractions, and epitope tagging with enhanced green fluorescent protein, have revealed that MENIN is located primarily in the nucleus *(31)*. Furthermore, enhanced green fluorescent protein-tagged MENIN deletional constructs have identified at least two independent nuclear localization signals that are located in the C-terminal quarter of the protein. Interestingly, none

---

Fig. 6. *(continued)* whereas the 40 members of group B were asymptomatic and were detected by biochemical screening. The 43 members of group C represent those individuals who are MEN1 mutant gene carriers (Fig. 5) and who remain asymptomatic and biochemically normal. The ages included for members of groups A, B and C are those at the onset of symptoms, at the finding of the biochemical abnormality, and at the last clinical and biochemical evaluation, respectively. Groups B and C contained members who were significantly younger than those in group A ($p < 0.001$). The younger age of the group C mutant gene carriers is consistent with an age-related penetrance for MEN1, and this was calculated **(B)** for the first 5 decades. The age-related penetrances (i.e., the proportion of mutant gene carriers with manifestations of the disease by a given age) rose steadily from 7% in the <10 yr group, to 52%, 87%, 98%, and 99%, by the ages of 20, 30, 40, and 50 yr, respectively. (Adapted with permission from ref. *18*.)

of the MEN1 germ-line missense or in-frame deletions *(15–20)* alter either of these putative nuclear localization signals. However, all of the truncated MEN1 proteins that would result from the nonsense and frameshift mutations, if expressed, would lack these nuclear localization signals. The nuclear localization of MENIN suggests that it may act either in the regulation of transcription, or DNA replication, or the cell cycle. However, the precise roles of MENIN in the nucleus and in the regulation of endocrine cell growth control remain to be elucidated.

Screening in MEN1

The detection by biochemical screening for the development of MEN1 tumors in asymptomatic members of families with MEN1 is of great importance, as earlier diagnosis and treatment of these tumors reduces morbidity and mortality. The age-related penetrance (i.e., the proportion of gene carriers manifesting symptoms or signs of the disease by a given age) has been ascertained (Fig. 6) and the mutation appears to be nonpenetrant below the age of 5 yr *(18)*. Thereafter the mutant MEN1 gene has a high penetrance, being >60% penetrant by 20 yr of age and >90% penetrant by 30 yr *(18)*. Screening for MEN1 tumors is difficult because the clinical and biochemical manifestations in members of any one family are not uniformly similar. The attempts to screen for the development of MEN1 tumors in the asymptomatic relatives of an affected individual have depended largely on measuring the serum concentrations of calcium, gastrointestinal hormones, and prolactin (reviewed in *2*). Parathyroid overactivity causing hypercalcemia is invariably the first manifestation of the disorder *(4)* and this has become a useful and easy biochemical screening investigation. However, it is suggested that DNA analysis should now be introduced in the screening program of MEN1 families *(2)*. The advantages of DNA analysis are that it requires a single blood sample and does not need to be repeated, unlike the biochemical screening tests *(1)*. This is because the analysis is independent of the age of the individual and provides an objective result. However, the great diversity together with the widely scattered locations of the MEN1 mutations (Fig. 4), and a lack of genotype-phenotype correlation will make such mutational screening time consuming, arduous, and expensive. Nevertheless, an integrated program of both mutational analysis, to identify mutant gene carriers, and biochemical screening, to detect the development of tumors, would be of advantage and is to be recommended *(32)*. Thus, a DNA test identifying an individual as a mutant gene carrier is likely to lead not to immediate medical or surgical treatment but to earlier and more frequent biochemical screening, whereas a DNA result that indicates that an individual is not at risk will lead to a decision for no further screening.

At present it is suggested that individuals at high risk of developing MEN1 (i.e., mutant gene carriers) should be screened at least once per annum. Screening should commence in early childhood, as the disease has developed in some individuals by the age of 8 yr, and should continue for life as some individuals have not developed the disease until the eighth decade. Screening history and physical examination should be directed toward eliciting the symptoms and signs of hypercalcemia, nephrolithiasis, peptic ulcer disease, neuroglycopenia, hypopituitarism, galactorrhea, and amenorrhea in women, acromegaly, Cushing's disease, visual field loss, and the presence of subcutaneous lipomata *(2,3,33–35)*. Biochemical screening should include serum calcium and prolactin estimations in all individuals, and measurement of gastrointestinal hormones and more specific endocrine function tests should be reserved for individuals who have symptoms or signs suggestive of a clinical syndrome. Thus, the recent advances in molecular biology which have enabled the localization of the gene causing MEN1 have helped in the clinical management of patients and their families with this disorder.

Summary

Combined clinical and laboratory investigations of MEN1 have resulted in an increased understanding of this disorder which may be inherited as an autosomal dominant condition. Defining the features of each disease manifestation in MEN1 has improved patient management and treatment, and has also facilitated a screening protocol to be instituted. The application of the techniques of molecular biology has enabled the identification of the gene causing MEN1 and the detection of mutations in patients. The function of the protein encoded by the MEN1 gene remains to be elucidated. However, these recent advances provide for the identification of mutant MEN1 gene carriers who are at a high risk of developing this disorder and thus require regular and biochemical screening to detect the development of endocrine tumors.

Acknowledgments

The author is grateful to the Medical Research Council (MRC), UK for support; to my colleagues J. D. H. Bassett, S. A. Forbes, and A. A. J. Pannett for helpful discussions; and to S. Kingsley for typing the manuscript.

References

1. Thakker, R. V. and Ponder, B. A. J. (1988) Multiple endocrine neoplasia, in *Clinical Endocrinology and Metabolism*, vol. 2, no. 4 (Shepphard, M. C., ed.), Balliere Tindall, London, pp.1031–1068.
2. Thakker, R. V. (1995) Multiple endocrine neoplasia type 1 (MEN1), in *Endocrinology* (DeGroot, L. J., Besser, G. K., Burger, H. G., Jameson, J. L., Loriaux, D. L., Marshall, J. C., et al., eds.), W. B. Saunders, Philadelphia, pp. 2815–2831.
3. Marx, S. J. (1998) Multiple endocrine neoplasia type 1, in *Genetic Basis of Human Cancer* (Vogelstein, B. and Kinzler, K. W., eds.), McGraw-Hill, New York, pp. 489–506.

4. Trump, D., Farren, B., Wooding, C., Pang, J. T., Besser, G. M., Buchanan, K. D., et al. (1996) Clinical studies of multiple endocrine neoplasia type 1 (MEN1) in 220 patients. *Q. J. Med.* **89,** 653–669.
5. Thakker, R. V. (1998) Multiple endocrine neoplasia: syndromes of the twentieth century. *J. Clin. Endocrinol. Metab.* **83,** 2617–2620.
6. Marx, S. J., Spiegel, A. M., Levine, M. A., Rizzoli, R. E., Lasker, R. D., Santora, A. C., et al (1982) Familial hypocalciuric hypercalcaemia: the relation to primary parathyroid hyperplasia. *N. Engl. J. Med.* **307,** 416–426.
7. Rizzoli, R., Green, J., and Marx, S. J. (1985) Primary hyperparathyroidism in familial multiple endocrine neoplasia Type 1. Long term follow–up of serum calcium levels after parathyroidectomy. *Am. J. Med.* **78,** 467–474.
8. Wolfe, M. M. and Jensen, R. T. (1987) Zollinger–Ellison syndrome. Current concepts in diagnosis and management. *N. Engl. J. Med.* **317,** 1200–1209.
9. Delcore, R., Hermreck, A. S., and Friesen, S. R. (1989) Selective surgical management of correctable hypergastrinemia. *Surgery* **106,** 1094–1102.
10. Sheppard, B. C., Norton, J. A., Dopmann, J. L., Maton, P. N., Gardner, J. D., and Jensen, R. T. (1989) Management of islet cell tumors in patients with multiple endocrine neoplasia: a prospective study. *Surgery* **106,** 1108–1118.
11. Thakker, R. V. (1993) The molecular genetics of the multiple endocrine neoplasia syndromes. *Clin. Endocrinol.* **39,** 1–14.
12. Larsson, C., Skogseid, B., Oberg, K., Nakamura, Y., and Nordenskjold M. C. (1988) Multiple endocrine neoplasia type I gene maps to chromosome 11 and is lost in insulinoma. *Nature* **332,** 85–87.
13. Thakker, R. V., Bouloux, P., Wooding, C., Chotai, K., Broad, P. M., Spurr, N. K., Besser, G. M. and O'Riordan, J. L. H. (1989) Association of parathyroid tumors in multiple endocrine neoplasia type 1 with loss of alleles on chromosome 11. *N. Engl. J. Med.* **321,** 218–224.
14. Byström, M. C., Larsson, C., Blomberg, C., Sandelin, F., Falkmer, U., Skogseid, B., et al. (1990) Localisation of the MEN1 gene to a small region within chromosome 11q13 by deletion mapping in tumors. *Proc. Natl. Acad. Sci.* **87,** 1968–1972.
15. Chandrasekharappa, S. C., Guru, S. C., Manickam P., Olufemi, S.-E., Collins, F. S., Emmert-Buck, M. R., et al. (1997 Positional cloning of the gene for multiple endocrine neoplasia-type 1. *Science* **276,** 404–407.
16. The European Consortium on MEN1. (1997) Identification of the Multiple Endocrine Neoplasia type 1 (MEN1) gene. *Hum. Mol. Genet.* **6,** 1177–1183.
17. Agarwal, S. K., Kester, M. B., Debelenko, L. V., Heppner, C., Emmert-Buck, M. R., Skarulis, M. C., et al. (1997) Germline mutations of the MEN1 gene in familial multiple endocrine neoplasia type 1 and related states. *Hum. Mol. Genet.* **6,** 1169–1175.
18. Bassett, J. H. D., Forbes, S. A., Pannett, A. A. J., Lloyd, S. E., Christie, P. T., Wooding, C., et al. (1998) Characterisation of mutations in patients with multiple endocrine neoplasia type 1 (MEN1). *Am. J. Hum. Genet.* **62,** 232–244.
19. Teh, B. T., Farnebo, F., Phelan, C., et al. (1998) Mutation analysis of the MEN1 gene in multiple endocrine neoplasia type 1, familial acromegaly and familial isolated hyperparathyroidism. *J. Clin. Endocrinol. Metab.* **83,** 2621–2626.
20. Giraud, S., Zhang, C. X., Sinilnikova, O., Waatot, V., Salandre, J., Buisson, N., Waterlot, C. et al. (1998) Germ-line mutation analysis in patients with multiple endocrine neoplasia type 1 and related disorders. *Am. J. Human Genet.* **63,** 455–467.

21. Thakkker, R. V., Pook, M. A., Wooding, C., Boscaro, M., Scanarini, M., and Clayton, R. N. (1993a) Association of somatotrophinomas with loss of alleles on chromosome 11 and with *gsp* mutations. *J. Clin. Invest.* **91,** 2815–2821.
22. Heppner, C., Kester, M. B., Agarwal, S. K., Debelenko, L. V., Emmert-Buck, M. R., Guru, S. C., et al. (1997) Somatic mutation of the MEN1 gene in parathyroid tumors. *Nat. Genet.* **16,** 375–378.
23. Zhuang, Z., Vortmeyer, A. O., Pack, S., Huang, S., Pham, T. A., Wang, C., et al. (1997) Somatic mutations of the *MEN1* tumor suppressor gene in sporadic gastrinomas and insulinomas. *Cancer Res.* **57,** 4682–4686.
24. Zhuang, Z., Ezzat, S. Z., Vortmeyer, A. O., Weil, R., Oldfield, E. H., Park, W.-S., et al. (1997) Mutations of the *MEN1* tumor suppressor gene in pituitary tumors. *Cancer Res.* **57,** 5446–5451.
25. Prezant, T. R., Levine, J., and Melmed, S. (1998) Molecular characterization of the *Men 1* tumor suppressor gene in sporadic pituitary tumors. *J. Clin. Endocrinol. Metab.* **83,** 1388–1391.
26. Debelenko, L.V., Brambilla, E., Agarwal, S.K., Swalwell, J. I., Kester, M. B., Lubensky, I. A., et al. (1997) Identification of *MEN1* gene mutations in sporadic carcinoid tumors of the lung. *Hum. Mol. Genet.* **6,** 2285–2290.
27. Vortmeyer, A. O., Böni, R., Pak, E., Pack, S., and Zhuang, Z. (1998) Multiple endocrine neoplasia 1 alterations in MEN1-associated and sporadic lipomas. *J. Nat. Cancer. Inst.* **90,** 398.
28. Farnebo, F., Teh, B. T., Kytölä, S., Svensson, A., Phelan, C., Sandelin, K., et al. (1998) Alterations of the *MEN1* gene in sporadic parathyroid tumors. *J. Clin. Endocrinol. Metab.* **83,** 2627–2630.
29. Carling, T., Correea. P., Hessman, O., et al. (1998) Parathyroid *MEN1* gene mutations in relation to clinical characteristics of non-familial primary hyperparathyroidism. *J. Clin. Endo. Metab.* **83,** 2951–2954.
30. Tanaka, C., Kimura, T., Yang, P., Moritani, M., Yamaoka, T., Yamada, S., et al. (1998) Analysis of loss of heterozygosity on chromosome 11 and infrequent inactivation of *MEN1* gene in sporadic pituitary adenomas. *J. Clin. Endocrinol. Metab.* **83,** 2631–2634.
31. Guru, S. C., Goldsmith, P. K., Burns A. L., Marx, S. J., Spiegel, A. M., Collins, F. S., and Chandrasekharappa, S. C. (1998) Menin, the product of the *MEN1* gene, is a nuclear protein. *Proc. Natl. Acad. Sci. USA* **95,** 1630–1634.
32. Thakker, R. V. (1994b) Molecular mechanisms of tumor formation in hereditary and sporadic tumors of the MEN1 type: the impact of genetic screening in the management of MEN1, in *Endocrinology and Metabolism Clinics of North America* (Gagel, R. F., ed.), W. B. Saunders, Philadelphia, pp.117–135.
33. Marx, S. J., Vinik, A. I., Santen, R. J., Floyd, J. C., Mills, J. L., and Green, J. (1986) Multiple endocrine neoplasia type 1: assessment of laboratory tests to screen for the gene in a large kindred. *Medicine* **65,** 226–241.
34. Benson, L., Ljunghall, S., Akerstrom, G., and Oberg, K. (1987) Hyperparathyroidism presenting as the first lesion in multiple endocrine neoplasia Type 1. *Am. J. Med.* **82,** 731–737.
35. Skogseid, B., Oberg, K., Benson, L., Lindgren, P. S., Lörelius, L. E., Lundquist, G., Wide, L., and Wilander, E. (1987). A standardized meal stimulation test of the endocrine pancreas for early detection of pancreatic endocrine tumors in multiple endocrine neoplasia type 1 syndrome: five years experience. *J. Clin. Endocrinol. Metab.* **64,** 1233–1240.
36. Pang, J. T. and Thakker, R. V. (1994) Multiple endocrine neoplasia type 1. *Eur. J. Cancer* **30A,** 1961–1968.

CHAPTER 15

The *Ret* Signaling System and Its Role in Hereditary Medullary Thyroid Carcinoma

Robert F. Gagel and Gilbert Cote

Introduction

The identification of mutations of the rearranged during transfection (*c-ret*) proto-oncogene causative for multiple endocrine neoplasia type 2 (MEN2) in 1993 was the first in a series of remarkable discoveries that have provided insight not only into the cause of medullary thyroid carcinoma (MTC), pheochromocytoma, and parathyroid neoplasia, but also the development of the neurologic and urogenital systems. It also illustrates one example of the frenetic and sometimes illogical process by which scientific knowledge has progressed over the past decade, mixing the use of molecular genetics, molecular biology, and animal model systems to identify and characterize a unique signaling system.

Mapping the Causative Gene for Multiple Endocrine Neoplasia Type 2

Efforts to map the causative gene for multiple endocrine neoplasia, type 2 (MEN2) by genetic linkage techniques began in the early 1980s. The clarity of the MEN2 phenotype and the availability of large and well-defined families with this neoplastic syndrome made it an excellent choice for early mapping studies. MEN2A or classic Sipple syndrome *(1)* is the most common variant and is characterized by the development of the thyroid cancer in nearly 100% of gene carriers, unilateral or bilateral pheochromocytoma in 50%, and hyperparathyroidism characterized by multiglandular hyperplasia or adenomas in 10–20%. MEN2B, a less common variant *(2–4)*, is characterized by the association of MTC, pheochromocytoma, oral and gastrointestinal neuromas, and bony changes similar to Marfan's syndrome

The Genetics of Osteoporosis and Metabolic Bone Disease
Ed.: M. J. Econs © Humana Press Inc., Totowa, NJ

(long thin arms, legs, and fingers and pectus abnormalities). Less common variants of MEN2A include familial MTC (hereditary MTC without other components of MEN2A) *(5)*, MEN2A with cutaneous lichen amyloidosis (a pruritic skin lesion located over the central upper back) *(6,7)*, and MEN2A and Hirschsprung disease (loss of neuronal innervation of the gastrointestinal tract) *(8)*. All variants are inherited in an autosomal dominant manner and the phenotypes suggested a gene that was involved in endocrine, neurologic, and bony development.

The identification of gene carriers in these kindreds was facilitated by the recognition that MTC produces a small peptide hormone, calcitonin, that made it possible to diagnose MTC during the first and second decades of life *(9)*. This observation not only led to improved diagnosis and treatment, but further enlarged the pool of well-defined genetic subjects available for mapping studies.

Although efforts to map the gene began in 1981, the causative gene was not mapped to a central chromosome 10 locus until 1987 *(10,11)*. The region containing the causative gene was progressively narrowed and mutations of the *Ret* proto-oncogene were identified in 1993 *(12,13)*.

The Ret *Proto-oncogene and the PTC Rearrangement*

The *Ret* proto-oncogene encodes a tyrosine kinase receptor (Fig. 1). The extracellular domain contains a cadherin-like region, whose function is unknown, and a cysteine-rich domain. The intracellular domains are similar to those found in other tyrosine kinase receptors. The gene was first identified as a potential oncogene in 1986 when a rearranged form of this receptor was shown to cause transformation in the NIH 3T3 cells, a model that identifies transforming activity based on cell growth and colony formation in soft agar *(14,15)*.

The first evidence that *Ret* could function naturally as an oncogene was the identification of a rearrangement in papillary thyroid carcinoma, now known as the papillary thyroid carcinoma (PTC) oncogene (Fig. 2). One-third to one-half of papillary thyroid carcinomas express one of three rearranged forms of *Ret* in which the promoter sequences from a constitutively expressed gene drive the expression of the downstream tyrosine kinase domain *(16)*. The breakpoint for each of these rearrangements occurs in intron 11, just downstream of the plasma membrane spanning region of the receptor (Fig. 2). In this particular type of rearrangement the tyrosine kinase is expressed intracellularly as a soluble factor, devoid of the plasma membrane and the extracellular sequences that normally regulate its function. The importance of this rearrangement in the development of PTC is underscored by the fact that one-third to one-half of thyroid carcinomas in children exposed to radiation from the Chernobyl nuclear power plant disaster express one of these three rearrangements *(17–19)*. For unclear reasons the PTC arrangement is unique to papillary thyroid carcinoma and is rarely found in other tumors.

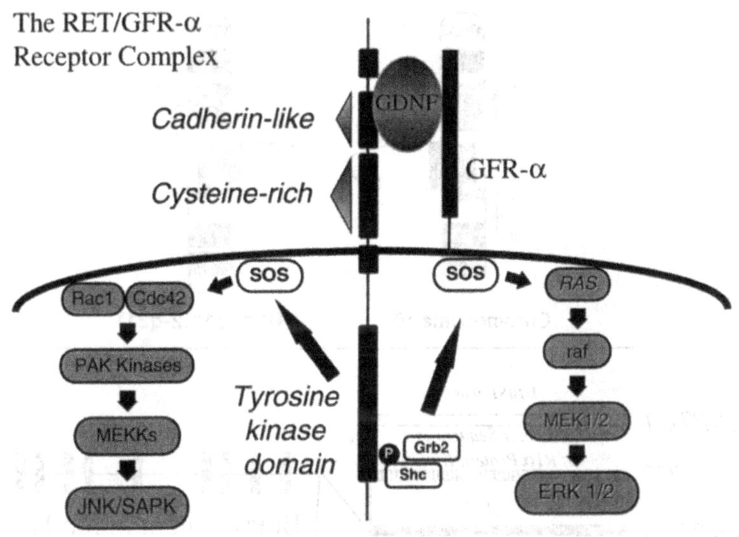

Fig. 1. The *Ret*/GFR receptor complex. *Ret* and GFR-a form the extracellular receptor for GDNF (glial cell-derived neurotrophic factor). GDNF activates the *Ret* tyrosine kinase receptor, activating the JNK/SAPK and ERK 1/2 pathways.

Activating Mutations of the c-ret Proto-oncogene in Hereditary Medullary Thyroid Carcinoma

Activating mutations of *c-ret* that cause hereditary medullary thyroid carcinoma fall into two broad categories, missense mutations within the cysteine-rich extracellular domain or mutations of the intracellular tyrosine kinase domain (Fig. 3).

Extracellular Domain Mutations

The extracellular domain mutations convert highly conserved cysteines to another amino acid. Mutations of codon 634 in exon 11 (Table 1) account for over 80% of all mutations in hereditary MTC *(20)*. The most common coding change is a cys634arg mutation that accounts for approximately one-half of all mutations in hereditary MTC (Fig. 3, *see* Table 1). Mutations of codons 630 (exon 11) and 609, 611, 618, and 620 (exon 10) account for approx 15% of the remaining mutations in hereditary MTC (Fig. 3, *see* Table 1) *(20)*. In general, mutations of codon 634 most commonly cause classic MEN2A and those in exon 10 (609, 611, 618, and 620) mutations cause FMTC, although overlap exists *(20)*. An important point in the clinical management of kindreds with hereditary MTC is that designation of an FMTC kindred should be based on assessment of 10 or more family members over several generations. Misclassification of death caused by pheochromocytoma in classic MEN2A kindreds was common prior to the recognition of MEN2A in 1961 and therefore older family history may be less than helpful in establishing the presence or absence of pheochromocytoma in the family.

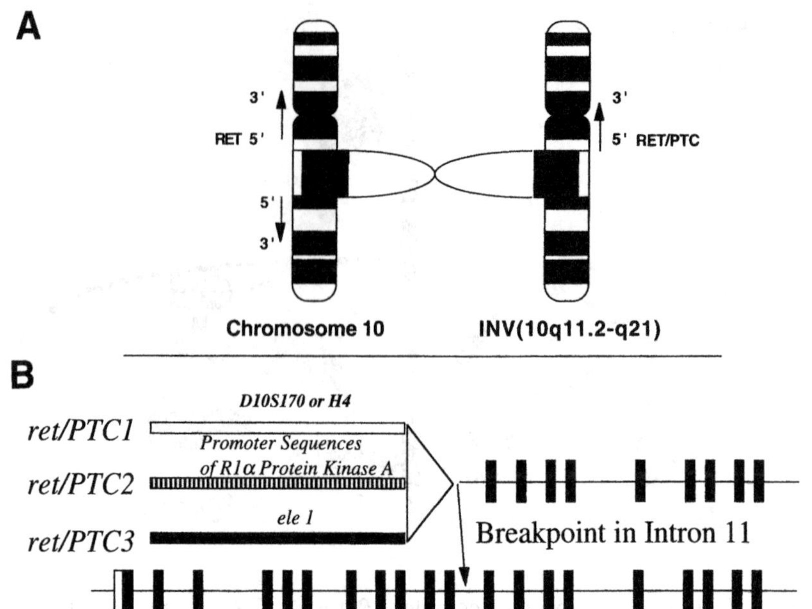

Fig. 2. The papillary thyroid carcinoma (PTC) oncogene. A chromosome 10 inversion (**A**) results in a rearranged form of Ret. At least 3 variants of the PTC oncogene with different promoters (*Ret/PTC1, Ret/PTC2,* and *Ret/PTC3)* have been identified. In each the breakpoint within *Ret* occurs in intron 11.

The mechanisms by which these mutant sequences cause transformation has, in part, been elucidated. Mutations of the extracellular domain affect highly conserved cysteines that regulate receptor dimerization. Convincing evidence from several laboratories has shown that a codon 634 mutation induces receptor dimerization *(21,22)* and activation of JNK/SAPK and ERK 1/2 pathways leading to transformation (Fig. 1) *(23,24)*.

Intracellular Domain Mutations

At least eight different intracellular missense mutations have been associated with hereditary MTC (Fig. 3, *see* Table 1). The most common is a codon 918 missense mutation that accounts for 3–5% of all germline mutations *(20,25)* and is found as a somatic mutation in approx 25% of all sporadic MTCs *(26)*. Mutations of codons 883 and 922 have been identified in a handful of MEN2B patients (Fig. 3, *see* Table 1). Codon 768, 791, and 891 mutations have been found in a few FMTC kindreds and codon 790 and 804 mutations have been identified in a few kindreds with either MEN2A or FMTC (Fig. 3, *see* Table 1) *(27)*. The numbers of kindreds identified with the intracellular domain mutations is small suggesting a larger experience will be required before definitive genotype-phenotype correlations can be made.

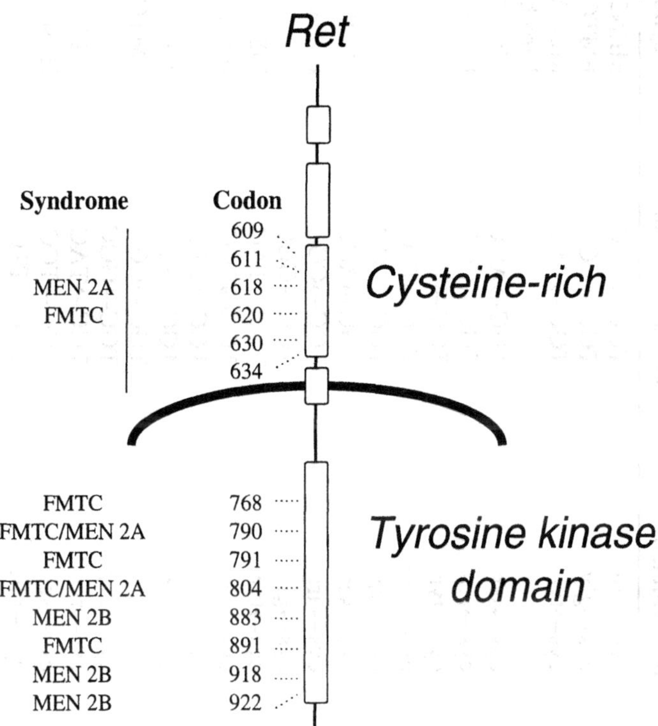

Fig. 3. Mutations of the *Ret* proto-oncogene causative for hereditary medullary thyroid carcinoma. The extracellular domain mutations (codons 609–634 in the cysteine-rich domain) are the most common and may be associated with either MEN2A or FMTC. The intracellular domain mutations (in the tyrosine kinase domain) cause a diverse group of indicated clinical syndromes. Abbreviations as described in the text.

The mechanism of transformation for an intracellular mutation (codon 918) differs from that observed for the extracellular domain mutations. Dimerization of the receptor does not seem to be involved in the activation event, although there is receptor autophosphorylation and phosphorylation of downstream proteins in the mitogen-activated protein-kinase (MAPK) cascade (Fig. 1) *(21,22)*.

The Identification of the *Ret* Ligand and the Recognition of a Second Receptor Component

At the time of its identification *Ret* was classified as an orphan (without known ligand) receptor. The first clue that one of the *Ret* ligands is glial cell-derived neurotrophic factor (GDNF), a small peptide identified as a survival factor for neurons *(28)*, developed from nearly identical phenotypes in mice in which the genes for *Ret (29)* or GDNF *(30,31)* were inactivated. In these mice

Table 1
Mutations of the Ret Proto-oncogene in Hereditary Medullary Thyroid Carcinoma

Exon	Affected codon	% of Hereditary mutations	Amino acid change normal→mutant	Nucleotide change normal→mutant	Clinical syndrome
10	609	0–1	cys→arg	TGC→CGC	MEN2A/
			cys→gly	TGC→GGC	FMTC
			cys→tyr	TGC→TAC	MEN2A/
					Hirschspring
10	611	2–3	cys→ser	TGC→AGC	MEN2A/
			cys→arg	TGC→CGC	FMTC
			cys→tyr	TGC→TAC	
			cys→phe	TGC→TTC	
			cys→trp	TGC→TGG	
			cys→ser	TGC→AGC	MEN2A/
			cys→arg	TGC→CGC	FMTC
10	618	3–5	cys→gly	TGC→GGC	
			cys→tyr	TGC→TAC	MEN2A/
			cys→ser	TGC→TCC	Hirschsprung
			cys→phe	TGC→TTC	
			cys→ser	TGC→AGC	MEN2A/
			cys→arg	TGC→CGC	FMTC
			cys→gly	TGC→GGC	
10	620	6–8	cys→tyr	TGC→TAC	MEN2A/
			cys→ser	TGC→TCC	Hirschsprung
			cys→phe	TGC→TTC	
			cys→trp	TGC→TGG	
			cys→tyr	TGC→TAC	MEN2A/

11	630	0–1	cys→ser	TGC→TCC	FMTC
			cys→phe	TGC→TTC	
			cys→ser	TGC→AGC	MEN2A
			cys→arg	TGC→CGC	
			cys→gly	TGC→GGC	MEN2A/
11	634	75–85	cys→tyr	TGC→TAC	CLA
			cys→ser	TGC→TCC	
			cys→phe	TGC→TTC	
			cys→trp	TGC→TGG	
11	635	rare	thr ser cys ala	ACGAGCTGTGCC	MEN2A
11	637	rare	cys arg thr	TGCCGCACG	MEN2A
13	768	0–1	glu→asp	GAG→GAC	FMTC
13	790	0–1	leu→phe	TTG→TTC	MEN2A/
			leu→phe	TTG→TTT	FMTC
13	791	0–1	tyr→phe	TAT→TTT	FMTC
13	804	0–1	val→met	GTG→ATG	MEN2A/
			val→leu	GTG→TTG	FMTC
15	883	rare	ala→phe	GCT→TTT	MEN2B
15	891	rare	ser→ala	TCG→GCG	FMTC
16	918	3–5	met→thr	ATG→ACG	MEN2B
16	922	rare	ser→tyr	TCC→TAC	MEN2B

there was lack of normal renal development, a Hirschsprung-like failure of gastrointestinal neuronal development, and suboptimal development of the sympathetic nervous system derived from somites one through five. Subsequent studies proved GDNF to be a ligand for the *Ret* receptor.

The third component of this receptor system was discovered by investigators looking for a receptor for GDNF. They identified an extracellular protein (GDNFR-α or GFR-α) with a glycosylphosphatidylinositol linkage to the cell membrane that functioned as a receptor for GDNF *(32)*. By combining their observations with others studying *Ret*-GDNF interactions, the model of GDNF-*Ret*/GFR-α shown in Fig. 1 has evolved. Support for this model of the GDNF/*Ret*/GFR-α receptor system is provided by the finding of nearly identical phenotypes for *Ret*, GDNF, and GFR-α mice.

Role of Receptor System in Embryonic Development

There is now compelling evidence that *Ret*/GFR and GDNF function as a signaling system to promote normal embryonic development of certain components of the enteric and sympathetic nervous system and normal renal development. Where this has been shown most clearly is in renal development (Fig. 4). GDNF (expressed in the developing metanephric blastema) interacts with the *Ret*/GFR-α receptor system in the developing ureteric bud leading to invasion and branching of the ureteric bud into the blastema with development of the collecting system (Fig. 4, upper panel). The absence of expression of either GDNF or *Ret* results in a failure of normal ingrowth (Fig. 4, lower panel) *(30,31,33)*. In the GDNF knockout mice, normal branching of the ureteric bud can be rescued by placing pellets containing GDNF into the embryonic kidney (Fig. 4, lower panel) *(31)*.

The importance of this interaction between ligand and receptor during development is underscored by the neuronal development of the gastrointestinal tract during development. *Ret*-expressing cells migrate from the neural crest derived from somites 1–5 into the developing gastrointestinal tract *(34)*. It is likely that *Ret*-expressing neural crest cells are enticed to migrate in response to the trophic effects of GDNF expression in the gastrointestinal tract. Thus it is the expression of a receptor by one cell type and the synchronous expression of the ligand by another that leads to the correct temporal and spatial organization of central and peripheral nervous system components.

The Ret/GFR Receptor Family

At least 3 different GFR receptors (GFR-α-1, GFR-α-2, and GFR-α-3) *(35–38)* and 3 ligands (GDNF, neurturin, and persephin) *(38)* have been identified (*see* Table 2). The interrelationships between the several ligands and receptor systems is currently being defined.

The components of the *Ret*/GFR receptor system and the several ligands are expressed widely throughout the nervous system and in a number of other tissues such as heart, lung, liver, and gonads, suggesting an important role for these receptor systems in normal embryonic development. In some cases there is coexpression of one of the three ligands with GFR and *Ret*; in other tissues some

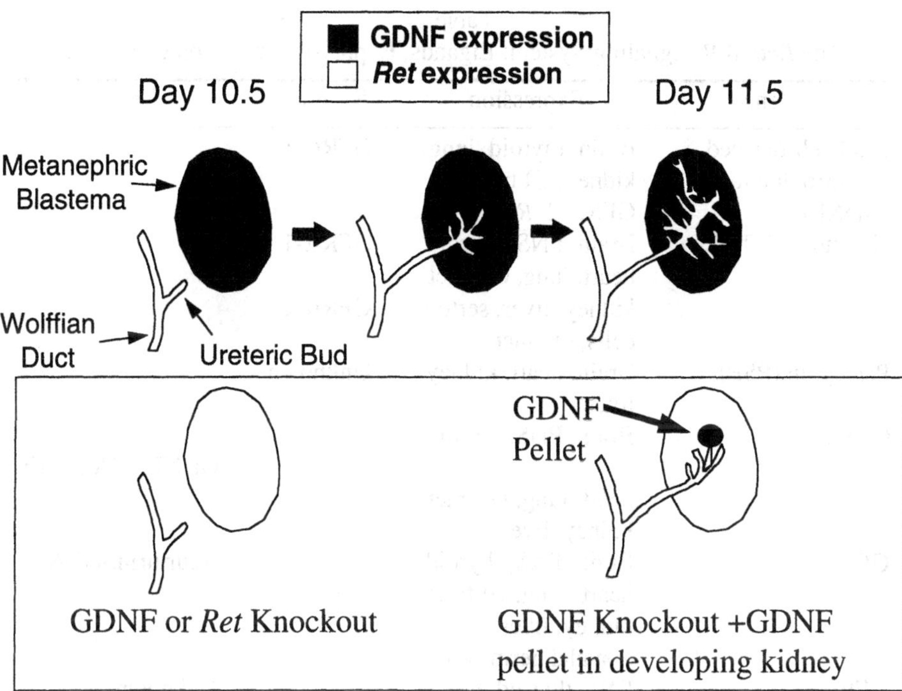

Fig. 4. Expression of *Ret* and GDNF in the developing kidney directs normal development of the collecting system. **(A)** GDNF, produced in the developing metanephric blastema, acts in a tropic manner to cause invasion by the ureteric bud. **(B)** In either a GDNF or *Ret* knockout mouse there is a failure of urogenital bud invasion into the developing metanephric blastema (left). This phenotype can be rescued by placing a pellet of GDNF into the developing kidney and maintaining it in organ culture (right).

components are not expressed, suggesting that there are other members of this receptor system or that not all components are required for functionality.

Mutations of the GDNF/Ret/GFR Signaling System in Hirschsprung Disease

Several important pieces of information came together in the early 1990s and led to the elucidation of *Ret* proto-oncogene mutations in Hirschsprung disease. The first is the identification of a proximal chromosome 10 deletion in a child with Hirschsprung disease *(39)* that led to localization of the causative gene. Subsequent reports documented a wide spectrum of mutations, mostly inactivating. There are, however, several reports of apparent germline activating mutations leading to a Hirschsprung phenotype in (mutations of codon 609 *(26)*, 618 *(40)* or 620) or outside of hereditary MTC. In addition, infrequent mutations of GDNF have been identified in Hirschsprung patients

Table 2
The *Ret*/GFR Signaling System: Ligands, Expression, and Nomenclature.

Gene	Expression	Receptor	Ligand
Glial cell-derived neurotrophic factor (GDNF)	Brain, thyroid, lung, kidney, GI tract, GFRα-2, *Ret*	GFRα-1	
Neurturin (NTN)	Brain, PNS, thyroid, heart, lung, GI tract	GFRα-1	
	kidney, liver, sertoli cells, oviduct	GFRα-2	
Persephin (PSP)	Brain, heart, kidney, liver	Unknown	
GFRα-1	Brain, PNS, thyroid, heart, lung, GI tract, kidney, liver		GDNF>>Neurturin
GFRα-2	Brain, PNS, thyroid, heart, lung, GI tract, kidney, liver, gonadal germ cells		Neurturin>GDNF
GFRα-3	PNS, thyroid, heart, lung, GI tract, kidney, liver,		Unknown
Ret proto-oncogene	Brain, PNS, thyroid, heart, lung, GI tract, kidney, liver		GDNF Neurturin

Abbreviations: GDNF, glial cell-derived neurotrophic factor; NTN, neurturin; GFRα-1, GDNFR-α; GFRα2, TmR-2, NTNR-α, *RET*L2, GDNFR-β; and PNS, peripheral nervous system.

(41). Mutations of the endothelin-B receptor gene (Online Mendelian Inheritance in Man [OMIM] accession #131244) *(42)* and its ligand, endothelin-3 (OMIM accession #131242) *(43)* have also been identified in Hirschsprung disease.

A Role for the Ret/GFR Receptor System in Bone Development?

The characteristic clinical features of MEN2B (long, thin fingers; and long legs and arms (leading to altered upper/lower body ratio, pectus abnormalities, and slipped femoral epiphysis) argue for a role of *Ret* in normal cartilaginous development. There have, to date, been no studies that focus on this aspect of bone development.

The Clinical Use of Ret Mutational Analysis in the Management of Hereditary MTC

The localization of *Ret* mutations causative for hereditary MTC into well-defined regions of the gene, the tight correlation between genotype and phenotype, and the knowledge that early intervention will alter the long-term course of this syndrome make it possible to utilize *Ret* testing for management of hereditary MTC. Approx 90% of all *Ret* mutations that cause MTC are located within a 100 nucleotide region. Several straightforward techniques have been utilized to identify mutations within this region, all based on polymerase chain reaction (PCR) amplification with analysis most commonly by direct DNA sequencing, restriction analysis *(44)*, or less commonly by denaturing gradient gel electrophoresis *(40)*. Additional PCR reactions are required to analyze exon 13, 14, 15, and 16 mutations (Table 1). Mutation analysis can be obtained from several commercial sources. (Information on availability of commercial genetic testing is available on the University of Texas M.D. Anderson Cancer Center Section of Endocrine Neoplasia Web Site at: http://endocrine.mdacc.tmc.edu/)

Users of this information should be aware of the potential for error. Sample mixup, contamination of the PCR reaction, failure of specific primers to amplify the mutant allele, or transcribing errors lead to an error rate estimated to be at least 5% *(45)*. Before a decision is made to consider surgical intervention in a gene carrier or to eliminate an MEN2 kindred member with a normal analysis from further screening, the test should be performed on a separately obtained and independently analyzed blood sample.

More than 90% of clinicians who care for children with MEN2 utilize genetic testing to make a decision to perform a total thyroidectomy around the age of 5 yr. There is convincing evidence from studies initiated 25 yr ago that early thyroidectomy results in cure of 80–85% of children who are gene carriers *(46)*. Since the mean age of surgery in these children was 13 yr, there is reason to believe that earlier thyroidectomy might further improve the cure rate. Earlier detection methods (using serum calcitonin measurments) did not detect MTC in a premalignant phase in over 50% of children, raising the possibility that metastasis might have occurred before thyroidectomy. It is less clear whether to perform early surgery on children who carry exon 13, 14, or 15 mutations (*see* Table 1), because of the generally accepted lower virulence of these tumors. Children with MEN2B and codon 918 mutations may have early metastasis and thyroidectomy should be performed early in life (within the first year). Genetic testing has not altered parathyroid gland and pheochromocytoma management other than the exclusion from screening of those family members who do not have a *Ret* mutation.

Summary and Conclusions

Mutations of the *Ret* proto-oncogene have been implicated in the causation of multiple endocrine neoplasia and Hirschsprung disease. The GDNF/*Ret*/GFR-α receptor system defines a unique system for neural crest and neural differentiation and its further study will undoubtedly lead to an understanding of the temporal and spatial organization of the nervous system.

References

1. Sipple, J. H. (1961) The association of pheochromocytoma with carcinoma of the thyroid gland. *Am. J. Med.* **31,** 163–166.
2. Carney, J. A., Go, V. L., Sizemore, G. W., and Hayles, A. B. (1976) Alimentary-tract ganglioneuromatosis. A major component of the syndrome of multiple endocrine neoplasia, type 2b. *N. Engl. J. Med.* **295,** 1287–1291.
3. Rashid, M., Khairi, M. R., Dexter, R. N., Burzynski, N. J., and Johnston, C. C., Jr. (1975) Mucosal neuroma, pheochromocytoma and medullary thyroid carcinoma: multiple endocrine neoplasia type 3. *Medicine (Baltimore)* **54,** 89–112.
4. Carney, J. A., Sizemore, G. W., and Hayles, A. B. (1978) Multiple endocrine neoplasia, type 2b. *Pathobiol. Ann.* **8,** 105–153.
5. Farndon, J. R., Leight, G. S., Dilley, W. G., Baylin, S. B., Smallridge, R. C., Harrison, T. S., and Wells, S. A., Jr. (1986) Familial medullary thyroid carcinoma without associated endocrinopathies: a distinct clinical entity. *Br. J. Surg.* **73,** 278–281.
6. Gagel, R. F., Levy, M. L., Donovan, D. T., Alford, B. R., Wheeler, T., and Tschen, J. A. (1989) Multiple endocrine neoplasia type 2a associated with cutaneous lichen amyloidosis. *Ann. Intern. Med.* **111,** 802–806.
7. Nunziata, V., Giannattasio, R., di Giovanni, G., D'Armiento, M. R., and Mancini, M. (1989) Hereditary localized pruritus in affected members of a kindred with multiple endocrine neoplasia type 2A (Sipple's syndrome). *Clin. Endocrinol.* **30,** 57–63.
8. Verdy, M., Weber, A. M., Roy, C. C., Morin, C. L., Cadotte, M., and Brochu P. (1982) Hirschsprung's disease in a family with multiple endocrine neoplasia type 2. *J. Pediatr. Gastroenterol. Nutr.* **1,** 603–607.
9. Melvin, K. E. W., Miller, H. H., and Tashjian, A. H., Jr. (1971) Early diagnosis of medullary carcinoma of the thyroid gland by means of calcitonin assay. *N. Engl. J. Med.* **285,** 1115–1120.
10. Simpson, N. E., Kidd, K. K., Goodfellow, P. J., McDermid, H., Myers, S., Kidd, J. R., Jackson, C. E., Duncan, A. M., Farrer, L. A., and Brasch, K. (1987) Assignment of multiple endocrine neoplasia type 2A to chromosome 10 by linkage. *Nature* **328,** 528–530.
11. Mathew, C. G., Chin, K. S., Easton, D. F., Thorpe, K., Carter, C., Liou, G. I., et al. (1987) A linked genetic marker for multiple endocrine neoplasia type 2A on chromosome 10. *Nature* **328,** 527–528.
12. Mulligan, L. M., Kwok, J. B., Healey, C. S., Elsdon, M. J., Eng, C., Gardner, E., et al. (1993) Germ-line mutations of the RET proto-oncogene in multiple endocrine neoplasia type 2A. *Nature* **363,** 458–460.
13. Donis-Keller, H., Dou, S., Chi, D., Carlson, K. M., Toshima, K., Lairmore, T. C., et al. (1993) Mutations in the RET proto-oncogene are associated with MEN2A and FMTC. *Hum. Mol. Genet.* **2,** 851–856.
14. Takahashi, M. and Cooper, G. M. (1987) Ret transforming gene encodes a fusion protein homologous to tyrosine kinases. *Mol. Cell. Biol.* **7,** 1378–1385.
15. Takahashi, M., Ritz, J., and Cooper, G. M. (1985) Activation of a novel human transforming gene, ret, by DNA rearrangement. *Cell* **42,** 581–588.

16. Grieco, M., Santoro, M., Berlingieri, M. T., Melillo, R. M., Donghi, R., Bongarzone, I., et al. (1990) PTC is a novel rearranged form of the ret proto-oncogene and is frequently detected in vivo in human thyroid papillary carcinomas. *Cell* **60,** 557–563.
17. Pisarchik, A. V., Ermak, G., Fomicheva, V., Kartel, N. A., and Figge J. (1998) The ret/PTC1 rearrangement is a common feature of Chernobyl-associated papillary thyroid carcinomas from Belarus. *Thyroid* **8,** 133–139.
18. Klugbauer, S., Lengfelder, E., Demidchik, E. P., and Rabes, H. M. (1995) High prevalence of RET rearrangement in thyroid tumors of children from Belarus after the Chernobyl reactor accident. *Oncogene* **11,** 2459–2467.
19. Bonn, D. (1996) RET oncogene puzzle in Chernobyl thyroid tumours [news]. *Lancet* **347,** 1176.
20. Eng, C., Clayton, D., Schuffenecker, I., et al. (1996) The relationship between specific RET proto-oncogene mutations and disease phenotype in multiple endocrine neoplasia type 2. International RET mutation consortium analysis. *JAMA* **276,** 1575–1579.
21. Asai, N., Iwashita, T., Matsuyama, M., and Takahashi, M. (1995) Mechansims of activation of the ret proto-oncogene by multiple endocrine neoplasia 2A mutations. *Mol. Cell. Biol.* **15,** 1613–1619.
22. Santoro, M., Carlomagno, F., Romano, A., Bottaro, D. P., Dathan, N. A., et al. (1995) Activation of RET as a dominant transforming gene by germline mutations of MEN2A and MEN2B. *Science* **267,** 381–383.
23. Xing, S., Furminger, T. L., Tong, Q., and Jhiang, S. M. (1998) Signal transduction pathways activated by RET oncoproteins in PC12 pheochromocytoma cells. *J. Biol. Chem.* **273,** 4909–4914.
24. Chiariello, M., Visconti, R., Carlomagno, F., Melillo, R., Bucci, C., Defranciscis, V., et al. (1998) Signalling of RET receptor tyrosine kinase through the C-Jun NH2-terminal protein kinases (JNKS)-evidence for a divergence of the erks and jnks pathways induced by RET. *Oncogene* **16,** 2435–2445.
25. Hofstra, R. M., Landsvater, R. M., Ceccherini, I., Stulp, R. P., Stelwagen, T., Luo, Y., et al. (1994) A mutation in the RET proto-oncogene associated with multiple endocrine neoplasia type 2B and sporadic medullary thyroid carcinoma. *Nature* **367,** 375–376.
26. Wohllk, N., Cote, G. J., Bugalho, M. M. J., Ordonez, N., Evans, D. B., Goepfert, H., et al. (1996) Relevance of RET proto-oncogene mutations in sporadic medullary thyroid carcinoma. *J. Clin. Endocrinol. Metab.* **81,** 3740–3745.
27. Bolino, A., Schuffenecker, I., Luo, Y., Seri, M., Silengo, M., Tocco, T., et al. (1995) RET mutations in exons 13 and 14 of FMTC patients. *Oncogene* **10,** 2415–2419.
28. Lin, L. F., Doherty, D. H., Lile, J. D., Bektesh, S., and Colline, F. (1993) GDNF: a glial cell line-derived neurotrophic factor for midbrain dopaminergic neurons. *Science* **260,** 1130–1132.
29. Schuchardt, A., D'Agati, V., Larsson-Blomberg, L., Costantini, F., and Pachnis, V. (1994) Defects in the kidney and enteric nervous system of mice lacking the tyrosine kinase receptor Ret. *Nature* **367,** 380–383.
30. Sanchez, M., Silos-Santiago, I., Frisen, J., He, B., Lira, S., and Barbacid, M. (1996) Newborn mice lacking GDNF display renal agenesis and absence of enteric neurons, but no deficits in midbrain dopaminergic neurons. *Nature* **382,** 70–73.
31. Pichel, J. G., Shen, L., Sheng, H. Z., Granholm, A.-C., Drago, J., Grinberg, A., et al. (1996) Defects in enteric innervation and kidney development in mice lacking GDNF. *Nature* **382,** 73–76.

32. Jing, S., Wen, D., Yu, Y., Holst, P. L., Luo, Y., Fang, M., et al. (1996) GDNF-induced activation of the Ret protein tyrosine kinase is mediated by GDNFR-α, a novel receptor for GDNF. *Cell* **85,** 1113–1124.
33. Moore, M. W., Klein, R. D., Farinas, I., Sauer, H., Armanini, M., Phillips, H., et al. (1996) Renal and neuronal abnormalities in mice lacking GDNF. *Nature* **382,** 76–79.
34. Tsuzuki, T., Takahashi, M., Asai, N., Iwashita, T., Matsuyama, M., and Asai J. (1995) Spatial and temporal expression of the *ret* proto-oncogene product in embryonic, infant and adult rat tissues. *Oncogene* **10,** 191–198.
35. Trupp, M., Raynoschek, C., Belluardo, N., and Ibanez, C. (1998) Multiple GPI-anchored receptors control GDNF-dependent and independent activation of the c-ret receptor tyrosine kinase. *Mol. Cell. Neurosci.* **11,** 47–63.
36. Baloh, R., Gorodinsky, A., Golden, J., Tansey, M., Keck, C., Popescu, N., Johnson, E., and Milbrandt J. (1998) GFR-alpha-3 is an orphan member of the GDNF/neurturin/persephin rececptor family. *Proc. Natl. Acad. Sci. USA* **95,** 5801–5806.
37. Baloh, R. H., Tansey, M. G., Golden, J. P., Creedon, D. J., Heuckeroth, R. O., Keck, C. L., et al. (1997) TrnR2, a novel receptor that mediates neurturin and GDNF signaling through Ret. *Neuron* **18,** 793–802.
38. Milbrandt, J., de Sauvage, F. J., Fahrner T. J., et al. (1998) Persephin, a novel neurotrophic factor related to GDNF and neurturin. *Neuron* **20,** 245–253.
39. Puliti, A., Covone, A. E., Bicocchi, M. P., Bolino, A., Lerone, M., Martucciello, G., Jasonni, V., and Romeo G. (1993) Deleted and normal chromosome 10 homologs from a patient with Hirschsprung disease isolated in two cell hybrids through enrichment by immunomagnetic selection. *Cytogenet. Cell. Genet.* **63,** 102–106.
40. Borst, M. J., Van Camp, J. M., Peacock, M. L., and Decker, R. A. (1995) Mutational analysis of multiple endocrine neoplasia type 2A associated with Hirschsprung's disease. *Surgery* **117,** 386–391.
41. Martucciello, G., Thompson, H., Mazzola, C., Morando, A., Bertagnon, M., Negri, F., et al. (1998) GDNF deficit in Hirschsprung's disease. *J. Pediatr. Surg.* **33,** 99–102.
42. Puffenberger, E., Hosoda, K., Washington, S., Nakao, K., deWit, D., Yanagisawa, M., and Chakravarti, A. (1994) A missense mutation of the endothelin-B receptor gene in multigenic Hirschsprung's disease. *Cell* **79,** 1257–1266.
43. Hofstra, R. M., Osinga, J., Tan-Sindhunata, G., Wu, Y., Kamsteeg, E. J., Stulp, R. P., et al. (1996) A homozygous mutation in the endothelin-3 gene associated with a combined Waardenburg type 2 and Hirschsprung phenotype (Shah-Waardenburg syndrome). *Nature Genet.* **12,** 445–447.
44. Khorana, S., Gagel, R. F., and Cote G. J. (1994) Direct sequencing of PCR products in agarose gel slices. *Nucleic Acids Res.* **22,** 3425–6.
45. Gagel, R. F., Cote, G. J., Martins Bugalho, M. J. G., Boyd, A. E., Cummings, T., Goepfert, H., et al. (1995) Clinical use of molecular information in the management of multiple endocrine neoplasia type 2A. *J. Intl. Med.* **238,** 333–341.
46. Gagel, R. F., Tashjian, A. H., Jr., Cummings, T., Papathanasopoulos, N., Kaplan, M. M., DeLellis, R. A., et al. (1988) The clinical outcome of prospective screening for multiple endocrine neoplasia type 2a: an 18–year experience. *N. Engl. J. Med.* **318,** 478–484.

Chapter 16

Genetics of Paget's Disease of Bone

Frederick R. Singer and Robin J. Leach

Introduction

In 1877, Sir James Paget described a localized skeletal disorder affecting five patients over 40 yr of age, which he termed osteitis deformans *(1)*. He chose this term for the disorder because of the deformities of his patients and the supposition that an unknown type of inflammatory process was responsible for its manifestations. His detailed and lucid description of the clinical and pathological characteristics of the disorder led to the use of the term Paget's disease of bone to represent this condition of abnormal skeletal remodeling. The primary underlying abnormality appears to be local activation of osteoclastic bone resorption which can proceed slowly to affect an entire bone. The osteoclasts, which are often quite large, contain nuclear and cytoplasmic inclusions which closely resemble nucleocapsids of the Paramyxoviridae virus family *(2)*. In response to the resorptive process, osteoblastic repair is initiated, but the resulting new bone formation is chaotic and excessive. This finally leads over many years to the enlarged, but fragile, bones that Paget noted in his patients.

Familial Aggregation of Paget's Disease

In 1882 Paget described an additional seven cases *(3)* and after having reported a total of 23 patients by 1889 *(4)*, Paget noted that "I have tried in vain to trace any hereditary tendency to the disease. I have not found it twice in the same family." He apparently was unaware of the brief reports of Pick *(5)* in 1883 and Lunn *(6)* in 1885, who described probable Paget's disease in a father and daughter and in two sisters, respectively. During the first 25 yr after the initial paper of Paget the disorder was recognized by the characteristic skeletal deformities it produced. The first description of the radiographic appearance of Paget's disease appeared in 1901 *(7)*. The use of radiographs then allowed earlier diagnosis and was to a considerable degree responsible for the recognition that the disease was not rare, as was first believed. When it was realized in 1929 that increased activity of the enzyme alkaline phosphatase in the circulation was associated with Paget's disease *(8)*, this blood test became another means of discovering previously unsuspected lesions after a radiographic survey was ordered. These diagnostic tests made Paget's disease more widely recognized. Thus, during the first half of the 20th century, large series of patients were published *(9,10)* and numerous reports appeared of families in which more than one case was present *(11)*. This led McKusick to state that "The hereditary nature of the process appears to be established *(11)*. He felt that the accumulated data indicated that the trait for Paget's disease was controlled by a simple autosomal Mendelian-dominant gene.

In the earlier reports of familial Paget's disease the average number of patients in an affected family was less than three. More recently, kindreds have been described with 10 *(12)* and 12 *(13)* affected family members. Paget's disease has also been described in five identical twins, although only in one pair of twins was molecular evidence of monozygosity reported *(14)*. Considering that one pair of identical twins is produced approximately every 300 births *(15)* it is somewhat surprising that so few examples have been reported.

Although there can be little doubt that there is a genetic basis for Paget's disease in some families, it is uncertain what proportion of the total population of patients with Paget's disease represents sporadic disease and what proportion represents familial. In large studies involving 100 index cases or more, the proportion of patients with a family history of Paget's disease was 1.1 to 13.8% *(16)*. A positive family history was generally defined as a known diagnosis of Paget's disease in at least one first degree relative. The two largest series were published by Sofaer and colleagues *(16)* (407 patients) and Siris and colleagues *(17)* (788 patients). Sofaer found that 13.8% of the patients had a positive family history and that there was a 10-fold higher prevalence of Paget's disease among parents and siblings of index cases compared with parents and siblings of unaffected spouses. Siris found that 12.3% of the patients had a positive family history and that first degree relatives of the patients had nearly seven times the prevalence of Paget's disease as did the relatives of the spouses.

It is quite possible that these studies underestimate the true proportion of familial Paget's disease since the diagnosis is usually not apparent until the age of 50 yr and in many affected individuals there are no signs or symptoms. In support of this is a study of first-degree relatives of index cases in Spain *(18)*. By utilizing bone scans, the most sensitive means of detecting Paget's disease, Morales-Piga and colleagues found a 40% prevalence of familial Paget's disease in a clinic population of 35 patients. This could be an overestimate because of the relatively small number of index cases. However, this study should give impetus to future studies which should more closely evaluate the familial grouping of Paget's disease in other populations.

Another finding by Sofaer and colleagues *(16)* was the diagnosis of three years earlier of Paget's disease in those with familial disease compared to sporadic patients. The disease was diagnosed nine years earlier in the patients described by Morales-Piga and colleagues *(18)*. Kanis *(19)* found no difference in age at diagnosis, but did observe that patients with a family history had more lesions detected by radiographs and bone scans as well as higher serum total alkaline phosphatase activity, reflecting more widespread disease. Morales-Piga and colleagues also found that familial Paget's disease patients had twice the number of affected bones as did sporadic patients. It is now generally accepted that patients with familial disease tend to have an earlier diagnosis and more severe manifestations of Paget's disease.

HLA Typing of Paget's Disease Patients

Because of known associations between disease susceptibility and histocompatibility loci on chromosome 6, numerous studies have been performed since 1975 to determine if there is any association between human leucocyte antigens (HLA) and Paget's disease. A variety of studies have been conducted. HLA typing in groups of patients has most frequently been performed *(19–24)*. The typing of Class 1 antigens has produced no significant results. However, in the only two studies in which Class II antigens were assessed, significant associations were found *(25,26)*. An increased incidence of HLA-DQW1 and HLA-DR2 was found in a preliminary report of 53 patients in Los Angeles *(25)*. A second study of 25 Ashkenazi Jews in Israel revealed an increased incidence of HLA-DR2 *(26)*. Another study relevant to HLA typing is a preliminary report of increased HLA DRB1*1104 (Class II) gene frequency in Ashkenazi Jews with Paget's disease living in Los Angeles and New York *(27)*. Since Asian populations have a very low frequency of the HLA DRB*1104 gene this could be related to the rarity of Paget's disease in people of Asian ancestry. However, the significance of all these observations is unclear. Two possibilities arise: these associations could be the result of an epistatic effect of these HLA loci with Paget's disease or, alternatively, these associations could be evidence of loose linkage of a predisposition for Paget's disease to a HLA DR locus. The latter interpretation would be consistent with a founder effect in these populations.

HLA Linkage Studies

In studies of families with Paget's disease, the results of linkage studies to the HLA loci have been variable. Studies in New York *(28)* and New Zealand *(29)* gave suggestive evidence of linkage using standard linkage analysis. In the study from New York, three families with 29 informative children (all over the age of 45) were utilized. These kindreds were typed at the HLA-A, -B, and -C loci. Using haplotype data, the investigators *(28)* obtained a maximum LOD score of 2.44 at a recombination fraction of 0.01. However, since a LOD score of 3 is needed to establish linkage, these data suggest but do not establish linkage between HLA and a Paget's disease predisposition locus. Likewise, the families studied in New Zealand were not sufficient to establish linkage between the HLA locus and a predisposition gene for Paget's disease. In those studies *(29)*, the investigators described two new kindreds. The first New Zealand kindred included four affected and four unaffected members. All four unaffected individuals were evaluated before the age of 45. In this kindred, only one recombinant was observed between the HLA loci and the putative Paget's disease predisposition locus. This "supposed" recombinant was in a 42-yr-old female who had the "affected" haplotype but did not appear to be affected based on a normal serum alkaline phosphatase level and no clinical signs of Paget's disease. In the second New Zealand kindred, no recombinants were observed between the Paget's disease predisposition locus and the HLA loci in the five informative loci. For the linkage analysis, the investigators *(29)* used the data from all five families [three from New York *(28)* and two from New Zealand *(29)*]. The peak LOD score obtained was 3.67 at a recombination fraction of 0.10. Thus, these combined data were sufficient for establishing a predisposition locus for Paget's disease on human chromosome 6 near, but not at, the HLA loci.

Two other family studies have been published which explored the linkage of Paget's disease to the HLA region with both studies concluding that there was no evidence for linkage to the HLA region in their kindreds *(30,31)*. One study used a family from Rochester, MN *(30)* which included six informative meioses. In this study, two recombinants were observed between the HLA loci and the Paget's disease predisposition gene. Although no LOD score calculations were presented, this pedigree does not appear to be sufficiently large to exclude linkage. Such an exclusion would require a -2 LOD score at the same locus. Similarly, a study was published on a single family from Korea involving five informative meioses *(31)*. One recombinant was observed in an affected individual without the "affected" haplotype. Once again, no LOD score calculations were presented. In summary, both of these studies found recombinants with the HLA loci. It should be noted that the original reports of the linkage *(28,29)* between HLA and a Paget's disease predisposition gene showed recombinants in their kindreds. The original investigations placed the Paget's disease predisposition gene within 10 recombination units from HLA. The exact location of this predisposition locus, i.e., proximal or distal, with respect to HLA loci is unclear since only HLA markers were typed in all of these kindred. Therefore, it is difficult to conclude whether the families from Minnesota and Korea are linked to a locus near HLA on chromosome 6 locus or map to another region of the genome, since precise genetic mapping of the original locus was never performed. These two families are not sufficiently large enough to prove the hypothesis that Paget's disease is genetically heterogeneous. However, more recent studies have shown that there is more than one Paget's disease predisposition locus in the genome.

Genetics of Familial Expansile Osteolysis

A remarkable kindred in Northern Ireland has been described in which 46 members over five generations have been found to have a skeletal disorder that resembles Paget's disease but exhibits some striking differences *(32)*. The disease is inherited through an autosomal dominant pattern of transmission and has been termed familial expansile osteolysis (FEO), emphasizing the dominance of the osteolytic process. Unlike typical Paget's disease, these patients usually have an onset of symptoms in the early adult years, the lesions are more generalized, and in contrast to Paget's disease sclerotic bone is not the characteristic radiographic finding *(33)*. However, the osteoclasts in lesions of FEO do exhibit inclusions similar to those in Paget's disease *(34)*.

To identify the locus involved in FEO, a genome-wide scan using genetic markers was performed. Over 300 polymorphic markers were typed through this family by Hughes and co-workers *(35)*. After excluding more than 95% of the genome, a locus for FEO was finally identified on 18q. A maximum LOD score of 11.5 with a recombination fraction of zero was obtained. Because of the similarities between Paget's disease and FEO, Hughes proposed that FEO could be an allelic variant of Paget's disease, i.e., these diseases could be caused by different mutations of the same gene. The identification of the FEO gene could therefore help gain an understanding of the etiology of Paget's disease *(32)*. If her hypothesis is true, then Paget's disease kindreds that link to chromosome 18 should exist.

Genetic Linkage of Paget's Disease to Chromosome 18q

Within the last few years, a number of pagetic families have been evaluated with genetic markers from the FEO region of chromosome 18. Cody and co-workers *(12)* evaluated 16 DNA samples from one large kindred, with eight individuals affected with Paget's disease over the age of 34. Their analysis of the data from chromosome 18 yields a two-point LOD score of 3.4 using a genetic marker known to be tightly linked to the FEO locus. Subsequently Haslam and colleagues found evidence of linkage to 18q in five families with Paget's disease *(36)*. A preliminary report of a French pedigree also found linkage to 18q *(37)*. These results supported Hughes' hypothesis that FEO may be an allelic variant of Paget's disease, and that both disorders are caused by the same gene. An alternative explanation, which cannot be eliminated at this time, is that this predisposition locus for Paget's disease could be caused by a different gene which is tightly linked to the FEO locus.

Strong evidence of genetic heterogeneity has been presented in one report *(36)* and three abstracts *(37–39)*. In six families no evidence of linkage to chromosome 18 was found. Data regarding HLA loci were not presented in any of

Table 1
Summary of Linkage Studies with Familial Paget's Disease

Authors (references)	No. of families studied	Region of genome evaluated	Conclusion of authors
Fontino et al. *(28)*	3	HLA	Suggestive linkage
Tilyard et al. *(29)*	2 + 3 from ref. *(30)*	HLA	Proof of linkage
Moore and Hoffman *(30)*	1	HLA	No evidence of linkage
Kim et al. *(31)*	1	HLA	No evidence of linkage
Cody et al. *(12)*	1	18q, near FEO locus	Proof of linkage
Haslam et al. *(36)*	8	18q, near FEO	5 families linked 3 families not linked
Lucotte *(37)*	1	18q, near FEO	Proof of linkage
Genuario et al. *(38)*	2	18q, near FEO	No evidence of linkage
Brown et al. *(39)*	1	18q, near FEO	No evidence of linkage

Osteosarcoma in Paget's Disease

The most feared complication of Paget's disease is osteosarcoma. Five of the 23 patients originally reported by Paget developed this deadly neoplasm *(1,3,4)*. The tumors develop in bone lesions previously affected by Paget's disease. The frequency of these malignant transformations in Paget's disease has been reported to range from 0.7% *(40)* to 5.5% *(41)*, with the lower frequency reported in studies in which both asymptomatic and symptomatic cases of Paget's disease were followed. Although there is clearly an increased risk for osteosarcoma in Paget's disease, the molecular basis for this finding remains unclear.

Paget's disease is primarily a disease of the osteoclast, although there are increased numbers of osteoblasts in pagetic lesions. In contrast, all osteosarcomas are of osteoblastic lineage. It has been suggested that the malignant change which occurs in association with Paget's disease is the result of prolonged abnormal cellular activity of the osteoblasts *(42)*. Thus, it may be hypothesized that the observed higher incidence of osteosarcoma in Paget's disease patients is related to highly active osteoblasts.

Of considerable interest from the genetic standpoint are four reports of familial osteosarcomas occurring in familial Paget's disease *(43–46)*. Barry described two male siblings with osteosarcoma who also had an uncle and aunt with Paget's disease *(43)*.Brenton and colleagues observed the combination in two male siblings who had another brother with Paget's disease *(44)*. Nassar and Gravanis *(45)* described a father and son who had both diseases. No other relatives were known to be affected by either problem. More recently, Wu and colleagues described a family in which a brother and a sister with Paget's disease died of osteosarcoma *(46)*. A second sister had Paget's disease only. These studies further demonstrate that Paget's disease families have a high incidence of osteosarcoma.

Recent evidence has indicated a molecular link between Paget's disease and osteosarcoma, which raises another possible explanation for the increased incidence of osteosarcoma in Paget's patients. In an attempt to identify tumor suppressor genes involved in the development of osteosarcoma, Nellisery and co-workers *(47)* have compared genetic analysis of osteosarcomas with matched normal controls. They have detected a tumor-specific loss of constitutional heterozygosity (also known as loss-of-heterozygosity, LOH) on 18q in 61/96sporadic osteosarcomas and in 6/7 osteosarcomas arising in Paget's disease. The region with highest loss on 18q is hypothesized to be the site of a tumor suppressor gene. The critical region for this putative tumor suppressor gene is completely contained within the critical region for both familial Paget's disease as defined by Cody *(12)* and the critical region for FEO *(32)*. This finding provides some molecular genetic evidence that the association between Paget's disease and osteosarcoma could be the result of a single gene or two tightly linked genes on chromosome 18. If it were the latter, than Paget's disease and osteosarcoma could be part of a contiguous gene syndrome. Identification of the gene(s) in this region will be critical for determining which hypothesis is correct.

Giant Cell Tumor in Paget's Disease

Giant cell tumors of bone can arise in pagetic lesions but appear to be less common than sarcomas as less than 100 cases have been reported since 1931 *(48)*. The only report in which the two problems occur in one family describes a mother, daughter, and a second cousin of the daughter with Paget's disease and a giant cell tumor *(49)*. However, subsequent review of the pathology by Upchurch and colleagues led to the opinion that these cases were more likely giant cell reparative granulomas *(50)*. At the present it appears uncertain whether giant cell tumors occur in Paget's disease on a familial basis.

Summary

By the middle of the 20th century it began to be appreciated that Paget's disease could be hereditary and that the trait was controlled by a simple autosomal Mendelian-dominant gene. Genetic linkage studies of a disorder similar to Paget's disease, FEO, revealed a locus for FEO on chromosome 18q. Studies in several Paget's disease kindreds have identified a similar locus on 18q but other families failed to demonstrate this linkage. Thus, it appears that there are two or more predisposition loci for Paget's disease.

Osteosarcoma is an uncommon complication of Paget's disease. Recent studies have indicated that tumor-specific loss of constitutional heterozygosity on 18q can be detected in osteosarcomas arising in pagetic lesions as well as in osteosarcomas arising in patients without Paget's disease. This suggests a tumor suppressor gene (contained within the critical region for both familial Paget's disease and FEO) may be involved in the development of osteosarcoma. The association between Paget's disease and osteosarcoma could be the result of a single gene or two tightly linked genes on chromosome 18.

References

1. Paget, J. (1877) On a form of chronic inflammation of the bones (osteitis deformans). *Med.-Chir. Trans.* **60,** 37–64.
2. Singer, F. R. (1996) Paget's disease of bone. Possible viral basis. *Trends Endocrinol. Metab.* **7,** 258–261.
3. Paget, J. (1882) Additional cases of osteitis deformans. *Trans. Roy. Med.-Chir. Soc., Glasgow* **65,** 225–236.
4. Paget, J. (1889) Remarks on osteitis deformans. *Illustr. Med. News* **2,** 181–182.
5. Pick, A. (1883) Osteitis deformans. *Lancet* **2,** 1125–1126.
6. Lunn, J. R. (1885) Four cases of osteitis deformans. *Trans. Clin. Soc. London* **18,** 272.
7. Beclere, A. (1901) Radiographie d'un cas de maladie de Paget. *Bull. Mem. Soc. Med. Hosp. Paris* **18,** 929–931.
8. Kay, H. D. (1929) Plasma phosphatase in osteitis deformans and in other diseases of bone. *Br. J. Exp. Pathol.* **10,** 253–259.
9. Gutman, A. B. and Kasabach, H. (1936) Paget's disease (osteitis deformans). Analysis of 116 cases. *Am. J. Med. Sci.* **191,** 361–380.
10. Dickson, D. D., Camp, J. D., and Ghormley, R. K. (1945) Osteitis deformans, Paget's disease of the bone. *Radiology* **44,** 449–470.
11. McKusick, V. A. (1956) *Heritable Disorders of Connective Tissue,* C. V. Mosby Co., St. Louis, MO, pp. 200–205.
12. Cody, J. D., Singer, F. R., Roodman, G. D., Otterud, B., Lewis, T. B., Leppert, M., and Leach, R. J. (1997) Genetic linkage of Paget disease of bone to chromosome 18q. *Am. J. Hum. Genet.* **61,** 1117–1122.
13. Morales-Piga, A., Gonzalez-Lanza, M., Arnaiz-Villena, A., Martinez-Escribano, B., Alonso-Ruiz, A., and Zea-Mendoza, A. (1983) Familial clustering in Paget's disease, etiopathologenic implications. Presentation of a family with 12 affected members. *Med. Clin. (Barcelona)* **18,** 43–36.
14. Melick R. A. and Martin T. J. (1975) Paget's disease in identical twins. *Aust. N. Z. J. Med.* **5,** 564–565.
15. Myrianthopoulos, N. C. (1970) An epidemiologic survey of twins in a large, prospectively studied population. *Am. J. Hum. Gen.* **22,** 611–629.
16. Sofaer, J. A., Holloway, S. M., and Emery A. E. H. (1983) A family study of Paget's disease of bone. *J. Epidemiol. Commun. Health* **37,** 226–231.
17. Siris, E. S., Ottman, R., Flaster, E., and Kelsey, J. L. (1991) Familial aggregation of Paget's disease of bone. *J. Bone Miner. Res.* 6, 495–500.

18. Morales-Piga, A. A., Rey-Rey, J. S., Corres-Gonzales, J., Garcia-Sagredo, J. M., and Lopez-Abente, G. (1995) Frequency and characteristics of familial aggregation in Paget disease of bone. *J. Bone. Miner. Res.* **10,** 663–670.
19. Kanis, J. A. (1991) *Pathophysiology and Treatment of Paget's Disease of Bone,* Martin Dunit Ltd., London.
20. Simon, L., Blotman, F., Seignalet, J., and Claustre, J. (1975) Etiologie de la maladie osseuse de Paget. *Rev. Rheum.* **42**, 535–544.
21. Roux, H., Mercier, P., Maestracci, D., Eisinger, J., and Recordier, A. M. (1975) HL-A et maladie de Paget. *Rev. Rheum.* **42**, 661–662.
22. Cullen, P., Russel, G. G., Walton, R. J., and Whiteley, J. (1976) Frequencies of HLA-A and HLA-B histocompatibility antigens in Paget's disease of bone. *Tissue Antigens* **7,** 55–56.
23. Singer, F. R., Schiller, A. L., Pyle, E. B., and Krane, S. M. (1978) Paget's disease of bone, in *Metabolic Bone Disease*, Vol. II. (Avioli, L. V., Krane, S. M., eds.), Academic Press, New York, pp. 489–575.
24. Gordon, M. T., Cartwright, E. J., Mercer, S., Anderson, D. C., and Sharpe, P. T. (1994) HLA polymorphisms in Paget's disease of bone. *Semin. Arthritis Rheum.* **23,** 229.
25. Singer, F. R., Mills, B. G., Park, M. S., Takemura, S., and Terasaki, P. I. (1985) Increased HLA-DQWI antigen pattern in Paget's disease of bone. *Clin. Res.* **33,** 574A.
26. Foldes, J., Shamir, S., Brautbor, C., Schermann, L., and Menczel, J. (1991) HLA-D antigens and Paget's disease of bone. *Clin. Orthop. Rel. Res.* **266,** 301–303.
27. Singer, F. R., Siris, E. S., Knirem, A., Gjertson, D., and Terasaki, P. I. (1996) The HLA DRB1*1104 gene frequency is increased in Ashkenazi Jews with Paget's disease of bone. *J. Bone Miner. Res.* **11(Suppl. 1),** S369.
28. Fotino, M., Haymovits, A., and Falk, C. T. (1971) Evidence for linkage between HLA and Paget's disease. *Transplant. Proc.* **9,** 1867,1868.
29. Tilyard, M. W., Gardner, R. J. M., Milligan, L., Cleary, T. A., and Stewart, R. D. H. (1982) A probable linkage between familial Paget's disease and the HLA loci. *Aust. N. Z. J. Med.* **12,** 498–500.
30. Moore, S. B. and Hoffman, D. L. (1988) Absence of HLA linkage in a family with osteitis deformans (Paget's disease of bone). *Tissue Antigens* **31,** 69,70.
31. Kim, G. S., Kim, S. H., Cho, J. K., Park, J. Y., Shin, M. J., Shong, Y. K., et al. (1997) Paget bone disease involving young adults in 3 generations of a Korean family. *Medicine* **76,** 157–169.
32. Hughes, A. E. and Barr, R. J. (1996) Familial expansile osteolysis, A genetic model of Paget's disease, in *The Molecular Biology of Paget's Disease* (Sharpe, P. T., ed.), R. G. Landes Co., Austin, TX, pp. 179–199.
33. Crone, M. D. and Wallace, R. G. (1990) The radiographic features of familial osteolytic osteolysis. *Skeletal Radiol.* **19,** 245–250.
34. Dickson, G. R., Shirodaria, P. V., and Kanis, J. A. (1991) Familial expansile osteolysis, a morphological, histomorphometric and serological study. *Bone* **12,** 331–338.
35. Hughes, A. E., Shearman, A. M., Weber, J. L., Barr, R. J., Wallace, R. G., Osterberg, P. H., Nevin, N. C., and Mollan, R. C. (1994) Genetic linkage of familial expansile osteolysis to chromosome 18q. *Hum. Mol. Genet.* **3,** 359–361.
36. Haslam, S. I., Van Hul, W., Morales-Piga, A., Balemans, W., San-Millan, J. L., Nakatsuka, K., et al. (1998) Paget's disease of bone, evidence for a susceptibility locus on chromosome 18q and for genetic heterogeneity. *J. Bone Miner. Res.* **13,** 911–917.
37. Lucotte, G. (1999) Genetic linkage of Paget's disease to chromosome 18q in a French pedigree. *Bone* **24(Suppl),** 31S.

38. Genuario, R., Scherpbier-Heddema, J. T., Pons-Estel, B., Soler, R. I., Parque, S., Reginato, et al. (1997) Exclusion of a chromosome 18q locus in two large families with Paget's disease of the bone. *Arthritis Rheum.* **40(Suppl),** S279.
39. Brown, J. P., Raymond, V., and Morissette, J. (1999) Genetic epidemiology of paget's disease of bone in eastern Québec. *Bone* **24(Suppl),** 15S.
40. Hadjipavlou, A., Lander, P., Srolovitz, H., and Enker, I. P. (1992) Malignant transformation in Paget disease of bone. *Cancer* **70,** 2802–2808.
41. Freydinger, J. E., Duhig, J. T., and McDonald, L. W. (1963) Sarcoma complicating Paget's disease of bone. A study of seven cases with report of one long survival after surgery. *Arch. Pathol.* **75,** 496–500.
42. Smith, B. J. and Eveson, J. W. (1981) Paget's disease of bone with particular reference to dentistry. *J. Oral Pathol.* **10,** 233–247.
43. Barry, H. C. (1969) *Paget's Disease of Bone*, E. & S. Livingstone, London.
44. Brenton, D. P., Isenberg, D. A., and Bertram, J. (1980) Osteosarcoma complicating familial Paget's disease. *Postgrad. Med. J.* **56,** 238–243.
45. Nassar, V. H. and Gravanis, M. B. (1981) Familial osteogenic sarcoma occurring in pagetoid bone. *Am. J. Clin. Pathol.* **76,** 235–239.
46. Wu, R. K., Trumble T. E., and Ruwe, P. A. (1991) Familial incidence of Paget's disease and secondary osteogenic sarcoma. A report of three cases from a single family. *Clin. Ortho. Rel. Res.* **265,** 306–309.
47. Nellissery, M. J., Padalecki, S. S., Brkanac, Z., Singer, F. R., Roodman, G. D., Unni, K. K., et al. (1998) Evidence for a novel osteosarcoma tumor–suppressor gene in the chromosome 18 region genetically linked with Paget disease of bone. *Am. J. Hum. Genet.* **63,** 817–824.
48. Singer, F. R. and Mills, B. G. (1993) Giant cell tumor arising in Paget's disease of bone. Recurrences after 36 years. *Clin. Orthop.* **293,** 293–301.
49. Jacobs, T. P., Michelsen, J., Poloy, J. S., D'Adomo, A. C. and Canfield, R. E. (1979) Giant cell tumor in Paget's disease bone. Familial and geographic clustering. *Cancer* **44,** 742–747.
50. Upchurch, K. S., Simon, L. S., Schiller, A. L., Rosenthal, D. I. Campion, E. W., and Krane, S. M. (1983) Giant cell reparative granuloma of Paget's disease of bone: a unique clinical entity. *Ann. Intern. Med.* **98,** 35–40.

Chapter 17

Osteopetrosis

L. Lyndon Key, Jr.

Introduction

Osteopetrosis results from a reduction in bone resorption relative to bone formation, leading to an accumulation of excessive amounts of bone. The relative decrease in resorption is a consequence of inadequate osteoclastic bone resorption. This imbalance leads to a thickening of the cortical region and a decrease in the size of the medullary space in the long bones, with sclerosis of the base of the skull *(1,2)* and vertebral bodies. There are a number of serious consequences resulting from the excessive accumulation of bone. A reduced marrow space results in decrease in hematopoiesis even to the point of complete bone marrow failure. Extramedullary hematopoiesis occurs, but is unable to compensate for the reduction in medullary blood cell production. A decrease in the caliber of the cranial nerve and vascular canals leads to nerve compression and vascular compromise. Dense bones are subject to fracture and are poorly vascularized, predisposing the bones to necrosis and infection.

An understanding of osteopetrosis in humans has been intertwined with the description and creation of a variety of animal mutations in osteoclastic function *(3)*. While the precise genetic defect in most patients remains to be established (one exception being the deficiency in carbonic anhydrase type II *[4,5]*), the animal models have contributed substantially to the understanding of osteoclastic function and dysfunction. The osteoclast biology learned from these mutants has led to a variety of treatment strategies that have been used in patients with osteopetrosis. An understanding of the genetic basis of the animal mutations has generated a list of candidate genes which may prove to be the basis for discovering the genetic defects in humans.

The Genetics of Osteoporosis and Metabolic Bone Disease
Ed.: M. J. Econs © Humana Press Inc., Totowa, NJ

Clinical Description

Classically, osteopetrosis has been divided into a fatal infantile malignant form, and a milder adult form of osteopetrosis with long-term survival *(6–9)*. Recently, a variety of intermediate forms have been described. Without knowledge of the genetic defect explaining the osteoclastic dysfunction, it has been difficult to delineate the mechanisms of these different forms.

Infantile Forms

A variety of presentations of osteopetrosis have been seen in infancy. In general, patients have had sporadic forms that appear to have an autosomal recessive inheritance. While the severe, malignant form predominates, milder forms and autosomal dominant inheritance patterns have also been observed in individuals diagnosed in the neonatal period *(9,10)*. In the absence of a known genetic defect in osteoclastic function, histomorphometric and clinical parameters have been established to describe the degree of severity.

Malignant

Patients with osteopetrosis presenting at birth or in early infancy are usually referred to as having the severe, malignant form. The implication is that these patients will have severe sequellae and death during the first decade of life. This has justified the use of treatment modalities, such as bone marrow transplantation, that carry a high risk of mortality and morbidity *(11–13)*. Patients with the malignant form are characterized by a diffusely sclerotic skeleton with little or no bone marrow space evident, even at birth (Fig. 1) *(14)*. In addition, there is evidence of a severe defect in bone resorption leading to the presence of the "bone in bone" appearance on radiographs (Fig. 2) and in cartilaginous islands within mineralized bone on histology (Fig. 3).

However, some patients with this phenotype will not have a fatal outcome. Indeed, up to 30% of patients diagnosed with severe, malignant osteopetrosis are still alive at age 6 yr with rare patients surviving into the second or third decade *(14)*. While the quality of life is reported to be poor, up to half of the surviving patients, despite a variety of skeletal and neurologic impairments have normal intelligence and are capable of attending school (Dr. Jane Charles, personal communication).

A subgroup of patients have an extremely malignant disease. In a group of 33 patients reported by Gerritsen et al., eight patients had hematological and visual impairment before three months of age *(14)*. All eight of these patients died before the age of 12 mo. Hematological impairment before 6 mo of life is prognostic of a markedly reduced survival rate; however, visual impairment alone does not correlate with an early fatal outcome.

Cytological evidence of large osteoclasts with increased numbers of nuclei and a markedly increased amount of ruffled border membrane correlates with a poor prognosis for cure with bone marrow transplantation *(13,15)*. While there is no exact explanation for the reduced success in cure by transplantation, the defect

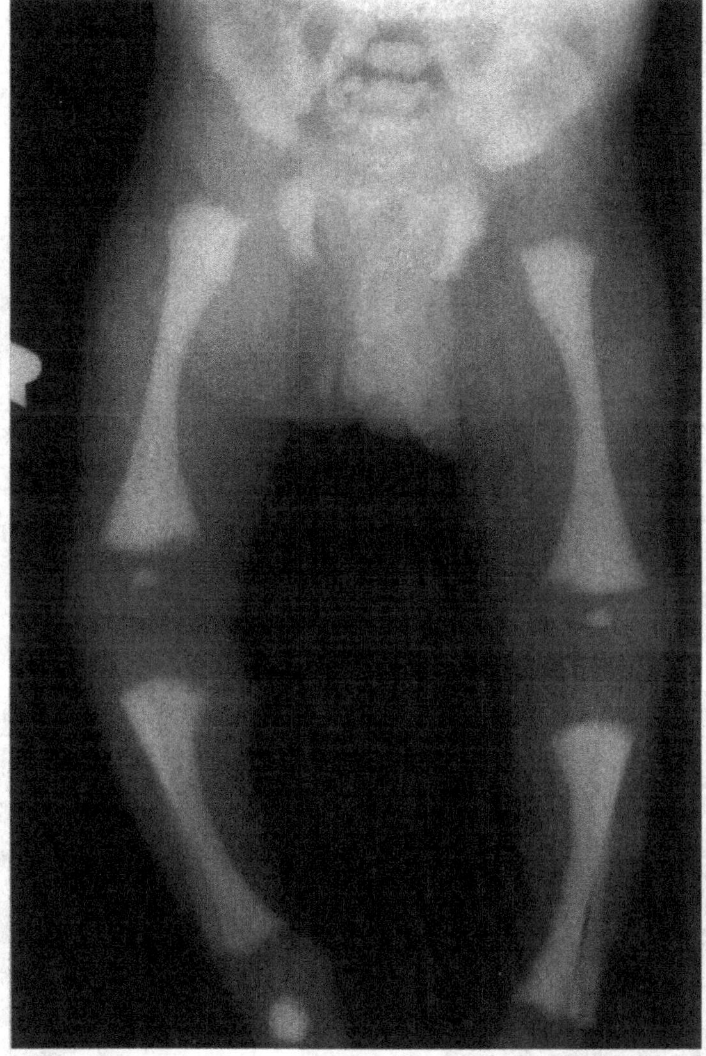

Fig. 1. The skeleton, both the long bones and the pelvis, are shown to be sclerotic in this radiograph of a 5-d-old infant with anemia and optic nerve compression. Patients with this severe presentation have a 100% chance of death before age 1 yr, if untreated. Note that no intramedullary space is seen in the long bones or the pelvis.

in bone resorption in these patients could be explained if the osteoclast itself were normal, but some other aspect of the bone rendered it less resorbable. Thus, histologic and electronmicroscopic analysis of osteoclasts is recommended before a transplantation is undertaken.

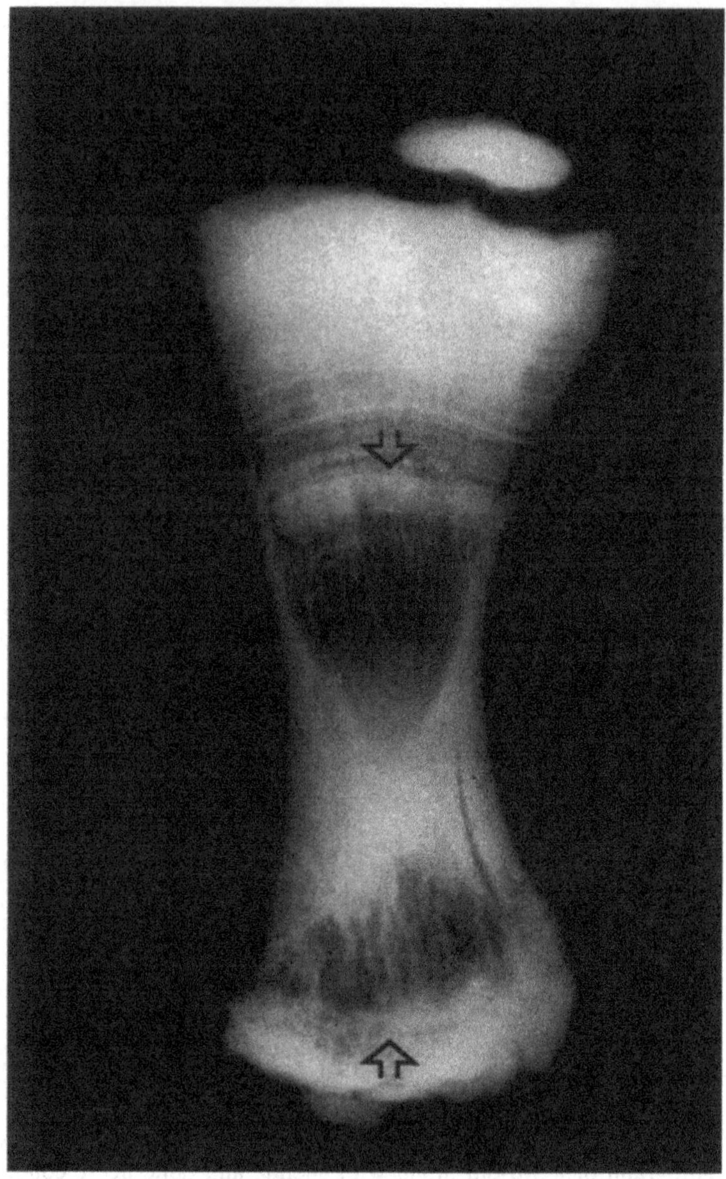

Fig. 2. This radiograph shows a phalangeal bone, obtained at autopsy from a 7-yr-old with malignant osteopetrosis treated with calcitriol. Note the presence of the original bony template (endobone, between the arrows) that was present at birth and never remodeled. The radiograph shows the presence of mineralized bone which has been laid down outside of this original bone/cartilage template without the underlying template having been resorbed.

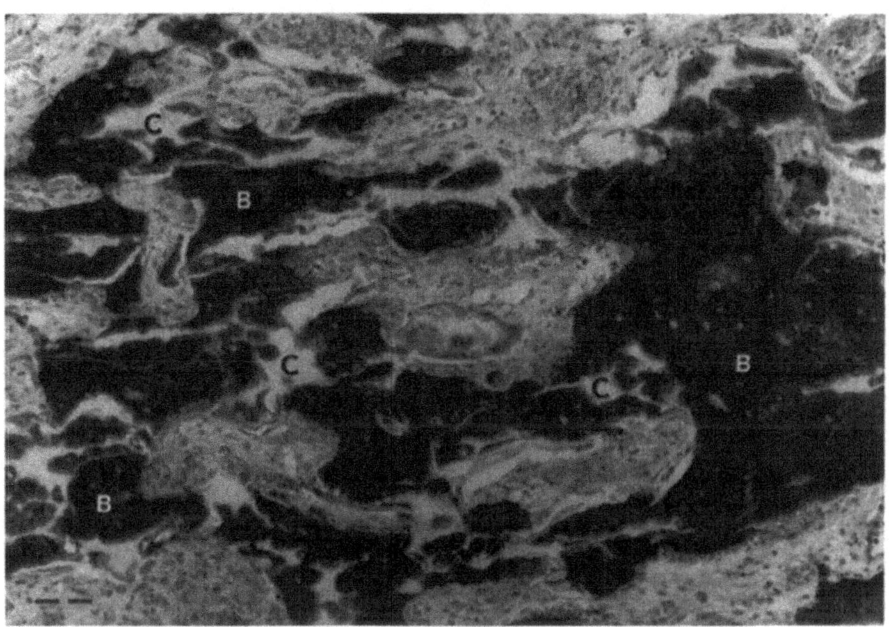

Fig. 3. The pathonomic feature of osteopetrosis at the histological level is the presence of unresorbed cartilage **(C)**. Around the cartilage, a highly cellular, embryonic bone **(B)** has been laid down. This combination of non-resorbed cartilage and poorly formed bone is the microscopic feature which results in the macroscopic appearance seen in the "bone in bone" appearance on radiographs (*see* Fig. 2). The bar denotes 80 μm.

Another form of osteopetrosis that has not responded to any therapeutic modality is associated with a neurodegenerative disease *(9)*. In some patients a neuronal storage disease has been suggested by cytoplasmic inclusions. In most patients, seizures, poor neurologic development, abnormalities in the cerebral cortex seen on magnetic resonance imaging, and early development of central apnea characterize this specific presentation. No therapy that has been tried in these patients (bone marrow transplantation, calcitriol, or interferon gamma) has resulted in any significant improvement of the disease. It is likely that even when the boney disease can be reversed (as has occurred using each of the modalities), the underlying neurologic disorder remains unaffected. Death usually occurs before 2 yr of age.

Intermediate

The intermediate form of osteopetrosis is frequently "silent" at birth with few or no obvious clinical abnormalities *(7,9)*. Some cases are diagnosed in infancy, when

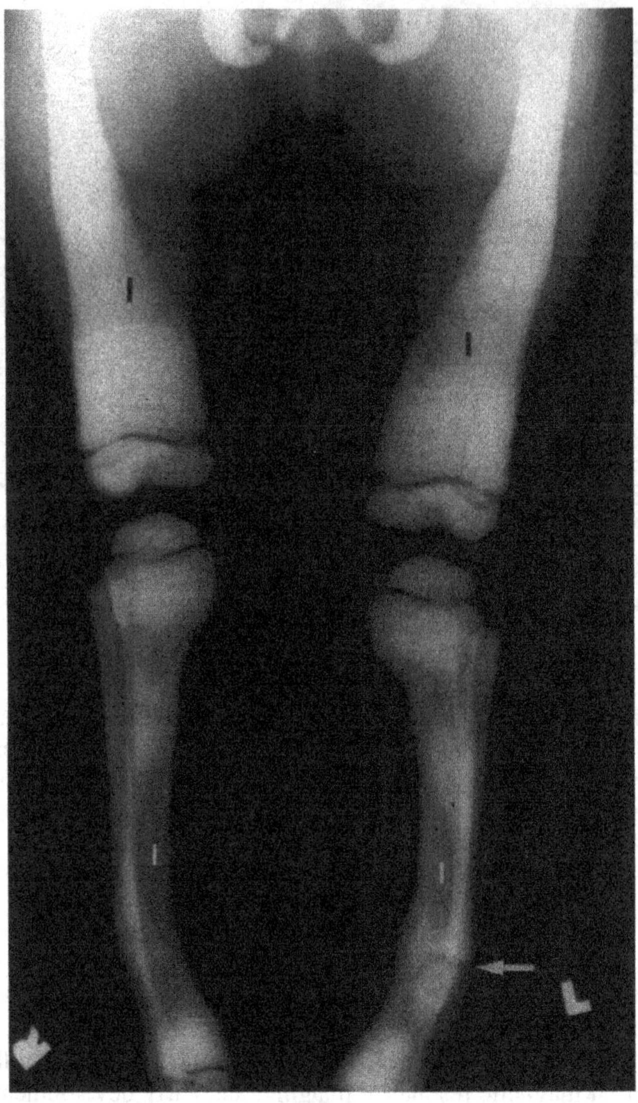

Fig. 4. A radiograph of the long bones of a 6-yr-old with an intermediate form of osteopetrosis shows the presence of some intramedullary space (denoted as "I"). The deformities of modeling result in bowing and thickening of the shaft and metaphyseal regions of the bone. Note a fracture, which was clinically not apparent, is present in the left tibia (arrow).

suspected, suggesting that the defect is present at a subclinical level even from birth. Of interest, the radiographs frequently demonstrate severe manifestation of osteosclerosis in this form of the disorder, quite similar to those seen in the malignant form (Fig. 4). These patients tend to have fractures toward the end of the first decade and frequently have repetitive fractures with very minor trauma. Infections of the bone can be difficult to irradicate, especially if the mandible is involved. Most patients survive into adulthood. While anemia and hepatosplenomegaly are rare, at least one patient has developed anemia and thrombocytopenia so severe that he was transfusion dependent. His anemia and thrombocytopenia were eliminated by splenectomy.

A subgroup of patients with the intermediate form of osteopetrosis have a carbonic anhydrase II deficiency *(4,5)*. These patients have a hyperchloremic metabolic acidosis. Several different mutations have been described in the more than 50 cases diagnosed. Patients tend to have delayed development with a reduction in intelligence as adults, short stature, fractures, cranial nerve compression, dental malocclusion, and cerebral calcifications. Patients usually have no defects in hematological function and no increased risk of infection.

Transient

Some patients with severe radiographic abnormalities and with anemia have had severe osteosclerosis early which resolves without specific therapy (*9*; personal observation). While long-term follow up is not available in these patients, no known sequellae resulted from the condition. The patients had no visual impairment, but did have anemia and thrombocytopenia. In one patient (personal experience), there was a history of acetazolamide administration. While osteopetrosis has not been widely associated with acetazolamide administration, the existence of osteopetrosis with naturally occurring mutations in carbonic anhydrase suggests that the therapy may be related to the osteoclastic dysfunction. In both cases, the resolution in the bone disease was apparent early (within one month). In addition, patients with other milder sclerosing boney dysplasias are frequently considered to have osteopetrosis in infancy. A classic case is seen in the natural history of severe craniometaphyseal dysplasia, where early radiographs are nearly indistinguishable from osteopetrosis (Fig. 5); however, there is no involvement of the vertebral bodies.

Adult Forms

In general patients with the adult forms of the disease have a family history suggesting an autosomal dominant inheritance pattern *(9)*. Anemia is not a common manifestation; however, fractures and cranial nerve dysfunction are frequently observed *(16,17)*. When defects have been looked for in infancy, radiographic abnormalities have been found which define the presence of the disease and portend the onset of symptoms in later life.

Severe

We have observed two patients who presented with severe neonatal disease who had a family history suggestive of the presence of an autosomal dominant disorder. In each of these cases, the children were diagnosed with the malignant

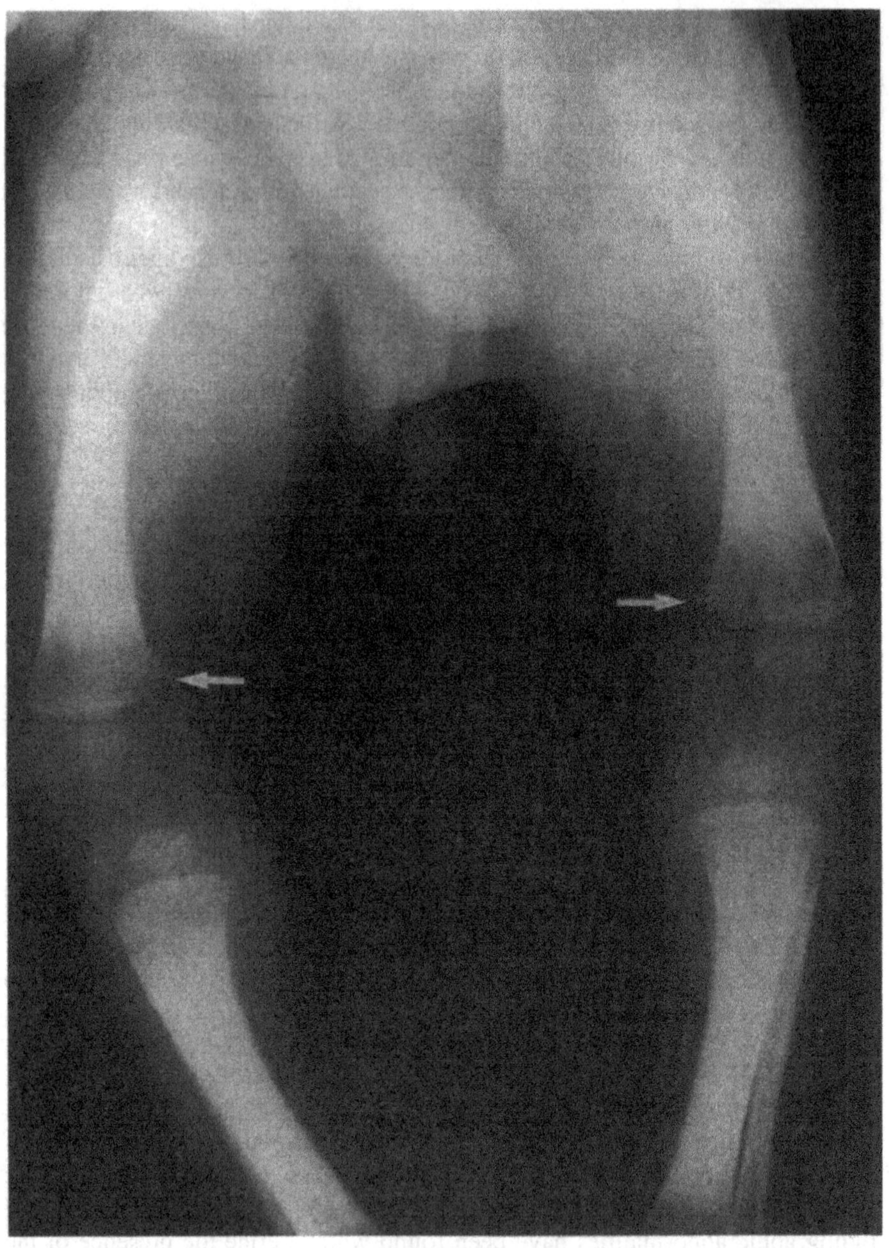

Fig. 5. This radiograph of a 1-mo-old with craniometaphyseal dysplasia demonstrates sclerotic long bones with little marrow space seen in the diaphyses. It should be noted that there is already some clearing of the bone in the distal metaphyseal region of both femurs (arrows, which had been sclerotic at birth).

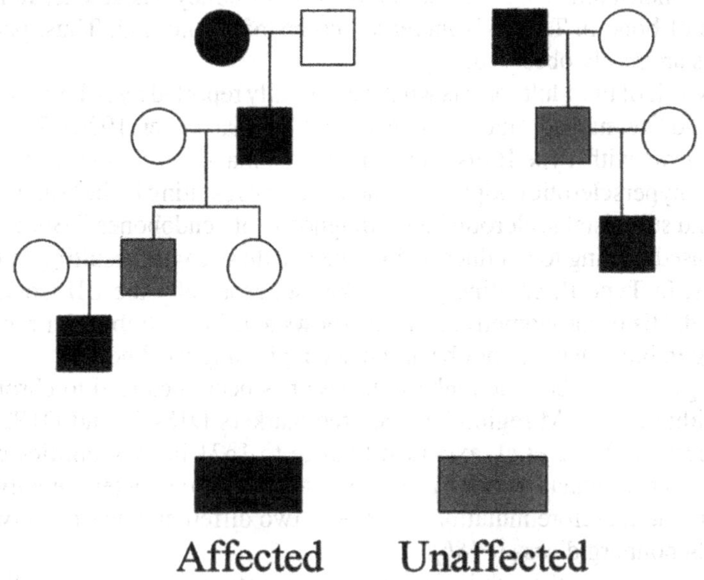

Fig. 6. This is the family tree of two patients with adult forms of osteopetrosis. The presentation of these patients was severe enough (sclerosis of the long bones in one; anemia, sclerosis of the long bones and blindness in the second) to result in an initial diagnosis of the severe malignant form.

form of the disease due to anemia and cranial nerve dysfunction presenting in infancy. In one patient, there was a history of severe infections and failure to thrive. Family members in each case had survived into the fifth and sixth decade (Fig. 6). In each case, the parent transmitting the disease was unaffected.

Mild

The "benign" adult form of osteopetrosis is frequently "silent" until later in life *(9,16,18)*. Two distinct subtypes have been described based upon radiographic appearance, symptoms, and biochemical characteristics. Each of these subtypes have been inherited in a variety of kindreds. Each subtype has a distinct natural history, resulting in differing symptomatic presentations. Both types have universal osteosclerosis, primarily involving the axial skeleton. Little or no modeling defects are seen in the long bones. Both types have been observed in some children in the identified families. Approximately 40% of patients with the adult form of osteopetrosis are symptom free regardless of type. Anemia is rare in either type. Bone pain is common to both types.

Type I is characterized radiographically, by massive osteosclerosis of the skull with increased thickness of the cranial vault. There is diffuse osteosclerosis of the spine and pelvis. Cranial nerve compression is common in Type I. There are few abnormalities seen in the remodeling of boney trabeculae. Indeed, the strength of bone in Type I is increased compared to normal. Thus, pathologic fractures are rarely observed.

Type II of the adult form is what was initially reported by Albers-Schonberg (1904) and later named "marble bone disease" by Karschner, 1926). Radiographs from patients with Type II disease demonstrate massive sclerosis of the base of the skull, hypersclerotic endplates of the vertebrae resulting in the "rugger jersey" spine, and subcristal scelerotic bands diagnostic of "endobones." Bone turnover is decreased leading to a reduction in bone tensile strength, resulting in frequent fractures. In Type II, creatine phosphokinase, especially the BB isoenzyme is increased. Histomorphometric analysis shows a defect in trabecular remodeling resulting in bone that had not been replaced, yielding weakness.

A gene for Albers-Schonberg disease has been localized to chromosome 1p21 within an 8.5cM region between the markers D1S486 and D1S2792 (?). More recently White et al. excluded linkage to 1p21 in two families with this disease from Indiana, demonstrating that there is locus heterogeneity of this disorder, and therefore mutations in at least two different genes can give rise to Albers-Schonberg disease *(18b)*.

In summary, the adult forms of osteopetrosis are usually diagnosed symptomatically in the second decade. These disorders rarely significantly alter hematopoiesis. Defects in Type I disease result in cranial nerve compression, but fractures are rare. In Type II disease, fractures are common, but nerve compression is rare.

Pathophysiology

Osteoclast Dysfunction

While animal models and a few patients have been found with a profoundly reduced number of osteoclasts, defective function rather than a reduction of formation appears to be the primary pathogenesis *(12)*. This holds true for malignant, intermediate, and benign forms. In the malignant form, there is the possibility of replacing the defective cell and curing the disease with bone marrow transplantation. However, defects in the osteoclasts' environment have also been suspected and may be the explanation for the greater than predicted rate of failure in bone marrow transplantation therapy in this disorder *(7,14)*. However, to date, no patient has been definitively diagnosed with the one clear-cut stromal defect, a defect in producing macrophage colony stimulating factor (M-CSF) seen in the op/op (osteopetrotic) mouse model *(20)*. One patient was reported with a decreased level of M-CSF after a failed transplantation; however, no data were available prior to the immunomodulation necessary for the transplantation.

A defect in white cell and osteoclastic superoxide production has been documented in the majority of patients with osteopetrosis *(12)*. The defect in superoxide generation in osteoclasts may represent a more generalized decrease in the ability of the osteoclast to resort bone. However, therapy with interferon gamma 1b, designed to increase superoxide production, increases white blood cell superoxide production, reducing infections; and increases bone resorption, enhancing hematopoiesis and enlarging cranial nerve foramina. The result is a reduction in the need for intravenous antibiotics, in the need for transfusions, and in a deceleration of cranial nerve damage. The net result is an improved survival with reduced morbidity.

Genetic Defects

There has been a marked increase in the understanding of bone biology and specific genetic defects that could result in osteopetrosis, no specific defect, other than carbonic anhydrase deficiency, has been found in humans. M-CSF production is normal *(21)*. There is no evidence of a defect in the c-src tyrosine kinase *(22)*, or abnormalities in vitamin D receptors. The answers to discerning the genetic defects may be nested in the current and growing list of animal models.

Animal Models

Classic

A variety of animal models for osteopetrosis have been explored. The M-CSF deficiency in the op/op mouse seems to be the most clearly related defect *(23–28)*; however, replacing the M-CSF with exogenous cytokine does not result in a complete remission *(29)*. Several possible explanations have been suggested. The timing of the administration may not be the most advantageous *(29–31)*. Alternatively, there may be other related factors which must interact. One of the most plausible ideas is that in addition to circulating levels of M-CSF, there is also the need for membrane bound M-CSF *(32)* on the osteoblast or embedded in the bone surface *(33)* to be presented to the osteoclast or its precursors. A less clear-cut defect, but a demonstrated role for M-CSF therapy in improving the phenotypic abnormalities in the tl/tl (toothless) rat *(34,35)*, has suggested some involvement with the M-CSF production or the M-CSF receptor in the genesis of this mutant phenotype as well. To date the precise defect has not been reported. Thus, animals or humans with few macrophages and osteoclasts may be found to have a defect in M-CSF production or response.

In the mi/mi mouse (microphthalmic), there is a defect in the production of a transcription factor *(36)*. This has led to the possibility that a variety of defects, all related to the presence of a defective transcription factor, could exist in the osteoclast and/or in other cells as well. One suggested defect is a decrease in the production of the c-kit receptor, necessary for stimulation of tyrosine kinase activity with the stem cell factor *(37)*. Stem cell factor and M-CSF activate similar receptor populations, c-kit and c-fms, which are quite similar in their binding regions. There is also data suggesting that possibly there is a defect in the ability of mi/mi stromal cells, failing to support osteoclastic function *(7)*, or possibly even inhibiting osteoclastic function in vitro.

Both M-CSF and/or interferon gamma have been shown to improve the defect in the mi/mi mouse *(20)*. Since these cytokines are not deficient in these animals, the studies suggest that these therapies circumvent the specific defects, rather than reversing the defects directly. Similar effects of these cytokines have been observed in patients with osteopetrosis where defects are unknown and not directly related to deficiencies in cytokine production or response elements.

Knock-out

Perhaps the greatest interest has been in the analysis of man-made knock-out mutations which have been found to yield an osteopetrotic phenotype. The most important and well-studied of these mutants is the *c-src* knock-out mutation *(24,38)*. In this mutation, the *c-src* tyrosine kinase is defective and yields a mutant with osteoclasts lacking ruffled borders. This appears to be due to the lack of production of phosphorylated proteins necessary to allow fusion of the membrane of endosomes with the cellular membrane within the sealed attachment of the osteoclast to bone. The result is an inactive cell with none of the machinery present at the basolateral membrane, necessary to resorb bone. The precise mechanism is not well understood and seems to be more complex than originally thought.

In the *c-fos* knock-out mutation *(39–42)*, there are few mature osteoclasts formed. In this mutation, there is a reduction in the number of osteoclasts and an increase in the number of macrophages. Thus, it appears that *c-fos* is related to the "switch point" in the osteoclast lineage which determines whether the progenitor moves in the direction of the osteoclast or the macrophage *(39)*.

In other more recent experiments, the association between osteoclast differentiation and PU.1, a myeloid- and B-cell-specific transcription factor, or NF-κB proteins was determined in knock-out mice which surprisingly also exhibited the classic hallmarks of osteopetrosis. These studies showed that both osteoclasts and macrophages were absent in PU.1-deficient *(43)* and NF-κB1/ NF-κB2 *(44)* double-knock-out mice. These results suggest that these transcription factors play essential roles in regulating development along the osteoclast/macrophage lineage. Additional studies are necessary to define osteoclast-specific target genes for these transcription factors and to understand how the transcriptional regulation of these genes controls the development along the osteoclast and macrophage lineage.

At the present time, knock-out mutations have been much more important in understanding osteoclastic function than in explaining the human osteopetrotic condition. However, these studies do provide a variety of candidate genes (both those already identified and possible defects in the same or related families of proteins) that may someday be found in one or more forms of osteopetrosis. Just as this review is considerably different from one published just two years ago, there is no doubt that we are on the brink of detecting a variety of genetic abnormalities which will unlock our understanding of this family of defects.

Summary

In summary, significant progress has been made in classifying osteopetrosis. There are at least three major categories (malignant, intermediate, benign) of the disease with a variety of subtypes. This classification allows prognostic information to be provided to the parent or patient, improving decision making concerning the appropriate therapy. The genetics of osteopetrosis have not been worked out, but the explosion of animal mutations expressing osteopetrotic phenotypes promises to lead to the identification of some, if not all, of the mutations in the near future. Finally, treatment is largely still directed toward enhancing osteoclastic function in general, rather than being targeted toward specific defects. Bone marrow transplantation remains the only hope of complete cure. The introduction of calcitriol, M-CSF, and Interferon gamma-1b provides promise for the future survival and hopefully, the cure of osteopetrosis. As in the past, this very interesting family of disorders continues to lead the way in developing our understanding of osteoclast function.

References

1. Elster, A. D., Theros, E. G., Key, L. L., and Chen, M. Y. M. (1992a) Cranial imaging in autosomal recessive osteopetrosis. Part I. Facial bones and calvarium. *Radiology* **183,**129–135.
2. Elster, A. D., Theros, E. G., Key, L. L., and Chen, M. Y. M. (1992b) Cranial imaging in autosomal recessive osteopetrosis. Part II. Skull base and brain. *Radiology* **183,** 137–144.
3. Seifert, M. F., Popoff, S. N., Jackson, M. E., Mackay, C. A., Cielinski, M., and Marks, S. C. (1993) Experimental studies of osteopetrosis in laboratory animals. *Clin. Orthop. Rel. Res.* **294,** 23–33.
4. Fathallah, D. M., Bejaoui, M., Sly, W. S., Lakhoua, R., and Dellagi, K. (1994) A unique mutation underlying carbonic anhydrase II deficiency syndrome in patients of Arab descent. *Hum. Genet.* **94,** 581–582.
5. Whyte, M. P. (1993a) Carbonic anhydrase II deficiency. *Clin. Orthop. Rel. Res.* **294,** 52–63.
6. Grodum, E., Gram, J., Broxen, K., and Bollerslev, J. (1995) Autosomal dominant osteopetrosis: Bone mineral measurements of the entire skeleton of adults in two different subtypes. *Bone* **16(4),** 431–434.
7. Key, L. L., Jr. (1987) Osteopetrosis: a genetic window into osteoclast function. A CPC series: cases in metabolic bone disease, Vol. 2, No. 3.
8. Shapiro, F. (1993) Osteopetrosis. *Clin. Rel. Res.* **94,** 34–44.
9. Whyte, M. P. (1993b) Sclerosing bone dysplasias, in *Primer on the Metabolic Bone Diseases and Disorders of Mineral Metabolism,* Raven Press, New York, pp. 327–331.
10. Manusov, E. G., Douville, D. R., Page, L. V., and Trivedi, D. V. (1993) Osteopetrosis (Marble Bone Disease) *Am. Fam. Physician* **47(1),** 175–180.
11. Gerritsen, E. J. A., Vossen, J. M., Fasth, A., Friedrich, W., Morgan, G., Padmos, A., et al. (1994b) Bone marrow transplantation for autosomal recessive osteopetrosis. *Pediatrics* 896–902.
12. Key, L. L., Jr. and Ries, W. L. (1993) Osteopetrosis: the pharmaco-physiologic basis of therapy. *Clin. Orthop. Rel. Res.* **294,** 85–89.

13. Schroeder, R. E., Johnson, F. L., Silberstein, M. J., Neuman, W. L., Hoag, J. M., Farber, R. A., and Noguchi, A. (1992) Longitudinal follow-up of malignant osteopetrosis by skeletal radiographs and restriction fragment length polymorphism analysis after bone marrow transplantation. *Pediatrics* **90,** 986–989.
14. Gerritsen, E. J. A., Vossen, J. M., van Loo, I. H. G., Hermans, J., Helfrich, M. H., Griscelli, C., and Fischer, A. (1994a) Autosomal recessive osteopetrosis: Variability of findings at diagnosis and during the natural course. *Pediatrics* **90,** 986–989.
15. Shapiro, F., Key, L. L., Jr., and Anast, C. (1988) Variable osteoclast appearance in human infantile osteopetrosis. *Calcif. Tissue Int.* **43,** 67–76.
16. Bollerslev, J. and Mosekilde, L. (1993) Autosomal Dominant Osteopetrosis. *Clin. Orthop. Rel. Res.* **294,** 45–51.
17. Bollerslev, J., Marks, S. C., Jr., Mosekilde, L., Lian, J. B., Stein, G. S., and Mosekilde, L. (1994) Cortical bone osteocalcin content and matrix composition in autosomal dominant osteopetrosis type I. *Eur. J. Endocrinol.* **130,** 592–594.
18. Johnston, C. C.,Jr., N. Lavy, T. Lord, F. Vellios, A. D. Merritt, and W. P. Deiss, Jr. (1968) Osteopetrosis. a clinical, genetic, metabolic, and morphologic study of the dominantly inherited, benign form. *Medicine* **47,** 149–167.
18b. Albers-Schonberg, H. (1904) Röntgenbilder einer selten Knochenkrankung. *Muenchener Med. Wschr.* **51,** 365.
19. White, K. E., Koller, D. L, Takacs, I., Foroud, T, Econs, M. J. (1999) Locus heterogeneity of autosomal dominant osteopetrosis (ADO) *J. Clin. Endocrinol Metab.* **84,** 1047–1051.
20. Key, L. L., Jr., Rodriguiz, R. M., and Wang, W. C. (1995a) Cytokines and Bone Resorption in Osteopetrosis. *Intl. J. Pediatr. Hematol./Oncol.* **2,** 143–149.
21. Orchard, P. J., Dahl, N., Aukerman, L., Blazar, B. R., and Key, L. L., Jr. (1992) Circulating macrophage colony-stimulating factor is not reduced in malignant osteopetrosis. *Exp. Hematol.* **20,** 103–105.
22. Meyerson, G., Dahl, N., and Pahlman, S. (1993) Malignant osteopetrosis: C-src kinase is not reduced in fibroblasts. *Calcif. Tissue Int.* **53,** 69–70.
23. Begg, S. K., Radley, J. M., Pollard, J. W., Chisholm, O. T., Stanley, E. R., and Bertoncello, I. (1993) Delayed hematopoietic development in osteopetrotic (op/op) mice. *J. Exp. Med.* **177,** 237–242.
24. Lowe, C., Yoneda, T., Boyce, B. F., Chen, H., and Mundy G. R. (1993) Osteopetrosis in Src-deficient mice is due to an autonomous defect of osteoclasts. *Proc. Natl. Acad. Sci. USA* **90,** 4485–4489.
25. Marks, S. C., Wojtowicz, A., Szperl, M., Urbanowska, E., Mackay, C. A., Wiktor-Jedrzejczak, W., et al. (1992) Administration of colony stimulating factor-1 corrects some macrophage, dental, and skeletal defects in an osteopetrotic mutation (toothless, tl) in the rat. *Bone* **13,** 89–93.
26. Nilsson, S. K., and Bertoncello. (1994) The development and establishment on hemopoiesis in fetal and newborn osteopetrotic (op/op) mice. *Dev. Biol.* **164,** 456–462.
27. Philippart, C., Tzehoval, E., Moricard, Y., Bringuier, A.-F., Seebold, C., Lemoine, F.-M., Arys, A., Dourov, N., Labat, M.-L. (1993) Immune cell defects affect bone remodelling in osteopetrotic op/op mice. *Bone Miner.* **23,** 317–332.
28. Wiktor-Jedrezejczak, W., Urbanowska, E., and Szperl, M. (1994) Granulocyte-macrophage colony-stimulating factor corrects macrophage deficiences, but not osteopetrosis, in the colony-stimulating factor-1-deficient op/op mouse*. *Endocrinology* **134(4),** 1932–1935.

29. Sundquist, K. T., Cecchini, M. G., and Marks, S. C. (1995) Colony-stimulating factor-1 injections improve but do not cure skeletal sclerosis in osteopetrotic (op) mice. *Bone* **16 (1),** 39–46.
30. Hofstetter, W., Wetterwald, A., Cecchini, M. G., Mueller, C., and Felix, R. (1995) Detection of transcripts and binding sites for colony-stimulating factor-1 during bone development. *Bone,* **17(2),** 145–151.
31. Lee, T. H., Fevold, K. L., Muguruma, Y., Lottsfeldt, J. L., and Lee, M. Y. (1994) Relative roles of osteoclast colony-stimulating factor and macrophage colony-stimulating factor in the course of osteoclast development. *Exp. Hematol.* **22,** 66–73.
32. Stanley, E. R., Berg, K. L., Einstein, D. B., Lee, P. S. W., and Yeung, Y. G. (1994) The biology and action of colony stimulating factor-1. *Stem Cells* **12(suppl 1),** 15–25.
33. Ohtsuki, T., Hatake, K., Suzu, S., Saito, K., Motoyoshi, K., and Miura, Y. (1995) Immunohistochemical identification of proteoglycan form of macrophage colony-stimulating factor on bone surface. *Calcif. Tissue Int.* **57,** 213–217.
34. Aharinejad, S., Marks, S. C., Jr., Bock, P., Mason-Savas, A., MacKay, C. A., Larson, E. K., Jackson, M. E., Luftensteiner, M., and Wiesbauer, E. (1995) Csf-1 treatment promotes angiogenesis in the metaphysis of osteopetrotic (toothless, tl) rats. *Bone* **6(3),** 315–324.
35. Marks, S. C., Mackay, C. A., Jackson, M. E., Larson, E. K., Cielinski, M. J., Stanley, E. R., and Aukerman, S. L. (1993) The skeletal effects of colony-stimulating factor-1 in toothless (osteopetrotic) rats: Persistent metaphyseal sclerosis and the failure to restore subepiphyseal osteoclasts. *Bone* **14,** 675–680.
36. Steingrimsson, E., Moore, K. J., Lamoreux, M. L., Ferré-D'Amaré, A. R., Burley, S. K., Zimring, D. C., Skow, L. C., Hodgkinson, C. A., Arnheiter, H., Copeland, N. G., and Jenkins, N. A. (1994) Molecular basis of mouse microphthalmia (ml) mutations helps explain their developmental and phenotypic consequences. *Nat. Genet.* **8,** 256–263.
37. Ebi, Y., Kanakura, Y., Jippo-Kanemoto, T., Tsujimura, T., Furitsu, T., Ikeda, H., et al. (1992) low c-kit expression of cultured mast cells of mi/mi genotype may be involved in their defective responses to fibroblasts that express the ligand for c-kit. *Blood* **80(6),** 1454–1462.
38. Boyce, B. F., Chen, H., Soriano, P., and Mundy, G. R. (1993) Histomorphometric and immunocytochemical studies of src- related osteopetrosis. *Bone* **14,** 335–340.
39. Jacento, O. (1995) c-fos and bone loss: a proto-oncogeneregulates osteoclast lineage determination. *BioEssays* **17(4),** 277–291.
40. Grigoriadis, A. E., Wang, Z., Cecchini, M. G., Hofstetter, W., Felix, R., Fleisch, H. A., and Wagner, E. F. (1994) c-Fos a key regulator of osteoclast-macrophage lineage determination and bone remodeling. *Science* **266,** 443–448.
41. Johnson, R. S., Spiegelman, B. M., and Papaioannou, V. (1992) Pleiotropic effects of a null mutation in the c-fos proto-oncogene. *Cell* **71,** 577–586.
42. Wang, Z., Ovitt, C., Grigoriadis, A. E., Mohle-Steinlein, U., Ruther, and Wagner, E. F. (1992) Bone and haematopoietic defects in mice lacking, c-fos. *Nature* **360,** 741–745.
43. Tondravi ,M. M., McKercher, S. R., Anderson, K., Erdmann, J. M., Quiroz, M., Maki, R., and Teitelbaum, S. L. (1997) Osteopetrosis in mice lacking haematopoietic transcription factor PU. 1. *Nature* **386,** 81–84.
44. Iotsova, V., Caamano, J., Loy, J.,Yang, Y., Lewin, A., and Bravo, R. (1997) Osteopetrosis in mice lacking NF–κB1 and NF–κB2. *Nat. Med.* **3,** 1285–1289.

CHAPTER 18

Hypophosphatasia

Michael P. Whyte

Introduction

Hypophosphatasia (McKusick #146300, #241500, #241510) is a heritable metabolic bone disease that establishes a critical (but as yet unspecified) role for alkaline phosphatase (ALP) in skeletal mineralization *(1,2)*. Subnormal activity of ALP in serum (hypophosphat*asemia*) is the biochemical hallmark of the disorder, and reflects a generalized deficiency of activity of the tissue-nonspecific (liver/bone/kidney) ALP isoenzyme (TNSALP) *(3)*. Catalysis by the tissue-specific ALP isoenzymes—intestinal, placental, and germ-cell (placental-like) ALP—is not diminished *(3)*. The impaired skeletal mineralization caused by the deficient TNSALP activity manifests clinically as rickets in infants and children and as osteomalacia in adults. In fact, the severity of the disease among patients with this inborn error of metabolism is extraordinarily variable *(1–3)*.

Reviewed below, the perinatal and infantile forms of hypophosphatasia, which are often lethal, are transmitted as autosomal recessive traits due to homozygosity or compound heterozygosity for a considerable number and variety of mutations in the TNSALP gene. Of interest, and now becoming understood, patients with the more mild childhood, adult, or odontohypophosphatasia forms of hypophosphatasia can have TNSALP mutations associated with more severe disease and also demonstrate autosomal recessive inheritance. Further intriguing aspects of hypophosphatasia include some kindreds with clinically mild disease manifesting autosomal dominant transmission, especially rare cases that may be caused by defective regulation of TNSALP gene expression or TNSALP enzyme processing, and a few patients who have *pseudo*hypophosphatasia.

This chapter provides first a brief overview of the molecular and biochemical nature of ALP, then describe the remarkable range of clinical expressivity for hypophosphatasia, and conclude with a summary of what has been reported concerning TNSALP gene defects and their biological sequelae.

Molecular Biology and Biochemistry of Alkaline Phosphatase

Alkaline phosphatase (*orthophosphoric-monoester phosphohydrolase, alkaline optimum, EC 3.1.3.1*) apparently is present in most plants and in all animals *(4)*. In humans, ALPs are encoded by at least four genes *(5–7)*. Three of the ALPs isoenzymes are expressed in a tissue-specific manner—intestinal, placental, and germ-cell (placental-like) ALP. The fourth isoenzyme is present in all tissues, but is especially rich in liver, bone, and kidney *(5,6)*. Hence, this "liver/bone/kidney" ALP is also called "tissue-nonspecific "ALP (TNSALP) *(3,6,7)*. It has been suggested that in humans there may also be a fetal intestinal ALP isoenzyme *(7)*.

The distinctive physicochemical properties separating the ALPs purified from human liver, bone, and kidney tissue disappear after digestion with glycosidases *(8)*. Thus, TNSALPs are actually a family of "secondary" isoenzymes (isoforms) which differ only by posttranslational modifications involving carbohydrate residues *(9)*.

The TNSALP gene (McKusick *171760) is located near the end of the short arm of chromosome 1 (1p36.1-34) *(10)*; the genes for intestinal, placental, and germ-cell ALP and perhaps fetal intestinal ALP (McKusick *171740, *171750, *171800, *171810, respectively) are located near the tip of the long arm of chromosome 2 (2q34-37) *(11)*. Unfortunately, the current human gene mapping symbol for the TNSALP locus is ALPL ("ALP-liver") although the function of the liver isoform of TNSALP is unknown *(7,12)*.

Each ALP locus has been sequenced *(13–15)*. The TNSALP gene is greater than 50 kb and contains 12 exons, 11 of which are translated to form the 507 amino acid nascent enzyme *(6,15)*. The promoter region for TNSALP is located within 610 nucleotides 5' to the major transcription start site *(16)*. TATA and Sp1 sequences may act as regulatory elements. Apparently, basal levels of TNSALP gene expression reflect inherent "housekeeping" promoter activity, whereas differential expression in various tissues may be mediated by a posttranscriptional mechanism *(16)*. In fact, the 5' untranslated region differs between the bone and liver TNSALP isoforms *(17)*.

The tissue-specific ALP genes are smaller than the TNSALP gene, primarily due to shorter introns. Amino acid sequences deduced from the cDNAs suggest 87% positional identity between placental and intestinal ALP, but only 50–60% identity between TNSALP and the tissue-specific ALPs *(5,6)*. Nevertheless, the active site of TNSALP, which is encoded by six exons and comprised of 15 amino acid residues *(18)*, reflects a nucleotide sequence that has been conserved in ALPs found throughout nature *(19)*. TNSALP seems to represent an ancestral gene, whereas the tissue-specific ALPs in man likely originated from a series of gene duplications *(5)*.

The ALPs are Zn^{2+}-metalloenzymes *(4,5)*. Catalytic activity requires a multimeric configuration of identical subunits ranging from 40–75 kDa *(6)*. Each monomer has one active site and binds two Zn^{2+} atoms that stabilize its tertiary structure *(20)*. The cDNA sequence of TNSALP predicts five potential N-linked glycosylation sites *(15)*. Indeed, N-glycosylation is necessary for enzymatic activity *(17)*. O-glycosylation involves the bone, but not the liver, isoform of TNSALP *(17)*.

The ALPs are generally regarded as homodimeric in the circulation *(4,6)*. However, in tissues ALPs are attached to cell surfaces probably as homotetramers *(21,22)*. TNSALP, in symmetrical dimeric form, has α/β topology for each subunit with a 10-stranded β-sheet at its center *(23)*.

ALP isoenzymes have broad substrate specificities and pH optima, which depend on the type and concentration of phosphocompound undergoing catalysis *(4)*. Catalytic activity requires Mg^{2+} as a cofactor *(4)*. Hydrolytic activity cleaves phosphoesters and inorganic pyrophosphate (PPi) *(24)*. The reaction involves phosphorylation-dephosphorylation of a serine residue and dissociation of covalently linked Pi seems to be the rate-limiting step. In fact, Pi is a potent competitive inhibitor of ALP activity *(4,20)*. Of interest, however, Pi may also stabilize the enzyme *(25)*.

Relatively little is established concerning the biosynthesis of ALP in higher organisms. Analysis of the human ALP isoenzyme gene sequences indicates that the nascent polypeptides have a short signal sequence of 17–21 amino acid residues *(5,6)* and a hydrophobic domain at their carboxy-termini *(13–15)*. These ALPs become tethered to the plasma membrane surface where they are bound to the polar head group of a phosphatidylinositol-glycan moiety and can be liberated by phosphatidylinositol-specific phospholipase *(22,23,26)*. However, the precise interaction with phosphatidylinositol may differ among the ALP isoenzymes *(26)*. Intracellular degradation of ALPs can involve proteosomes *(27)*.

Although lipid-free ALP circulates in the blood, how it is released from cell surfaces is poorly understood *(28)*. In healthy men and women, most of the ALP in serum apparently consists of equal amounts of TNSALP from liver and bone tissue *(29)*. However, in infants and children, and particularly during the growth spurt of puberty, the circulation is enriched in the bone isoform of TNSALP *(4)*. Placental ALP normally enters the blood only in women during the latter stages of pregnancy *(3)*.

With the discovery in 1988 that a deactivating mutation in the TNSALP gene could cause hypophosphatasia came unequivocal evidence that TNSALP acts critically during mineralization of the skeleton in man *(30)*. However, the seemingly undisturbed function of other organs/tissues in hypophosphatasia patients questions the biological significance of TNSALP elsewhere in the human body *(1–3,6)*.

Hypophosphatasia

More than a half century ago, in 1948, J.C. Rathbun, a Canadian pediatrician, coined the term hypophosphatasia when he published his description of an infant

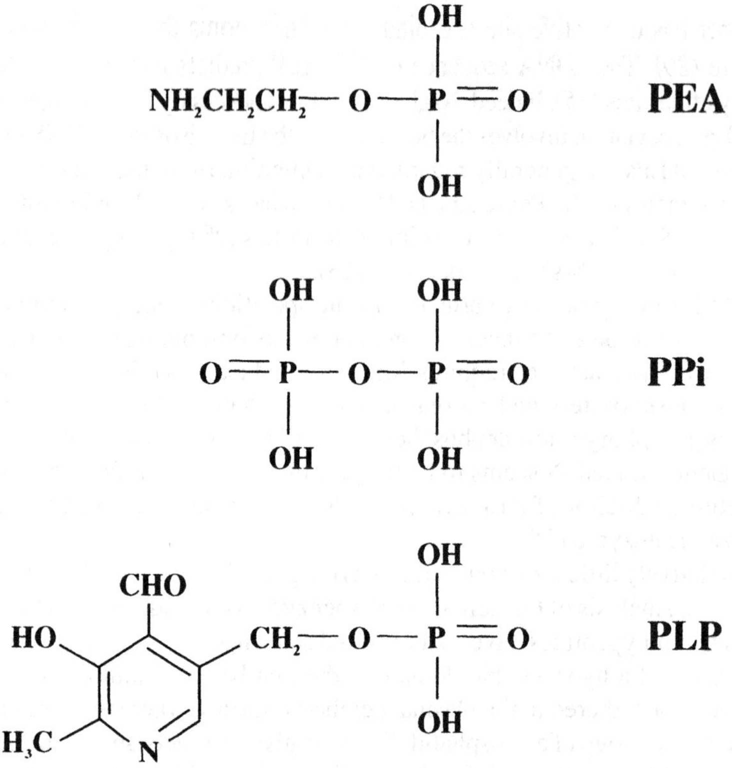

$$NH_2CH_2CH_2-O-P(=O)(OH)_2 \quad \textbf{PEA}$$

$$O=P(OH)_2-O-P(=O)(OH)_2 \quad \textbf{PPi}$$

Fig. 1. Three phosphocompounds seem to be natural substrates for TNSALP, because each accumulates endogenously in hypophosphatasia:phosphoethanolamine (PEA), inorganic pyrophosphate (PPi), and pyridoxal 5'-phosphate (PLP).

boy who died from severe rickets, weight loss, and seizures, yet whose ALP activity in serum, bone, and other tissues was paradoxically subnormal *(32)*. Several hundred patients have since been described in the medical literature *(3)*.

Major advances in our understanding of hypophosphatasia included the discoveries of elevated levels endogenously of three phosphocompounds (Fig. 1). Each accumulation clarifies the metabolic basis of this disorder and the physiological role of TNSALP *(3)*. The origin of the PEA excess may reflect a disturbance in the degradation of the cell surface anchors for ALPs and other proteins. Excess PPi, an inhibitor of hydroxyapatite crystal growth, may explain the defective skeletal mineralization *(33)*. Markedly elevated plasma PLP levels indicate that TNSALP acts physiologically as an ectoenzyme *(1–3,34)*.

Clinical Features

Hypophosphatasia occurs worldwide. However, it is especially common in the Mennonite population of Manitoba, Canada. In these often inbred families,

1 in 2500 newborns suffers severe disease and about 1 in 25 individuals is a carrier for the disorder *(35)*. The incidence of severe hypophosphatasia in Toronto, Canada, is understandably lower, and was estimated in 1957 to be 1 per 100,000 live births *(36)*.

Although relatively high levels of TNSALP activity are found in bone, liver, kidney, and adrenal tissue in healthy individuals, and at least some TNSALP is present in other cell types throughout the body, hypophosphatasia disturbs primarily the skeleton and the dentition *(1–3)*. Nevertheless, clinical expression varies remarkably among patients and ranges from death *in utero* to problems only with dentition during adult life *(36–40)*. In fact, some individuals who manifest characteristic biochemical abnormalities (see below) may never become symptomatic *(38,39)*. Although within sibships hypophosphatasia generally breeds true, significant differences in disease severity can occasionally occur in this setting as well (see later) *(38,39,41,42)*.

Because the genetic basis for hypophosphatasia is now being rapidly elucidated *(3,7)*, there is promise for a better understanding of this variable disease severity and a molecular nosology in the near future. Nevertheless, the current classification of patients for prognostication and recurrence risk estimates, and so on, remains a clinical one. Several such schemes have been proposed that attempt to deal with this inborn error of metabolism's remarkable range of expression *(36,37)*. Six forms of hypophosphatasia constitute a useful separation. The age at which lesions in bone are first documented distinguish the perinatal, infantile, childhood, and adult form of hypophosphatasia *(36,40)*. Patients who have dental manifestations alone are regarded as having "odontohypophosphatasia." An extremely rare variant, pseudohypophosphatasia, resembles infantile hypophosphatasia, but serum ALP activity is normal or elevated in routine assays used in clinical laboratories *(3)*.

The prognoses for these six types of hypophosphatasia reflect the severity of the skeletal disorder which, in turn, reflects the age at which the bone disease presents itself. Generally, the younger a patient becomes symptomatic, the more severe the condition lifelong *(1,2,36)*. Levels of ALP in serum (adjusted for patient age) and levels of substrate accumulation endogenously also reflect disease severity *(3)*.

Although the above nosology is useful, there is considerable variability within each form of hypophosphatasia, no clear-cut separations between them, and prognostication is imprecise.

Perinatal (lethal) Hypophosphatasia

Perinatal hypophosphatasia is the most severe form. It manifests *in utero* and often causes stillbirth. Neonates have *caput membraneceum* and short, deformed limbs that reflect soft bones from profound skeletal hypomineralization. Some affected newborns survive for a few days, but then suffer increasing pulmonary compromise from rachitic defects of the thorax and from hypoplastic lungs *(43)*. They may fail to gain weight and can have a high-pitched cry, periodic apnea with cyanosis and bradycardia,

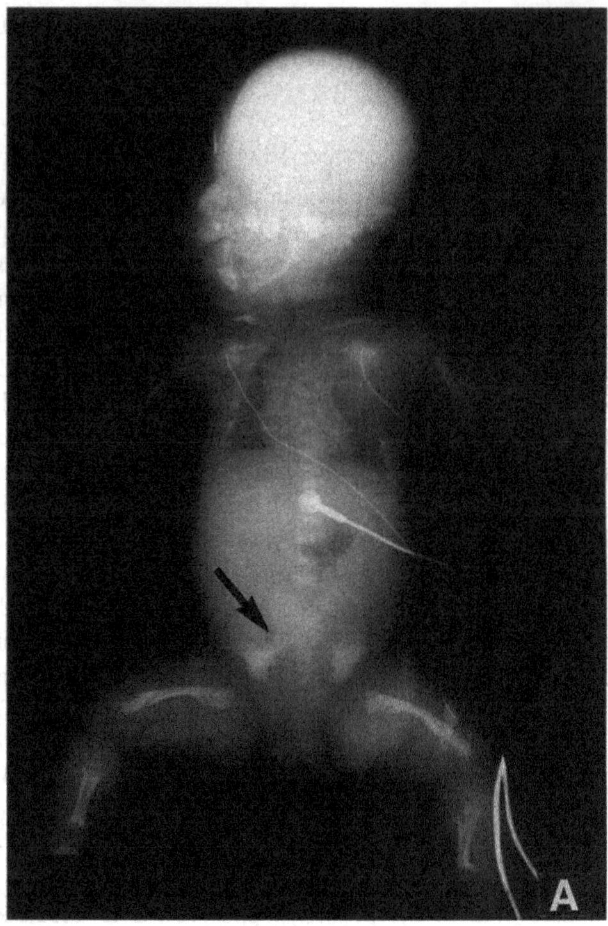

Fig. 2. (**A**) Variable expression of hypophosphatasia in siblings. Perinatal hypophosphatasia manifested in this stillborn girl with profound skeletal hypomineralization, femoral fractures, and "missing" vertebrae. A plastic umbilical cord clip (arrow) has similar density to the skeleton.

irritability, unexplained fever, myelophthisic anemia, intracranial hemorrhage, and seizures *(37,40)*. Very rarely there is prolonged survival *(44)*. Radiographic study distinguishes perinatal hypophosphatasia from even the most severe types of osteogenesis imperfecta and other forms of congenital dwarfism. In fact, the X-ray findings at birth are essentially diagnostic *(45,46)*. Nevertheless, the radiographic changes can be diverse *(46)*. In some patients, the skeleton appears almost totally unmineralized. In other patients, there is marked bony undermineralization and severe rachitic changes (Fig. 2A,B). Cranial bones

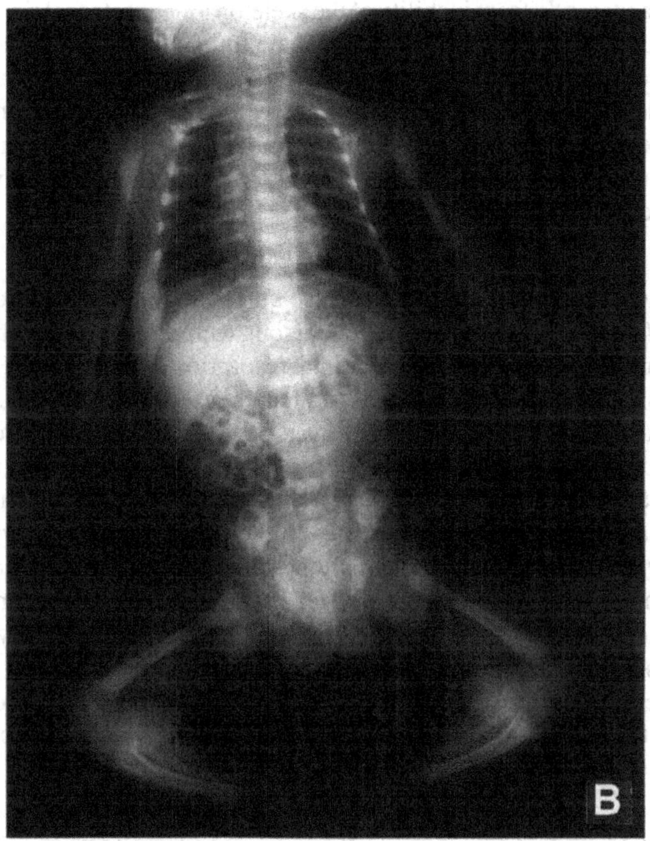

Fig. 2. **(B)** Infantile hypophosphatasia had been diagnosed in her brother at $3^{1/2}$ mo of age. He died at 8 mo of age. His skeleton is much better mineralized, as shown here at 4 mo of age, compared with his sister's.

may seem calcified only centrally, giving the illusion that the sutures are widely separated, and individual vertebrae may appear to be missing.

Infantile Hypophosphatasia

Infantile hypophosphatasia manifests before 6 mo of age *(36)*. Growth and development often seem normal until poor feeding, inadequate weight gain, and clinical signs of rickets are noted. The cranial sutures feel wide, but the ossification abnormality in the calvarium can cause a functional craniosynostosis with increased intracranial pressure. True premature bony fusion of the cranial sutures sometimes occurs if the patient survives infancy *(45)*. A flail chest from rachitic deformity, rib fractures, scoliosis, etc. may fatigue patients, make feeding difficult, and predispose them to pneumonia. Hypercalcemia and hypercalciuria, apparently from inability of the skeleton to sequester calcium absorbed from the diet, is common and can contribute to inanition, recurrent vomiting, nephrocalcinosis, and renal compromise *(36,47,48)*. The radiographic features of infantile hypophosphatasia are distinctive and resemble the perinatal form, although less severe *(45)*. Sequential X-ray studies may disclose not only rachitic disease, but gradual skeletal demineralization that is an especially worrisome prognostic sign *(48)*.

Childhood Hypophosphatasia

Childhood hypophosphatasia is also quite variable in its clinical expression *(36,43,49)*. Typically, several deciduous teeth are lost prematurely (i.e., earlier than 5 yr of age) with only minimal resorption of their roots. Hypoplasia or dysplasia of dental cementum fails to anchor the tooth root *(50,51)*. However, the prognosis for the permanent dentition is generally better *(52)*. Rickets often causes short stature and delays walking. Patients may complain of joint pain and stiffness, as well as isolated episodes of joint swelling. They can have considerable weakness in their limbs (especially the thighs) consistent with a static myopathy *(53)*. There is a characteristic waddling gait *(36,47)*. Beading of the costochondral junctions; either bowed legs or knock-knees; enlargement of the wrists, knees, and ankles from flared metaphyses; and occasionally a brachycephalic skull are additional physical findings. Radiography of the wrists and knees often demonstrates characteristic focal bony defects—"tongues" of radiolucency that project from the physes into the metaphyses. Functional or true craniosynostosis can occur.

Adult Hypophosphatasia

Adult hypophosphatasia typically presents during middle age *(38,39)*. Not infrequently, however, patients recall being told that as children they had rickets and suffered premature loss of deciduous teeth. Osteomalacia in adult life manifests with painful feet due to recurrent, poorly healing metatarsal stress fractures. Sometimes, there is discomfort in the thighs or hips caused by proximal femoral pseudofractures. Early loss or extraction of adult teeth is not uncommon *(38,39,54)*. Calcium pyrophosphate dihydrate deposition, occasionally with attacks of arthritis (pseudogout), troubles some patients. Others have PPi arthropathy *(38,39)*. In some kindreds, there is periarticular deposition of calcium phosphate that manifests clinically with "calcific periarthritis" *(55,56)*.

Odontohypophosphatasia

Odontohypophosphatasia is diagnosed when the only clinical manifestation stems from the dentition and radiographic or biopsy studies exclude skeletal disease *(3)*.

Pseudohypophosphatasia

Pseudohypophosphatasia is a particularly intriguing form of hypophosphatasia that has been documented convincingly in only two infants *(57,58)*. The clinical, radiographic, and biochemical findings resemble infantile hypophosphatasia, except that serum ALP activity is consistently normal or increased in routine assays *(57,58)*. The enzymatic defect apparently involves a mutant TNSALP that retains or has enhanced catalytic activity under the nonphysiological conditions of clinical ALP assay procedures, but has diminished hydrolytic activity endogenously *(59)*.

Laboratory. Diagnosis

Hypophosphatasia is diagnosed with confidence when a compatible clinical history, physical findings, and radiographic changes occur with clearly and consistently subnormal serum ALP activity *(3)*. In general, the more severe the disease the lower the serum ALP activity adjusted for age *(3)*. Also differing from other types of rickets or osteomalacia, neither calcium nor Pi levels in serum are low in hypophosphatasia. In fact, hypercalcemia occurs frequently in the infantile form of the disease *(37,60)*, and in childhood and adult hypophosphatasia serum Pi levels are above the mean value for controls and approx 50% of patients are distinctly hyperphosphatemic due to enhanced renal reclamation of Pi (increased tubular maximum for Pi/glomerular filtration rate; i.e., TmP/GFR) *(61)*. Several patients reportedly have had elevated serum PTH levels, but renal compromise from hypercalcemia with retention of immunoreactive PTH fragments, perhaps, is the explanation. Conversely, low circulating levels of PTH occur also *(62)*.

TNSALP Deficiency

Early on, autopsy studies of perinatal and infantile cases elucidated the enzymatic defect underlying hypophosphatasia and inferred its etiology. Profound deficiency of ALP activity was documented in liver, bone, and kidney tissue, yet ALP activity was not diminished in intestine or in placenta (fetal trophoblast) *(63,64)*. This observation concurred with amino acid sequences and other data obtained from ALPs purified from healthy human tissues *(1,2,6)* and indicated a defect which selectively diminished the catalytic activity of the secondary isoforms comprising the TNSALP isoenzyme family.

Investigation of the cardinal biochemical feature of hypophosphatasia, hypophosphatasemia, supports the autopsy studies. There is subnormal activity of both the liver and bone isoforms of TNSALP in serum *(29,65)*. Coincubation experiments with mixtures of serum (as well as cell coculture and heterokaryon studies using fibroblasts) exclude the presence of an inhibitor or the absence of an activator of TNSALP *(36,38,66,67)*. Instead, the hypophosphatasemia seems to reflect a more fundamental disturbance of bone and liver TNSALP activity in the circulation *(65)*.

Preliminary observations using autopsy specimens and a polyclonal antibody to the liver isoform of TNSALP suggest that normal amounts of TNSALP protein can be found in tissues in severe hypophosphatasia *(68,69)*. However, a monoclonal antibody-based immunoassay measuring dimeric TNSALP demonstrated low levels of the bone and the liver TNSALP isoforms in the serum of patients representing all clinical forms of hypophosphatasia except pseudohypophosphatasia *(65)*. Accordingly, sequestration of TNSALP within cells or disruption of TNSALP dimeric structure subsequent to release from plasma membrane surfaces could be occurring in hypophosphatasia patients *(65)*. Recently, there is evidence from studies of a few TNSALP gene mutations that aberrant TNSALP can indeed accumulate with cells (*see* below).

Some ALP activity is detectable by especially sensitive methods in liver, bone, and kidney tissue and in skin fibroblasts in culture in severely affected patients *(70,71)*. However, the enzyme in fibroblasts has different physicochemical properties compared with the enzyme in normal cells, though it is TNSALP-like *(70)*. Furthermore, the physicochemical and immunological properties of these TNSALPs differ from patient to patient *(72)*.

Inheritance

The first evidence that hypophosphatasia has a genetic basis came when affected siblings were described in 1950 *(73)*. Early on, family studies of severe disease in infants or children indicated autosomal recessive inheritance. Consanguinity was reported in some kindreds. Parents of patients were sometimes noted to have low or low-normal levels of ALP activity in serum and PEA was sometimes detected in their urine *(36,60)*.

For the milder forms of hypophosphatasia, the inheritance pattern has been less clear. In some reports, the childhood and adult forms, as well as odontohypophosphatasia, are regarded as autosomal recessive conditions *(74–76)*. Indeed, generation-to-generation transmission of clinically apparent disease seems to be unusual *(38,39)*, yet biochemical abnormalities and mild disease have been reported as dominant traits *(38,39,52,77–79)*. Occasionally, mild and severe disease occur in different generations of the same family *(38,79,80)*.

Identification of carriers for hypophosphatasia by biochemical methods can be difficult—necessitating quantitation of several biochemical markers including urinary PPi levels *(81)*. Pyridoxine loading, followed by assay of plasma PLP levels, distinguishes patients from controls especially well *(82)*, and can help to identify carriers as demonstrated in studies involving the Mennonite population in Canada *(83)*.

TNSALP Gene Defects

Chromosomal defects have been rarely reported in hypophosphatasia. In 1970, a common D/D translocation (nonbanded methodology) seems to have been a coincidental finding in one affected adult *(66)*. Complex phenotypes are also unusual. Phenylketonuria was described in one infant with low serum ALP activity, phosphoethanolaminuria, and generalized skeletal demineralization *(84)*. Morquio syndrome together with hypophosphatasia occurred in a Hutterite family in Canada. Here, coincidence of two autosomal recessive conditions appears to be the explanation *(85)*.

In 1984, a brief preliminary report based upon skin fibroblast heterokaryon studies involving 10 unrelated patients with perinatal or infantile disease described absence of complementation (i.e., persistently low cellular ALP activities) indicating a single defective gene locus in hypophosphatasia *(67)*.

In 1987, linkage studies by Chodirker and co-workers of the Rh blood group to hypophosphatasia in six Mennonite kindreds from Manitoba provided evidence that the "candidate" TNSALP gene would be altered in this Canadian population *(86)*.

In 1988, characterization of the gene encoding TNSALP by Weiss and colleagues *(15)* provided the basis for understanding of the molecular pathology of hypophosphatasia *(15,87)*. Indeed, that same year, these investigators discovered a missense mutation within the TNSALP gene in an infant boy with perinatal hypophosphatasia born to second cousins *(30)*. The patient was homozygous and both parents were carriers of a single base transition. Transfection analysis confirmed that the gene defect diminished the altered enzyme's catalytic activity. Furthermore, information derived from X-ray crystallography of *E. coli* ALP *(20)* suggested that in the patient's TNSALP the spatial relationship of metal ligands to an important arginine residue at the catalytic pocket had been disrupted *(30)*.

In 1992, Henthorn and workers sequenced TNSALP cDNAs from four additional unrelated patients with perinatal or infantile hypophosphatasia *(87)*. A different missense mutation was documented in the eight TNSALP alleles examined, suggesting that there would be considerable molecular heterogeneity causing this inborn error of metabolism. Notably, allele-specific oligonucleotide screening of leukocyte DNA from 50 unrelated hypophosphatasia patients disclosed 23 individuals harboring one of these defects, several of whom had relatively mild disease — including the childhood, adult, or even the odonto form of hypophosphatasia. However, the nature of the other TNSALP allele in these individuals was not known at that time. Also noted in this report, two sibs with typical childhood hypophosphatasia and one unrelated elderly woman with typical adult hypophosphatasia were compound heterozygotes for the identical combination of TNSALP gene missense mutations. Hence, it was demonstrated that childhood and adult hypophosphatasia can be the same disorder, and that these more mild forms of hypophosphatasia can be transmitted as autosomal recessive traits *(87)*. Further analysis showed that each of the nine TNSALP gene missense mutations identified by 1992 altered an amino acid residue conserved in mammalian TNSALPs, including some residues that are conserved in bacteria *(19)*. The three-dimensional structure of *E. coli* ALP *(19,20)* indicated that some of the nucleotide substitutions would disturb metal ligand binding in the mature enzyme, but how the other mutations were deleterious was not understood *(19)*.

In 1993, Greenberg and colleagues reported that homozygosity for a tenth TNSALP missense mutation accounted for the severe hypophosphatasia that is prevalent in Canadian Mennonites, presumably explained by a founder effect and inbreeding *(35)*.

Table 1
TNSALP Gene Mutations in Hypophosphatasia

Reference	Amino Acid Change	Exon
(18,92)	S-1F	
Precursor		
(87)	A16V	3
(18,92)	A23V	3
(18,94)	M45L	4
(87)*	R54C	4
(87)	R54P	4
(92)	G58S	4
(18,95)	A94T	5
(18,92)	G103R	5
(95)	A111T	5
(18,92)	G112R	5
(18,94)	R119H	5
(18,94)	G145V	6
(18,92)	N153D	6
(18,94)	H154Y	6
(95)	A160T	6
(98)	A162T	6
(18,92)	R167W	6
(95)	E174G	6
(18,87)	E174K	6
(95)	A177T	6
(30)	A179T	6
(18,94)	C184Y	6
(87)*	Q190P	6
(95)	E191G	6
(18,92)	R206W	7
(18)	G232V	7
(18,92)	W253X	8
(90)	L272F	9
(18,92)	E274K	9
(87)	D277A	9
(88)	E281K	9
(94)	D289V	9
(90)	L289F	9
(18,94)	D289V	9
(27,44)	F310L	9
(18,35,99)	G317D	10
(95)	F327L	10
(35)	G334D	10
(87,101)*	D361V	10

(95)	V365I	10
(18)	R374C	10
(95)	V382I	11
(18,94)	R411X	11
(87)*	Y419H	11
(18,92)	S428P	12
(18,92)	R433C	12
(44)	G439R	12
(18,92)	G456S	12
(18,94)	E459K	12
(18,92)	G474R	12
(18)	648+1A**	n.a.
(94)	862+5A**	n.a.
(18)	997+3C**	n.a.
(18,94)	delG544**	n.a.
(89)	delCTT1154-1156**	9
(18,94)	delC1172**	n.a.
(27,96)	delT1735**	12

*Allele also contains Y246H amino-acid change.
**Nucleotide changes instead of amino-acid changes.

Subsequent studies from 1994 to 1998 by Ozono et al. *(44)*, Orimo et al. *(88, 89)*, Sugimoto et al. *(90)*, and Cai et al. *(27)* characterized additional TNSALP gene mutations in the Japanese population — including nonsense, donor splice site, and frame shift deletions.

In 1998, Mumm et al. detected additional missense mutations in North America *(91)*. Also in 1998, Mornet and co-workers reported 18 TNSALP gene mutations in 13 European families with the perinatal, infantile, or childhood forms of hypophosphatasia *(92)*. Among these mutations, 15 were novel and, once again, most were missense *(92)*. These investigators found that 24 of the 26 alleles harbored a defect responsible for severe hypophosphatasia. In two patients, however, only one mutation was found. This observation seemed consistent, therefore, with a possible dominant negative effect or a functional role for some polymorphisms in the TNSALP gene *(92,93)*. Computer-assisted modeling of the mutated TNSALPs in this study did not reveal any obvious modification in the predicted enzyme structure, except for mutation R206W that possibly abolished a turn between two β-sheets *(92)*.

In 1999, Taillandier and colleagues reported 11 additional mutations in European patients with severe hypophosphatasia *(94)*.

In summary, 58 different molecular defects have been reported at the time of this writing in the TNSALP gene in hypophosphatasia patients (Table 1). The mutations include missense, nonsense, donor splice site, and frame shift deletions *(30,35,44,87,91,92,94,95)*. We now know that all major clinical forms of hypophosphatasia can involve TNSALP gene defects. Furthermore, all principal forms of hypophosphatasia, even the clinically most mild form, odonto-hypophosphatasia, can be inherited as autosomal recessive traits *(96)*. Hence, it is now apparent that in outbred populations worldwide, molecular diagnosis of hypophosphatasia will require extensive analysis of the TNSALP gene *(87,92,93)*.

Exceptionally rare cases of hypophosphatasia, however, could be due to a regulatory defect in the biosynthesis of TNSALP. In one boy with the infantile form of hypophosphatasia, a series of intravenous infusions of pooled normal plasma was followed by a 4-mo correction of hypophosphatasemia. Normalization of his serum ALP activity was due to skeletal synthesis of the bone isoform of TNSALP *(97)*. Remarkable transient remineralization of osseous tissue occurred during this period of ALP correction. The significant but brief clinical, radiographic, and biochemical improvement could not simply be attributed to the infused ALP, because the circulating half-life of the ALPs is just a few days *(97)*.

The molecular basis of pseudohypophosphatasia is unknown, but the inheritance pattern seems to be autosomal recessive *(3,59)*.

Genotype/Phenotype Correlations

In 1998, several groups of investigators using transfection studies reported that mutations associated with severe hypophosphatasia can impair intracellular transport leading to TNSALP enzyme aggregation within cells *(92,94,96,98,99)*. Also, some TNSALP gene defects may diminish expression of the mutated TNSALP allele or alter TNSALP mRNA stability *(44,100)*.

In 1999, Zurutuza and colleagues reported on genotype/phenotype correlations in European patients with hypophosphatasia *(18)*. Disease severity, assessed by a lethal outcome (typically within the first year of life), was contrasted with ALP activity in renal MDCK cells transfected with patient TNSALP cDNA containing missense mutations. Missense mutations that caused profound reductions in MDCK ALP activity (<4.1% wild-type activity) were associated with lethal outcome. Nonlethal disease was predicted by higher transfected cellular ALP activity. Computer-assisted modeling (Fig. 3) provided insight concerning how the molecular defects could affect TNSALP catalytic activity. [Programs on the internet for TNSALP modeling include Chemscape Chime™ Version 1.02 by MDL Information Systems, Inc. (San Leandro, CA) at http://www.mdli.com and RasWin Molecular Graphics, Windows Version 2.6 by Roger Sayle, Glaxo-Wellcome Research & Development (Stevenage, Hertfordshire, UK) at http://www.umass.edu/microbio/rasmo/index.html] Depending upon the altered amino acid, there appeared to be interference with the active site, metal ligand binding, or dimer interaction *(18)*.

Indeed, variation in the phenotypic expression of hypophosphatasia may be due to additional genetic or epigenetic effects. This is illustrated in some sibships in which there is significantly different severity of hypophosphatasia (Fig. 2A,B). Regulation of TNSALP biosynthesis could affect the expression of hypo-

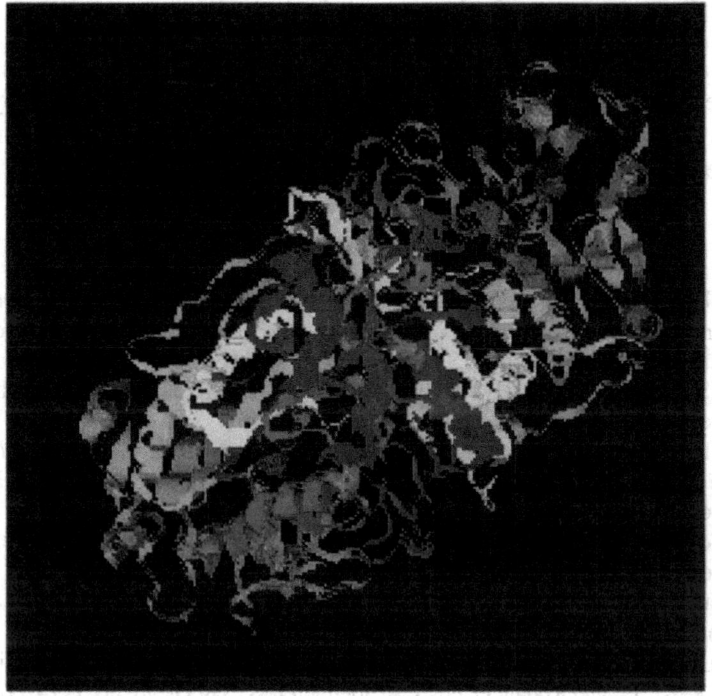

Fig.3. Structure of TNSALP monomer. The RasMol "ribbons" display with "group" color scheme. This shows a smooth, solid, ribbon surface, between each amino acid whose alpha carbon is currently selected, passing along the backbone of the TNSALP protein. The color scheme codes residues by their position in a macromolecular chain. Each chain is drawn as a smooth spectrum from blue through green, yellow, and orange to red. The N terminus of the protein is colored red, and the C terminus is drawn in blue.

phosphatasia. In the childhood form, absolute levels of ALP activity are greater than in adult-onset cases. Perhaps, the physiological decrease in skeletal ALP levels during the adult years explains the clinical re-expression of the disorder in some patients. However, it is noteworthy that the degree of hypophosphatasemia (relative to the serum ALP level that is appropriate for age) is similar in affected children and adults and perhaps helps to explain the "overlap" in defining these two clinical forms of hypophosphatasia.

Biochemical assessments using clinical specimens from patients or obligate heterozygotes (e.g., serum ALP activity and PEA, PPi, and PLP accumulation) vs genotype has not been reported. However, we now seem to be on the verge of considerable improvement in our understanding of the molecular pathology of hypophosphatasia.

Acknowledgments

I am grateful to Michelle N. Podgornik for skilled research assistance. Darlene Harmon provided expert secretarial help. Supported in part by Grant #15958 from the Shriners Hospitals for Children and The Clark and Mildred Cox Inherited Metabolic Bone Disease Research Fund.

References

1. Whyte, M. P. (1996) Hypophosphatasia, nature's window on alkaline phosphatase function in man, in *Principles of Bone Biology* (Bilezikian, J., Raisz, L., and Rodan, G., eds.), Academic Press, San Diego, pp. 951–968.
2. Whyte, M. P. (1994) Hypophosphatasia and the role of alkaline phosphatase in skeletal mineralization. *Endocr. Rev.* **15,** 439–461.
3. Whyte, M. P. Hypophosphatasia, in *The Metabolic and Molecular Bases of Inherited Disease,* 8th ed. (Scriver, C. R., Beaudet, A. L., Sly, W. S., and Vale, D. eds.), McGraw–Hill, New York, in press.
4. McComb, R. B., Bowers, G. N., Jr., and Posen, S. (1979) *Alkaline Phosphatase,* Plenum, New York.
5. Harris, H. (1989) The human alkaline phosphatases: what we know and what we don't know. *Clin. Chim. Acta* **186,** 133–150.
6. Henthorn, P. S. (1996) Alkaline phosphatase, in *Principles of Bone Biology* (Bilezikian, J., Raisz, L., and Rodan, G. eds.), Academic Press, San Diego, pp. 197–206.
7. McKusick, V. A. (1998) *Mendelian Inheritance in Man, A Catalog of Human Genes and Genetic Disorders,* 12th ed., Johns Hopkins University Press, Baltimore.
8. Moss, D. W. and Whitaker, K. B. (1985) Modification of alkaline phosphatases by treatment with glycosidases. *Enzyme* **34**, 212–216.
9. Harris, H. (1980) *The Principles of Human Biochemical Genetics*, 3rd ed., Elsevier, Amsterdam, The Netherlands.
10. Smith, M., Weiss, M. J., Griffin, C. A., Murray, J. C., Buetow, K. H., Emanuel, B. S., et al. (1988) Regional assignment of the gene for human liver/bone/kidney alkaline phosphatase to human chromosome 1p36.1-p34. *Genomics* **2,** 139–143.
11. Griffin, C. A., Smith, M., Henthorn, P. S., Harris, H., Weiss, M. J., Raducha, M., and Emanuel, B. S. (1987) Human placental and intestinal alkaline phosphatase genes map to 2q34-q37. *Am. J. Hum. Genet.* **41,** 1025–1034.
12. Human gene mapping (1986) *Cytogenet. Cell Genet.* **40,** 1.
13. Berger, J., Garattini, E., Hua, J.-C., and Udenfriend, S. (1987) Cloning and sequencing of human intestinal alkaline phosphatase cDNA. *Proc. Natl. Acad. Sci. USA* **84,** 695–698.
14. Henthorn, P. S., Raducha, M., Edwards, Y. H., Weiss, M. J., Slaughter, C., Lafferty, M. A., and Harris, H. (1987) Nucleotide and amino acid sequences of human intestinal alkaline phosphatase. Close homology to placental alkaline phosphatase. *Proc. Natl. Acad. Sci. USA* **84,** 1234–1238.
15. Weiss, M. J., Ray, K., Henthorn, P. S., Lamb, B., Kadesch, T., and Harris, H. (1988) Structure of the human liver/bone/kidney alkaline phosphatase gene. *J. Biol. Chem.* **263,** 12,002–12,010.
16. Kiledjian, M. and Kadesch, T. (1990) Analysis of the human liver/bone/kidney alkaline phosphatase promoter in vivo and in vitro. *Nucleic Acids Res.* **18,** 957–961.

17. Nosjean, O., Koyama, I., Goseki, M., Roux, B., and Komoda, T. (1997) Human tissue non-specific alkaline phosphatases: sugar-moiety-induced enzymic and antigenic modulations and genetic aspects. *Biochem. J.* **321,** 297–303.
18. Zurutuza, L., Muller, F., Gibrat, J. F., Taillandier, A., Simon-Bouy, B., Serre, J. L., and Mornet, E. (1999) Correlations of genotype and phenotype in hypophosphatasia. *Hum. Mol. Genet.* **8,** 1039–1046.
19. Henthorn, P. S. and Whyte, M. P. (1991) Missense mutations of the tissue-nonspecific alkaline phosphatase gene in hypophosphatasia. *Clin. Chem.* **38,** 2501–2505.
20. Kim, E. E. and Wyckoff, H. W. (1991) Reaction mechanism of alkaline phosphatase based on crystal structures. Two-metal ion catalysis. *J. Mol. Biol.* **218,** 449–464.
21. Hawrylak, K. and Stinson, R. A. (1987) Tetrameric alkaline phosphatase from human liver is converted to dimers by phosphatidylinositol pospholipase C. *FEBS Lett.* **212,** 289–291.
22. Fedde, K. N., Lane, C. C., and Whyte, M. P. (1988) Alkaline phosphatase is an ectoenzyme that acts on micromolar concentrations of natural substrates at physiologic pH in human osteosarcoma (SAOS–2) cells. *Arch. Biochem. Biophys.* **264,** 400–409.
23. Hoylaerts, M. F. and Millan, J. L. (1991) Site-directed mutagenesis and epitope-mapped monoclonal antibodies define a catalytically important conformational difference between human placental and germ cell alkaline phosphatase. *Eur. J. Biochem.* **202,** 605–616.
24. Xu, Y., Cruz, T. F., and Pritzker, K. P. (1991) Alkaline phosphatase dissolves calcium pyrophosphate dihydrate crystals. *J. Rheumatol.* **18,** 1606–1610.
25. Farley, J. R. (1991) Phosphate regulates the stability of skeletal alkaline phosphatase activity in human osteosarcoma (SaOS-2) cells without equivalent effects on the level of skeletal alkaline phosphatase immunoreactive protein. *Calcif. Tissue Int.* **57,** 371–378.
26. Seetharam, B., Tiruppathi, C., and Alpers, D. H. (1987) Hydrophobic interactions of brush border alkaline phosphatases. The role of phosphatidyl inositol. *Arch. Biochem. Biophys.* **253,** 189–198.
27. Cai, G., Michigami, T., Yamamoto, T., Yasui, N., Satomura, K., Yamagata, M., et al. (1998) Analysis of localization of mutated tissue–nonspecific alkaline phosphatase proteins associated with neonatal hypophosphatasia using green fluorescent protein chimeras. *J. Clin. Endocrinol. Metab.* **83,** 3936–3942.
28. Anh, D. J., Dimai, H. P., Hall, S. L., and Farley, J. R. (1998) Skeletal alkaline phosphatase activity is primarily released from human osteoblasts in an insoluble form, and the net release is inhibited by calcium and skeletal growth factors. *Calcif. Tissue Int.* **62,** 332–340.
29. Millan, J. L., Whyte, M. P., Avioli, L. V., and Fishman, W. H. (1980) Hypophosphatasia (adult form): quantitation of serum alkaline phosphatase isoenzyme activity in a large kindred. *Clin. Chem.* **26,** 840–845.
30. Weiss, M. J., Cole, D. E., Ray, K., Whyte, M. P., Lafferty, M. A., Mulivor, R. A., and Harris, H. (1988) A missense mutation in the human liver/bone/kidney alkaline phosphatase gene causing a lethal form of hypophosphatasia. *Proc. Natl. Acad. Sci. USA* **85,** 7666–7669.
31. Weiss, M. J., Cole, D. E., Ray, K., Whyte, M. P., Lafferty, M. A., Mulivor, R., and Harris, H. (1989) First identification of a gene defect for hypophosphatasia, evidence that alkaline phosphatase acts in skeletal mineralization. *Connect. Tissue Res.* **21,** 99–104.

32. Rathbun, J. C. (1948), Hypophosphatasia: a new developmental anomaly. *Am. J. Dis. Child.* **75,** 822–831.
33. Anderson, H. C., Hsu, H. H. T., Morris, D. C., Fedde, K. N., and Whyte, M. P. (1997) Matrix vesicles in osteomalacic hypophosphatasia bone contain apatite-like mineral crystals. *Am. J. Pathol.* **151,** 1555–1561.
34. Whyte, M. P., Mahuren, D. J., Vrabel, L. A., and Coburn, S. P. (1985) Markedly increased circulating pyridoxal-5'-phosphate levels in hypophosphatasia: alkaline phosphatase acts in vitamin B_6 metabolism. *J. Clin. Invest.* **76,** 752–756.
35. Greenberg, C. R., Taylor, C. L., Haworth, J. C., Seargeant, L. E., Philipps, S., Triggs-Raine, B., and Chodirker, B. N. (1993) A homoallelic Gly317—Asp mutation in ALPL causes the perinatal (lethal) form of hypophosphatasia in Canadian Mennonites. *Genomics* **17,** 215–217.
36. Fraser, D. (1957) Hypophosphatasia. *Am. J. Med.* **22,** 730–746.
37. Taillard, F., Desbois, J. C., Delepine, N., Gretillat, F., Allaneau, C., and Herrault, A. (1984) L'hypophosphatasie affection polymorphe de frequence peut-etre sous estimee. *Med. Inform. (Lond)* **91,** 559–576.
38. Whyte, M. P., Teitelbaum, S. L., Murphy, W. A., Bergfeld, M., and Avioli, L. V. (1979) Adult hypophosphatasia, clinical, laboratory, and genetic investigation of a large kindred with review of the literature. *Medicine (Baltimore)* **58,** 329–347.
39. Whyte, M. P., Murphy, W. A., and Fallon, M. D. (1982) Adult hypophosphatasia with chondrocalcinosis and arthropathy, Variable penetrance of hypophosphatasemia in a large Oklahoma kindred. *Am. J. Med.* **72,** 631–641.
40. Terheggen, H. G. and Wischermann, A. (1984) Congenital hypophosphatasia. *Monatsschr. Kinderheilkd.* **132,** 512–522.
41. Moore, C. A., Ward, J. C., Rivas, M. C., Magill, H. L., and Whyte, M. P. (1990) Infantile hypophosphatasia: autosomal recessive transmission to two related sibships. *Am. J. Med. Genet.* **36,** 15–22.
42. Macfarlane, J. D., Kroon, H. M., and van der Harten, J. J. (1992) Phenotypically dissimilar hypophosphatasia in two sibships. *Am. J. Med. Genet.* **42,** 117–121.
43. Silver, M. M., Vilos, G. A., and Milne, K. J. (1988) Pulmonary hypoplasia in neonatal hypophosphatasia. *Pediatr. Pathol.* **8,** 483–493.
44. Ozono, K., Yamagata, M., Michigami, T., Nakajima, S., Sakai, N., Cai, G., et al. (1996) Identification of novel missense mutations (Phe310Leu and Gly439Arg) in a neonatal case of hypophosphatasia. *J. Clin. Endocrinol. Metab.* **81,** 4458–4461.
45. Kozlowski, K., Sutcliffe, J., Barylak, A., Harrington, G., Kemperdick, H., Nolte, K., et al. (1976) Hypophosphatasia, Review of 24 cases. *Pediatr. Radiol.* **5,** 103–117.
46. Shohat, M., Rimoin, D. L., Gruber, H. E., and Lachman. R. S. (1991) Perinatal lethal hypophosphatasia; clinical, radiologic, and morphologic findings. *Pediatr. Radiol.* **21,** 421–427.
47. Teree, T. M. and Klein, L. R. (1968) Hypophosphatasia: clinical and metabolic studies. *J. Pediatr.* 72**,** 41–50.
48. Whyte, M. P., Valdes, R. Jr., Ryan, L. M., and McAlister, W. H. (1982) Infantile hypophosphatasia, Enzyme replacement therapy by intravenous infusion of alkaline phosphatase-rich plasma from patients with Paget bone disease. *J. Pediatr.* **101,** 379–386.
49. Fallon, M. D., Teitelbaum, S. L., Weinstein, R. S., Goldfischer, S., Brown, D. M., and Whyte, M. P. (1984) Hypophosphatasia: clinicopathologic comparison of the infantile, childhood, and adult forms. *Medicine (Baltimore)* **63,** 12–24.

50. Kjellman, M., Oldfelt, V., Nordenram, A., and Olow-Nordenram, M. (1973) Five cases of hypophosphatasia with dental findings. *Int. J. Oral Surg.* **2,** 152–158.
51. Lundgren, T., Westphal, O., Bolme, P., Modeer, T., and Noren, J. G. (1991) Retrospective study of children with hypophosphatasia with reference to dental changes. *Scand. J. Dent. Res.* **99,** 357–364.
52. Lepe, X., Rothwell, B. R., Banich, S., and Page, R. C. (1997) Absence of adult dental anomalies in familial hypophosphatasia. *J. Periodontal Res.* **32,** 375–380.
53. Seshia, S. S., Derbyshire, G., Haworth, J. C., and Hoogstraten, J. (1990) Myopathy with hypophosphatasia. *Arch. Dis. Child.* **65,** 130–131.
54. Wendling, D., Cassou, M., and Guidet, M. (1985) Hypophosphatasia in adults. Apropos of 2 cases. *Rev. Rhum. Mal. Osteoartic.* **52,** 43–50.
55. Chuck, A. J., Pattrick, M. G., Hamilton, E., Wilson, R., and Doherty, M. (1989) Crystal deposition in hypophosphatasia: a reappraisal. *Ann. Rheum. Dis.* **48,** 571–576.
56. Lassere, M. N. and Jones, J. G. (1990) Recurrent calcific periarthritis, erosive osteoarthritis and hypophosphatasia: a family study. *J. Rheumatol.* **17,** 1244–1248.
57. Scriver, C. R. and Cameron, D. (1969) Pseudohypophosphatasia. *N. Engl. J. Med.* **281,** 604–606.
58. Moore, C. A., Wappner, R. S., Coburn, S. P., Mulivor, R. A., Fedde, K. N., and Whyte, M. P. (1990) Pseudohypophosphatasia, clinical, radiographic, and biochemical characterization of a second case. (abstr.) *Am. J. Hum. Genet.* **47,** A-68.
59. Fedde, K. N., Cole, D. E. C., and Whyte, M. P. (1990) Pseudohypophosphatasia, Aberrant localization and substrate specificity of alkaline phosphatase in cultured skin fibroblasts. *Am. J. Hum. Genet.* **47,** 776–783.
60. Currarino, G., Neuhauser, E., Reyersback, G., and Sobel, E. (1957) Hypophosphatasia. (abstr.) *Am. J. Roentgenol.* **78,** 392.
61. Whyte, M. P. and Rettinger, S. D. (1987) Hyperphosphatemia due to enhanced renal reclamation of phosphate in hypophosphatasia (abstr. 399). *J. Bone Miner. Res.* **(Suppl 1),** 2.
62. Taillard, F., Desbois, J.-C., Gueris, J., Delepine, N., Lacour, B., Gretillat, F., and Wyart, D. (1985) Pyrophosphates inorganiques et parathormone dans l'hypophosphatasie. Etude d'une famille. *Biomed. Pharmacother.* **39,** 236–241.
63. Vanneuville, F. J. and Leroy, J. G. (1981) Enzymatic diagnosis of congenital lethal hypophosphatasia in tissues, plasma, and diploid skin fibroblasts. *J. Inherit. Metab. Dis.* **4,** 129–130.
64. Mueller, H. D., Stinson, R. A., Mohyuddin, F., and Milne, J. K. (1983) Isoenzymes of alkaline phosphatase in infantile hypophosphatasia. *J. Lab. Clin. Med.* **102,** 24–30.
65. Whyte, M. P., Walkenhorst, D. A., Fedde, K. N., Henthorn, P. S., and Hill, C. S. (1996) Hypophosphatasia, Levels of bone alkaline phosphatase isoenzyme immunoreactivity in serum reflect disease severity. *J. Clin. Endocrinol. Metab.* **81,** 2142–2148.
66. O'Duffy, J. D. (1970) Hypophosphatasia associated with calcium pyrophosphate dihydrate deposits in cartilage. *Arthritis Rheum.* **13,** 381–388.
67. Whyte, M. and Vrabel, L. (1984) Infantile hypophosphatasia: complementation analysis with skin fibroblast heterokaryons suggests a defect(s) at a single gene locus. (abstr.) *Am. J. Hum. Genet.* **26,** 209–S.
68. Fallon, M. D., Whyte, M. P., Weiss, M. J., and Harris, H. (1989) Molecular biology of hypophosphatasia, A point mutation or small deletion in the bone/liver/kidney alkaline phosphatase gene results in an intact but functionally inactive enzyme. (abstr.) *J. Bone Miner. Res.* **4,** S-304.

69. Goseki, M., Oida, S., Takagi, Y., Okuyama, T., Watanabe, J., and Sasaki, S. (1990) Immunological study on hypophosphatasia. *Clin. Chim. Acta* **190,** 263–268.
70. Whyte, M. P., Rettinger, S. D., and Vrabel, L. A. (1987) Infantile hypophosphatasia, Enzymatic defect explored with alkaline phosphatase-deficient patient skin fibroblasts in culture. *Calcif. Tissue Int.* **40,** 244–252.
71. Whyte, M. P., Mahuren, J. D., Fedde, K. N., Cole, F. S., McCabe, E. R., and Coburn, S. P. (1988) Perinatal hypophosphatasia, Tissue levels of vitamin B_6 are unremarkable despite markedly increased circulating concentrations of pyridoxal-5'-phosphate (evidence for an ectoenzyme role for tissue-nonspecific alkaline phosphatase). *J. Clin. Invest.* **81,** 1234–1239.
72. Fedde, K. N., Michell, M. P., Henthorn, P. S., and Whyte, M. P. (1996) Aberrant properties of alkaline phosphatase in patient fibroblasts correlate with clinical expressivity in severe forms of hypophosphatasia. *J. Clin. Endocrinol. Metab.* **81,** 2587–2594.
73. Schneider, R. W. and Corcoran, A. C. (1950) Familial nephrogenic osteopathy due to excessive tubular reabsorption of inorganic phosphate: a new syndrome and a novel mode of relief. *J. Lab. Clin. Med.* **36,** 985–986.
74. Pimstone, B., Eisenberg, E., and Silverman, S. (1966) Hypophosphatasia, genetic and dental studies. *Ann. Intern. Med.* **65,** 722–729.
75. Harris, B. and Robson, E. B. (1959) A genetical study of ethanolamine phosphate excretion in hypophosphatasia. *Hum. Genet.* **23,** 421–441.
76. McCance, R. A., Fairweather, D. V. I., Barrett, A. M., and Morrison, A. B. (1956) Genetic, clinical, biochemical and pathological features of hypophosphatasia. *Q. J. Med.* **25,** 523–537.
77. Eberle, F., Hartenfels, S., Pralle, H., and Kabisch, A. (1984) Adult hypophosphatasia without apparent skeletal disease, "Odontohypophosphatasia" in four heterozygote members of a family. *Klin. Wochenschr.* **62,** 371–376.
78. Silverman, J. L. (1962) Apparent dominant inheritance of hypophosphatasia. *Arch. Intern. Med.* **110,** 191–198.
79. Eastman, J. R. and Bixler, D. (1983) Clinical, laboratory, and genetic investigations of hypophosphatasia, Support for autosomal dominant inheritance with homozygous lethality. *J. Craniofac. Genet. Dev. Biol.* **3,** 213–234.
80. Eastman, J. and Bixler, D. (1982) Lethal and mild hypophosphatasia in half-sibs. *J. Craniofac. Genet. Dev. Biol.* **2,** 35–44.
81. Sorensen, S. A., Flodgaard, H. and Sorensen, E. (1978) Serum alkaline phosphatase, serum pyrophosphatase, phosphorylethanolamine and inorganic pyrophosphate in plasma and urine: a genetic and clinical study of hypophosphatasia. *Monogr. Hum. Genet.* **10,** 66–69.
82. Whyte, M. P. (1989) Alkaline phosphatase, physiologic role explored in hypo–phosphatasia. *Bone Mineral Research,* 6th ed. (Peck, W. A., ed.), Elsevier Science, Amsterdam, The Netherlands, pp. 175–218.
83. Chodirker, B. N., Coburn, S. P., Seargeant, L. E., Whyte, M. P., and Greenberg, C. R. (1990) Increased plasma pyridoxal-5'-phosphate levels before and after pyridoxine loading in carriers of perinatal/infantile hypophosphatasia. *J. Inherit. Metab. Dis.* **13,** 891–896.
84. Blaskovics, M. E. and Shaw, K. N. (1974) Hypophosphatasia with phenylketonuria. *Eur. J. Pediatr.* **117,** 265–273.

85. Lowry, R. B., Snyder, F. F., Wesenberg, R. L., Machin, G. A., Applegarth, D. A., Morgan, K., et al. (1985) Morquio syndrome (MPS IVA) and hypophosphatasia in a Hutterite kindred. *Am. J. Med. Genet.* **22,** 463–475.
86. Chodirker, B. N., Evans, J. A., Lewis, M., Coghlan, G., Belcher, E., Philipps, S., et al. (1987) Infantile hypophosphatasia-linkage with the RH locus. *Genomics* **1,** 280–282.
87. Henthorn, P. S., Raducha, M., Fedde, K. N., Lafferty, M. A., and Whyte, M. P. (1992) Different missense mutations at the tissue-nonspecific alkaline phosphatase gene locus in autosomal recessively inherited forms of mild and severe hypophosphatasia. *Proc. Natl. Acad. Sci. USA* **89,** 9924–9928.
88. Orimo, H., Hayashi, Z., Watanabe, A., Hirayama, T., Hirayama, T., and Shimada, T. (1994) Novel missense and frameshift mutations in the tissue-nonspecific alkaline phosphatase gene in a Japanese patient with hypophosphatasia. *Hum. Mol. Genet.* **3,** 1683–1684.
89. Orimo, H., Goseki-Sone, M., Sato, S., and Shimada, T. (1997) Detection of deletion 1154-1156 hypophosphatasia mutation using TNSALP exon amplification. *Genomics* **42,** 364–366.
90. Sugimoto, N., Iwamoto, S., Hoshino, Y. and Kajii, E. (1998) A novel missense mutation of the tissue-nonspecific alkaline phosphatase gene detected in a patient with hypophosphatasia. *J. Hum. Genet.* **43,** 160–164.
91. Mumm, S., Jones, J., Henthorn, P. S., Eddy, M. C., and Whyte, M. P. (1998) Mutational analysis of the bone alkaline phosphatase gene in hypophosphatasia (Abstr.). *Bone* **5(Suppl 1),** S28.
92. Mornet, E., Taillandier, A., Peyramaure, S., Kaper, F., Muller, F., Brenner, R., et al. (1998) Identification of fifteen novel mutations in the tissue-nonspecific alkaline phosphatase (TNSALP) gene in European patients with severe hypophosphatasia. *Eur. J. Hum. Genet.* **6,** 308–314.
93. Henthorn, P., Ferrero, A., Fedde, K., Coburn, S., and Whyte, M. (1996) Hypophosphatasia mutation D361V exhibits dominant effects both in vivo and in vitro. (abstr.) *Am. J. Hum. Genet.* **59,** A199.
94. Taillandier, A., Zurutuza, L., Muller, F., Simon-Bouy, B., Serre, J. L., Bird, L., et al. (1999) Characterization of eleven novel mutations (M45L, R119H, 544delG, G145V, H154Y, C184Y, D289V, 862+5A, 1172delC, R411X, E459K) in the tissue-nonspecific alkaline phosphatase (TNSALP) gene in patients with severe hypophosphatasia. *Hum. Mutat.* **13,** 171,172.
95. Goseki–Sone, M., Orimo, H., Iimura, T., Takagi, Y., Watanabe, H., Taketa, K., et al. (1998) Hypophosphatasia, identification of five novel missense mutations (G507A, G705A, A748G, T1155C, G1320A) in the tissue-nonspecific alkaline phosphatase gene amoung Japanese patients. *Hum. Mutat.* **(Suppl 1),** S263–S267.
96. Goseki-Sone, M., Orimo, H., Iimura, T., Miyazaki, H., Oda, K., Shibata, H., et al. (1998) Expression of the mutant (1735T–DEL) tissue–nonspecific alkaline phosphatase gene from hypophosphatasia patients. *J. Bone Miner. Res.* **13,** 1827–1834.
97. Whyte, M. P., Magill, H. L., Fallon, M. D., and Herrod, H. G. (1986) Infantile hypophosphatasia, normalization of circulating bone alkaline phosphatase activity followed by skeletal remineralization. Evidence for an intact structural gene for tissue nonspecific alkaline phosphatase. *J. Pediatr.* **108,** 82–88.
98. Shibata, H., Fukushi, M., Igarashi, A., Misumi, Y., Ikehara, Y., Ohashi, Y., and Oda, K. (1998) Defective intracellular transport of tissue-nonspecific alkaline phos-

phatase with an Ala$^{162\vee}$–Thr mutation associated with lethal hypophosphatasia. *J. Biochem.* **123,** 968–977.

99. Fukushi, M., Amizuka, N., Hoshi, K., Ozawa, H., Kumagai, H., Omura, S., et al. (1998) Intracellular retention and degradation of tissue-nonspecific alkaline phosphatase with a Gly^{317}–Asp substitution associated with lethal hypophosphatasia. *Biochem. Biophys. Res. Commun.* **246,** 613–618.
100. Weiss, M. J., Ray, K., Fallon, M. D., Whyte, M. P., Fedde, K. N., Lafferty, M. A., et al. (1989) Analysis of liver/bone/kidney alkaline phosphatase mRNA, DNA, and enzymatic activity in cultured skin fibroblasts from 14 unrelated patients with severe hypophosphatasia. *Am. J. Hum. Genet.* **44,** 686–694.
101. Henthorn, P. S. and Whyte, M. P. (1995) Infantile hypophosphatasia, successful prenatal assessment by testing for tissue-non-specific alkaline phosphatase isoenzyme gene mutations. *Prenat. Diagn.* **15,** 1001–1006.

CHAPTER 19

Jansen and Blomstrand

Two Human Chondrodysplasias Caused by PTH/PTHrP Receptor Mutations

Harald Jüppner and Caroline Silve

Introduction

Genetic linkage studies and positional cloning strategies have led with increasing frequency to the identification of molecular defects, often in unforeseen candidate genes or in novel genes with yet unknown biological relevance. Similar advances in understanding the physiological importance of a variety of proteins have been achieved through gene ablation techniques and through the targeted expression of genes using tissue-specific promoters. Since they often provided unanticipated results, these studies using gene manipulation techniques have proved to be of considerable importance for determining the biological role(s) of some known gene products, frequently redirecting the search for abnormalities in these proteins in human or other mammalian disorders. This is illustrated, as outlined in this chapter, by the identification of activating and inactivating PTH/PTHrP receptor mutations as the cause of two rare genetic disorders in humans.

Parathyroid Hormone (PTH) and PTH-Related Peptide (PTHrP)

The most important endocrine regulators of mineral ion homeostasis in mammals are PTH and 1,25$(OH)_2$ vitamin D_3 *(1)*. PTH is expressed almost exclusively in the parathyroid glands [only small amounts were identified in rat hypothalamus *(2)*], where its synthesis and secretion are inhibited by elevated concentrations of extracellular calcium and 1,25$(OH)_2$ vitamin D_3, but enhanced

The Genetics of Osteoporosis and Metabolic Bone Disease
Ed.: M. J. Econs © Humana Press Inc., Totowa, NJ

by low calcium concentrations. The amino-terminal portion of PTH acts primarily on kidney and bone to maintain blood calcium (and phosphate) concentrations within narrow limits, but different portions of the intact PTH molecule may serve a variety of additional biological functions *(3)*.

PTHrP was first discovered as the major cause of the humoral hypercalcemia of malignancy syndrome *(4–8)*. Shortly after its initial isolation from several different tumors, however, PTHrP and its mRNA were found in large variety of fetal and adult tissues, suggesting that PTHrP has an important biological role throughout life *(9,10)*. Within its amino-terminal portion, PTHrP shares partial amino acid sequence homology with PTH, and as a result of these limited structural similarities, amino-terminal fragments of both peptides have largely indistinguishable biological properties, at least with regard to the regulation of adult mineral ion homeostasis *(11–14)*. Additional mid/carboxyl-terminal fragments of either peptide are generated through alternative splicing and/or posttranslational processing. These PTH and PTHrP fragments have little or no importance for the regulation of adult mineral ion homeostasis and it appears likely that their actions are mediated through different, as yet unidentified receptors *(3)*.

PTHrP Is Important for Endochondral Bone Formation

The most prominent biological role of PTHrP, besides its importance in the humoral hypercalcemia of malignancy syndrome, was revealed when both alleles of its gene were ablated through homologous recombination in mice *(15)*. Homozygous PTHrP gene-ablated animals die during the perinatal period and show striking skeletal changes which include domed skulls, short snouts and mandibles, and disproportionately short extremities, yet no obvious developmental defects in other organs. These skeletal changes are caused by a dramatic acceleration of chondrocyte differentiation that leads to premature growth plate mineralization, providing compelling evidence for an important role of PTHrP in chondrocyte differentiation *(15)*. In contrast, heterozygous animals, lacking only one copy of the PTHrP gene, show normal growth and development, and are fertile, but develop, despite apparently normal calcium and phosphorus homeostasis, mild osteopenia later in life *(16)*.

Growth plate abnormalities that are, in many respects, the opposite of those found in PTHrP-ablated mice are observed in animals that overexpress PTHrP under the control of the α1(II) collagen promoter *(17)*. Throughout life these animals are smaller in size than their wild-type litter mates, and show a disproportionate foreshortening of limbs and tail, which is most likely due to a severe delay in chondrocyte differentiation and endochondral ossification. Thus, too little or too much PTHrP leads to short-limbed dwarfism, although through entirely different mechanisms.

From these and other studies, it is now well established that PTHrP facilitates the continuous proliferation of chondrocytes in the growth plate, and that it postpones their programmed differentiation into hypertrophic chondrocytes. Consistent with this role of PTHrP in endochondral bone formation, earlier in vitro studies had shown that PTH (used in earlier studies instead of PTHrP) affects chondrocyte maturation and activity *(18,19)*. More recent studies confirmed these findings by showing that PTH and PTHrP stimulate, presumably through cAMP-dependent mechanisms *(20)*, the proliferation of fetal growth plate chondrocytes, inhibit the differentiation of these cells into hypertrophic chondrocytes, and furthermore stimulate the accumulation of cartilage-specific proteoglycans that are thought to act as inhibitors of mineralization *(21–23)*. In the absence of these cartilage-specific PTHrP effects, growth plates of homozygous PTHrP gene-ablated mice have a thinner layer of proliferating chondrocytes, while the layer of hypertrophic chondrocytes is relatively normal in thickness, but somewhat disorganized. Taken together these findings suggested that the lack of PTHrP accelerates the normal differentiation process of growth plate chondrocytes, i.e., resting and proliferating chondrocytes undergo fewer cycles of cell division and differentiate prematurely into hypertrophic cells which then undergo apoptosis before being replaced by invading osteoblasts.

The PTH/PTHrP Receptor: A Receptor for Two Ligands

The actions of amino-terminal PTH and PTHrP fragments are mediated through the common PTH/PTHrP receptor which belongs to a distinct family of G protein-coupled receptors *(24)*. Recombinant PTH/PTHrP receptors, when expressed by mammalian cells, bind amino-terminal fragments of PTH and PTHrP with similar or indistinguishable affinity, and both ligands stimulate with similar potency the formation of at least two second messengers, cAMP and inositol phosphate *(25–29)*. Similar to the widely expressed PTHrP, the mRNA encoding the PTH/PTHrP receptor is found in a surprisingly large variety of fetal and adult tissues *(30–34)*. The most abundant expression, however, is found in renal tubular cells and in osteoblasts, where the PTH/PTHrP receptor mediates the endocrine actions of PTH, and in prehypertrophic chondrocytes of metaphyseal growth plate, where it mediates the autocrine/paracrine actions of PTHrP *(15,17)*.

A second PTH-receptor, termed the PTH2-receptor, which belongs to the same family of G protein-coupled receptors as the PTH/PTHrP receptor, has been recently isolated *(35,36)*. However, unlike the common PTH/PTHrP receptor, this novel receptor is expressed only in few tissues, and at least the human PTH2R interacts with PTH *(35,37,38)* and with a recently isolated hypothalamic peptide TIP39) *(39)*, but not with PTHrP. Due to this ligand specificity and due to its limited expression, it appears unlikely that the PTH2-receptor mediates any of the PTHrP-dependent autocrine/paracrine processes *(15,40)*. Consistent with this notion, mice in which both alleles encoding the PTH/PTHrP receptor are ablated, show growth plate abnormalities that are similar to, but more severe than, those observed in PTHrP-ablated animals *(40)*.

As outlined above, the PTH/PTHrP receptor mediates directly the actions of PTH and PTHrP, but indirectly it mediates also the actions of *Indian Hedgehog* (*Ihh*) *(40,41)*. This developmentally important protein is abundantly expressed in growth plate chondrocytes that are about to differentiate into hypertrophic cells, and its ectopic expression in chicken wing cartilage blocks the normal chondrocyte differentiation program *(41)*. The aberrant expression of *Ihh* thus leads to growth plate changes that are similar to those observed in transgenic mice overexpressing PTHrP under the control of the α1(II) collagen promoter *(17)*, and are the opposite of those found in mice in which the genes encoding PTHrP or its PTH/PTHrP receptor had been disrupted through homologous recombination *(15,40)*. PTHrP, which acts through the PTH/PTHrP receptor, and *Ihh*, which acts through the membrane-associated proteins *patched* and *smoothened*, are thus critically important components of a negative feed-back loop within the growth plate *(40,41)*.

It is unusual that a single receptor mediates the actions of two distinct ligands, PTH and PTHrP, that have entirely different biological functions. This made it difficult to identify in humans, or other mammals, disorders that are caused by either activating or inactivating mutations in the PTH/PTHrP receptor. Inactivating mutations in the PTH-receptor, e.g., the PTH/PTHrP receptor, were initially thought to cause pseudohypoparathyroidism type Ib *(42,43)*. However, such mutations were not identified in any of the coding and noncoding exons of the PTH/PTHrP receptor gene, and recent linkage studies have mapped the genetic locs of the disease to a region onchromosome 20q (20q13.3), which comprises the *GNAS1* gene that encodes the stimulatory G protein *(44–48)*. Moreover, due to its prominent expression in three different tissues, kidney, bone, and growth plates, and due to its obvious importance in mineral ion homeostasis and bone elongation, it became apparent that PTH/PTHrP receptor mutations (activating or inactivating mutations) would affect growth plate development as well as calcium/phosphorus homeostasis. This was demonstrated by the identification of defects in the PTH/PTHrP receptor gene in patients with Jansen's and Blomstrand's chondrodysplasia.

Jansen's Metaphyseal Chondrodysplasia (JMC)

JMC, first described in 1934 *(49)*, is a rare autosomal dominant form of short-limbed dwarfism associated with laboratory abnormalities that are typically observed only in patients with either primary hyperparathyroidism or with the humoral hypercalcemia of malignancy syndrome [reviewed in *(50,51)*]. These biochemical changes, i.e., hypercalcemia, renal phosphate wasting, and increased urinary cAMP excretion, occur despite low or undetectable concentrations of circulating PTH and PTHrP. Radiological studies in younger patients with JMC show severe metaphyseal changes, especially of the long bones (Fig. 1). These metaphyseal areas are enlarged and expanded, and give a club-like appearance to the ends of the long bones. There are patches of partially calcified cartilage that protrude into the diaphyses, and that appear relatively radiolucent on X-rays. Histologically, the growth plates show a severe delay in endochondral ossification of the metaphyses, including a lack of the regular columnar arrangement of the maturing cartilage cells, a lack of excess osteoid (which is usually indicative

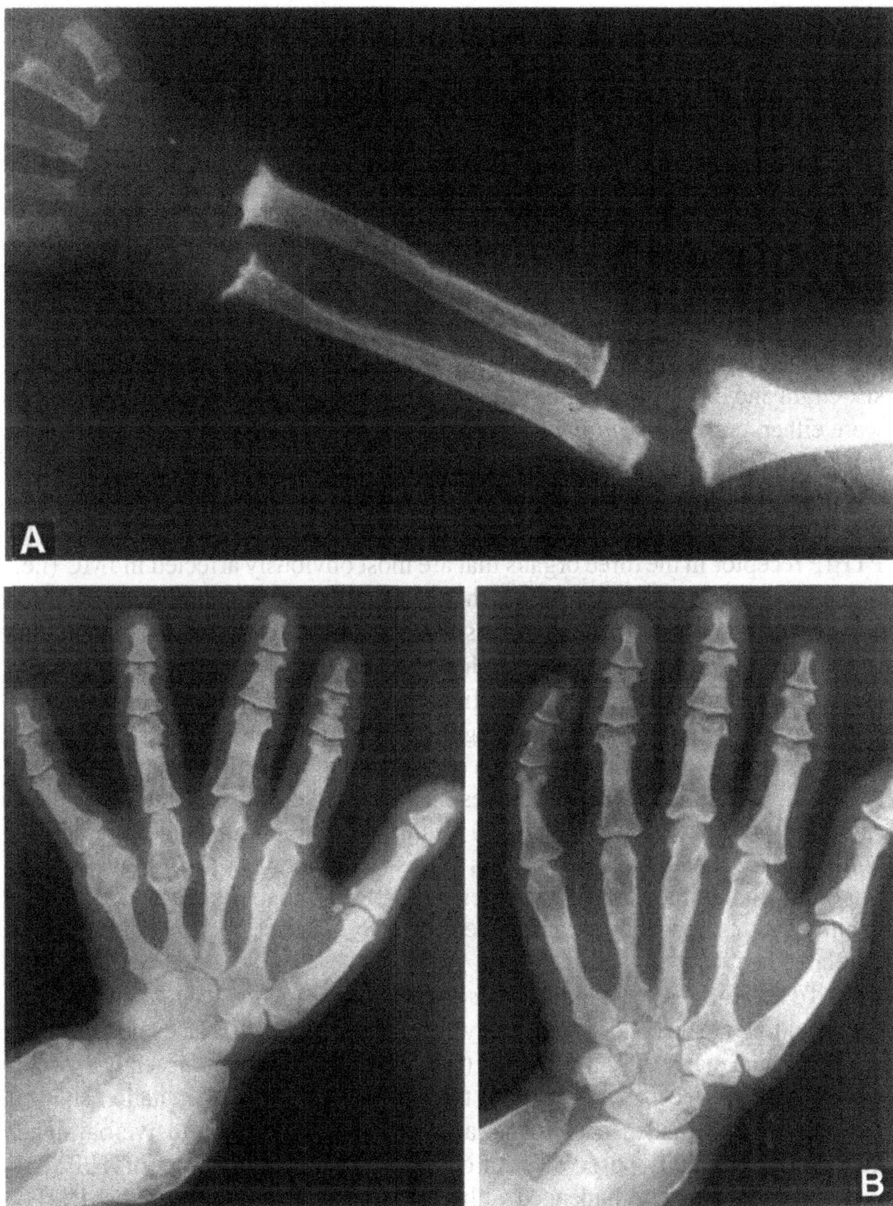

Fig. 1. Hand radiographs of a patient with Jansen's disease. Note that the metaphyseal ends at 5 wk of age (upper panel) are irregular and have an appearance that resembles rickets; at age 10 (lower left panel) there is irregular calcification, the metaphyseal areas are severely enlarged and expanded; at age 22 (lower right panel) the abnormalities in zones of calcification have completely disappeared, from *(95)* with permission.

of active rickets or osteomalacia), little or no vascularization of cartilage, and no evidence for osteitis fibrosa *(52,53)*. In contrast, bone specimens from adult JMC patients can show significant fibrosis, increased activity of osteoblasts and osteoclasts, leading to an exaggerated loss of cortical bone, despite preservation of cancellous bone *(51,52,54)*.

Jansen's Disease Is Caused by Activating PTH/PTHrP Receptor Mutations

To explain the obvious association between the abnormal regulation of endochondral bone formation and the profound changes in mineral ion homeostasis, Gram and colleagues suggested that the changes in calcium and phosphorus were either *"secondary to the underlying bone defect,"* or related to *"an undefined metabolic disorder that gave rise to both metaphyseal and biochemical changes." (54)* Because of the findings in the different genetically manipulated mice described previously, and because of the abundant expression of the PTH/PTHrP receptor in the three organs that are most obviously affected in JMC (i.e., kidney, bone, and metaphyseal growth plate), activating receptor mutations were considered as the cause of this rare disease. Indeed, in several unrelated patients with this disorder, a heterozygous nucleotide exchange, which changes a histidine at position 223 to arginine, was identified in exon M2 of the PTH/PTHrP receptor gene *(50,55–57)*. A second heterozygous nucleotide exchange, which changes threonine at position 410 to proline in exon M5, was identified so far only in one JMC patient (Fig. 2)*. Both mutated residues are predicted to be located at or close to the intracellular surface of the cell membrane, and both residues are strictly conserved in all mammalian members of this receptor family *(24)*, suggesting an important functional role for both residues. Both mutations were excluded in healthy parents and siblings, and in genomic DNA from a significant number of unrelated healthy individuals.

To test in vitro the functional consequences of the missense mutations in JMC, the two different nucleotide exchanges were introduced into the cDNA encoding the wild-type human PTH/PTHrP receptor (50, 55-57). COS-7 cells transiently expressing PTH/PTHrP receptors with either the H223R or the T410P mutation showed constitutive, ligand-independent cAMP accumulation that was three to fivefold higher than the basal activity observed with cells expressing the wild-type PTH/PTHrP receptor (Fig. 3). When challenged with increasing concentrations of either PTH or PTHrP, cells expressing the mutant receptor showed submaximal cAMP accumulation, in comparison to cells expressing the wild-type receptor. Furthermore, the two mutant PTH/PTHrP receptors showed no evidence for increased basal inositol phosphate accumulation, indicating that neither mutation leads to a constitutive activation of the phosphoinositol pathway *(55,56)*.

*A third activating PTH/PTHrP recpetor mutaion was recently identified *(96)*.

Activating mutations in other G protein-coupled receptors have been implicated in several other human diseases. These disorders include rare forms of retinitis pigmentosa or congenital stationary blindness (activating mutations in rhodopsin) *(58,59)*, thyroid adenomas or nonautoimmune hyperthyroidism (activating TSH receptor mutations) *(60–65)*, gonadotropin-independent male precocious puberty (activating mutations in the luteinizing hormone receptor) *(66–69)*, and autosomal dominant forms of familial hypocalcemia (activating calcium-sensing receptor mutations) *(70–75)*.

To prove that the growth plate abnormalities in Jansen's disease are indeed caused by constitutively active PTH/PTHrP receptors, transgenic mice were recently generated that express the H223R mutant under the control of the rat α1(II) collagen promoter, thereby targeting receptor expression to proliferating chondrocytes *(76)*. Two transgenic mouse lines were established, both of which showed delayed mineralization and decelerated conversion of proliferative chondrocytes into hypertrophic chondrocytes, a delay in vascular invasion and a prolonged presence of hypertrophic chondrocytes. In one of these mouse lines, the defect in endochondral bone formation was only apparent at the microscopic level, while the second line showed shortened and deformed limbs that are reminiscent of the findings in patients with Jansen's disease. Based on these results it appears likely that the growth abnormalities in JMC are caused by the expression of mutant, constitutively active PTH/PTHrP receptor in growth plate chondrocytes.

In an attempt to prolong the survival of mice that are homozygous for the PTHrP-gene ablation, the transgenic "Jansen" animals were crossed with heterozygous "PTHrP-knock-out" mice. Inbred offspring that lack both copies of the PTHrP gene, yet express the "Jansen" transgene show no obvious developmental defect at birth. Subsequently, however, these "rescued" mice fail to grow normally, and die at the age of about 2 mo for yet unknown reasons *(76)*. These findings demonstrate that the early lethality of mice lacking both copies of the PTHrP gene is caused by the drastically accelerated process of endochondral bone formation.

Blomstrand's Lethal Chondrodysplasia (BLC)

Based on the findings in patients with Jansen's disease and in mutant mice in which the alleles encoding PTHrP or the PTH/PTHrP receptor had been ablated, it was speculated that inactivating receptor mutations would lead to a recessive human disorder characterized by early lethality, advanced bone maturation and accelerated chondrocyte differentiation, and most likely severe abnormalities in mineral ion homeostasis. Such a lethal chondrodysplasia characterized by markedly increased bone density, and advanced bone age, was first described by Blomstrand and colleagues in 1985 *(77)*, and subsequently by others *(78–82)*. The disorder was shown to occur in families of different ethnic backgrounds and appears to affect males and females equally. Furthermore, affected infants are typically born to consanguineous parents [only in one instance did unrelated parents have two

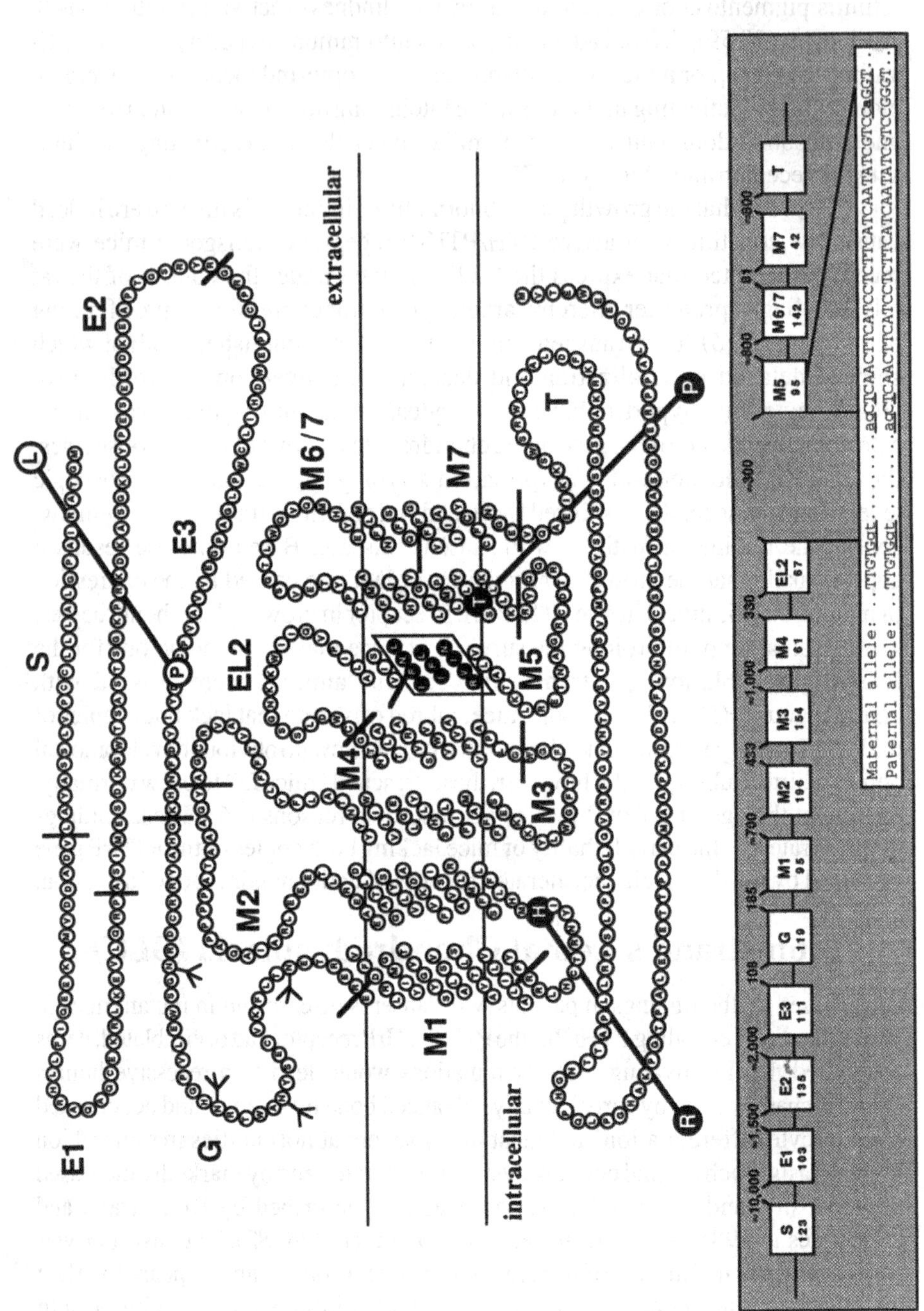
E1
S
G
E2
E3
M1
M2
M3
M4
M5
M6/7
M7
EL2
T
extracellular
intracellular
Maternal allele:
Paternal allele:

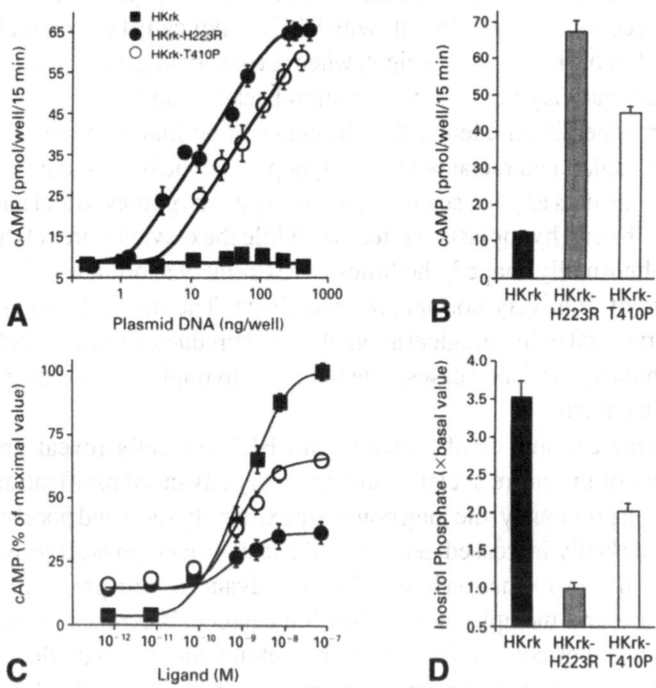

Fig. 3. Functional characterization of constitutively active PTH/PTHrP receptors identified in patients with Jansen's disease. The properties of wild-type (HKrk) and mutant PTH/PTHrP receptors (HKrk-H223R and HKrk-T410P) transiently expressed in COS-7 cells are shown. Basal cAMP accumulation of COS-7 cells that express increasing concentrations of wild-type or mutant PTH/PTHrP receptors **(A)**; basal **(B)** and PTH-stimulated **(C)** cAMP accumulation; and PTH-stimulated inositol phosphate accumulation **(D)** using COS-7 cells expressing maximal concentrations of wild-type or mutant PTH/PTHrP receptors. Wild-type human PTH/PTHrP receptor, HKrk ■; HKrk-H223R ●; HKrk-T410P ○. From *(56)* with permission.

Fig. 2. *(See opposite page)* Amino acid sequence of the human PTH/PTHrP receptor (upper panel) and schematic representation of the organization of its gene (lower panel). The locations of the missense mutations that lead to constitutive receptor activation (●) or loss-of-function (○) are shown; the receptor region that is deleted due to the nucleotide exchange that introduces a novel splice acceptor site into the maternal allele is delineated by a solid line. Nucleotide sequences encoding portions of exons M5 and M6/7, and the splice sites that were identified in wild-type PTH/PTHrP receptor gene are shown; consensus nucleotides of splice-acceptor and splice-donor sites are underlined *(44)*. The nucleotide exchange identified in the maternal allele of one patient with Blomstrand's disease is indicated in bold; it introduces a novel splice-acceptor site in exon M5; the normal paternal allele is shown for comparison.

offspring that are affected by Blomstrand's disease *(80)*], suggesting that BLC is an autosomal recessive disease. Infants with BLC are typically born prematurely and die shortly after birth. The birth weight, when corrected for gestational age, appears to be normal, but may be an overestimation because most infants are hydroptic with severe generalized edema; the placenta can be immature and edematous. Nasal, mandibular, and facial bones are hypoplastic, the base of the skull is short and narrow, the ears are low set, the thoracic cage is hypoplastic and narrow with short thick ribs and hypoplastic vertebrae. While the clavicles are relatively long and often abnormally shaped, the limbs are extremely short, and only the hands and feet are of relatively normal size and shape. The internal organs show no apparent structural or histological anomalies, but preductal aortic coarctation was observed in most published cases. The lungs are hypoplastic, and the protruding eyes show cataracts.

Radiological studies of patients with BLC typically reveal pronounced hyperdensity of the entire skeleton and markedly advanced ossification (Fig. 4). As mentioned previously, the long bones are extremely short and poorly modeled, and show markedly increased density, and a lack of metaphyseal growth plates. Endochondral bone formation is dramatically advanced, with premature fusion of the epiphyseal and metaphyseal ossification centers. The zones of chondrocyte proliferation and of column formation are lacking, and the zone that comprises normally the layer of hypertrophic chondrocytes is poorly defined, narrow and irregular. Capillary ingrowth, bone resorption, and bone formation are reported by some authors to be unaltered *(79)*, while others describe the bone remodeling events as deficient *(80)*.

Blomstrand's Disease Is Caused by Inactivating PTH/PTHrP Receptor Mutations

The recent identification of defects in the PTH/PTHrP receptor gene established the role of this receptor in BLC. Thus far, three different defects in the PTH/PTHrP receptor have been reported in two patients with Blomstrand's disease (Fig. 2). The first reported case, a product of nonconsanguineous parents, was shown to have two distinct abnormalities in the PTH/PTHrP receptor gene *(83)*. Through a nucleotide exchange in exon M5 of the maternal PTH/PTHrP receptor allele, a novel splice acceptor site is introduced that leads to a mutant mRNA that encodes an abnormal receptor lacking portions of the fifth membrane-spanning domain. This receptor mutant fails, despite seemingly normal cell surface expression, to respond to PTH or PTHrP with an accumulation of cAMP and inositol phosphate. For yet unknown reasons, the paternal PTH/PTHrP receptor allele from this patient is only extremely poorly expressed, suggesting an unidentified mutation in one of the different promoter regions or in a putative enhancer element.

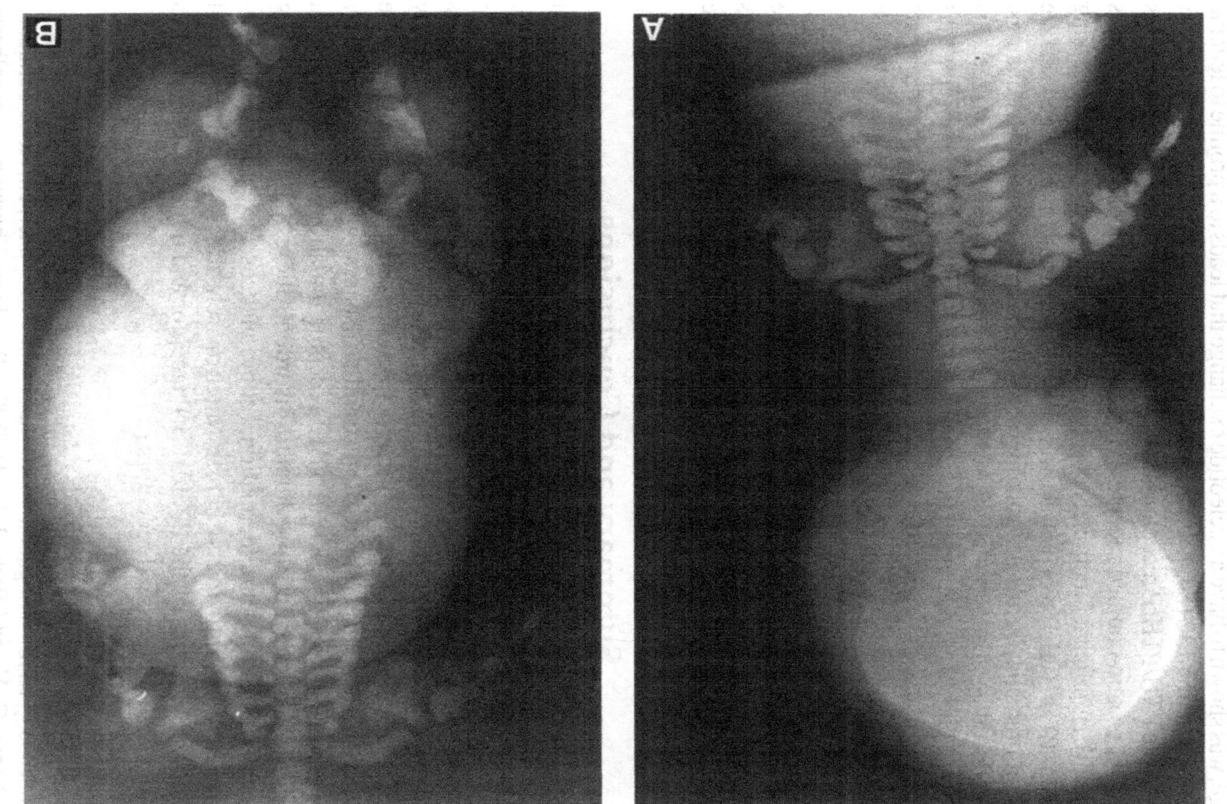

Fig. 4. Radiological findings in a patient with BLC; from *(79)* with permission. Note the dramatic acceleration of endochondral bone formation of all skeletal elements, the extremely short limbs, despite the comparatively normal size and shape of hands and feet. Furthermore, note that the clavicles are relatively long and abnormally shaped.

A second patient with Blomstrand's disease, the product of a consanguineous marriage, was shown to have a nucleotide exchange that leads to a proline to leucine mutation at position 132 *(84,97)*. This residue in the amino-terminal, extracellular domain of the PTH/PTHrP receptor is invariant in all mammalian members of this family of G protein-coupled receptors, indicating that the identified mutation is likely to have significant functional consequences. Indeed, COS-7 cells expressing this mutant PTH/PTHrP receptor showed, despite apparently normal cell surface expression, dramatically impaired binding of radiolabeled PTH and PTHrP analogs, greatly reduced agonist-stimulated cAMP accumulation, and showed no measurable inositol phosphate response (Fig. 5). The findings in both BLC patients thus provided a plausible explanation for the severe abnormalities in endochondral bone formation, and suggest that this rare human disease is the equivalent of the mouse PTH/PTHrP receptor "knock-out."

Inactivating mutations have been described in other G protein-coupled receptors. For example, genetic forms of growth hormone deficiency were shown to be caused by mutations in the growth hormone-releasing hormone receptor in humans *(85)* and in mice (*little* mouse) *(86)*, and mutations in the thyrotropin receptor are the cause of inherited hypothyroidism in mice *(87,88)*.

Summary and Conclusions

Recent findings in transgenic and gene-ablated mice provided novel insights into the complicated autocrine/paracrine mechanisms that regulate growth and differentiation of growth plate chondrocytes, and thus bone elongation. The characteristic abnormalities in these genetically manipulated animals provided important clues in the search for human disorders that are caused by mutant PTH/PTHrP receptors, and led to the molecular definition of two rare genetic disorders, Jansen's and Blomstrand's diseases, which are caused by activating and inactivating PTH/PTHrP receptor mutations, respectively. In addition to resolving puzzling human disorders, these naturally occurring mutations, each having unique functional consequences, have provided important new insights into the structure/function relationship and the signal transduction properties of the PTH/PTHrP receptor and other members of this family of G protein-coupled receptors *(89–94)*.

References

1. Kronenberg, H. M., Bringhurst, F. R., Nussbaum, S., Jüppner, H., Abou-Samra, A. B., Segre, G. V., and Potts, J. T., Jr. (1993) Parathyroid hormone: biosynthesis, secretion, chemistry, and action, in *Handbook of Experimental Pharmacology: Physiology and Pharmacology of Bone* (Mundy, G. R. and Martin, T. J., eds.) Springer-Verlag, Heidelberg, Germany, pp. 185–201.
2. Nutley, M. T., Parimi, S. A., and Harvey, S. (1995) Sequence analysis of hypothalamic parathyroid hormone messenger ribonucleic acid. *Endocrinology* **136,** 5600–5607.

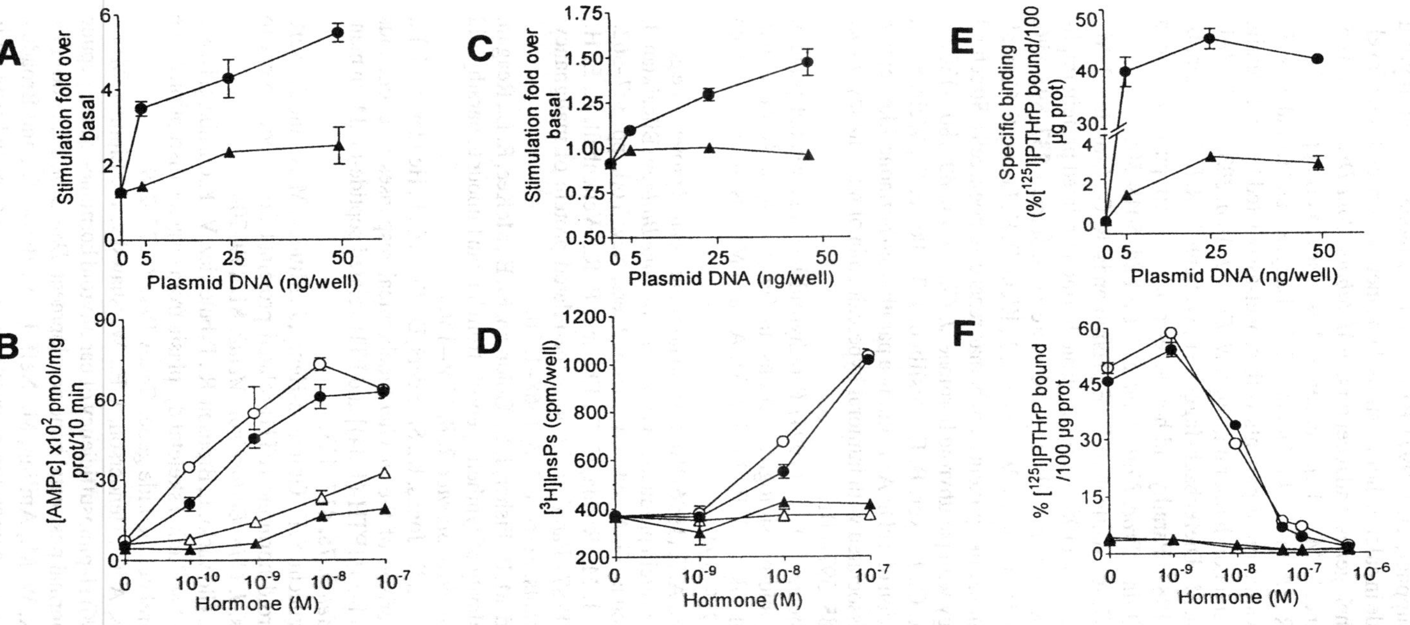

Fig. 5. Functional evaluation of the wild-type and P132L PTH/PTHrP receptors expressed in COS-7 cells. In panels **(A)**, **(C)**, and **(E)**, results are shown for cells transiently transfected with the indicated doses of plasmid DNA encoding the wild-type (circles) or mutant (triangles) PTH/PTHrP receptors. Cyclic AMP **(A)** and inositol phosphate accumulation **(C)** in response to 10^{-7} *M* hPTH(1–34). **(E)**: specific binding of radiolabeled ligand (total binding of [^{125}I]PTHrP(1–36)amide minus binding observed in the presence of 5 ¥ 10^{-7} *M* unlabeled PTH). Panels **(B)**, **(D)** and **(F)** show the results obtained for cells transiently transfected with 50 ng/well of plasmid DNA coding for wild-type (circles) or mutant (triangles) PTH/PTHrP receptors, and incubated in the presence of increasing concentrations of hPTH(1–34) (closed symbols) and PTHrP(1–34) (open symbols); stimulation of cAMP **(B)** and inositol phosphate accumulation **(D)**; competitive inhibition of the binding of [^{125}I]PTHrP(1–36)amide by the indicated concentrations of unlabeled hPTH(1–34) and PTHrP(1–34), respectively. Adapted with permission from *ref. (84)*.

3. Potts, J. T., Jr. and Jüppner, H. (1997) Parathyroid hormone and parathyroid hormone-related peptide in calcium homeostasis, bone metabolism, and bone development: the proteins, their genes, and receptors, in *Metabolic Bone Disease*, 3rd ed. (Avioli, L. V. and Krane, S. M., eds.), Academic Press, New York, pp. 51–94.
4. Stewart, A. F., Horst, R., Deftos, L. J., Cadman, E. C., Lang, R., and Broadus, A. E. (1980) Biochemical evaluation of patients with cancer-associated hypercalcemia. Evidence for humoral and non-humoral groups. *N. Engl. J. Med.* **303,** 1377–1381.
5. Moseley, J. M., Kubota, M., Diefenbach-Jagger, H., Wettenhall, R. E. H., Kemp, B. E., Suva, L. J., et al. (1987) Parathyroid hormone-related protein purified from a human lung cancer cell line. *Proc. Natl. Acad. Sci. USA* **84,** 5048–5052.
6. Suva, L. J., Winslow, G. A., Wettenhall, R. E., Hammonds, R. G., Moseley, J. M., Diefenbach-Jagger, H., et al. (1987) A parathyroid hormone-related protein implicated in malignant hypercalcemia: cloning and expression. *Science* **237,** 893–896.
7. Strewler, G. J., Stern, P. H., Jacobs, J. W., Eveloff, J., Klein, R. F., Leung, S. C., et al. (1987) Parathyroid hormone-like protein from human renal carcinoma cells. Structural and functional homology with parathyroid hormone. *J. Clin. Invest.* **80,** 1803–1807.
8. Mangin, M., Webb, A. C., Dreyer, B. E., Posillico, J. T., Ikeda, K., Weir, E. C., et al. (1988) Identification of a cDNA encoding a parathyroid hormone-like peptide from a human tumor associated with humoral hypercalcemia of malignancy. *Proc. Natl. Acad. Sci. USA* **85,** 597–601.
9. Broadus, A. E. and Stewart, A. F. (1994) Parathyroid hormone-related protein: Structure, processing, and physiological actions, in *The parathyroids. Basic and Clinical Concepts* (Bilezikian, J. P., Levine, M. A., and Marcus, R., eds.) Raven Press, New York, pp. 259–294.
10. Yang, K. H. and Stewart, A. F. (1996) Parathyroid hormone-related protein: the gene, its mRNA species, and protein products, in *Principles of Bone Biology* (Bilezikian, J. P., Raisz, L. G., and Rodan, G. A., eds.) Academic Press, New York, pp. 347–362.
11. Kemp, B. E., Mosely, J. M., Rodda, C. P., Ebeling, P. R., Wettenhall, R. E. H., Stapleton, D., et al. (1987) Parathyroid hormone-related protein of malignancy: active synthetic fragments. *Science* **238,** 1568–1570.
12. Horiuchi, N., Caulfield, M. P., Fisher, J. E., Goldman, M. E., McKee, R. L., Reagan, J. E., et al. (1987) Similarity of synthetic peptide from human tumour to parathyroid hormone *in vivo* and *in vitro*. *Science* **238,** 1566–1568.
13. Fraher, L. J., Hodsman, A. B., Jonas, K., Saunders, D., Rose, C. I., Henderson, J. E., et al. (1992) A comparison of the *in vivo* biochemical responses to exogenous parathyroid hormone-(1-34) [PTH-(1-34)] and PTH-related peptide-(1-34) in man. *J. Clin. Endocrinol. Metab.* **75,** 417–423.
14. Everhart-Caye, M., Inzucchi, S. E., Guinness-Henry, J., Mitnick, M. A., and Stewart, A. F. (1996) Parathyroid hormone (PTH)-related protein(1-36) is equipotent to PTH(1–34) in humans. *J. Clin. Endocrinol. Metab.* **81,** 199–208.
15. Karaplis, A. C., Luz, A., Glowacki, J., Bronson, R., Tybulewicz, V., Kronenberg, H. M., and Mulligan, R. C. (1994) Lethal skeletal dysplasia from targeted disruption of the parathyroid hormone-related peptide gene. *Genes Dev.* **8,** 277–289.
16. Amizuka, N., Karaplis, A. C., Henderson, J. E., Warshawsky, H., Lipman, M. L., Matsuki, Y., et al. (1996) Haploinsufficiency of parathyroid hormone-related peptide (PTHrP) results in abnormal post-natal bone development. *Dev. Biol.* **175,** 166–176.
17. Weir, E. C., Philbrick, W. M., Amling, M., Neff, L. A., Baron, R., and Broadus, A. E. (1996) Targeted overexpression of parathyroid hormone-related peptide in

chondrocytes causes skeletal dysplasia and delayed endochondral bone formation. *Proc. Natl. Acad. Sci. USA* **93,** 10,240–10,245.

18. Lebovitz, H. E. and Eisenbarth, G. S. (1975) Hormonal regulation of cartilage growth and metabolism. *Vitam. Horm.* **33,** 575–648.
19. Smith, D. M., Roth, L. M., and Johnston, C. C., Jr. (1976) Hormonal responsiveness of adenylate cyclase activity in cartilage. *Endocrinology* **98,** 242–246.
20. Jikko, A., Murakami, H., Yan, W., Nakashima, K., Ohya, Y., Satakeda, H., et al. (1996) Effects of cyclic adenosine 3',5'-monophosphate on chondrocyte terminal differentiation and cartilage-matrix calcification. *Endocrinology* **137,** 122–128.
21. Takano, T., Takigawa, M., Shirai, E., Suzuki, F., and Rosenblatt, M. (1985) Effects of synthetic analogs and fragments of bovine parathyroid hormone on adenosine 3',5'-monophosphate level, ornithine decarboxylase activity, and glycosaminoglycan synthesis in rabbit costal chondrocytes in culture: structure-activity relations. *Endocrinology* **116,** 2536–2542.
22. Koike, T., Iwamoto, M., Shimazu, A., Nakashima, K., Suzuki, F., and Kato, Y. (1990) Potent mitogenic effects of parathyroid hormone (PTH) on embryonic chick and rabbit chondrocytes. Differential effects of age on growth, proteoglycan, and cyclic AMP responses of chondrocytes to PTH. *J. Clin. Invest.* **85,** 626–631.
23. Iwamoto, M., Jikko, A., Murakami, H., Shimazu, A., Nakashima, K., Iwamoto, M., et al. (1994) Changes in parathyroid hormone receptors during chondrocyte cytodifferentiation. *J. Biol. Chem.* **269,** 17,245–17,251.
24. Jüppner, H. (1994) Molecular cloning and characterization of a parathyroid hormone (PTH)/PTH-related peptide (PTHrP) receptor: a member of an ancient family of G protein-coupled receptors. *Curr. Opin. Nephrol. Hypertens.* **3,** 371–378.
25. Jüppner, H., Abou-Samra, A. B., Freeman, M. W., Kong, X. F., Schipani, E., Richards, J., et al. (1991) A G protein-linked receptor for parathyroid hormone and parathyroid hormone-related peptide. *Science* **254,** 1024–1026.
26. Abou-Samra, A. B., Jüppner, H., Force, T., Freeman, M. W., Kong, X. F., Schipani, E., et al. (1992) Expression cloning of a common receptor for parathyroid hormone and parathyroid hormone-related peptide from rat osteoblast-like cells: a single receptor stimulates intracellular accumulation of both cAMP and inositol triphosphates and increases intracellular free calcium. *Proc. Natl. Acad. Sci. USA* **89,** 2732–2736.
27. Abou-Samra, A. B., Jüppner, H., Khalifa, A., Karga, H., Kong, X. F., Schiffer-Alberts, D., et al. (1993) Parathyroid hormone (PTH) stimulates adrenocorticotropin release in AtT-20 cells stably expressing a common receptor for PTH and PTH-related peptide. *Endocrinology* **132,** 801–805.
28. Schipani, E., Karga, H., Karaplis, A. C., Potts, J. T., Jr., Kronenberg, H. M., Segre, G. V., et al. (1993) Identical complementary deoxyribonucleic acids encode a human renal and bone parathyroid hormone (PTH)/PTH-related peptide receptor. *Endocrinology* **132,** 2157–2165.
29. Smith, D. P., Zang, X. Y., Frolik, C. A., Harvey, A., Chandrasekhar, S., Black, E. C., et al. (1996) Structure and functional expression of a complementary DNA for porcine parathyroid hormone/parathyroid hormone-related peptide receptor. *Biochim. Biophys. Acta* **1307,** 339–347.
30. Tian, J., Smorgorzewski, M., Kedes, L., and Massry, S. G. (1993) Parathyroid hormone-parathyroid hormone related protein receptor messenger RNA is present in many tissues besides the kidney. *Am. J. Nephrol.* **13,** 210–213.

31. Urena, P., Kong, X. F., Abou-Samra, A. B., Jüppner, H., Kronenberg, H. M., Potts, J. T., Jr., et al. (1993) Parathyroid hormone (PTH)/PTH-related peptide (PTHrP) receptor mRNA are widely distributed in rat tissues. *Endocrinology* **133,** 617–623.
32. Lee, K., Deeds, J. D., Chiba, S., Un-no, M., Bond, A. T., and Segre, G. V. (1994) Parathyroid hormone induces sequential *c-fos* expression in bone cells in vivo: *in situ* localization of its receptor and *c-fos* messenger ribonucleic acids. *Endocrinology* **134,** 441–450.
33. Lee, K., Deeds, J. D., and Segre, G. V. (1995) Expression of parathyroid hormone-related peptide and its receptor messenger ribonucleic acid during fetal development of rats. *Endocrinology* **136,** 453–463.
34. Lee, K., Brown, D., Urena, P., Ardaillou, N., Ardaillou, R., Deeds, J., and Segre, G. V. (1996) Localization of parathyroid hormone/parathyroid hormone-related peptide receptor mRNA in kidney. *Am. J. Physiol.* **270,** F186–F191.
35. Usdin, T. B., Gruber, C., and Bonner, T. I. (1995) Identification and functional expression of a receptor selectively recognizing parathyroid hormone, the PTH2 receptor. *J. Biol. Chem.* **270,** 15,455–15,458.
36. Usdin, T. B., Bonner, T. I., Harta, G., and Mezey, E. (1996) Distribution of PTH-2 receptor messenger RNA in rat. *Endocrinology* **137,** 4285–4297.
37. Gardella, T. J., Luck, M. D., Jensen, G. S., Usdin, T. B., and Jüppner, H. (1996) Converting parathyroid hormone-related peptide (PTHrP) into a potent PTH-2 receptor agonist. *J. Biol. Chem.* **271,** 19,888–19,893.
38. Behar, V., Nakamoto, C., Greenberg, Z., Bisello, A., Suva, L. J., Rosenblatt, M., and Chorev, M. (1996) Histidine at position 5 is the specificity "switch" between two parathyroid hormone receptor subtypes. *Endocrinology* **137,** 4217–4224.
39. Usdin, T. B. (1999) Tip39: a new neuropeptide and PTH2-receptor agonist from hypothalamus. *Nat. Neurosci.* **2,** 941–943.
40. Lanske, B., Karaplis, A. C., Luz, A., Vortkamp, A., Pirro, A., Karperien, M., et al. (1996) PTH/PTHrP receptor in early development and Indian hedgehog-regulated bone growth. *Science* **273,** 663–666.
41. Vortkamp, A., Lee, K., Lanske, B., Segre, G. V., Kronenberg, H. M., and Tabin, C. J. (1996) Regulation of rate of cartilage differentiation by Indian hedgehog and PTH-related protein. *Science* **273,** 613–622.
42. Silve, C., Santora, A., Breslau, N., Moses, A., and Spiegel, A. (1986) Selective resistance to parathyroid hormone in cultured skin fibroblasts from patients with pseudohypoparathyroidism type Ib. *J. Clin. Endocrinol. Metab.* **62,** 640–644.
43. Levine, M. A. and Aurbach, G. D. (1989) Pseudohypoparathyroidism, in *Endocrinology* (DeGroot. L. J., ed.) Saunders, Philadelphia, pp. 1065–1079.
44. Schipani, E., Weinstein, L. S., Bergwitz, C., Iida-Klein, A., Kong, X. F., Stuhrmann, M., et al. (1995) Pseudohypoparathyroidism type Ib is not caused by mutations in the coding exons of the human parathyroid hormone (PTH)/PTH-related peptide receptor gene. *J. Clin. Endocrinol. Metab.* **80,** 1611–1621.
45. Suarez, F., Lebrun, J. J., Lecossier, D., Escoubet, B., Coureau, C., and Silve, C. (1995) Expression and modulation of the parathyroid hormone (PTH)/PTH-related peptide receptor messenger ribonucleic acid in skin fibroblasts from patients with type Ib pseudohypoparathyroidism. *J. Clin. Endocrinol. Metab.* **80,** 965–970.
46. Fukumoto, S., Suzawa, M., Takeuchi, Y., Nakayama, K., Kodama, Y., Ogata, E., and Matsumoto, T. (1996) Absence of mutations in parathyroid hormone (PTH)/PTH-related protein receptor complementary deoxyribonucleic acid in patients with pseudohypoparathyroidism type Ib. *J. Clin. Endocrinol. Metab.* **81,** 2554–2558.

47. Jüppner, H., Schipani, E., Bastepe, M., Cole, D. E. C., Lawson, M. L., Mannstadt, M., Hendy, G. N., Plotkin, H., Koshiyama, H., Koh, T., Crawford, J. D., Olsen, B. R., and Vikkula, M. (1998) The gene responsible for pseudohypoparathyroidism type Ib is paternally imprinted and maps in four unrealted kindreds to chromosome 2-q13.3. *Proc. Natl. Acad. Sci. USA* **95,** 11,798–11,803.
48. Bettoun, J. D., Minagawa, M., Kwan, M. Y., Lee, H. S., Yasuda, T., Hendy, G. N., et al. (1997) Cloning and characterization of the promoter regions of the human parathyroid hormone (PTH)/PTH-related peptide receptor gene: analysis of deoxyribonucleic acid from normal subjects and patients with pseudohypoparathyroidism type Ib. *J. Clin. Endocrinol. Metab.* **82,** 1031–1040.
49. Jansen, M. (1934) Über atypische Chondrodystrophie (Achondroplasie) und über eine noch nicht beschriebene angeborene Wachstumsstörung des Knochensystems: Metaphysäre Dysostosis. *Zeitschr. Orthop. Chir.* **61,** 253–286.
50. Jüppner, H. (1996) Jansen's metaphyseal chondrodysplasia: A disorder due to a PTH/PTHrP receptor gene mutation. *Trends Endocrinol. Metab.* **7,** 157–162.
51. Parfitt, A. M., Schipani, E., Rao, D. S., Kupin, W., Han, Z.-H., and Jüppner, H. (1996) Hypercalcemia due to constitutive activity of the PTH/PTHrP receptor. Comparison with primary hyperparathyroidism. *J. Clin. Endocrinol. Metab.* **81,** 3584–3588.
52. Jaffe, H. L. (1972) Certain other anomalies of skeletal development, in *Metabolic, Degenerative, and Inflammatory Diseases of Bones and Joints,* Lea and Febiger, Philadelphia, pp. 222–226.
53. Cameron, J. A. P., Young, W. B., and Sissons, H. A. (1954) Metaphysial dysostosis. Report of a case. *J. Bone Joint Surg.* **36B,** 622–629.
54. Gram, P. B., Fleming, J. L., Frame, B., and Fine, G. (1959) Metaphyseal chondrodysplasia of Jansen. *J. Bone Joint Surg.* **41A,** 951–959.
55. Schipani, E., Kruse, K., and Jüppner, H. (1995) A constitutively active mutant PTH-PTHrP receptor in Jansen-type metaphyseal chondrodysplasia. *Science* **268,** 98–100.
56. Schipani, E., Langman, C. B., Parfitt, A. M., Jensen, G. S., Kikuchi, S., Kooh, S. W., et al. (1996) Constitutively activated receptors for parathyroid hormone and parathyroid hormone-related peptide in Jansen's metaphyseal chondrodysplasia. *N. Engl. J. Med.* **335,** 708–714.
57. Minagawa, M., Arakawa, K., Minamitani, K., Yasuda, T., and Niimi, H. (1997) Jansen-type metaphyseal chondrodysplasia: analysis of PTH/PTH–related protein receptor messenger RNA by the reverse transcription-polymerase chain method. *Endocr. J.* **44,** 493–499.
58. Robinson, P. R., Cohen, G. B., Zhukovsky, E. A., and Oprian, D. D. (1992) Constitutively active mutants of rhodopsin. *Neuron* **9,** 719–725.
59. Dryja, T. P., Berson, E. L., Rao, V. R., and Oprian, D. D. (1993) Heterozygous missense mutation in the rhodopsin gene as a cause of congenital stationary night blindness. *Nat. Genet.* **4,** 280–283.
60. Parma, J., Duprez, L., Van Sande, J., Cochaux, P., Gervy, C., Mockel, J., et al. (1993) Somatic mutations in the thyrotropin receptor gene cause hyperfunctioning thyroid adenomas. *Nature* **365,** 649–651.
61. Duprez, L., Parma, J., Van Sande, J., Allgeier, A., Leclere, J., Schvartz, C., et al. (1994) Germline mutations in the thyrotropin receptor gene cause non-autoimmune autosomal dominant hyperthyroidism. *Nat. Genet.* **7,** 396–401.

62. Paschke, R., Tonacchera, M., van Sande, J., Parma, J., and Vassart, G. (1994) Identification and functional characterization of two new somatic mutations causing constitutive activation of the TSH receptor in hyperfunctioning autonomous adenomas of the thyroid. *J. Clin. Endocrinol. Metab.* **79,** 1785–1789.
63. Kopp, P., van Sande, J., Parma, J., Duprez, L., Gerber, H., Joss, E., et al. (1995) Brief report: Congenital hyperthyroidism caused by a mutation in the thyrotropin-receptor gene. *N. Engl. J. Med.* **332,** 150–154.
64. Tonacchera, M., van Sande, J., Cetani, F., Swillens, S., Schvartz, C., Winiszewski, P., et al. (1996) Functional characterisitics of three new germline mutations of the thyrotropin receptor gene causing autosomal dominant toxic thyroid hyperplasia. *J. Clin. Endocrinol. Metab.* **81,** 547–554.
65. Grüters, A., Schöneberg, T., Biebermann, H., Krude, H., Krohn, H. P., Dralle, H., and Gudermann, T. (1998) Severe congenital hyperthyroidism caused by a germline *neo* mutation in the extracellular portion of the thyrotropin receptor. *J. Clin. Endocrinol. Metab.* **83,** 1431–1436.
66. Shenker, A., Laue, L., Kosugi, S., Merendino, J. J., Jr., Minegishi, T., and Cutler, G. B. (1993) A Constitutively activating mutation of the luteinizing hormone receptor in familial male precocious puberty. *Nature* **365,** 652–654.
67. Latronico, A. C., Anasti, J., Arnhold, I. J. P., Mendonca, B. B., Domenice, S., Albano, M. C., et al. (1995) A novel mutation of the luteinizing hormone receptor gene causing male gonadotropin-independent precocious puberty. *J. Clin. Endocrinol. Metab.* **80,** 2490–2494.
68. Kraaij, R., Post, M., Kremer, H., Milgrom, E., Epping, W., Brunner, H. G., et al. (1995) A missense mutation in the second transmembrane segment of the luteinizing hormone receptor causes familial male-limited precocious puberty. *J. Clin. Endocrinol. Metab.* **80,** 3168–3172.
69. Shenker, A. (1998) Disorders caused by mutations of the lutropin/choriogonadotropin receptor gene, in *G Proteins, Receptors, and Disease* (Spiegel, A. M., ed.), Humana Press, Totowa, New Jersey, pp. 139–152.
70. Pollak, M. R., Brown, E. M., Estep, H. L., McLaine, P. N., Kifor, O., Park, J., et al. (1994) Autosomal dominant hypocalcaemia caused by a Ca^{2+}-sensing receptor gene mutation. *Nat. Genet.* **8,** 303–307.
71. Pearce, S. (1995) Calcium-sensing receptor mutations in familial benign hypercalcaemia and neonatal hyperparathyroidism. *J. Clin. Invest.* **96,** 2683–2692.
72. Pearce, S. H. S. and Brown, E. M. (1996) Calcium-sensing receptor mutations: insights into a structurally and functionally novel receptor. *J. Clin. Endocrinol. Metab.* **81,** 1309–1311.
73. Baron, J., Winer, K., Yanovski, J., Cunningham, A., Laue, L., Zimmerman, D., and G Cutler, J. (1996) Mutations in the Ca^{2+} sensing receptor cause autosomal dominant and sporadic hypoparathyroidism. *Hum. Mol. Genet.* **5,** 601–606.
74. Pearce, S. H., Williamson, C., Kifor, O., Bai, M., Coulthard, M. G., Davies, M., et al. (1997) A familial syndrome of hypocalcemia with hypercalciuria due to mutations in the calcium-sensing receptor. *N. Engl. J. Med.* **335,** 1115–1122.
75. Brown, E. M., Pollak, M., Bai, M., and Hebert, S. C. (1998) Disorders with increased or decreased responsiveness to extracellular Ca^{2+} owing to mutations in the Ca^{2+}-sensing receptor, in *G Proteins, Receptors, and Disease* (Spiegel, A. M., ed.), Humana Press, Totowa, NJ.

76. Schipani, E., Lanske, B., Hunzelman, J., Kovacs, C. S., Lee, K., Pirro, A., et al. (1997) Targeted expression of constitutively active PTH/PTHrP receptors delays endochondral bone formation and rescues PTHrP–less mice. *Proc. Natl. Acad. Sci. USA* **94,** 13,689–13,694.
77. Blomstrand, S., Claësson, I., and Säve-Söderbergh, J. (1985) A case of lethal congenital dwarfism with accelerated skeletal maturation. *Pediatr. Radiol.* **15,** 141–143.
78. Young, I. D., Zuccollo, J. M., and Broderick, N. J. (1993) A lethal skeletal dysplasia with generalised sclerosis and advanced skeletal maturation: Blomstrand chondrodysplasia. *J. Med. Genet.* **30,** 155–157.
79. Leroy, J. G., Keersmaeckers, G., Coppens, M., Dumon, J. E., Roels, H. (1996) Blomstrand lethal chondrodysplasia. *Am. J. Med. Genet.* 63**,** 84–89.
80. Loshkajian, A., Roume, J., Stanescu, V., Delezoide, A. L., Stampf, F., and Maroteaux, P. (1997) Familial Blomstrand chondrodysplasia with advanced skeletal maturation: further delineation. *Am. J. Med. Genet.* **71,** 283–288.
81. den Hollander, N. S., van der Harten, H. J., Vermeij-Keers, C., Niermeijer, M. F., and Wladimiroff, J. W. (1997) First-trimester diagnosis of Blomstrand lethal osteochondrodysplasia. *Am. J. Med. Genet.* **73,** 345–350.
82. Oostra, R. J., Baljet, B., Dijkstra, P. F., and Hennekam, R. C. M. (1998) Congenital anomalies in the teratological collection of museum Vrolik in Amsterdam, The Netherlands. II: Skeletal dysplasia. *Am. J. Med. Genet.* **77,** 116–134.
83. Jobert, A. S., Zhang, P., Couvineau, A., Bonaventure, J., Roume, J., LeMerrer, M., and Silve, C. (1998) Absence of functional receptors parathyroid hormone and parathyroid hormone-related peptide in Blomstrand chondrodysplasia. *J. Clin. Invest.* **102,** 34–40.
84. Zhang, P., Jobert, A. S., Couvineau, A., and Silve, C. (1998) A homozygous inactivating mutation in the parathyroid hormone/parathyroid hormone-related peptide receptor causing Blomstrand chondrodysplasia. *J. Clin. Endocrinol. Metab.* **83,** 3365–3368.
85. Wajnrajch, M. P., Gertner, J. M., Harbison, M. D., Chua, S. C., Jr., and Leibel, R. L. (1996) Nonsense mutation in the human growth hormone-releasing hormone receptor causes growth failure analogous to the little (*lit*) mouse. *Nat. Genet.* **12,** 88–90.
86. Godfrey, P., Rahal, J. O., Beamer, W. G., Copeland, N. G., Jenkins, N. A., and Mayo, K. E. (1993) GHRH receptor of little mice contains a missense mutation in the extracellular domain that disrupts receptor function. *Nat. Genet.* **4,** 227–232.
87. Stein, S. A., Oates, E. L., Hall, C. R., Grumbles, R. M., Fernandez, L. M., Taylor, N. A., et al. (1994) Identification of a point mutation in the thyrotropin receptor of the *hyt/hyt* hypothyroid mouse. *Mol. Endocrinol.* **8,** 129–138.
88. Gu, W. X., Du, G. G., Kopp, P., Rentoumis, A., Albanese, C., Kohn, L. D., et al. (1995) The thyrotropin (TSH) receptor transmembrane domain mutation (Pro556-Leu) in the hypothyroid hyt/hyt mouse results in plasma membrane targeting but defective TSH binding. *Endocrinology* **136,** 3146–3153.
89. Gardella, T. J., Luck, M. D., GS, G. S. J., Schipani, E., Potts, J. T., Jr., and Jüppner, H. (1996) Inverse agonism of amino-terminally truncated parathyroid hormone (PTH) and PT-related peptide (PTHrP) analogs revealed with constitutively active mutant PTH/PTHrP receptors linked to Jansen's metaphyseal chondrodysplasia. *Endocrinology* **137,** 3936–3941.
90. Heller, R. S., Kieffer, T. J., and Habener, J. F. (1996) Point mutations in the first and third intracellular loops of the glucagon-like peptide-1 receptor alter intracellular signaling. *Biochem. Biophys. Res. Commun.* **223,** 624–632.

91. Tseng, C. C. and Lin, L. (1997) A point mutation in the glucose-dependent insulinotropic peptide receptor confers constitutive activity. *Biochem. Biophys. Res. Commun.* **232,** 96–100.
92. Cohen, D. P., Thaw, C. N., Varma, A., Gershengorn, M. C., and Nussenzveig, D. R. (1997) Human calcitonin receptors exhibit agonist-independent (constitutive) signaling activity. *Endocrinology* **138,** 1400–1405.
93. Hjorth, S. A., Ørskov, C., and Schwartz, T. W. (1998) Constitutive activity of glucagon receptor mutants. *Mol. Endocrinol.* **12,** 78–86.
94. Gaudin, P., Maoret, J. J., Couvineau, A., Rouyer-Fessard, C., and Laburthe, M. (1998) Constitutive activation of the human vasoactive intestinal peptide 1 receptor, a member of the new class II family of G protein-coupled receptors. *J. Biol. Chem.* **273,** 4990–4996.
95. Frame, B. and Poznanski, A. K. (1980) Conditions that may be confused with rickets, in *Pediatric Diseases Related to Calcium* (DeLuca, H. F. and Anast, C. S., eds.), Elsevier, New York, pp. 269–289.
96. Schipani, E., Langman, C. B., Hunzelman, J., LeMerrer, M., Loke, K. Y., Dillon, M. J., Silve, C., and Juupper, H. (1999) A novel PTH/PTHrP receptor mutation in Jansen's metaphysical chondrodysplasia. *J. Clin. Endocrinol. Metab.* **84,** 3052–3057.
97. Karaplis, A. C., Bin He, M. T., Nguyen, A., Youbg, I. D., Semeraro, D., Ozawa, H., and Amizuka, N. (1998) Inactivation mutation in the human parathyroid hormone receptor type I gene in Blomstrand chondrodysplasia. *Endocrinology* **139,** 5255–5258.

CHAPTER 20

Genetic Linkage Analysis in Human Disease

Suzanne M. Leal and Marcy C. Speer

Introduction

Linkage analysis is a powerful tool for identifying and characterizing the genetic basis for human disease. Most successes have been in the localization of diseases whose inheritance is known to follow simple patterns of Mendelian inheritance like X-linked hypophosphatemic rickets, neurofibromatosis, and Duchenne muscular dystrophy. For these diseases, linkage analysis follows a standard approach — identifying the chromosomal location of the disease gene, determining the minimum candidate interval by the identification of critical recombination events, and systematically narrowing the interval to as small a region as possible by typing additional markers and individuals. This approach is well established: if enough informative meioses are available, the diagnosis is correctly assigned and the power of the available pedigree material is sufficient, the locus *will* be mapped.

For complex traits, however, the approach is less straightforward but still has the ability to identify and characterize the genetic component of these complex traits. For these diseases, the true genetic model is unknown and is usually due to the combination of many different genes. Parametric linkage analysis is not always feasible. For complex traits, a useful strategy is to utilize methods that examine the proportion of alleles shared identical-by-descent or identical-by-state. Since identifying true recombination events is less clear-cut and frequently cannot be done with certainty, identifying the minimum candidate interval is not always possible, complicating molecular efforts to identify the underlying disease gene.

Regardless of the trait under study, the first question to address involves determining whether it has an underlying genetic basis.

The Genetics of Osteoporosis and Metabolic Bone Disease
Ed.: M. J. Econs © Humana Press Inc., Totowa, NJ

What Evidence Suggests a Trait Is Genetic?

Evidence in favor of a genetic component can come from several different sources: twin studies, segregation analysis, comparisons of prevalence of disease in relatives of affecteds and the prevalence in the general population, and association with other known genetic disorders. In addition, clustering of a disease or trait within a family "familial aggregation" is often a hallmark of a genetic contribution to disease; however, it is important to recognize that familial aggregation can be due to a variety of nongenetic factors including a common environmental exposure (e.g., infection, lead poisoning) or chance (*see* Chapter 2). The ultimate proof that a disease has a genetic component is the identification of a gene that has an allele that leads to an increase in risk. For some diseases, the evidence that a disease trait is genetic from one type of study is so overwhelming that evidence from other types of studies, although useful, may be redundant. For instance, in diseases which are transmitted in a clear Mendelian pattern such as Huntington disease (autosomal dominant), cystic fibrosis (autosomal recessive), or X-linked hypophosphatemic rickets (X-linked dominant), visual inspection of pedigree data is frequently enough to give a general gestalt of the genetic basis, although this is clearly not statistical proof.

Interestingly, geneticists frequently make the argument that understanding the genetic basis of the rare familial cases of common disease will allow insight into the pathogenesis of the more common sporadic cases. Although this may be true in some diseases, it may be false in others. A recent example of differences in mutation rates between familial cases and sporadic cases of a disease is found in holoprosencephaly, a midfacial clefting defect. Roessler et al. *(1)* found mutations in the sonic hedgehog gene (SHH) in 23% of familial cases, but in fewer than 1% of sporadic cases.

Twin Studies

Studies of disease in monozygotic (MZ; identical) and dizygotic (DZ; fraternal) twins have long been a mainstay in genetic analysis. In humans, twins provide a unique opportunity to consider the relative effects of genetic and environmental factors that may play a role in disease development. Because MZ twins are derived from the same egg and sperm that splits very soon after fertilization, they share 100% of their genes in common. In contrast, DZ twins occur when two eggs are fertilized independently by separate sperm. Therefore, DZ twins share approx 50% of their genetic material in common, just like other types of siblings. Unlike other siblings, however, DZ twins share a more similar intrauterine and extrauterine environment than nontwin siblings.

Twin studies are performed by studying the occurrence of a disease in MZ and DZ twins, perhaps raised under different environmental conditions. The disease concordance rates provide insight into the relative importance of genetic and environmental effects on disease. A typical design is to compare the concordance rates for a disease between MZ twins raised together and DZ twins raised together. There are subtle differences in the "environment" of MZ and DZ twins; for instance, MZ twins are more likely to look alike than DZ twins and thus will be treated differently as a pair. However, the environment can be considered to have a negligible effect under this design. If the trait is clearly genetic, then the expectation is that the MZ concordance rate will be significantly higher than the DZ concordance rate. If the trait is autosomal dominant with complete penetrance, then the expected MZ concordance rate would be 100% and DZ concordance rate would be 50%. An MZ concordance rate less than 100% might suggest a gene with incomplete or age-dependent penetrance; alternatively, it might suggest the contribution of a significant common environmental factor. The utility of twin studies has been recently reviewed in Martin et al. *(2)*.

Segregation Analysis

The purpose of segregation analysis is to test if transmission patterns within families are consistent with genetic models of transmission *(3–5)*. Segregation analysis was originally designed to test consistency with the hypothesis of a single gene. It has been expanded to test models that include polygenic and oligogenic inheritance *(6)*.

The goal of segregation analysis is to identify the best fitting model. In a segregation analysis, various mathematical models of genetic transmission are analyzed (i.e., dominant, recessive, polygenic, and environmental). Unlike epidemiologic studies where the null hypothesis is no association, in segregation analysis the null hypothesis is that the data fit some mode of inheritance (either genetic or nongenetic). In segregation analysis low power can lead to the situation where although a model (null hypothesis) is incorrect it is not rejected. If all candidate models are inadequate and even the best fitting model does not fit the data adequately, the best model cannot be detected by simply comparing maximum likelihoods. For "complex" traits, so many parameters must be estimated, the models that are compared may be almost saturated and consequently, the data fit all models equally well. Segregation analysis alone can never prove that a particular genetic model is correct or even if a trait is genetic. It can only be used to determine whether observed patterns of a trait are consistent with a specific model compared to a more general model.

A major obstacle in segregation analysis is ascertainment bias. Not only can ascertainment bias influence estimates of segregation probabilities, but it may also make the data appear consistent with a single gene model when this is not the case *(7)*.

Pedigrees collected may be biased in the ways they were sought, thus leading to ascertainment bias. In the case of complete selection, ascertainment is done through random sampling of parents without regard to their offspring. In most cases complete selection (i.e., for recessive traits both parents are unaffected) is not possible and pedigrees are sampled via incomplete selection. For incomplete selection pedigrees are ascertained through one or more affected individuals in a sibship instead of through parental matings. This simplistic example will demonstrate how the segregation proportion can be biased by sampling through affected offspring. If two heterozygotes for an autosomal recessive trait (AaxAa), do not produce any affected offspring the probability that they will be included in a sample is 0. For this mating type, the probability of not being collected for sibship sizes of 1, 2, and 3 are 75, 56.3, and 42.2%, respectively. Sampling through affected offspring leads to truncation of the binomial distribution. The more affected children within a kindred, the higher the probability that the kindred is ascertained. When families are collected without controlling for ascertainment bias, the segregation probability can be biased upward.

Segregation analysis has been successful in confirming genetic transmission in a number of Mendelian disorders, e.g., von Willebrand disease *(8)* and von Hippel-Lindau disease *(9)*. Major gene effects for continuous traits have also been demonstrated using segregation analysis: blood and urine glucose *(10)*, chronic atrophic gastritis *(11)*, and alpha-N-acetyl-d-glucosaminidase levels *(12)*.

The major methods of segregation analysis in use today are the mixed model *(6,13,14)* and the transmission probability model of Elston and Stewart *(15)*. The unified model of Lalouel et al. *(16)*, incorporates the transmission probabilities from the model of Elston and Stewart *(15)* into the mixed model. To allow for the inclusion of environmental covariates, Bonney *(17)* developed regressive models.

Sophisticated analytical computer packages (SAGE, PAP, etc.) have been developed that use maximum likelihood techniques to determine the best underlying model, genetic or otherwise, for the observed pedigree data. All approaches to segregation analysis are subject to significant biases as a result of the way the data were ascertained. In fact, the ascertainment "problem" may be intractable in some circumstances *(18,19)*.

This tool is somewhat controversial in the genetic epidemiology community. If segregation analysis identifies the existence of a major genetic component to a disease, it provides solid evidence for pursuing a genomic screen to identify the underlying genes. However, many geneticists feel that a negative segregation analysis in the presence of familial aggregation would not prevent them from initiating a genomic screen. For example, an appropriately designed segregation analysis may fail to identify an underlying major gene in the presence of extensive heterogeneity, phenocopies, or the interaction of genes with other genes or the environment. Ultimately, the proof that a disease has a genetic component comes only from identifying the gene itself.

Increased Relative Risk

The amount of increase in risk to different types of relatives for genetic disease is well established in Mendelian disease. Since Mendelian diseases are usually rare, the risk to first degree relatives of an affected proband is significantly higher than the risk to a random person in the general population. For example, the population incidence of cystic fibrosis is 1/1600 in American Caucasians. The risk to siblings of a patient with cystic fibrosis is 1/4, and thus the risk for a sibling of an affected individual is 400-fold higher than the risk for a random individual in the general population. Characterizing the strength of the genetic component in a disease was extended by Risch to complex disease *(20)*. The strength of the genetic component is measured by the relative risk λ_i, where ι represents the type of relative. The relative risk is the ratio of the recurrence risk for a particular relative type of a proband to the general population prevalence. In general, the higher the λ-value, the stronger the genetic component. It should be noted that this ratio is extremely sensitive to the frequency of the disease in the population—the more prevalent the disease, the lower the λ will be. The λ value tends to be higher the more closely related individuals are. When a variety of λ's for differing relatives of the proband can be compared within a disease, the patterns can be used to develop hypotheses about underlying genetic mechanisms *(20)*.

Association with Other Known Genetic Diseases

If a trait is inherited in tandem with a disease known to have a genetic effect, this provides evidence in favor of a gene influencing development of the disease. Similarly, diseases which occur together with a chromosomal rearrangement suggest an underlying genetic component and also provide clues into the possible location of the underlying gene. For instance, the co-occurrence of X-chromosome rearrangements with Duchenne muscular dystrophy (DMD) was responsible in large part for the identification of the dystrophin gene *(21)*.

What Is a Phenotype, and How Is It Defined?

A phenotype is the physical manifestation of a disease. For instance, the phenotype of osteoporosis is low bone mass and microarchitectural deterioration of the skeleton, which results in an increased risk of atraumatic fractures. The phenotype of a female with X-linked hypophosphatemic rickets (XLH) is renal phosphate wasting and inappropriate calcitriol concentration that results in rickets with corresponding lower extremity deformity, tooth abscesses, bone pain, enthesopathy (calcification of tendons, ligaments and joint capsule), and short stature.

Phenotypes can be characterized as either qualitative (discrete) or quantitative (continuous). Qualitative phenotypes are those which are scored as present or absent. Quantitative traits are those which are scored along a continuous spectrum. Examples of qualitative phenotypes include cystic fibrosis, Huntington disease, and muscular dystrophy. Even for qualitative traits, the phenotype may not predict genotype.

Examples of quantitative traits include bone density, weight, and blood pressure. Some phenotypes can be scored as either discrete or quantitative traits. For instance, osteoporosis can be scored in terms of bone mineral density (a quantitative trait) or by establishing a threshold above which individuals are "affected" with osteoporosis (those with bone mineral density t score ≤ 2.5 are "affected," those above are "unaffected"). It is generally thought that quantitative traits are due to the effect of multiple genes as well as environmental factors. Although it may be possible to define a cut off point along a spectrum to determine who is "unaffected " and "affected" this is usually not advisable due to a resultant loss of information and increase in misclassification error.

A phenotype is often further characterized by its *penetrance* and its *expression*. The expression of an allele is characterized by the clinical signs and symptoms that it produces. For instance, the expression of myotonic dystrophy may include myotonia, frontal balding, cataracts, and narcolepsy. Expression of a disease allele is often variable, in that different individuals who carry the same disease allele—even within families!—may show different components of the disease. Formally, penetrance is the conditional probability of observing the phenotype given the genotype. In many cases penetrance is dependent on age. For example, the probability that an individual expresses the disease given that he or she carries the disease allele may increase with age.

For diseases with reduced or incomplete penetrance an individual can be unaffected even though he carries the disease allele. In the situation where the disease genotype is not known unequivocally from the observed disease phenotype, probabilities can be calculated for the various disease genotypes, and these probabilities can be incorporated in linkage analysis.

With incomplete penetrance, although an individual carries a disease allele he may not become affected within his lifetime. For example, 15% of females who carry the BRCA1 mutation will not become affected with breast cancer within their lifetimes *(22,23)*. Penetrance of the tuberous sciensis gene is estimated at 90%; therefore, heterozygotes for the disease allele have a 90% chance of becoming affected *(24)*. When disease etiology involves incomplete penetrance, other factors, either environmental or genetic, must be involved in the development of the disease etiology.

Some genetic traits display a variable age of onset, e.g., Huntington's disease *(25)*. Individuals are not affected at birth, but instead become affected later in life. For Huntington's disease most disease allele carriers become affected between 35–50 yr of age. Almost all disease allele carriers are affected by age 65 *(26)*. Huntington's disease displays variable age of onset, but not incomplete penetrance, since if an individual lives long enough he will eventually become affected *(27)*.

An individual may express the disease phenotype although he does not carry the disease allele. These cases are known as sporadics or phenocopies. For instance, the majority of breast cancer cases are not due to the BRCA1 *(28)* or BRCA2 *(29,30)* loci, but to other genetic and/or environmental causes *(22)*. Phenocopies can also be due to disease misdiagnosis as is the case in 10% of all unautopsied cases of Alzheimer disease *(31)*.

Linkage Concepts: Recombination Fraction and Map Length

Two genes are *linked* to one another when the recombination fraction between the two loci is less than 50%. *Linkage* implies a physical connection between two loci and requires that the two loci are on the same chromosome; however, not all loci that are on the same chromosome are linked. Loci on the same chromosome are syntenic; however, syntenic loci with a recombination fraction of 50% between them are not linked.

In order to localize genetic loci, linkage analysis uses information on how frequently recombination occurs between two loci. When two loci are close to each other they segregate together, violating Mendel's law of independent assortment. During meiosis, genes in close proximity to each other have a very small chance of recombination. In this case the recombination fraction (θ) between the two loci is ≈ 0. The further apart two loci are the more frequently recombination occurs until it reaches a maximum of 50%. Fifty percent recombination can occur when two loci are either located far apart on the same chromosome or are located on different chromosomes.

The genetic map distance (in Morgans) between two loci is defined as the expected number of crossovers occurring between them on a gamete. One centiMorgan (cM) is defined as the amount of DNA between loci exhibiting 1% recombination. The physical measurement of DNA in 1 cM will vary across regions of the chromosome, since recombination is more frequent at the telomere and less frequent at the centromere. In general, 1 cM of DNA is approximately equal to 1 million base pairs of DNA. For large distances recombination fractions are not additive, due to the occurrence of multiple crossovers between loci. If no multiple crossovers between loci occur (complete interference); map distance (x) equals the recombination fraction.

A number of map functions can be used to convert recombination fractions to map distance, which, unlike the recombination fraction, can be added. The Haldane map function makes the assumption that crossovers in different intervals occur independently of each other according to Poisson probability law (no interference). The various map functions make different assumptions on the nature of interference ranging from complete interference to no interference.

Family Ascertainment: Mendelian Traits

Which individuals are ascertained for a linkage study involving a Mendelian trait depends on the mode of inheritance and the penetrance model. Unaffected individuals under the average age of onset for a given disease do not give any linkage information; however, in the situation in which these unaffected individuals have affected sibs and a parent is not available for genotyping they may be helpful to reconstruct the parental genotype. In diseases where most true genetic cases have an early age of onset, older affected individuals may be more likely to be phenocopies and therefore contribute less linkage information than their counterparts with an earlier age of onset. Ideally all individuals who are informative for linkage should be ascertained; however, the cost of doing so may be prohibitive. Therefore it is important to be aware *a priori* how much information different family members are contributing in order to make educated decisions about whom to ascertain. Likewise, when undertaking a genome scan, individuals who give only a small amount of linkage information may be excluded from the genome scan and only genotyped later for regions which are suggestive of linkage for the disease locus or in order to refine the genetic region.

Autosomal Recessive Inheritance

For families with autosomal recessive (AR) inheritance, an affected offspring gives five times the amount of linkage information as unaffected individuals when the disease and marker locus are completely linked and all meioses are fully informative. For this situation in kindreds where the parents are unrelated, the first affected individual gives no linkage information, as the first affected individual is used to set linkage phase. Subsequently, each additional affected individual contributes an additional 0.6 to the LOD score and each additional unaffected individual contributes 0.125 to the LOD score *(32)*. For the pedigree in Fig. 1 individuals II.1, II. 2, and III.1-6 should be ascertained; however, the affected individuals (III.1 and III.3) have a higher priority for ascertainment then their unaffected sibs (III.2 and III.4–6). The grandparents I.1 and I.2 should not be ascertained since they give no linkage information, unless II.1 could not be ascertained. For an autosomal recessive trait the grandparents do not give any phase information, since it is not possible to tell which of the grandparents carry the disease allele.

In the pedigree in Fig. 2. parents (III.1 and III.2) and their offspring (IV.1.–4.) should be ascertained. However for this consanguineous kindred the grandparents (II.1–4) and also, if they were available, the great-grandparents should be ascertained since they give linkage information. For autosomal recessive diseases affected children who are products of consanguineous matings have a higher probability of having received two disease genes from the same common ancestor. This probability increases the rarer the disease allele is.

For consanguineous matings, there is linkage information even when only one affected individual is available. For example one affected offspring of a first cousin mating gives a LOD score of 1.2 under the following special conditions: the recombination fraction between the marker and disease locus is 0.0, the marker is infinitely polymorphic and the disease allele is infinitely rare. Each additional affected and unaffected offspring supply an additional 0.6 and 0.125 LOD score, respectively. The reason why one affected offspring in this situation gives 1.2 LOD score are that the grandparents' genotypes at the disease locus and phase is known in this situation (heterozygous disease allele carriers) and thus both the grandparents and parents of the affected offspring are fully informative.

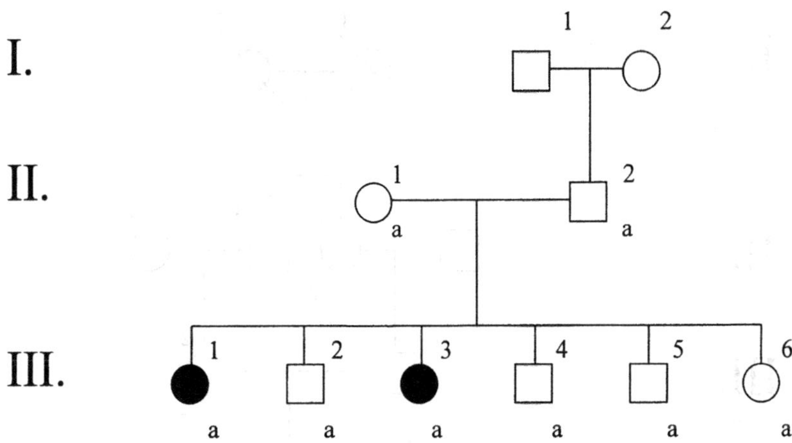

Fig. 1. Ascertainment scheme for autosomal recessive pedigree. Circles are females; squares are male. Shaded individuals are affected with the trait and unshaded individuals are unaffected with the trait. Individuals marked with an 'a' subscript are appropriate for ascertainment for linkage studies.

It is true that the same amount of linkage information can be obtained with or without the grandparents' genotypes. When the parents and grandparents are unavailable, the analysis is totally dependent on the specified allele frequencies and is not robust to error in the allele frequencies.

Autosomal Dominant Inheritance

For a disease trait that is fully penetrant with no phenocopies, affected individuals and their unaffected sibs give the same amount of linkage information. Each phase known meiotic event for a marker with no recombination between the disease and marker loci contributes 0.3 to the LOD score. For the autosomal dominant pedigree in Fig. 3 , individuals I.3, I.4, II.1, II.2, III.1–5, and IV.1–3 all give linkage information. Individuals I.3. and I.4 help to establish linkage phase. Individuals III.2–5 and IV.1–3, if the marker is fully informative, each add 0.3 to the LOD score. Individual I.1–2 do not carry a copy of the disease allele and therefore should not be ascertained since they give no linkage information. Likewise, individuals III.6 and IV.4–6 do not give linkage information. Since individual III.5 is unaffected she cannot pass a disease allele to her offspring.

X-Linked Traits

For X-linked recessive traits, expression of the phenotype is generally limited to males. For some traits, the carrier females also express a milder phenotype and therefore it is possible to determine which females are carriers even if they don't have any affected sons. In the pedigree in Fig. 4 the carrier females do not express the

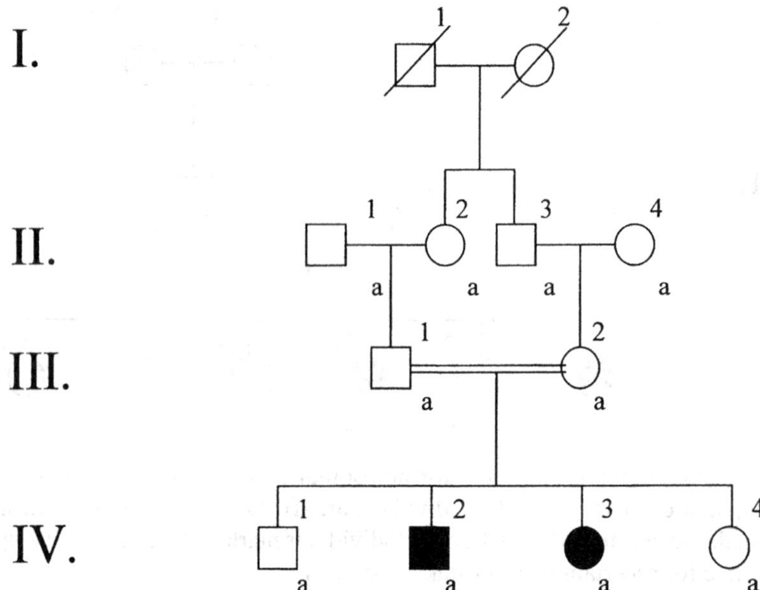

Fig. 2. Ascertainment scheme for an autosomal recessive pedigree with a consanguineous mating. Individuals marked with an "a" subscript are appropriate for linkage analysis.

phenotype and it is only possible to tell unequivocally that they are carriers if they have an affected son. For this kindred individuals I.1–2 and their offspring II. 1,2,5,6,8 should be ascertained. It is not possible to determine if II.4. is a carrier or not since she has no offspring; this individual will not provide linkage information. Individuals II.9 and III. 7, III.8, III.9 should not be ascertained since the father II.8 cannot pass on his X chromosome to his sons and individual III.8 is an obligate carrier. In addition, individual II.3 and his daughter III.3. should not be ascertained. It is not necessary to ascertain the father since he can not pass an X-chromosome to his sons.

Family Ascertainment: Complex Traits

Depending on the types of pedigrees available, it is often worthwhile to develop an ascertainment scheme that will capitalize on a variety of analysis strategies. Frequently, studies are limited — usually by funds — to a single ascertainment scheme such as ascertaining affected sib pairs.

Multiplex Families

Multiplex pedigrees are those in which two or more family members are affected with a disease. Ascertainment of these pedigrees involves sampling the affected individuals and all connecting relatives. Often with complex diseases, probands will report that a distant relative is affected. The rule of thumb for

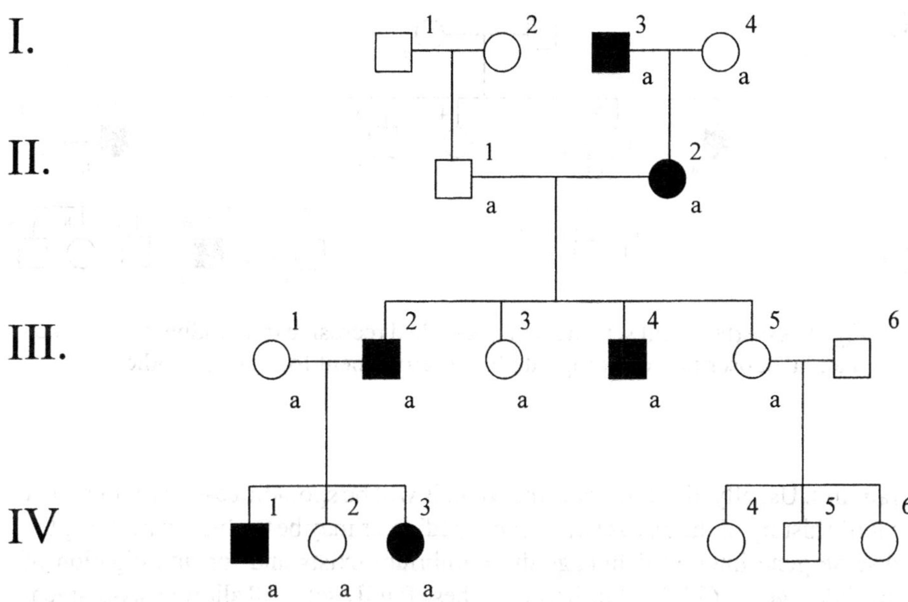

Fig. 3. Ascertainment scheme for a fully penetrant, autosomal dominant trait. Individuals marked with an "a" subscript are appropriate for ascertainment for linkage studies.

determining whether or not the affected relative is more likely due to a common genetic factor or to chance alone (the general population risk) is based on comparing the probability that the affected relative pair shares an allele identical by descent (IBD) to the general population risk for disease. For instance, an avuncular pair (aunt/uncle with nephew/niece) share on average 1/8 of their genes IBD. As long as the general population disease frequency is less than 1/8 (12.5%), it is worthwhile to sample this affected relative pair.

Sib Pairs

When a large number of affected sibling pairs are easy to obtain, Hauser et al. *(33)* demonstrated that an efficient sampling design for genomic screening involves typing only the affected sibling pairs, without other family members, for a series of markers spaced about 10–20 cM apart. When the study design is limited to affected sibling pairs, it is frequently useful to sample their parents when they are available so that identity-by-descent status can be determined with as much certainty as possible. Decisions about including more than two affected siblings and/or unaffected siblings are often based on availability and cost of recruitment *(33)*.

Trios (for Linkage Disequilibrium Testing)

When possible, it is useful to collect a series of trios including an affected individual and his or her parents independent from the collection of multiplex

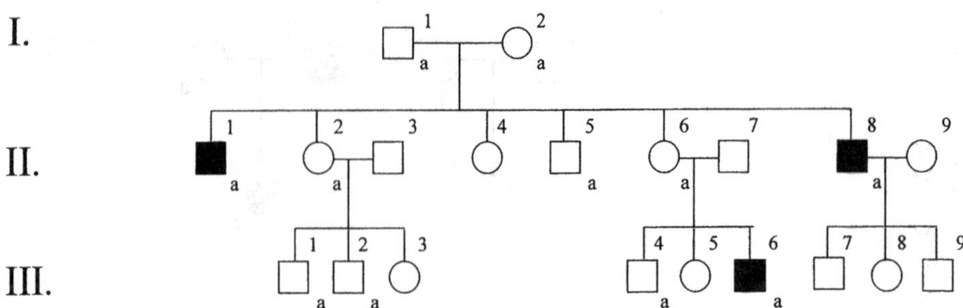

Fig. 4. Ascertainment scheme for an X-linked recessive trait. Individuals marked with an 'a' subscript are appropriate for ascertainment for linkage studies.

families. Usually, these affected individuals will be sporadic cases, without other family history of the disease trait. These pedigrees may be useful in narrowing the disease gene interval if linkage disequilibrium exists and for investigation of candidate genes *(34,35)*. Furthermore, these family sets will allow an assessment as to whether or not the genes underlying a disease in multiplex pedigrees are the same as those in the usually more frequent sporadic families. However, in many late-onset diseases, the parents of the affected individual are unavailable and therefore it may be advisable to collect additional siblings of the proband.

Evaluating the Number of Families Necessary to Establish Linkage

Before embarking on a linkage study it is first necessary to know if it will be possible to ascertain a large enough sample to detect linkage. Alternatively, if a sample of families has already been ascertained or identified, this sample can be evaluated to determine if the sample size is large enough to detect linkage or whether additional families should be ascertained. The minimum required information for assessing power is the family structure, affection status of individuals in the families (i.e., who is affected and who is not affected), and parameters of the underlying genetic model (mode of inheritance, penetrance, and allele frequencies).

Power Studies for Mendelian Disease

For Mendelian traits, simulation studies can determine whether a given sample set will be able to identify linkage. Simulation studies are often done after a family or set of families has been identified and the phenotype has been determined for family members. In order to evaluate if a given data set can be used to establish linkage, the power and expected LOD score (ELOD) are estimated.

For each replicate, alleles at a linked marker locus are generated conditional on the observed pedigree structure and disease phenotype at a given recombination fraction. The penetrance model and disease allele frequency used to generate the replicates are based upon the estimates obtained from epidemiological studies. In general for the marker allele frequency, a highly polymorphic marker is used, for example a marker with 5 alleles of equal frequency (heterozygosity = 0.80). A number of replicates are generated, usually between 50–200. One of two programs are often used to simulate marker genotypes conditional on the disease phenotype, SLINK *(36,37)* and SIMLINK *(38,39)*. The replicates are analyzed with the same parameter values used to generated them (i.e., penetrance model, disease allele frequency, etc). The power and ELOD are calculated from the replicates. The ELOD is the average LOD score at the recombination fraction at which the pedigrees were simulated. The power is the probability of establishing linkage. It is the proportion of replicates where the LOD score is equal to or greater than a given threshold (3 for autosomal traits and 2 for X-linked traits [these are the values necessary to establish linkage]). A maximum LOD score of ±3 is often considered proof that it is possible to detect linkage for a given data set, due to the abundance of polymorphic markers which will result in all meioses being genetically informative. The use of the maximum LOD score in power studies is advisable only for traits where reduced penetrance and phenocopies are not present (Ott, personal communication). In the presence of phenocopies and reduced penetrance, a much more reliable measure is the ELOD, the average LOD score. Generally power of 80% or above is considered sufficient to establish linkage for a given data set.

Reduced Penetrance

The maximum amount of information with respect to the LOD score will be obtained when the phenotype at the trait locus can be scored with as much precision as possible. The ideal situation is where all individuals can be accurately classified as either affected or unaffected for the disease trait. Any loss of precision through the presence of reduced penetrance or phenocopies will reduce the expected LOD score (ELOD). Ott *(40)* demonstrated that 20% and 32% more data are necessary to obtain the same ELOD when penetrance for genetic cases is reduced by 5% and 10%, respectively.

Heterogeneity

For many traits linkage heterogeneity (i.e., mutations in different genes may result in the same phenotype) is present, which can be taken into consideration when evaluating the power to detect linkage with a given data set. Not all of the families within a data set may be segregating the same locus. Therefore the power to detect linkage and the ELOD should be evaluated for various values of θ, the proportion of families segregating the same locus. The simulation studies should be carried out with a proportion of the families unlinked to the disease locus and analyzed allowing for heterogeneity using a program like ELODHET *(41)*.

Using Simulation Studies to Evaluate the p*-Value*

Previously it was discussed how simulation studies could be used to establish whether or not a given data set is sufficient to establish linkage. Simulation studies can also be used to determine the empirical *p*-value for a given analysis *(42)*. Using simulation studies to determine the empirical *p*-value is useful in a variety of situations: when the distribution of the null hypothesis is unknown for a test statistic; and when multiple models are tested.

The data are simulated under the null hypothesis of no linkage. The number of times a given critical value is achieved or exceeded out of the total number of replicates is counted. In order to obtain a reasonable estimate of the *p*-value, a large number of replicates must be simulated. The number of replicates that should be simulated is dependent on the how small a *p*-value one wishes to estimate. For $p = 0.001$ at least 10,000 replicates should be simulated.

Power Studies for Complex Traits

For complex traits it is very difficult, if not impossible, to accurately estimate the number of families necessary to establish linkage. Simulation studies as described previously are not an option since the mode of inheritance is unknown and therefore it is not only unknown under what model to carry out the analysis, but also what model to use to simulate the pedigree data.

However, alternate approaches are possible. For sib-pair analysis based upon the relative risk and the number of hypothesized loci it is possible to estimate the number of sib-pairs necessary to detect linkage. For instance it is usually possible to estimate the relative risk or λs value and use this to perform estimates of power *(35)*. For instance, to detect a single locus with a λs of 3.0 with 80% power, approx 100 pairs of affected siblings are required. These calculations further assume a fully informative marker linked at 0% recombination with the disease locus. As λs decreases, the number of affected sibling pairs required to detect linkage increases (Table 1). Risch and Merikangas *(35)* provide formulas for calculations of powerz for sib-pair studies. It should be noted that the number of sib-pairs necessary to establish linkage can vary greatly depending on the number of hypothesized loci. In addition, the calculations of approximate sample size are based on the assumed value of λs at a given locus. In practice, the number of underlying loci is never known and the locus-specific λs is also unknown.

Parametric ("LOD SCORE") Linkage Analysis

Various methods for statistical analysis of human linkage data have been proposed including Bernstein's y-statistic *(43)*, sib-pair analysis *(44–46)*, and the probability ratio test of Haldane and Smith *(47)*. Current likelihood-based methods utilize the sequential linkage test proposed by Morton *(48)*. This test combines Haldane and Smith's probability ratio test *(47)* and Wald's sequential probability ratio test *(49)*. To assess the statistical significance, instead of reporting likelihoods *(47)* that are

Table 1
Approximate Number of Affected Sibling Pairs Required to Detect Linkage[a]

	Probability of correctly identifying linkage (power)	
λ_s	0.80	0.95
2.0	200	300
5.0	60	80

[a]Calcuations assume a fully informative marker linked at 0% recombination with the disease locus at $\alpha = 0.05$. (Adapted with permission from ref. *94*.)

difficult to interpret, the base 10 logarithm of the likelihood ratio (LOD score [Z(θ)] is used. Besides being easier to interpret, log likelihoods have the advantage that they can be summed across families for a given recombination fraction, as opposed to working with the likelihood which must be multiplied across families for a given recombination fraction. Even with these advantages, Morton's sequential linkage test *(48)* has limited use, since it is generally limited to two-generation pedigrees. The Elston and Stewart *(15)* algorithm and its extension *(50)* made it possible to calculate the likelihood for more complex pedigrees.

To calculate a two-point LOD score, the likelihood of the pedigree and the marker data is calculated under the null hypothesis ($\theta = 0.50$, i.e., free recombination) between the disease and marker loci. This likelihood is compared to the likelihood calculated at various increments of θ, (0.00 – 0.49) between the marker and disease loci. The LOD score is calculated as follows:

$$Z(\theta) = \log_{10} L\,(\text{pedigree}, \theta < 0.5)/L(\text{pedigree}, \theta = 0.5) \qquad (1)$$

The value of the recombination fraction, θ, at which the LOD score is at its highest value is the best estimate of the recombination fraction.

Morton *(48)* suggested that a $Z(\theta) \geq 3.0$ (1000:1 odds in favor of linkage) be considered conclusive evidence in favor of linkage. A $Z(\theta) \leq -2$ is considered conclusive evidence against the linkage of two loci. $Z(\theta)$ between –2 and 3 are considered inconclusive and warrant more testing in the region before a decision can be made. These values were selected to represent an approximate false positive rate of 5%.

For a genome scan where hundreds of markers are tested, the statistical issue of inflated type 1 error from these multiple comparisons becomes an issue. To counteract this, current recommendations suggest *(51)* using a LOD score (3.6 as the threshold for significance for genome wide scans due to multiple testing. Using a less stringent criterion could result in a >5% chance of reporting false positive findings.

In order to examine the variability of the recombination fraction, a support interval is calculated around the point estimate of θ. It is preferable to calculate a support interval instead of a confidence interval when working in a likelihood framework *(52)*. For example a 2.3-unit support interval (note: 2.3 $\log_e = 1 \log_{10}$) can be constructed around the estimate of θ *(53)* by graphing the LOD score curve, estimating the maximum LOD score, subtracting 1 LOD unit from the maximum LOD score, and graphically obtaining those estimates of θ leading to $Z_{max} - 1$. These results are approximately equivalent to a 95% confidence interval. In order to ensure that the disease gene is within the support interval, Ott *(40)* suggests that a three $\log_{10}$ unit support interval be constructed around the disease gene localization.

For Mendelian traits, multipoint linkage analysis has been shown to be more efficient than two-point mapping *(54–56)*. By using a series of linked markers within families or highly polymorphic markers, virtually all meioses will be fully informative at one or more loci. Multipoint linkage analysis also increases the precision of the estimated location of a locus on a genetic map. However, misspecification of parameters can have an even greater effect in biasing the estimate of the recombination fraction for multipoint analysis than for two-point analysis *(57)*. Multipoint mapping works as follows: Given a fixed genetic map of marker loci, a disease locus can sequentially be moved through the map, estimating multipoint LOD scores at each map location. Formally, the multipoint LOD score is calculated as:

$$Z(\theta) = \log_{10} L(x = \theta_0, \theta_{23}, \theta_{34}... / L(x = 0.5, \theta_{23}, \theta_{34}...) \quad (2)$$

where x is locus 1, which is to be mapped relative to a fixed map of marker loci of known distance. θ_0 is the distance between locus x and the fixed map, and θ_{23}, θ_{34}, ... represent the recombination fractions between loci 2 and 3, loci 3 and 4, and so forth.

Calculation of LOD Scores

The examples given here are limited to two-point analysis. It should be noted that these are simple examples that can easily be calculated with pencil and paper. When carrying out an actual linkage analysis, pedigree structures are more complex and analysis is usually not limited to fully penetrant Mendelian traits. In addition all of the family members may not be available for study. Therefore the probabilities of all possible genotypes based on the marker allele frequencies must be incorporated into the likelihood and generally must be calculated with the assistance of computer programs.

Calculation of the LOD Score for a Phase-Known Autosomal Dominant Kindred

The LOD score will be calculated for the pedigree shown in Fig. 5. For ease of calculation the assumption is made that individual I.1. is heterozygous for the disease trait, a reasonable assumption for rare diseases. Upon examination of the pedigree it can be seen that individual II.1 received the disease allele (D) and the marker allele 2 from his father. It should be noted that although II.1. received alleles D and 2 from his father, it is not known if the disease and marker loci are closely linked or on different chromosomes. Nonetheless, this observation allows us to

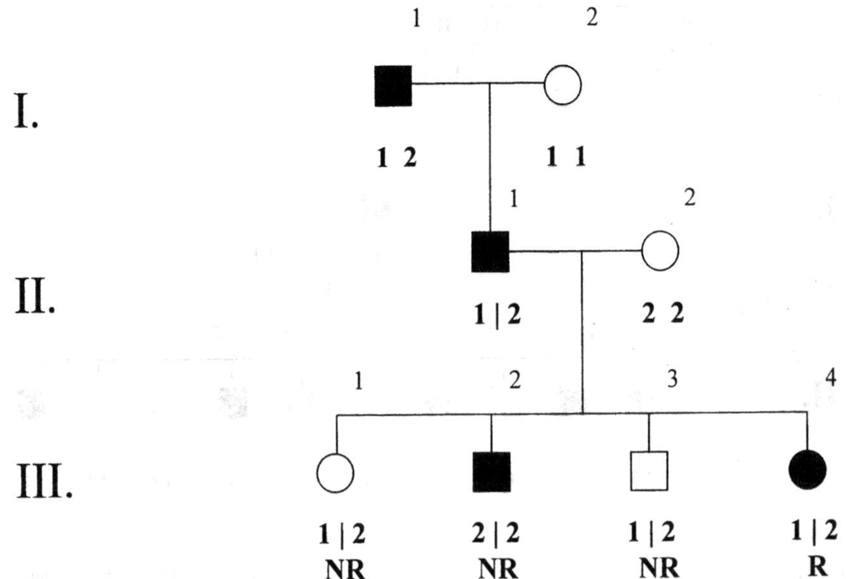

Fig. 5. Pedigree for calculation of the LOD score for fully penetrant autosomal dominant trait in a phase known pedigree. Unordered genotypes are shown beneath individuals I.1 and I.2. Once transmission of allele 2 from affected grandparent I.1 to his affected son II.1 is established, the linkage phase between the trait and marker locus is established, and genotypes listed beneath individuals are considered ordered for scoring purposes. NR indicates a nonrecombinant individual and R indicates a recombinant individual.

"set linkage phase" to allow scoring of recombination events in subsequent meioses. Since II.1's mother is unaffected, he must have received from her the wild-type allele or nondisease allele (+) at the disease locus and the marker allele 1. By examining the disease status and marker genotypes of II.1's children (III.1–4) we can see that III.1.–3 are products of gametes where recombination has not occurred. However individual III.4. is the product of a gamete where a recombination event has occurred. It can be seen that she received the 1 and D allele from her father II.1. The LOD score for this pedigree can be calculated for various values of theta using the following equation:

$$Z(\theta) = \log_{10}[\theta\,(1 - \theta)^3][1/2^1\,(1 - 1/2)^3] \tag{3}$$

where the term θ in the numerator is raised to the power of the number of recombinants and the term (1 – θ) is raised to the power of the number of nonrecombinants. For this pedigree in which all meioses result from phase-known matings, the estimate of the recombination fraction is

$$\theta = R/NR^{+}{}_{R} \tag{4}$$

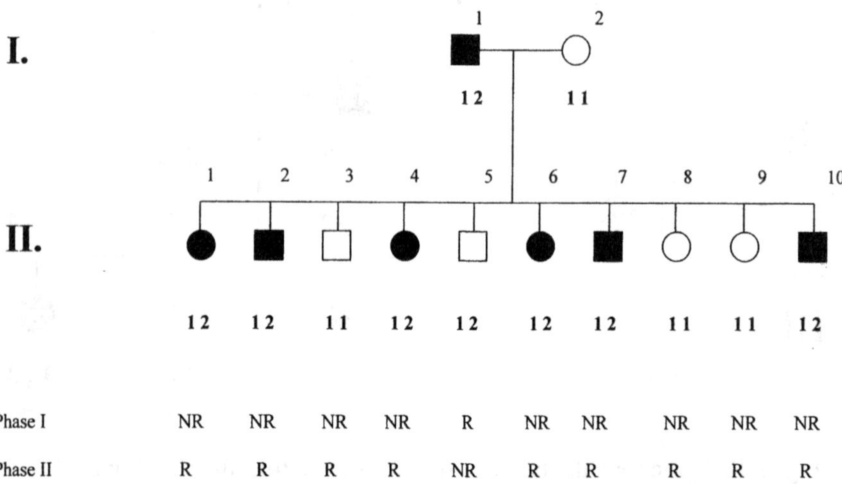

	1	2	3	4	5	6	7	8	9	10
Phase I	NR	NR	NR	NR	R	NR	NR	NR	NR	NR
Phase II	R	R	R	R	NR	R	R	R	R	R

Fig. 6. Pedigree for calculation of LOD score for fully penetrant autosomal dominant trait in a phase unknown pedigree. Two linkage phases (phase I and phase II) are *a priori* equally likely. Recombinant (R) and nonrecombinant (NR) individuals are scored separately for each of the two phases.

where R is the number of recombinants and NR is the number of nonrecombinants. For this example, θ equals 0.25. The maximum LOD score is $Z(\theta) = 0.227$ obtained at $\theta = 0.25$. From this one small pedigree it is not possible to say whether or not the disease and the marker locus are linked to each other. In order to establish linkage, the maximum LOD score must be ≥ 3.0; thus 14 of these pedigrees would be needed in order to establish linkage.

Calculation of the LOD Score for a Phase-Unknown Autosomal Dominant Kindred

The pedigree in Fig. 6 is a phase-known autosomal dominant pedigree. The parents of I.1. are unavailable for study. It is not known whether I.1. inherited the 2 or 1 allele at the marker locus with the disease allele (D) from his affected parent. Therefore two phases are possible with equal probability (1/2), phase 1 that he inherited the D and 2 allele together and the other possibility under phase 2 that he inherited the D and 1 allele together. The designation of phase 1 and phase 2 is arbitrary. Under phase 1, all offspring except II.5 are nonrecombinants; individual II.5. is a recombinant. Under phase 2 the reverse is true, all offspring

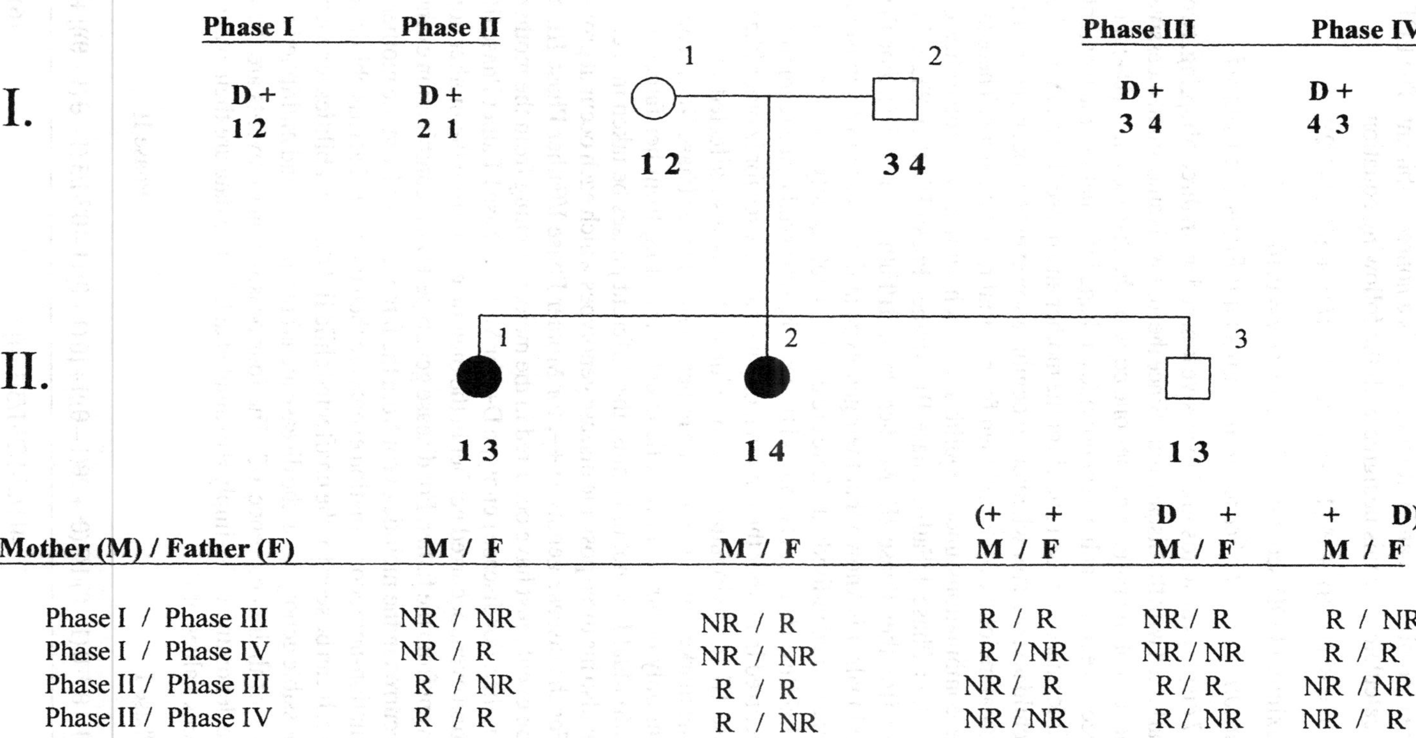

Mother (M) / Father (F)	M / F	M / F	(+ + M / F	D + M / F	+ D) M / F
Phase I / Phase III	NR / NR	NR / R	R / R	NR / R	R / NR
Phase I / Phase IV	NR / R	NR / NR	R / NR	NR / NR	R / R
Phase II / Phase III	R / NR	R / R	NR / R	R / R	NR / NR
Phase II / Phase IV	R / R	R / NR	NR / NR	R / NR	NR / R

Fig. 7. Pedigree for calculation of LOD score for fully penetrant autosomal recessive trait. Each parent has two possible linkage phases which are *a priori* equally likely. Recombinant (R) and nonrecombinant (NR) individuals are indicated for each of the possible phases.

except II.5 are recombinants and individual II.5. is a nonrecombinant. The LOD score can be calculated for this pedigree with the following equation.

$$Z(\theta) = \theta^1 (1 - \theta)^9 + \theta^9 (1 - \theta)^1 / 1/2^1 (1 - 1/2)^9 + 1/2^9 (1-1/2)^1 \quad (5)$$

The maximum LOD score of 1.3 occurs at $\theta = 0.10$.

Calculation of a LOD Score for an Autosomal Recessive Kindred

Figure 7 displays an autosomal recessive kindred, with three offspring, two of whom are affected with the disease trait. Since the disease is autosomal recessive we know that each of the parents carries one copy of the disease allele (D+). For autosomal recessive traits each parent provides linkage information. Each parent has two possible phases, phase I and II for the mother and phase III and IV for the father. Each child is scored for whether a recombination event has occurred or not, first for maternal meiotic events and then for paternal meiotic events. There are four possible combinations under equilibrium, each with a 1/4 probability of occurring (Mother Phase 1/Father Phase III, Mother Phase I/Father Phase IV, Mother Phase II/Father Phase III, Mother Phase II/Father Phase IV). For the affected individuals it is known that their genotype at the disease locus must be DD. For the unaffected individuals there are three possible genotypes each occurring with probability 1/3 (++, D+, and +D). It can be observed that a recombination event occurred in neither the maternal or paternal meioses for Mother Phase I/Father Phase III for individual II.1. Individual II.2. is also affected but her genotype at the marker locus is 1 4. For Mother Phase I/Father Phase III a recombination event only occurred in meiotic event originating from her father. For unaffected individual II.3, not only must the different phases be taken into consideration but also his three possible disease genotypes which each occur at probability 1/3. For the disease genotype ++, for Mother Phase I/Father Phase III, a recombination event must have occurred in the meiosis coming from the mother and from the father. For disease genotype D+, for Mother Phase I/Father Phase III a recombination event occurred neither in the meiotic event from the mother nor the meiotic event from the father. For disease genotype +D a recombination event must have occurred in the meiotic event from the father but not from the mother. The recombination-nonrecombination events are then multiplied across children for each phase. It can be seen for the unaffected child II.3 the probabilities for each of the three possible genotypes at the disease locus are summed and multiplied by the probability of their occurrence 1/3. The four possible phase events are then summed. The denominator is simply θ evaluated at 0.5. The data are then evaluated for various values of θ.

Phase I Phase II

$$Z(\theta) = \log_{10} \frac{[(1-\theta)^2 \cdot \theta (1-\theta) \cdot 1/3 (\theta^2 + 2\theta(1-\theta))] + [\theta (1-\theta) \cdot (1-\theta)^2 \cdot 1/3 (1-\theta (1-\theta))] +}{4[1/2^2 \cdot 1/2^2 \cdot 1/3\ 3/4)]} \quad (6)$$

Phase III Phase IV

$$[\theta(1-\theta)\cdot \theta^2\cdot 1/3\ (1-\theta(1-\theta))] + [\theta 2\cdot\theta(1-\theta)\cdot 1/3((1-\theta)^2+2\theta(1-\theta))]$$

The LOD score for this kindred at $\theta = 0.1$ is $Z(\theta) = -0.36$.

Allele Frequencies/Effects of Incorrect Model

Inaccurate allele frequencies for genetic markers have been well established to lead to false linkages, false exclusions, and inaccurate estimates of the recombination fraction *(58,41)*. These problems are encountered only in pedigrees in which genotypes on critical individuals are missing. Allele frequencies for a variety of genetic markers are available from either the CEPH database (http://www.genethon. fr), Marshfield Medical Research Laboratories database (http://www.marshmed.org/genetics), Genome Data Base (http://gdbwww.gdb.org) or on the web at http://www2.mc.duke.edu/depts/medicine/medgen. When utilizing allele frequencies from databases, it is important to ensure that standard genotypes listed in the databases are consistent with those obtained in local genotyping efforts. This is most easily accomplished by genotyping 2 or 3 CEPH family members for a marker or set of markers that have been genotyped by the reference laboratory. Another caveat is that the allele frequencies in the database might not reflect the allele frequencies within the population being studied. This can occur if the population under study is ethnically different from those used to estimate the allele frequencies in the CEPH pedigrees *(59)*.

The specification of the disease allele frequency plays into LOD score calculations in determining the probability that apparently unaffected founding individuals carry the disease allele. Methodological studies have demonstrated that LOD score linkage analysis is relatively robust to incorrect specification of the disease allele frequency as long as it is relatively close to the true value. Gross mis-specification of the disease allele frequency can lead to incorrect estimates of the LOD score and the recombination fraction, particularly when a common allele for a genetic marker is incorrectly made rare. In the worst-case scenario, it can lead to false positive findings.

Haplotyping and Identification of the Minimum Candidate Region

After the initial chromosomal localization, the next step is to determine the minimum candidate region (MCR). This process involves genotyping as many polymorphic genetic markers within the support interval for the disease locus as available. Then, the most likely linkage phase for the genotyped markers is established, and recombination events identified. An example of this process is shown in Fig. 8. (Computer programs [SIMWALK2, GENEHUMTER] are available for automated haplotyping.) Individuals involved in critical recombination events are resampled and regenotyped to ensure accuracy of results.

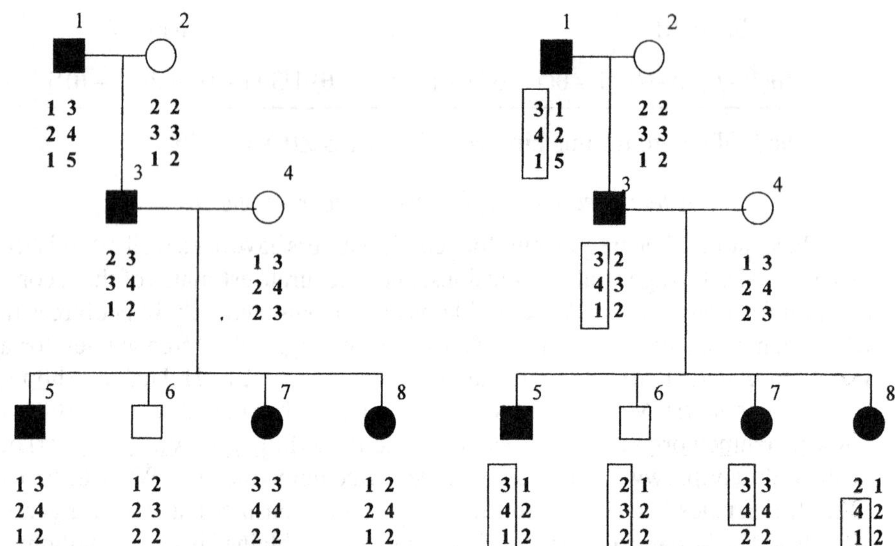

Marker Order

Marker 1
Marker 2
Marker3

Fig. 8. Haplotype analysis of an autosomal dominant disease linked to genetic markers, ordered from telomere to centromere. **(A)** Raw genotypes at the marker loci. **(B)** Most likely linkage phase established, and recombination events identified. Note that individual 7 is the result of a recombination event which places the disease gene distal to Marker 1 and individual 8 is the result of a recombination event which places the disease gene proximal to Marker 3. Marker 2 shows no recombination with the disease gene. Thus, the minimum candidate interval for the disease gene lies between Marker 1 and Marker 3.

Typically, the recombination events utilized for determining the MCR are limited to affected individuals as these are usually the family members whose diagnostic status is most certain. Although unaffected individuals can be utilized for determining the MCR, the diagnostic status of these individuals is usually not certain since incomplete penetrance is the rule rather than the exception. Recombination events in unaffected individuals should thus be used with care.

Linkage Heterogeneity

Linkage heterogeneity indicates that different genes are responsible for the same phenotype. Examples of disease etiology displaying locus heterogeneity include

Charcot-Marie-Tooth disease, *(60)*, tuberous sclerosis *(61,62)*, nonsyndromic hearing loss *(63)* and polycystic kidney disease *(64)*. It is possible to detect linkage heterogeneity using linkage analysis since the recombination fraction between the disease phenotype and a set of markers will not be consistent between families. Other types of heterogeneity include *clinical* where the disease presentation varies among affected individuals; *genetic*, where clinically identical diseases show different patterns of inheritance; and *allelic*, where different alleles at a locus can lead to clinically similar phenotypes. Two issues are addressed in this section, detecting linkage in the presence of heterogeneity and the ability to detect linkage heterogeneity.

Tests for Linkage Heterogeneity

The Predivided Sample Test (PS-Test)

The predivided sample test, also known as the M-test or K-test, can be used to test for homogeneity of data when there are recognizable classes of families *(65)*. Examples of criteria to divide a data set into classes, c, include country of origin, investigator, or each family can be considered a separate class. For this test, the null hypothesis, H_0 of linkage and homogeneity specifies that the recombination fraction is the same for each class, $\theta_1 = \theta_2 = \ldots \theta_c < 1/2$. Under the alternative hypothesis, H_1, the recombination fractions for each class are not equal and can be different for every class. To test for homogeneity, the likelihood ratio test is

$$X^2_{c-1} = 2 \ln (10) \times [\Sigma Zi\, (\hat{\theta} i) - Z(\hat{\theta})] \tag{7}$$

where Z (θ) is the maximum LOD-score that occurs at a recombination fraction of θ_i, for the *i*th class ($i = 1,\ldots,c$). For example, if each family is a class, this would simply be the sum of the maximum LOD score for each family at the θ value where the maximum LOD score occurred $Z(\hat{\theta})$ is the maximum LOD score that occurs at a specific value of θ for all families combined, in other words, the maximum LOD score under linkage homogeneity. The expression $X^2_{c-1} = 2 \ln (10) \times [\Sigma Z_i (\hat{\theta}_i) - Z (\hat{\theta})]$ is transformed from the base 10 logarithm to natural log and then multiplied by two. This X^2 test has c – 1 degrees of freedom, where *c* is the number of classes. The PS-test performs poorly when classification is by family, which may be due in part to the large number of degrees of freedom *(66)*.

The predivided sample test can be carried out using the MTEST computer program *(40)*.

Admixture Test

For the PS-test the alternative hypothesis is that the recombination fraction is potentially different in every family or class. In many testing situations a more credible alternative hypothesis is that there are two family types, a proportion of families (α) with linkage (θ < 1/2) and a proportion of families (1– α) without linkage (θ = 1/2) *(66,67)*.

The test of homogeneity of linkage (H_0:$\alpha = 1, \theta_r < 1/2$; H_1: $\alpha < 1, \theta_1 < 1/2$) is given by:

$$X_1^2 = 2[\log e\, L(\alpha, \theta 1) - \log e\, L(1, \theta r) \quad (8)$$

$\log e\, L(1, \theta r)$ is the maximum value of the LOD score under homogeneity converted to a natural log likelihood. The expression $[\log e\, L(\alpha, \theta 1)$ is the natural log likelihood maximized over α and θ. This X^2 test has 1 degree of freedom.

The A-test can also be used to test for linkage and heterogeneity, where the null hypothesis is there is no linkage (H_{00}: θ = 1/2) and the alternative hypothesis (H_1: α < 1, θ < 1/2) is that both linkage and heterogeneity are present. The test statistic is:

$$A = 2\, [\log e\, L(\alpha, \theta 1)] \quad (9)$$

Terwilliger and Ott *(68)* suggest that the criterion of a likelihood ratio above 2000:1 (LOD score of 3.3) should be used to declare that significant evidence exists for linkage in some proportion of families within the data set. The criterion of a likelihood ratio of 2000:1 is based on the likelihood ratio of 1000:1 required in a test for linkage and the allowance for a second free parameter α in the numerator of the odds ratio.

The A-test is robust to error in the specification of genetic parameters provided that the recombination fraction is not fixed a *priori* (i.e., when there is a candidate gene and θ is set to 0). In this situation heterogeneity can falsely be concluded. In other situations when genetic parameters are misspecified, neither linkage nor linkage heterogeneity can be falsely concluded, however, the estimates of both the recombination fraction and proportion of "linked" families may be strongly biased. When parameter values are incorrect, there may also be loss of power to detect linkage heterogeneity *(68)*.

The Admixture test can be carried out using the HOMOG computer program *(40)*.

Methods for Complex Disease

Nonparametric linkage analysis methods do not require the specification of the underlying genetic model (i.e., dominant vs recessive, frequency and penetrance of disease allele, etc.). A significant distinction between the various nonparametric linkage analysis methods is whether the method relies on characterizing identity-by-descent (IBD) relationships between affected relatives or identity-by-state (IBS) relationships.

For an allele to be identical-by-descent (IBD) between two relatives, it must have been inherited from a common ancestor (Fig. 9). Alleles that are identical by state (IBS) are alleles that are scored the same between individuals. Alleles that are IBS may or not be IBD; in fact, alleles may be IBS between totally unrelated individuals! An allele that is IBD is always IBS.

In general, methods based on IBD relationships are more powerful than IBS relationships; however, IBD relationships can sometimes be difficult to characterize accurately due to the nature of the disease. For instance, in late-onset

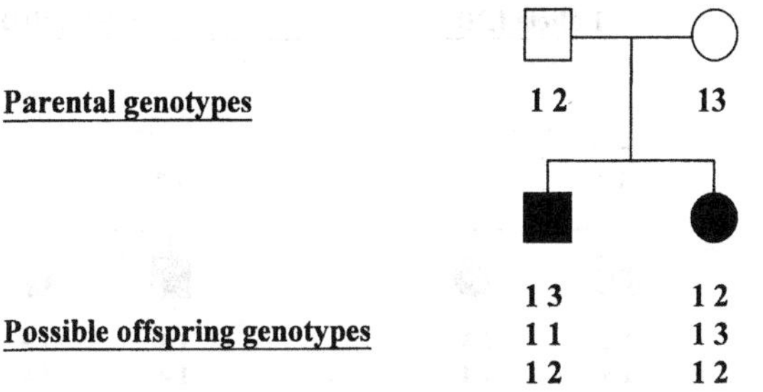

	Father	Mother
Parental genotypes	1 2	13
Possible offspring genotypes	1 3	1 2
	1 1	1 3
	1 2	1 2

Number of Alleles Shared	
IBD	**IBS**
0	1
1	1
2	2

Fig. 9. Calculation of number of alleles shared identical-by-descent (IBD) and identical-by-state (IBS) for a pair of affected siblings.

diseases when parents are frequently unavailable, the parental genotypes may not always be able to be inferred and IBD relationships between alleles shared by siblings cannot always be determined with certainty.

For purposes of brevity, discussion of nonparametric methods of linkage analysis will assume that the relative pairs under study are all affected (concordant) pairs. Most of the methods can be extended to include discordant pairs, where one member of the pair is affected and the other is unaffected or have measurements that are either concordant or discordant for a quantitative trait locus (QTL). This approach generally involves a prior belief by the investigator that the penetrance of the disease is relatively high, so that unaffected relatives are nongene carriers with a reasonably high probability.

Sib-Pair Analysis

For qualitative traits, sib-pair analysis involves studying a series of affected sibling pairs and determining what proportion of the pairs share 0, 1, or 2 alleles at a marker locus IBD. These proportions can be compared (using a variety of different test statistics) to those expected under the null hypothesis of no linkage between the disease and marker. These proportions assume Mendelian transmission of parental alleles and for sibling pairs, the proportions of siblings sharing 0, 1, or 2 alleles IBD are 1/4, 1/2, and 1/4, respectively. If the observed proportions of sharing deviate from these expected proportions either toward sharing 1 allele IBD or 2 alleles IBD, then the results are consistent with linkage.

Figure 10 shows an example of a hypothetical study involving 100 affected sibling pairs whose parents are fully informative for two markers unlinked to one another, marker A and marker B. For the sake of illustration, all family members are genotyped, with the genotypes of the parents being heterozygous with no allele shared between them. The possible genotypes of the offspring are listed below their pedigree symbols for the outcomes of the sibling sharing 0, 1, or 2 alleles IBD. Note that results for marker A are consistent with nonlinkage between the disease and marker locus since the observed proportion of sibling pairs sharing

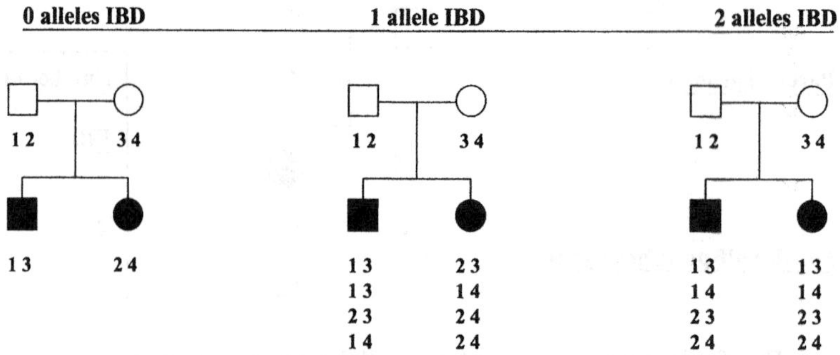

0 alleles IBD		1 allele IBD		2 alleles IBD	
1 2	3 4	1 2	3 4	1 2	3 4
1 3	2 4	1 3	2 3	1 3	1 3
		1 3	1 4	1 4	1 4
		2 3	2 4	2 3	2 3
		1 4	2 4	2 4	2 4

	# sibling pairs observed		
Study	**0 alleles IBD**	**1 allele IBD**	**2 alleles IBD**
Marker A	27	47	26
Marker B	10	60	30

Marker A

$$\chi^2_2 = \frac{(27-25)^2}{25} + \frac{(47-50)^2}{50} + \frac{(26-25)^2}{25} = 0.189; p = 0.90^*$$

Marker B

$$\chi^2_2 = \frac{(10-25)^2}{25} + \frac{(60-50)^2}{50} + \frac{(30-25)^2}{25} = 7.79; p = 0.02^*$$

Fig. 10. Example calculation of nonparametric affected sibling pair analysis for two hypothetical studies. *Note that the *p*-values associated with the χ^2_1 value are one-sided.

0, 1, and 2 alleles IBD is not different from the 1/4, 1/2, 1/4 proportions expected under nonlinkage. Marker B, however, demonstrates a significant skew away from sibling pairs sharing 0 alleles IBD, consistent with the disease and marker B being linked to one another. Note that in contrast to the LOD score approach, this X^2 statistic allows identification of linkage but no estimate of the associated recombination fraction.

Multiple Affected Siblings in a Sib-Pair

It is important to understand that not all sibling pairs are created equal. Specifically, estimates of IBD sharing for sibling pairs within a nuclear family with > 2 siblings are not independent, violating one of the assumptions underlying sib-pair linkage analysis. Once it has been established the sibling pair consisting of children 1 and 2 shares 0 alleles IBD and the sibling pair consisting of children 1 and 3 shares 2 alleles IBD, then the third pair (including children 2 and 3) *must* share 0 alleles IBD. Corrections can be performed by two different approaches – first, by weighting the relative contributions of each of the "dependent" sibling pairs *(70)* or alternatively by performing post hoc simulations designed to generate empiric *p* -values associated with a particular result. In very large samples, including all sibling pairs when nuclear families have >2 affected sibling pairs will not bias the results; however, the sample size may not be large enough to minimize this bias.

Use of Parametric Methods for Complex Traits

It is possible and frequently desirable to analyze complex traits using parametric methods. The majority of current methods localize one disease locus at a time. It has been shown for both Mendelian and multilocus traits *(71,58,57)* that analysis under the wrong model parameters retains much of the linkage information, but results in biased (inflated) estimates for the recombination fraction. When analyzing complex traits, analysis is often done using two-point linkage analysis and then testing for admixture *(72,66,67)*. When mapping susceptibility genes for complex traits the inheritance model is often unknown, and thus various models (e.g., dominant and recessive) are frequently tested *(73)*.

Parametric methods have been described and implemented which allow for analysis of two loci simultaneously *(74,75)*, however, these methods are computationally intensive and extensions for additional loci are computationally prohibitive.

Affected Relative Pair Studies

Frequently, pedigrees in complex diseases contain affected relative pairs other than siblings. In complex diseases, the investigator must capitalize on any type of pedigree material available. Thus, the affected sibling pair study design was extended to allow for the consideration of other types of affected relative pairs. The general idea is the same—to identify genes contributing to the phenotype by determining whether the proportion of genes shared in affected relatives is greater than that expected by chance alone. In siblings, the expected proportion of genes shared identical by descent is 50% while in cousins it is 1/8. Although in theory this extension seems very simple, in practice it is quite complex. For instance, the affected sibling pair study design benefits when the parents of the affected siblings are available for genotyping. Then, the proportion of genes a pair of siblings shares IBD is characterized with certainty. Complete sampling of all relatives connecting a pair of nonsibling affected relatives is frequently impossible and usually at best provides a logistic difficulty. Thus, the studies of traits in affected relative pairs utilize an approach which approximates the IBD approach, but requires a less stringent criteria. Instead of alleles being scored as identical by descent, they are scored simply as identical by state or not. Using IBS instead of IBD tends to increase the rate of false positive results. This very novel approach was originally described by Weeks and Lange *(76)* and programmed as the APM program ("affected pedigree member"), and its availability in large part helped to implicate the region on chromosome 19 ultimately identified as harboring the single most significant risk factor for late-onset Alzheimer disease, the "4" allele of APOE.

Recent extensions to this approach implemented in a program called SimIBD have allowed the closer approximation of the IBS approach to the IBD approach, thus rendering studies with extended affected relatives even more powerful *(77)*.

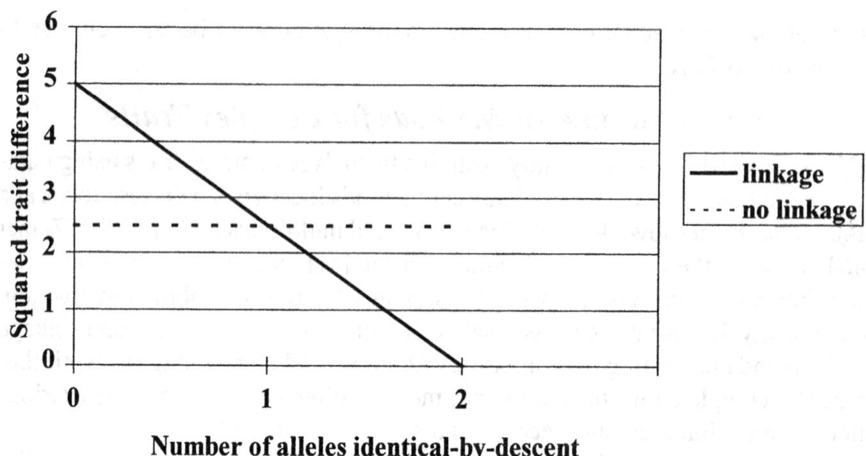

Fig. 11. Under linkage, the squared difference of trait values between sibling pairs is inversely related to the number of alleles shared identical-by-descent. Under nonlinkage, there is no relationship between the squared difference of trait values between siblings and the number of alleles shared identical-by-descent.

Quantitative Traits in Sib–Pair Analysis

The linkage approach for quantitative traits is similar to that for qualitative traits. Here, the difference in the quantitative trait values for the siblings is squared *(46)*. Under the alternate hypothesis of linkage between the disease and marker locus, the expectation is that the squared trait difference will be inversely related to the number of alleles shared IBD at the marker locus (Fig. 11). In other words, siblings whose trait values are similar to one another will tend to share more alleles IBD than siblings with very different trait values.

Association Studies

Case-control studies are a well-established method in epidemiology that have recently come into fashion once again as geneticists begin to look more closely at disease-marker associations. In a traditional association study, epidemiologists score the frequency of an exposure in disease and nondisease samples to determine whether the frequency of exposure is different in cases when compared to controls. For geneticists, the "exposure" is an allele at a genetic marker locus or candidate gene. The question that association studies answer for geneticists is: Is the risk for disease higher in individuals with a specific allele or not? In their simplest form, these analyses are performed with 2×2 contingency tables and are assessed with odds ratios.

As with all association studies, those applied in genetics face a series of formidable challenges *(78)*, the most significant of which is that the identification of a genetic association between two loci does not imply a causal relationship between the loci. Critical to the success of these studies is the availability of a well-matched control group. Given the known differences in allele frequencies between individuals in different ethnic groups, achieving a well-matched control population can be a prohibitive challenge. Differences between case and control frequencies can be due to different allele frequencies in the case and control populations or to admixture, a mixture of individuals from different ethnic (genetic) background. Admixture can either occur at an individual level (an individual's ancestors came from different population groups) or at the population level (the case and control populations are ethnically mixed). Admixture is a problem when the allele frequencies are different in cases and controls. The identification of a significant association between a genetic marker and a disease phenotype does not prove that the marker (candidate gene) is causative in its effect. A significant finding can be due to different allele frequencies in case and control populations.

For example, if American Caucasian and African-American populations are inadvertently included in the same analysis and the allele frequencies are different between the two populations, a false positive association between a marker allele and trait phenotype could be found, due solely to the differences in allele frequencies between the ethnic groups. Even if the analysis were limited to African-American cases vs African-American-controls, a spurious result may still be identified if, for instance, the case group had a higher proportion of Caucasian admixture than the control group.

A recently developed theory has allowed the use of family based controls to consider linkage disequilibrium *(79–82)*. These tests assess evidence for linkage in the presence of association. They involve the collection of mother-father-affected child trios (Fig. 12). Recent extensions have allowed the consideration of highly polymorphic microsatellite repeat markers *(83)*.

Such an approach may be realistic for birth defects or for diseases with early onset. Diseases with adult onset, however, may remain relatively intractable to this approach since one or both parents may be unavailable. New methods (Sib-TDT) have recently been developed *(84,85)* that utilize genotypic information from unaffected siblings to help to obviate the loss of parental data. Additional complications underlying the use of this approach include underlying genetic and allelic heterogeneity, or high rates of mutation at either the disease or marker locus, which will dilute evidence for linkage disequilibrium.

Linkage disequilibrium studies have been proposed for use in genomic screening *(35)*, following the availability of single nucleotide repeat polymorphisms (SNPs). They may be useful in fine mapping or in the initial identification of a region of interest. Although linkage disequilibrium may span a substantially large region of the chromosome in isolated populations, it is unlikely to extend more than one cM in heterogeneous populations like American Caucasians and may not be a useful approach in such a population.

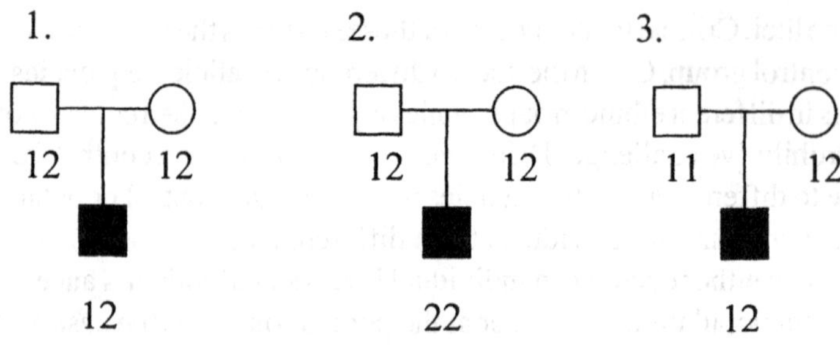

	Transmitted allele		
Non		**1**	**2**
Transmitted	**1**	A	B
Allele	**2**	C	D

Fig. 12. Sample pedigrees appropriate for use with the transmission disequilibrium test. Pedigree 1 contributes 1 count to cell B and 1 count to cell C; pedigree 2 contributes 2 counts to cell B; and pedigree 3 con tributes 1 count to cell A and 1 count to cell B. Statistical analysis is performed using the McNemar test: $\chi^2_1 = (B-C)^2/(B+C)$.

Available Programs for Linkage Analysis

The majority of computer programs that are discussed in this chapter are available free of charge. A complete listing of programs which implement parametric and nonparametric methods can be found at the web site of the Laboratory of Statistical Genetics at The Rockefeller University (http://linkage.rockefeller.edu). This web page <http://linkage.rockefeller.edu/soft/list.html> gives direct links to web sites where the program can either be downloaded or provide information on how the program can be obtained. Summaries of some common linkage analysis programs are provided as follows.

LINKAGE/FASTLINK

This suite of programs LINKAGE/FASTLINK *(86,54)* incorporates the Elston-Stewart Algorithm *(15)* and its extension *(50)* to carry out two-point (MLINK) and multipoint linkage analysis (LINKMAP). Although it is possible to perform linkage analysis on large pedigrees, the LINKAGE programs are limited in the number of marker loci they can handle in multipoint analysis, since the Elston-Stewart algorithm scales exponentially with the number of loci and linearly with the number of nonfounders (those individuals whose parents are included in the pedigree). It is possible to perform linkage analysis for both quantitative and qualitative traits with the LINKAGE programs. In addition, ILINK allows for the estimation of various parameters including recombination fractions, allele frequencies, and penetrances. Algorithmic improvements were implemented in FASTLINK *(86)* to speed up the LINKAGE programs by an order of magnitude for medium to large size problems.

VITESSE

VITESSE *(87)* is a program available for parametric linkage analysis. VITESSE is able to run quickly and efficiently due an algorithm which recodes each person's genotype and uses "fuzzy inheritance" to infer transmission probabilities. A major advantage of VITESSE over LINKAGE/FASTLINK *(86,54)* is its speed and its ability to handle problems which are beyond the memory constraints of LINKAGE/FASTLINK. These differences are important for performing multipoint linkage analysis, particularly for a large number of markers, markers with many alleles, and for pedigrees with many untyped individuals. VITESSE calculates exact multipoint likelihoods. One drawback of VITESSE is that the current version is unable to handle pedigrees of complex structure, i.e., those with consanguineous matings.

GENEHUNTER

GENEHUNTER *(88)* performs both parametric and nonparametric analysis on extended pedigrees. The parametric analysis provides an exact rapid calculation of multipoint LOD scores through the implementation of hidden Markov models (HMM). This approach scales linearly with the number of loci, but exponentially with the number of nonfounders. Therefore, although it can handle a large number of marker loci, GENEHUNTER can only handle pedigrees of small to moderate size. GENEHUNTER also allows for testing of linkage under heterogeneity by implementing the admixture test *(66,67,72)*.

The nonparametric linkage (NPL) analysis method that is implemented in GENEHUNTER counts the number of alleles share IBD. When more than two affected relatives are available within a kindred, GENEHUNTER measures the sharing among a set of relatives. When there is ambiguous IBD sharing, GENEHUNTER averages overall possible IBD sharing configurations. The *p*-value is based on the distributions formed by all possible IBD sharing schemes for a given set of pedigrees or can also be based on the normal approximation. A helpful feature of the program is that it provides graphs of multipoint LOD score and NPL score curves.

SIBPAL

SIBPAL is one member of SAGE, a suite of programs that performs affected sib–pair analysis. The Affected Sib Pair (ASP) means test implemented in SIBPAL does well for a variety of disease models. It has also been shown that it is robust when used with data with untyped parents as long as additional unaffected sibs are typed *(89–91)*.

MAPMAKER/SIBS

MAPMAKER/SIBS *(92)* was the first multipoint sib-pair analysis program available. It allows the evaluation of both quantitative and qualitative traits and is useful for both exclusion mapping and initial disease gene localization. Other multipoint sib-pair analysis programs have also been described *(33)*. The algorithm for MAPMAKERS/SIBS is now implemented in GENEHUNTER2.

Extended Relative Pair Analysis

The extended relative pair analysis (ERPA) *(93)* uses risk calculation to calculate the probability that each pair of affected relatives within a pedigree shares alleles IBD. ERPA is limited to problems involving few loci due to the aforementioned limitations of LINKAGE.

Summary

The identification and isolation of genes for Mendelian traits has been very successful. Diseases that are caused by single genes, however, make up only a small proportion (2–3%) of all human genetic diseases. The majority of human diseases with a genetic component are complex in nature. The analysis of complex traits brings new challenges in isolating the susceptibility genes. Current research has demonstrated the difficulties of finding genes with smaller effects. Often linkage/association studies cannot be replicated and to date only a few susceptibility genes have been isolated as a result of these studies.

The challenge of the 21st century is not only to isolate the genes involved in complex disease etiology, but also to elucidate gene-gene and gene-environment interactions. In order to meet these challenges, it is clear that new statistical genetic methods must be developed in order to map susceptibility genes and elucidate the interactions between genes and between genes and environmental factors. Geneticists have been extremely successful in identifying genes responsible for Mendelian disease and recent findings in complex diseases demonstrate that the future of genetics for these common diseases of significant public health concern is encouraging.

References

1. Roessler, E., Belloni, E., Gaudenz, K., Vargas, F., Scherer, S. W., Tsui, L.-C., and Muenke, M. (1997) Mutations in the C-terminal domain of Sonic Hedgehog cause holoprosencephaly. *Hum. Mol. Genet.* **6,** 1847–1853.
2. Martin, N., Boomsma, D., and Machin, G. (1997) A twin-pronged attack on complex traits. *Nat. Genet.* **17,** 387–392.

3. Lalouel, J. M. (1984) Segregation analysis: a gene or not a gene, in *Genetic Epidemiology of Coronary Heart Disease: Past, Present, and Future*, Alan R. Liss, pp. 217–243.
4. Morton, N. E. (1982) Segregation and linkage analysis, in *Human Genetics, Part B: Medical Aspects* (Rao, D. C., et al., eds.), Alan R. Liss, pp. 3–14.
5. Elston, R. C. (1981) Segregation analysis. *Adv. Hum. Genet.* **11,** 63–120.
6. Rutter, M., Yule, W., Berger, M., Yule, B., Morton, J., and Bagley, C. (1974) Children of West Indian immigrants. I. Rates of behavioural deviance and of psychiatric disorder. *J. Child Psychol. Psychiatr. Allied Disciplines*, **15,** 241–262.
7. Greenberg, D. A. (1986) The effect of proband designation on segregation analysis. *Am. J. Hum. Genet.* **39,** 329–339.
8. Goldin, L. R., Elston, R. C., Graham, J. B., and Miller, C. H. (1980) Genetic analysis of von Willebrand's disease in two large pedigrees: a multivariate approach. *Am. J. Med. Genet.* **6,** 279–293.
9. Go, C. P., Lamiell, J. M., Hsia, Y. E., and Yuen, W.-M. P. Y. (1984) Segregation and linkage analyses of von Hippel Lindau disease among 220 descendants from one kindred. *Am. J. Hum. Genet.* **36,** 142
10. Elston, R. C., Namboordiri, K. K., and Nino, H. V. P. W. S. (1974) Studies on blood and urine glucose in Seminole Indians: Indications for segregation of a major gene. *Am. J. Hum. Genet.* **26,** 13–33.
11. Bonney, G. E., Elston, R. C., Correa, P., Haenszel, W., Zavala, S. E., Zarama, G., et al. (1986) Genetic etiology of gastric carcinoma: chronic atrophic gastritis. *Genet. Epidemiol.* **3,** 213–224.
12. Pericak-Vance, M. A., Vance, J. M., Elston, R. C., Namboodiri, K. K., and Fogle, T. A. (1985) Segregation and linkage analysis of alpha-N-acetyl-D-glucosaminidase (NAG) levels in a black family. *Am. J. Med. Genet.* **20,** 295–306.
13. Lalouel, J. M. and Morton, N. E. (1981) Complex segregation analysis with pointers. *Hum. Hereditary.* **31,** 312–321.
14. MacLean, C. J., Morton, N. E., and Yee, S. (1984) Combined analysis of genetic segregation and linkage under an oligogenic model. *Comput. Biomed. Res.* **17,** 471–4806.
15. Elston, R. C. and Stewart, J. (1971) A general model for the genetic analysis of pedigree data. *Hum. Hered.* **21,** 523–542.
16. Lalouel, J. M., Rao, D. C., Morton, N. E., and Elston, R. C. (1983) A unified model for complex segregation analysis. *Am. J. Hum. Genet.* **35,** 816–826.
17. Bonney, G. E. (1984) On the statistical determination of major gene mechanisms in continuous human traits: regressive models. *Am. J. Hum. Genet.* **18,** 731–749.
18. Vieland, V. J. and Hodge, S. E. (1995) Inherent intractability of the ascertainment problem for pedigree data: a general likelihood framework. *Am. J. Hum. Genet.* **56,** 33–43.
19. Elston, R. C. (1995) Invited editorial. Twixt cup and lip: how intractable is the ascertainment problems? *Am. J. Hum. Genet.* **56,** 15–17.
20. Risch, N. (1990) Linkage strategies for genetically complex traits I. Multilocus models. *Am. J. Hum. Genet.* **46,** 222–228.
21. Worton, R. G. and Thompson, M. W. (1988) Genetics of Duchenne muscular dystrophy, in *Annual Review of Genetics* (Campbell, A., Baker, B. S., and Herskowitz, I. eds.), Annual Reviews Inc., Palo Alto, CA, pp. 601–630.
22. Easton, D. F., Bishop, D. T., Ford, D., Crockford, G. P., and Breast Cancer Linkage Consortium. (1993) Genetic linkage analysis in familial breast and ovarian cancer: results from 217 families. *Am. J. Hum. Genet.* **52,** 678–701.

23. Bowcock, A. M., Anderson, L. A., Friedman, L. S., Black, D. M., Osborne-Lawrence, S., Rowell, S. E., et al. (1993) THRA1 and D17S183 flank an interval of <4 cM for the breast-ovarian cancer gene (BRCA1) on chromosome 17q21. *Am. J. Hum. Genet.* **52,** 718–722.
24. Baraitser, M. and Pallon, M. A. (1985) Reduced penetrance in tuberous sciensis. *J. Med. Genet.* **22,** 29–31.
25. Folstein, M. F. (1989) Heterogeneity in Alzheimer's disease. *Neurobiol. Aging*. **10,** 434–435.
26. Farrer, L. A. and Conneally, P. M. (1985) A genetic model for age at onset in Huntington disease. *Am. J. Hum. Genet.* **37,** 350–357.
27. Pericak-Vance, M. A., Elston, R. C., Conneally, P. M., and Dawson, D. V. (1983) Age-of-onset heterogeneity in Huntington disease families. *Am. J. Med. Genet.* **14,** 49–59.
28. Futreal, P. A., Liu, Q., Shattuck–Eidens, D., Cochran, C., Harshman, K., Tavtigian, S., et al. (1994) BRCA1 Mutations in Primary Breast and Ovarian Carcinomas. *Science* **266,** 120–126.
29. Wooster, R., Bignell, G., Lancaster, J., Swift, S., Seal, S., Mangion, J., et al. (1995) Identification of the breast cancer susceptibility gene BRCA2. *Nature* **378,** 789–792.
30. Tavtigian, S. V., Simard, J., Rommens, J., Couch, F., Shattuck-Eidens, D., Neuhausen, S., et al. (1996) The complete BRCA2 gene and mutations in chromosome 13q–linked kindreds. *Nature Genet.* **12,** 333–337.
31. Pericak-Vance, M. A., Bebout, J. L., Gaskell, P. C., Yamaoka, L. H., Hung, W.-Y., Alberts, M. J., et al. (1991) Linkage studies in familial Alzheimer's disease: evidence for chromosome 19 linkage. *Am. J. Hum. Genet.* **48,** 1034–1050.
32. Leal, S. M. and Ott, J. (1990) Expected lod scores in linkage analysis of autosomal recessive traits for affected and unaffected offspring. *Am. J. Hum. Genet.* **47,** A188.
33. Hauser, E. R., Boehnke, M., Guo, S. W., and Risch, N. (1996) Affected-sib–pair interval mapping and exclusion for complex genetic traits– sampling considerations. *Genet Epidemiol.* **13,** 117–137.
34. Hacia, J. G., Brody, L. C., Chee, M. S., Fodor, S. P. A., and Collins, F. S. (1996) Detection of heterozygous mutations in BRCA1 using high density oligonucleotide arrays and two-colour fluorescence analysis. *Nat. Genet.* **14,** 441–447.
35. Risch, N. and Merikangas, K. (1996) The future of genetic studies of complex human disorders. *Science* **273,** 1516–1517.
36. Ott, J. (1989) Computer simulation methods in human linkage analysis. *Proc. Natl. Acad. Sci. USA* **86,** 4175–4178.
37. Weeks, D. E., Ott, J., and Lathrop, G. M. (1990) SLINK: A general simulation program for linkage analysis. *Am. J. Hum. Genet.* **47,** A204
38. Boehnke, M. (1986) Estimating the power of a proposed linkage study: a practical computer simulation approach. *Am. J. Hum. Genet.* **39,** 513–527.
39. Ploughman, L. M. and Boehnke, M. (1989) Estimating the power of a proposed linkage study for a complex genetic trait. *Am. J. Hum. Genet.* **44,** 543–551.
40. Ott, J. (1991) *Analysis of Human Genetic Linkage.* Johns Hopkins University Press, Baltimore.
41. Ott, J. (1992) Strategies for characterizing highly polymorphic markers in human gene mapping. *Am. J. Hum. Genet.* **51,** 283–290.
42. Weeks, D. E., Lehner, T., Squires-Wheeler, E., Kaufmann, C., and Ott, J. (1990) Measuring the inflation of the lod score due to its maximization over model parameter values in human linkage analysis. *Genet. Epidemiol.* **7,** 237–243.

43. Bernstein, F. (1931) Zur grundlegung der chromosomentheorie der vererbung beim menschen. *Z. Abst. Vererb.* **57,** 113–138.
44. Weinberg, W. (1912) Zur verebung der anlage der bluterkrankheit mit methodologischen ergaenzungen meiner geschwistermethode. *Arch. Rass. Ges. Biol.* **6,** 694–709.
45. Penrose, L. S. (1935) The detection of autosomal linkage in data which consists of pairs of brothers and sisters of unspecified parentage. *Ann. Eugen.* **6,** 133–138.
46. Haseman, J. K. and Elston, R. C. (1972) The investigation of linkage between a quantitative trait and a marker locus. *Behav.Genet.* **2,** 3–19.
47. Haldane, J. B. S. and Smith, C. A. B. (1947) A new estimate of the linkage between the genes for color blindness and hemophilia in man. *Ann. Eugen.* **14,** 10–31.
48. Morton, N. E. (1955) Sequential tests for the detection of linkage. *Am. J. Hum. Genet.***7,** 277–318.
49. Wald, A. (1947) *Sequential Analysis* John Wiley, New York.
50. Lange, K. and Elston, R. C. (1975) Extension to pedigree analysis. I. Likelihood calculations for simple and complex pedigrees. *Hum. Hered.* **25,** 95–105.
51. Lander, E. S. and Kruglyak, L. (1995) Genetic dissection of complex traits: guidelines for interpreting and reporting linkage results. *Nat. Genet.* **11,** 241
52. Edwards, A. W. F. (1992) *Likelihood (expanded ed.)*, Johns Hopkins University Press, Baltimore.
53. Conneally, P. M., Edwards, J. H., and Kidd, K. K. (1985) Report of the commitee on methods of linkage analysis reporting. Eighth International Workshop on Human Gene Mapping. *Cytogenet. Cell Genet.* **40,** 356–359.
54. Lathrop, G. M., Lalouel, J. M., Julier, C., and Ott, J. (1984) Strategies for multilocus linkage analysis in humans. *Proc. Natl. Acad. Sci. USA* **81,** 3443–3446.
55. Lander, E. S. and Botstein, D. (1986) Strategies for studying heterogeneous genetic traits in humans by using a linkage map of restriction fragment length polymorphisms. *Proc. Natl. Acad. Sci. USA* **83,** 7357
56. Lander, E. S. and Botstein, D. (1987) Homozygostiy mapping: a way to map human recessive traits with the DNA of inbred children. *Science* **236,** 1567–1570.
57. Risch, N. and Giuffra, L. (1992) Model misspecification and multipoint linkage analysis. *Hum. Hered.* **42,** 77–92.
58. Knowles, J. A., Vieland, V. J., and Gilliam, T. C. (1992) Perils of gene mapping with microsatellite markers. *Am. J. Hum. Genet.* **51,** 905–909.
59. Dausset, J., Cann, H., Cohen, D., Lathrop, M., Lalouel, J. M., and White, R. (1990) Centre d'etude du polymorphisme humanin (CEPH): collaborative genetic mapping of the human genome. *Genomics* **6,** 575–577.
60. Bird, T. D., Ott, J., and Giblett, E. F. (1982) Evidence for linkage of Charcot–Marie–Tooth neuropathy to the Duffy locus on chromosome 1. *Am. J. Hum. Genet.* **34,** 388–394.
61. Fryer, A. E., Connor, J. M., Povey, S., Yates, J. R. W., Chalmer, A., Fraser, I., et al. (1987) Evidence that the gene for tuberous sclerosis is on chromosome 9. *Lancet* **1,** 659–661.
62. Kandt, R. S., Haines, J. L., Smith, M., Northrup, H., Gardner, R. J., Short, M. P., et al. (1992) Linkage of an important gene locus for tuberous sclerosis to a chromosome 16 marker for polycystic kidney disease. *Nat. Genet.* **2,** 37–41.
63. Van Camp, G., Willems, P. J., and Smith, R. J. H. (1997) Nonsyndromic hearing impairment: unparalleled heterogeneity. *Am. J. Hum. Genet.* **60,** 758–764.
64. Reeders, S. T., Breuning, M. H., Ryynaenen, M. A., Wright, A. F., Davies, K. E., King, A. W., et al. (1987) A study of genetic linkage heterogeneity in adult polycystic kidney disease. *Hum. Genet.* **76,** 348–351.

65. Morton, N. E. (1956) The detection and estimation of linkage between the genes for elliptocytosis and the Rh blood type. *Am. J. Hum. Genet.* **8,** 80–96.
66. Ott, J. (1983) Linkage analysis and family classification under heterogeneity. *Ann. Hum. Genet.* **47,** 311–320.
67. Smith, C. A. B. (1961) Homogeneity test for linkage data. *Proc. Sec. Int. Cong. Hum. Genet.* 212–213.
68. Terwilliger, J. D. and Ott, J. (1994) *Handbook of Genetic Linkage*, Johns Hopkins University Press, Baltimore.
69. Clerget-Darpoux, F., Babron, M., and Bonaiti-Pellie, C. (1987) Power and robustness of the linkage homogeneity test in genetic analysis of common disorders. *J. Psychiatr. Res.* **21,** 625–630.
70. Hodge, S. E. (1984) The information contained in multiple sibling pairs. *Genet. Epidemiol.* **1,** 109–122.
71. Clerget-Darpoux, F., Bonaiti-Pellie, C., and Hochez, J. (1986) Effects of misspecifying genetic parameters in lod score analysis. *Biometrics* **42,** 393–399.
72. Smith, C. A. B. (1963) Testing for heterogeneity of recombination fractions values in human genetics. *Ann. Hum. Genet.* **27,** 175–182.
73. Berrettini, W. H., Ferraro, T. N., Goldin, L. R., Weeks, D. E., Detera-Wadleigh, S., Nurnberger, J. I., Jr., and Gershon, E. S. (1994) Chromosome 18 DNA markers and manic-depressive illness: evidence for a susceptibility gene. *Proc. Natl. Acad. Sci.USA* **91,** 5918–5921.
74. Lathrop, G. M. and Ott, J. (1990) Analysis of complex diseases under oligogenic models and intrafamilial heterogeneity by the LINKAGE program. *Am. J. Hum. Genet.* **47,** A188.
75. Schork, N. J., Boehnke, M., Terwilliger, J. D., and Ott, J. (1993) Two trait locus linkage analysis: a powerful strategy for mapping complex genetic traits. *Am. J. Hum. Genet.* **53,** 1127–1136.
76. Weeks, D. E. and Lange, K. (1988) The affected–pedigree member method of linkage analysis. *Am. J. Hum. Genet.* **42,** 315–326.
77. Davis, S., Schroeder, M., Goldin, L. R., and Weeks, D. E. (1996) Nonparametric simulation-based statistics for detecting linkage in general pedigrees. *Am. J. Hum. Genet.* **58,** 867–880.
78. Econs, M. J. and Speer, M. C. (1998) Genetic studies of complex diseases: let the reader beware. *J Bone Miner. Res.* **11,** 1835–1839.
79. Spielman, R. S., McGinnis, R. E., and Ewens, W. J. (1993) Transmission test for linkage disequilibrium: the insulin gene region and insulin-dependent diabetes mellitus (IDDM). *Am. J. Hum. Genet.* **52,** 506–516.
80. Schaid, D. J. and Sommer, S. S. (1994) Comparison of statistics for candidate-gene association studies using cases and parents. *Am. J. Hum. Genet.* **55,** 402–409.
81. Terwilliger, J. D. and Ott, J. (1992) A haplotype–based "haplotype relative risk" approach to detecting allelic associations. *Hum. Heredity* **42,** 337–346.
82. Falk, C. T. and Rubinstein, P. (1987) Haplotype relative risks: an easy reliable way to construct a proper control sample for risk calculations. *Ann. Hum. Genet.* **51,** 227–233.
83. Kaplan, N. L., Martin, E. R., and Weir, B. S. (1997) Power studies for the transmission/disequilibrium tests with multiple alleles. *Am. J. Hum. Genet.* **60,** 691–702.
84. Monks, S. A., Martin, E. R., Weir, B. S., and Kaplan, N. L. (1997) A sibship test of linkage in the absence of parental information. *Am. J. Hum. Genet.* **61,** A286(Abstract).

85. Boehnke, M. and Langefeld, C. D. (1998) Genetic association mapping based on discordant sib pairs: the discordant alleles test (DAT). *Am. J. Hum. Genet.* **62,** 950–961.
86. Cottingham, R. W. Jr., Idury, R. M., and Schaffer, A. A. (1993) Faster sequential genetic linkage computations. *Am. J. Hum. Genet.* **53,** 252–263.
87. O'Connell, J. R. and Weeks, D. E. (1995) The VITESSE algorithm for rapid exact multilocus linkage analysis via genotype set-recording and fuzzy inheritance. *Nat. Genet.* **11,** 402–408.
88. Kruglyak, L., Daly, M. J., Reeve-Daly, M. P., and Lander, E. S. (1996) Parametric and nonparametric linkage analysis:– a unified multipoint approach. *Am. J. Hum. Genet.* **58,** 1347–1363.
89. Blackwelder, W. C. and Elston, R. C. (1985) A comparison of sib-pair linkage tests for disease susceptibility loci. *Genet. Epidemiol.* **2,** 85–98.
90. Knapp, M., Seuchter, S., and Bauer, M. (1994) Linkage analysis in nuclear families. 1. Optimality criteria for affected sib–pair test. *Hum. Heredity* **44,** 37–43.
91. Davis, S. and Weeks, D. E. (1997) Comparison of nonparametric statistics for detection of linkage analysis in nuclear families: single marker evaluation. *Am. J. Hum. Genet.* **61,** 1431–1444.
92. Kruglyak, L. and Lander, E. S. (1995) Complete multipoint sib-pair analysis of qualitative and quantitative traits. *Am. J. Hum. Genet.* **57,** 439–454.
93. Curtis, D. and Sham, P. C. (1994) Using risk calculation to implement an extended relative pair analysis. *Am. J. Hum. Genet.* **58,** 151–162.
94. Speer, M. C. (1998) Sample size and power, in *Gene Mapping in Complex Human Disease* (Haines, J. L. and Pericak-Vance, M., eds.), Wiley-Liss, New York, pp. 161–200.

Chapter 21

The Identification of Disease Genes in a Candidate Region

Fiona Francis and Tim M. Strom

Abstract

The approaches used for positionally cloning a disease gene from a defined chromosomal region are rapidly evolving. In the past this step began with the screening of yeast artificial chromosome (YAC) libraries, followed by the identification of smaller clones propagated in *Escherichia coli*. With increasing amounts of resources generated by large-scale approaches, and advertised over the World Wide Web, this step in a positional cloning procedure may no longer be necessary. Transcripts can be identified using a variety of different methods, including those performed at the bench and those performed "in silico." Each of the genes identified need to be assessed for involvement in the disease. After the correct disease gene has been cloned, further functional analyses are often necessary to understand the role of the encoded protein and the pathophysiological mechanisms involved in the disease process.

Introduction

The identification of genes from candidate regions is these days greatly aided by the extensive resources which have been generated as a consequence of the Human Genome Project. This is a vast international collaboration which has the aim of mapping and sequencing the complete human genome *(1)*. As such, this project provides a catalogue of mapped genes for not only the elucidation and understanding of human diseases, but also developmental processes, and the maintenance of the organism. Early objectives of this project were to produce a high density of genetic markers spaced evenly throughout the genome and physical maps which show the locations of expressed genes. Although not yet complete, such genetical, physical, and transcriptional maps have revolutionized positional

The Genetics of Osteoporosis and Metabolic Bone Disease
Ed.: M. J. Econs © Humana Press Inc., Totowa, NJ

cloning strategies for the isolation of disease genes *(2–6)*. Whereas a few years ago, positional cloning needed many years of work, nowadays disease genes can be isolated within months. Nevertheless the cloning of rare disease genes and particularly the cloning of genes for polygenic diseases remains a challenge.

It is not only the resources and results from the Human Genome Project which benefit the positional cloners, but also the evolution of the techniques involved. Specifically with respect to the identification of expressed sequences, early attempts most often relied upon a search for CpG islands *(7)* and for sequences which are conserved between species. The development of exon-trapping and cDNA selection (for descriptions see below) has supplemented these techniques, and in some cases they have been adopted to produce transcriptional maps of large genomic regions *(8)*. More recently the sequencing and mapping of expressed sequence tags (ESTs; *9*), and large-scale genomic sequencing, have made the prospect of positional cloning in silico a reality *(10–12)*. Nevertheless, there may still be a need for a combination of the above-mentioned techniques, since one alone is unlikely to easily reveal all genes. In this chapter we will elaborate on the techniques, past and present, used for disease gene isolation.

Cloning the Region of Interest: Clone Libraries and Physical Mapping

Whether genetic linkage analyses or translocation breakpoints are used to define the region of interest, the methods used for gene identification remain the same. Translocation breakpoints nevertheless allow a much greater resolution of the candidate region: A small genomic fragment can be shown to cross the breakpoint, leading to an efficient identification of the relevant gene. Genetic linkage analyses define much larger regions requiring a more extensive cloning effort.

Clone libraries are produced by the breakage of chromosomes into smaller fragments, which are cloned and individually propagated in bacterial or yeast cells. The reconstruction of the order of these fragments results in a clone-based physical map or contig. Contigs are principally constructed in two ways: by hybridization approaches *(13)* in which case clones are assayed for probe content, or by sequence tagged site (STS) mapping *(6,14)*. In the latter case polymerase chain reactions (PCRs) are used to assay for short sequences within the clones using specific primer sets. Efficient screening approaches require arrayed libraries: the clones are distributed individually in microtiter dish wells, and stored as a frozen stock, such that each clone is a renewable source. For hybridization, clones can be gridded in an ordered pattern on Nylon membranes, and hybridization performed with a DNA probe therefore requiring no prior knowledge of the probe sequence *(13)*. Several genome centers and commercial companies worldwide, distribute such library filters (*see* Table 1 for Web addresses). Alternatively, primer sequences derived from STSs or ESTs can be used to isolate clones by PCR screening (*see* Table 1).

Table 1
Useful Web Addresses

Reference in text	Web address
Libraries	http://www.rzpd.de/
	http://www.hgmp. mrc.ac.uk./index.html
	http://www.genomesystems.com/
Sanger Centre	http://www.sanger.ac.uk/Software/Image/fingerprinting
NCBI	http://www.ncbi.nlm.nih.gov
Genemap	http://www.ncbi.nlm.nih.gov/genemap
BLAST	http://www.ncbi.nlm.nih.gov/BLAST
Unigene	http://www.ncbi.nlm.nih.gov/Unigene
MZEF	http://www.cshl.org/genefinder
GenScan	http://CCR-081.mit.edu/GENSCAN.html
FGENEH	http://dot.imgen.bcm.tmc.edu:9331/gene-finder/gf.html
Grail http://compbio.orml.gov/	
Genie	http://www..cse.ucsc.edu/~dkulp/cgi-bin/genie
GeneParser	http://beagle.colorado.edu/~eesnyder/GeneParser.html
Genome guide	http://www.ncbi.nlm.nih.gov/genome/guide
RepeatMasker	http://ftp.genome.washington.edu/RM/RepeatMasker.html
EST_cloned	http://www.ncbi.nlm.nih.gov/dbEST/dBEST_genes/
Nix(offered by the MRC after registration)	http://www.hgmp.mrc.ac.uk/
Rummage(not publically available)	http://genome.imb-jena.de
Genotator	http://www-hgc.lbl.gov/inf/annotation.html
Beauty	http://dot.imgen.bcm.tmc.edu:9331/seq-search/nucleic_acid-search.html

The yeast artificial chromosome (YAC) system *(15)* has a large cloning capacity and YAC clones range in size from several hundred kilobases to over a megabase of DNA. Because of their large size YACs have been chosen to map large chromosomal regions. YAC libraries are screened with markers from the region of interest, and the resulting clones are characterized further by screening with more markers to determine overlaps, and by rescuing the ends of clones for the same purpose, or to perform more library screens. Pulsed field gel electrophoresis (PFGE, *16*) allows the sizing of a YAC insert and in combination with rare cutter enzyme digestions can lead to the development of a restriction map. One important consideration when using YAC clones is that they can be chimeric, i.e., containing DNA from noncontiguous parts of the genome. For this reason it is advisable to perform fluorescence *in situ* hybridization (FISH) analysis to confirm that a clone contains DNA only from the region of interest, before pursuing an intensive characterization. An alternative approach to detect chimerism is the hybridization of end probes derived from a YAC, to DNA from somatic cell hybrids which contain individual chromosomes or parts of chromosomes.

Whole-genome, and individual chromosome YAC mapping efforts have been carried out by various laboratories, which often means that a YAC contig has already been constructed across the region of interest. Indeed for some chromosomes quite detailed maps are available *(17–22)*. However, the large-scale nature of these projects means that in most cases there are still gaps in the maps, and contigs which are available, generally need verification. Nevertheless this represents an invaluable resource which obviates the need to start with the isolation of YACs from a YAC library.

After a YAC contig has been constructed or verified, it is generally used to isolate smaller clones propagated in *E. coli*, which are easier to manipulate, and allow the production of DNA in larger amounts. Cosmid inserts have a maximum size of approx 40 kb, and cosmid libraries made from relatively pure individual chromosome preparations are available (*see* Table 1). Cloned cosmid DNA is easily isolated from *E. coli*, which makes this a useful system to derive starting material in the search for expressed sequences and for genomic sequencing projects. Contig building with this system alone has its limitations, such as the large number of clones which need to be processed, and the relatively small size of the initial contigs. For this reason cosmid clones are often isolated by screening YAC inserts against cosmid library filters. Alternatively new cosmid libraries can be generated from individual YAC clones. This latter strategy has the disadvantage that any problems associated with the YAC clone e.g., deletions or rearrangements, will be propagated in the cosmid clones.

Several other cloning systems have been developed, designed to accommodate pieces of DNA which are larger than cosmids, but also propagated in *E. coli* for ease of growth and manipulation. These are the P1 *(23)*, P1-derived artificial chromosome (PAC; *24*) and bacterial artificial chromosome (BAC; *25*) systems. These clones are of an intermediate size between YACs and cosmids, and in some cases they may be more stable than cosmids since they are maintained at a lower copy number. Like YAC libraries, P1, PAC, and BAC libraries are usually prepared from total genomic DNA, and are commonly available for screening (*see* Table 1). Due to the fact that PAC and BAC clones are larger than cosmids, they are often used for direct assembly into contigs (*see* Table 1) without the need for previously identifying YAC clones. As with cosmid clones, PACs and BACs can be initially identified by hybridization of probes or by PCR with specific primers. End sequences of identified PACs and BACs can be easily generated by direct sequencing *(26)*. Plasmid DNA should be purified using commercially available columns, and subjected to automated sequencing procedures using 1–2 µg DNA per end. Primers designed from end sequences are immediately useful for the identification of new clones in order to extend contigs or to close gaps between contigs.

In many cases in large-scale sequencing projects of individual chromosomes, efforts are being made to generate PAC, BAC, and cosmid contigs as a prerequisite. PACs and BACs especially are now a popular substrate for these projects, and they are also amenable to the gene identification methods described.

Methods for Gene Identification

In both positional cloning projects and projects aimed at producing whole chromosome transcriptional maps, an essential aspect has involved the methods used to identify coding sequences from the cloned genomic DNA. One earlier method for gene identification took advantage of the fact that many genes show evolutionary conservation. Therefore identification of cross-hybridizing sequences in other species by hybridization of genomic fragments to ''zoo'' blots, which contain digested genomic DNA from different organisms, led to the successful cloning of several disease genes *(27,28)*. A second classical method involves the identification of CpG islands within the cloned DNA *(7)*. CpG islands are highly GC-rich regions which are often associated with the 5' ends of genes (mainly housekeeping genes). They are detected within genomic DNA by a clustering of rare cutter enzyme sites which have GC-rich recognition sequences, for example *Not* I, *Eag* I, and *Sac* II. If a number of such sites are detected within a 1 – 2 kb region, then this could indicate the presence of the 5' end of a gene. In both the above methods genomic fragments containing potential sequences of interest can be used to screen cDNA libraries, or can be directly sequenced to identify putative coding sequences.

More recently several strategies were devised, which are better applicable to the isolation of genes from large stretches of genomic DNA. Exon-trapping *(29)* is a method for isolating exons by cloning genomic DNA, e.g., from a cosmid, PAC, or BAC clone, into a vector which contains functional 5' and 3' splice sites flanking the cloning site. DNA is transfected into mammalian COS-7 cells where an SV40 early promoter present in the vector drives high levels of transcription. If an exon is present within the cloned genomic fragment, splicing will occur removing intragenic DNA, leaving only exonic sequences cloned in the vector.

RNA is rescued from the COS-7 cells and exons are amplified by RT-PCR using vector primers, and the resulting products are cloned. Cosmid, PAC, and BAC clones from a contig can be individually cloned in the exon-trapping vector to derive exons from the region of interest, with no prior knowledge of the tissue specificities of the gene(s). Alternatively, all overlapping clones from a contig can be used in one exon-trapping experiment. This may however, result in a lower representation of cloned exons, depending on the size of the region and the quality of the exon-trap libraries produced. In the case of multi-exon genes this may not cause a problem because even one exon is sufficient as a tag for that particular gene, allowing the screening of Northern blots and cDNA libraries to isolate the remainder of the coding sequence. It is not however, possible to trap terminal exons because they have only one functional splice site. Some ''false-positives'' can be generated in the exon-trapping system, due to the recognition of cryptic splice sites within genomic DNA. Nevertheless this system remains extremely useful, and may always be required to identify functional transcriptional units even in regions which are in the process of being completely sequenced.

cDNA selection offers an alternative strategy *(30–33)*, and involves the immobilization of biotinylated genomic template DNA (which can be an individual clone, or a contig of clones) onto magnetic beads (or Nylon membranes) to act as a target for hybridization with cDNA libraries. Nonspecific cDNAs are washed away, and region-specific cDNAs are eluted. Two rounds of enrichment are usually performed before finally eluting and cloning the selected cDNAs. Obviously the success of this method relies on the presence of the relevant cDNAs in the starting cDNA library, and hence libraries are generally selected from tissue sources which are most likely to express the disease gene.

Both selected cDNA libraries and exon libraries can be transferred to membranes in order to generate clone filters for hybridization. In most cases randomly plated clones should be picked into microtiter dishes containing media, and regrown overnight. The saturated cultures can be spotted onto Nylon membranes, which are then placed on well-dried agar plates and grown overnight again. The following day hybridization membranes can be prepared using *in situ* colony lysis protocols *(34,35)*. Such filter membranes can be screened in a systematic fashion using genomic fragments derived from cosmids, PACs, and BACs. Positively hybridizing clones can be sequenced using vector primers, and mapped back onto the clones from the region. Such hybridizations can help reveal previously unidentified overlaps between genomic clones (although since cDNAs and trapped exons can often contain more than one exon, two hybridizing genomic clones may not necessarily overlap), and also allows an ordering of cDNAs across a genomic region. This information is useful to assess potential gene models, that is which exons are likely to be contained in the same gene. RT-PCRs can be performed between the adjacent transcriptional units to confirm their presence in the same gene. Sequence data generated from new cDNAs and trapped exons should immediately be screened against the sequence databases (*see* below). Not only can this generate information regarding the potential function of a gene, but also overlapping sequences in the form of ESTs can be used to reconstruct full-length gene sequences.

Cloning "In Silico"

All the aforementioned transcript identification methods can be extremely useful when trying to isolate genes from a cloned genomic contig. Over the last few years, all have been used in many successful positional cloning projects. However, disease gene isolation has entered a new era, where either "in silico" or "clone by phone" approaches are largely superceding the earlier strategies.

Once a disease locus has been established in a particular chromosome region, it is highly recommendable to search the Internet to find the resources which are already available. This includes genomic clone contigs, which, as described previously, are an ideal starting point for gene transcript identification. Other resources include mapped ESTs *(4)*, which make the "positional candidate" approach *(36)* a possibility, and ultimately the full genomic sequence of a region, which is amenable to exon prediction procedures. Identifying a gene using these resources can still be an arduous task if the region of interest is large, potentially containing many different genes, or if it is not clear what are the characteristics of an ideal candidate gene for a given disease. The expected expression pattern is usually the safest measure of candidate gene suitability, obviously one expects a candidate gene for a brain developmental disorder to be expressed in fetal brain and so on. Ubiquitously expressed genes are not as easily recognizable for their implication in a disease process, and occasionally the pattern of expression of a disease gene can be surprising. The same is true for disease gene function, which is not always as predicted from earlier biochemical experiments.

ESTs

Expressed sequence tags (ESTs) are short end sequences derived from cDNA clones *(9)*. Huge efforts have been made to quickly end sequence (usually 3' end) large numbers of clones from many different tissue sources. The IMAGE Consortium *(37)* in particular have provided high quality cDNA libraries for this purpose. More importantly all data from IMAGE libraries have been made publicly available. Large numbers of ESTs have also been produced by The Institute for Genomic Research (TIGR; *38*), although with limited access to the public. The dbEST database which is separate from the non redundant (nr) nucleotide sequence database, contains the collection of EST sequences from a variety of different organisms. This represents a very powerful resource, indeed, there are now over 120,000 human entries in dbEST (December 1998). Many sequences are redundant since a single gene may have been sequenced multiple times. Nevertheless, it is possible to walk through the EST database in order to build up a gene sequence: When an EST sequence is identified it can be rescreened back against the database in order to look for identical overlapping sequences, this procedure can then be repeated with a new sequence which extends the furthest, and so on. dbEST hence represents a very powerful resource for cloning "in silico."

With the aim of assimilating and managing this vast deposit of transcriptional information, an attempt has been made to cluster the redundant gene sequences in Genbank and dbEST, by the creation of the Unigene database (*see* Table 1; *39*). Each cluster contains sequences that represent a unique gene, and at the present time (December 1998) there are over 50,000 clusters, each of which is represented in the database by the longest sequence. Further information such as the mRNA sources from which the cDNA sequences were derived, and the genomic localization when known, have been included.

There are currently over 30,000 gene sequences positioned in precise genetic intervals on human chromosomes, and these are summarized in a separate database, the "genemap" (*see* Table 1; *4*). This is a whole genome map containing genes and ESTs which have been localized using irradiation hybrid panels. It is possible to search this map by specifying a particular region, and an ordered list of genes and ESTs encompassed in that region can be viewed. "Genemap" is hence an ideal starting place for a gene search when a particular genomic region has been pinpointed. However if the region is large, searching for a candidate gene may still be like looking for an elusive needle in a haystack. It is of course, impossible to predict for certain, how many genes have not yet made it onto the map.

The sequence databases (Genbank, DDBJ, EMBL, dbEST, and so on) can be searched with EST sequences using the BLAST algorithm *(40,41)*, either by email or using the WWW (*see* Table 1). A description of the different blast programs (e.g., blastn for searching a nucleotide query sequence against a nucleotide sequence database, blastp for searching a protein query sequence against a protein sequence database, etc) and advice on the interpretation of results, has been recently reviewed Brenner et al. *(42)*.

Why Not Wait for Genomic Sequence Data?

The availability of large amounts of genomic sequence deposited in the sequence databases and on various Web sites (reviewed in ref. *43*) has revolutionized the field of gene discovery. The human genome has been largely divided up between various Genome Centers interested in sequencing either whole chromosomes, large parts of chromosomes, or even the whole genome *(44)*. Within the near future the full genomic sequence will become available. Its analysis, not only the identification of genes but also functional elements involved in gene regulation and transcription, represents a huge challenge. Gene expression patterns, recognition of known protein domains, identification of interacting proteins, and understanding the pathway in which a gene product belongs, are further essential data which need to be obtained. Biologists interested in specific genes, pathways, and physiological processes, and willing to use the bioinformatics tools available, will play a fundamental role in the interpretation of sequence data. At present, the problem is knowing where to find the data, however with the commitment of the international sequencing community and curators of databases, this information should in time become more clearly displayed. The information of which sequencing center is sequencing which region of the human genome is available from the National Center for Biotechnology Information (NCBI) Web site (*see* Table 1), from their genome guide page (*see* Table 1). It is worth contacting a sequencing center that has staked a claim on a chromosome of interest to inquire about the priorities across the chromosome. In some cases, offering to supply a reliable BAC, or PAC contig may greatly speed up the sequencing process. Furthermore, genome centers have offered to sequence regions of interest preferentially.

Shotgun Sequencing

Genomic sequence data is released to the public at various levels of completeness. In the sequencing of a PAC or BAC clone the starting template DNA is divided randomly into smaller pieces (e.g., 2 kb in size) using a process such as sonication. A random sub-library or "shotgun library" is made from these pieces, and the resulting clones are end sequenced. Large numbers of clones are usually processed, and the resulting sequence data is assembled in order to try and recreate the original PAC or BAC clone sequence. At this stage the data is generally very redundant in certain regions, where for example, greater than 10 sequences are derived from the same piece of DNA. In other regions there are gaps in the sequence, where no clone has been sequenced containing that region. These local differences in coverage reflect the statistical nature of the process of randomly selecting shotgun clones for sequencing. However, it is possible to very quickly generate greater than 90% of the sequence of a PAC or BAC clone using this method. In the second phase of sequencing a more directed approach is used to try and close the gaps in the sequence and to verify problematic or unreliable sequences. The finished sequence then becomes available in the sequencing databases. The unfinished sequence nevertheless represents a very valuable resource, and the international sequencing community has agreed to also release this data to the public, although it currently exists in either a separate division of the sequence databases (high throughput genomic, HTG, sequences; *45*), or at individual sequencing center Web sites (summarized by the NCBI, and recently reviewed in ref. *43*).

Analysis of Genomic Sequence Data

Once genomic sequence has been located or generated across a region of interest it should be subjected to a systematic analysis, to assess the gene content. Large pieces of genomic sequence can themselves be searched back against the databases if a suitable repeat masking program is used. There are mainly two programs: RepeatMasker *(46)* is accessible on the Internet by Web browsers and Censor *(47)* by email server (censor@charon.lpi.org). Sequences must be masked separately and can then be used to search against the sequence databases. Some sites allow sequences to be processed by repeat masking programs, prior to database screening. This feature is offered by Powerblast *(48)*. Powerblast output contains an alignment of the query and the database sequences and allows the very rapid screening of cDNA and protein hits.

EST, mRNA, and protein matches found within the searched sequence can be further investigated, for example, the EST and mRNA matches should be scrutinized for evidence of splicing. The cDNA clones from which matching ESTs are derived can be obtained and fully sequenced, a comparison with the genomic sequence will reveal further evidence of the gene structure.

In some cases searches of genomic sequence against the sequence databases will not reveal any significant matches. In these cases the use of a variety of different gene and exon prediction programs becomes essential. Use of these programs is anyway recommended in order to fully assess the gene content of a genomic clone. Some of the programs available include MZEF, GenScan, FGENEH, Grail, Geneparser, and Genie (reviewed in ref. *49*; for WWW references, *see* Table 1). Since the programs use a variety of different methods to recognize exon sequences *(49)* it is not surprising that there are variations in the results generated. It is generally advisable to compare the results from several different programs to maximize the chances of recognizing as many exons as possible. At the same time, exons that are identified by more than one program are less likely to be false positives, and can be further characterized with priority. Predicted exon sequences should be compared with EST, gene and protein matches already identified within the sequence, or alternatively by performing new individual exon screens. Reverse transcriptase-polymerase reaction (RT-PCR) should be used to validate potential exons, in the absence of any other transcriptional data.

As the amount of available information increases, it becomes more difficult for the user to interpret the results. Database-searching "workbenches" attempt to address this problem by postprocessing search and analyses results and displaying them graphically (reviewed in ref. *50*). Examples of these strategies include Powerblast, Beauty, Genotator *(51)*, NIX, and Rummage (*see* Table 1).

Verification of Genes

The identification of exons, or parts of exons provides a handle by which an entire gene can be isolated. There are several criteria which allow one to distinguish between artefacts and real genes. As mentioned previously RT-dependent PCR is essential to prove the presence of a transcript in the RNA derived from a particular tissue. RT-PCR between two adjacent exons not only provides information that they are part of the same gene, but differences between genomic DNA and RT-PCR products will confirm the presence of an intron and hence rule out an unspliced pseudogene. Sequencing of RT-PCR products allows one to search for an open reading frame (ORF), which is an essential component of a protein coding gene. These sequences will also provide useful gene structure data by comparison to genomic DNA sequence. Some 3' untranslated regions (UTRs) are large: If a number of ESTs are available in a particular region where there is no apparent ORF, it may be that there are more exons present upstream. Northern blot screens are essential for determining the size of a transcript, and its tissue distribution. RT-PCR products can be used to screen both Northern blots and cDNA libraries in an attempt to obtain the full-length cDNA sequence.

Full-Length Sequences

In most cases, only a partial gene sequence will have been obtained by all the aforementioned screening procedures. Since most genes contain multiple exons, it is rare to obtain a full-length cDNA sequence using the procedures of exon-trapping and cDNA selection which generally result in small products. Additionally ESTs by their very nature are short sequences and since they are often derived from the 3' ends of genes, they might only contain 3' UTR sequences. 5' ends of genes are difficult to predict from genomic sequence data alone. If by screening of dbEST, or by screening available cDNA libraries (at the bench), has not revealed the ends of the gene, alternative methods are usually required especially to identify the 5' ends which represent the biggest challenge. 5' or 3' RACE (rapid amplification of cDNA ends, *52*) are extremely useful techniques to accomplish this, based on RT-PCR. 5' RACE is the annealing (to the full-length mRNA) of a gene-specific primer directed toward the 5' end of the gene, followed by extension using RT to generate first strand cDNA. An artificial tail is attached to the 5' end and PCR using this annealing site can thus be performed. 3' race starts with oligo dT priming and PCR is then performed on the resulting cDNA in combination with a gene specific primer. Obviously this technique depends heavily on the quality of the mRNA used.

At the 5' coding end of the sequence one expects to identify a start methionine codon (ATG), ideally surrounded by a particular sequence termed a Kozak consensus sequence *(53)*, which is the substrate of the mammalian translation machinery. Upstream of this one expects no further in-frame methionines, and the presence of stop codons is a good indication that the 5' end of the coding sequence has at least been identified. Identifying the transcriptional start site is not as straightforward and involves the use of techniques such as primer extension *(34)*, correlated with 5' RACE results to verify that the 5' end of the sequence has indeed been reached. This latter goal is not usually a priority in the cloning of a new gene: The full coding sequence is the major goal, since most mutations implicated in a particular disease will change amino acids or splice sites. 3' ends of genes are usually more easy to recognize: The 3' terminal exon usually contains the stop codon followed by all 3' UTR sequences. The presence of 3' ESTs or 3' RACE products generated from oligo dT derived cDNA, often means the position of a poly A tail is easily recognized. In comparison with genomic sequence, such data can be used to indicate the polyadenylation signal (usually AATAAA). Several such signals can be found in genes which are alternatively spliced at their 3' ends.

Even before the full-length sequence has been obtained, verification that the cloned gene is the one involved in the disease can begin. Hybridizations of cDNAs to patient DNA panels and searching for mutations by methods such as SSCP are the way to begin addressing this point and these methods are the subject of Chapter 22.

Conclusions and Perspectives

The identification of some disease genes can be rather challenging. There are those genes which are represented in dbEST (*see* Table 1) but for example have no known function. Obviously a lot more work is required to understand their involvement in a particular disease process. There are also those genes for which there exist no ESTs in the databases, either because they are highly tissue specific and present in a tissue not subjected to large amounts of EST sequencing, or because they are present at a very low abundance in all tissues. For the same reasons it is in some cases difficult to obtain Northern blot results. Under these conditions it is difficult to be convinced that a 'real' gene has actually been identified. One thing which is clear is that each gene-hunt is a different adventure. Ultimately the availability of genomic sequence and suitable ways to analyze it, will reveal all genes.

References

1. Collins, F. and Galas, D. (1993) A new five year plan for the US Human Genome Project. *Science* **262**, 43–46.
2. Chumakov, I., Rigault, P., Le Gall, I., et al. (1995) A YAC contig map of the human genome *Nature* **377(Suppl.),** 174–297
3. Bellanne-Chantelot, C., Lacroix, B., Ougen, P., Billault, A., Beaufils, S., Bertrand, S., et al.(1992) Mapping the whole human genome by fingerprinting yeast artificial chromosomes. *Cell* **70,** 1059–1068.
4. Deloukas, P., Schuler, G. D., Gyapay, G., Beasley, E. M., Soderlund, C., Rodriguez-Tome, P., et al. (1998) A physical map of 30,000 human genes. *Science* **282,** 744–746.
5. Dib, C., Faure, S., Fizames, C., Samson, D., Drouot, N., Vignal, A., et al. (1996) A comprehensive genetic map of the human genome based on 5,264 microsatellites *Nature* **380,** 152–154.
6. Hudson, T., Stein, L., Gerety, S., Ma, J., Castle, A., Silva, J., et al. (1995) An STS-based map of the human genome. *Science* **270,** 1945–1954.
7. Bird, A. P. CpG-rich islands and the function of DNA methylation. (1986) *Nature* **321,** 209–13.
8. Yaspo, M. L., Gellen, L., Mott, R., Korn, B., Nizetic, D., Poustka, A. M., and Lehrach, H.(1995) Model for a transcript map of human chromosome 21: isolation of new coding sequences from exon and enriched cDNA libraries. *Hum. Mol. Genet.* **4,** 1291–1304.

9. Adams, M. D., Kelley, J. M., Gocayne, J. D., Dubnick, M., Polymeropoulos, M. H., Xiao, H., et al. (1991) Complementary-DNA sequencing-expressed sequence tags and human genome project. *Science* **252,** 1651–1656.
10. Sauer, C. G., Gehrig, A., Warneke-Wittstock, R., Marquardt, A., Ewing, C. C., Gibson, A. et al. (1997) Positional cloning of the gene associated with X-linked juvenile retinoschisis. *Nat. Genet.* **17,** 164–70.
11. Strom, T. M., Nyakatura, G., Apfelstedt-Sylla, E., Hellebrand, H., Lorenz, B., Weber, B. H., et al. (1998) An L-type calcium-channel gene mutated in incomplete X-linked congenital stationary night blindness. *Nat. Genet.* **19,** 260–263.
12. Strom, T. M., Hortnagel, K., Hofmann, S., Gekeler, F., Scharfe, C., Rabl, W., et al. (1998) Diabetes insipidus, diabetes mellitus, optic atrophy and deafness (DIDMOAD) caused by mutations in a novel gene (wolframin) coding for a predicted transmembrane protein. *Hum. Mol. Genet.* **7,** 2021–2028.
13. Lehrach, H., Drmanac, R., Hoheisel, J., Larin, Z., Lennon, G., Monaco, A. P., et al. (1990) Hybridization fingerprinting in genome mapping and sequencing. *Genome Anal.* **1,** 39–81.
14. Olson, M., Hood, L., Cantor, C., and Botstein, D. (1989) A common language for physical mapping of the human genome. *Science* **245,** 1434–1435.
15. Burke, D. T., Carle, G. F., and Olson, M. V. (1987) Cloning of large segments of exogenous DNA into yeast by means of artificial chromosome vectors. *Science* **236,** 806–812.
16. Schwartz, D. C. and Cantor, C. R. (1984) Separation of yeast chromosome-sized DNAs by pulsed field gradient gel electrophoresis. *Cell* **37,** 67–75.
17. Chumakov, I., Rigault, P., Guillou, S., Ougen, P., Billaut, A., Guasconi, G., et al. (1992) Continuum of overlapping clones spanning the entire human chromosome-21q. *Nature* **359,** 380–387.
18. Foote, S., Vollrath, D., Hilton, A., and Page, D. C. (1992) The human Y-chromosome-overlapping DNA clones spanning the euchromatic region. *Science* **258,** 60–66.
19. Krauter, K., Montgomery, K., Yoon, S. J., LeBlanc-Straceski, J., Renault, B., Marondel, I., et al. (1995) A second–generation YAC contig map of human chromosome 12. *Nature* **377(Suppl.),** 321–333.
20. Gemmill, R. M., Chumakov, I., Scott, P., Waggoner, B., Rigault, P., Cypser, J., et al. (1995) A second-generation YAC contig map of human chromosome 3. *Nature* **377(Suppl.),** 299–319.
21. Collins, J. E., Cole, C. G., Smink, L. J., Garrett, C. L., Leversha, M. A., Soderlund, C. A. et al. (1995) A high-density YAC contig map of human chromosome 22. *Nature* **377(Suppl.),** 367–79.
22. Roest Crollius, H., Ross, M. T., Grigoriev, A., Knights, C. J. Holloway, E., Misfud, J., et al. (1996) An integrated YAC map of the human X chromosome. *Genome Res.* **6,** 943–955.
23. Sternberg, N. (1990) Bacteriophage-P1 cloning system for the isolation, amplification, and recovery of DNA fragments as large as 100 kilobase pairs. *Proc. Natl. Acad. Sci. USA* **87,** 103–107.
24. Ioannou, P. A., Amemiya, C. T., Garnes, J., Kroisel, P. M., Shizuya, H., Chen, C., et al. (1994) A new bacteriophage P1-derived vector for the propagation of large human DNA fragments. *Nat. Genet.* **6,** 84–89.
25. Shizuya, H., Birren, B., Kim, U. J., Mancino, V., Slepak, T., Tachiiri, Y., and Simon, M. (1992) Cloning and stable maintenance of 300-kilobase-pair fragments of human DNA in Escherichia-coli using an F-factor-based vector. *Proc. Natl. Acad. Sci. USA* **89,** 8794–8797.

26. Boysen, C., Simon, M. I., and Hood, L. (1997) Fluorescence-based sequencing directly from bacterial and P1-derived artificial chromosomes. *Biotechniques* **23,** 978–82.
27. Monaco, A. P., Neve, R. L., Collettifeener, C., Bertelson, C. J., Kurnit, D. M., and Kunkel, L. M. (1986) Isolation of candidate cDNAs for portions of the Duchenne muscular-dystrophy gene. *Nature* **323,** 646–650.
28. Rommens, J. M., Iannuzzi, M. C., Kerem, B. S., Drumm, M. L., Melmer, G., Dean, M., et al. (1989) Identification of the cystic-fibrosis gene—chromosome walking and jumping. *Science* **245,** 1059–1065.
29. Buckler, A. J., Chang, D. D., Graw, S. L., Brook, J. D., Haber, D. A., Sharp, P. A., and Housman, D. E. (1991) Exon amplification : a strategy to isolate mammalian genes based on RNA splicing. *Proc. Natl. Acad. Sci. USA* **88,** 4005–4009.
30. Lovett, M., Kere, J. H., and Hinton, L. M. (1991) Direct selection—a method for the isolation of cDNAs encoded by large genomic regions. *Proc. Natl. Acad. Sci. USA* **88,** 9628–9632.
31. Parimoo, S., Patanjali, S. R., Shukla, H., Chaplin, D. D., and Weissman, S. M. (1991) cDNA selection: efficient PCR approach for the selection of cDNAs encoded in large chromosomal DNA fragments. *Proc. Natl Acad. Sci. USA* **88,** 9623–9627.
32. Korn, B., Sedlacek, Z., Manca, A., Kioschis, P., Konecki, D., Lehrach, H., and Poustka, A. (1992) A strategy for the selection of transcribed sequences in the Xq28 region. *Hum. Mol. Genet.* **1,** 235–242.
33. Lovett, M. (1994) Fishing for complements : finding genes by direct selection. *Trends Genet.* **10,** 352–357.
34. Sambrook, J., Fritsch, E. F., and Maniatis, T. (eds.) (1989) *Molecular Cloning: A Laboratory Manual.* Cold Spring Harbor Laboratory Press, Cold Spring Harbor, NY.
35. Nizetic, D., Zehetner, G., Monaco, A. P., Gellen, L., Young, B. D., and Lehrach, H. (1991) Construction, arraying, and highdensity screening of large insert libraries of human chromosomeX and chromosome21their potential use as reference libraries. *Proc. Natl. Acad. Sci. USA* **88,** 3233–3237.
36. Ballabio, A. (1993) The rise and fall of positional cloning. *Nat. Genet.* **3,** 277–279.
37. Lennon, G., Auffray, C., Polymeropoulos, M., and Soares, M. B. (1996) The I.M.A.G.E. Consortium: an integrated molecular analysis of genomes and their expression. *Genomics* **33,** 151–152.
38. Adams, M. D., Kerlavage, A. R., Fleischmann, R. D., Fuldner, R. A., Bult, C. J., Lee, N. H., et al. (1995) Initial assessment of human gene diversity and expression patterns based upon 83 million nucleotides of cDNA sequence. *Nature* **377(Suppl.),** 3–174.
39. Schuler, G. D., Boguski, M. S., Stewart, E. A., Stein, L. D., Gyapay, G., Rice, K., et al. (1996) A gene map of the human genome. *Science* **274,** 540–546.
40. Altschul, S. F., Gish, W., Miller, W., Myers, E. W., and Lipman, D. J. (1990) Basic local alignment search tool. *J. Mol. Biol.* **215,** 403–410.
41. Altschul, S. F. (1998) Fundamentals of database searching, in *Trends Guide to Bioinformatics. Trends Supplement 1998* (Patterson, M. and Handel, M., eds.), Elsevier Science, London, pp. 7–9.
42. Brenner, S. (1998) Practical database searching, in *Trends Guide to Bioinformatics Trends Supplement 1998* (Patterson, M. and Handel, M., eds.), Elsevier Science, London, pp. 9–12.
43. Pruitt, K. D. (1997) WebWise: Navigating the Human Genome Project. *Genome Res.* **7,** 1038–1039.

44. Venter, J. C., Adams, M. D., Sutton, G. G., Kerlavage, A. R., Smith, H. O., and Hunkapiller, M. (1998) Shotgun sequencing of the human genome. *Science* **280,** 1540–1542.
45. Ouellette, B. F. F. and Boguski, M. S. (1997) Database divisions and homology search files: a guide for the perplexed. *Genome Res.* **7,** 952–955.
46. Smit, A. F. A. (1996) Origin of interspersed repeats in the human genome. *Curr. Opin. Genet. Dev.* **6,** 743–749.
47. Jurka, J., Klonowski, P., Dagman, V., and Pelton, P. (1996) CENSOR– A program for identification and elimination of repetitive elements from DNA sequences. *Comput. Chem.* **20,** 119–122.
48. Zhang, J. and Madden, T. L. (1997) PowerBLAST: a new network BLAST application for interactive or automated sequence analysis and annotation. *Genome Res.* **7,** 649–656.
49. Haussler, D. (1998) Computational genefinding, in *Trends Guide to Bioinformatics. Trends Supplement 1998* (Patterson, M. and Handel, M., eds.), Elsevier Science, London, pp. 12–15.
50. Baxevanis, A. D. and Ouellette, B. F. F. (1998) *Bioinformatics: A Practical Guide to the Analysis of Genes and Proteins,* John Wiley, New York.
51. Harris, N. L. (1997) Genotator: a workbench for sequence annotation. *Genome Res.* **7,** 754–762
52. Frohman, M. A., Dush, M. K., and Martin, G. R. (1988) Rapid production of full-length cDNAs from rare transcripts: amplification using a single gen--specific oligonucleotide primer. *Proc. Natl. Acad. Sci. USA* **85,** 8998–9002.
53. Kozak, M. (1987) An analysis of 5' noncoding sequences from 699 vertebrate messenger RNAs. *Nucleic Acid Res.* **15,** 8125–8148.

CHAPTER 22

Finding Mutations in Disease Genes

Peter S. N. Rowe

Introduction

Recent advances in the field of human molecular genetics have resulted in an exponential increase in the number of disease genes isolated and characterized. The identification of these disease genes has been the result of the development of specific strategies coupled with powerful and new technologies. Pivotal to these new technologies was the discovery and refinement of the polymerase chain reaction (PCR), and its application to linkage studies, mutation screening, and clone isolation. *Mendelian Inheritance in Man* lists all the known inherited human disorders and the defective genes associated with them, and to date there are 6000 traits listed *(1)*. Most of the genes identified are those responsible for single-gene disorders. The more common and complex ''disease-genes'' to identify are those that act in combination to cause disease. These multigene diseases are called polygenic or multifactorial. In view of the advances made in the study of single-gene disorders, there is justifiable optimism that new methods in statistical analysis and laboratory methodologies will be developed to tackle this new challenge. An important stage in any cloning strategy is the generation of candidate clones. This stage is the end-point of one of four optional strategies:

1. Positional cloning (PC), based on knowing nothing except subchromosomal location of the disease gene.
2. Cloning based on an aspect of deduced or known function (CFK), dependent on the gene product being known or a functional assay being available.
3. Cloning based on suggested animal homologues (CAH) or gene family similarities and independent of subchromosomal location.
4. Cloning based on database searches (CDS) and known chromosomal location of *the* disease ("positional candidate"). The positional candidate approach, is becoming increasingly important as more human genes are being mapped to specific chromosomal locations.

The Genetics of Osteoporosis and Metabolic Bone Disease
Ed.: M. J. Econs © Humana Press Inc., Totowa, NJ

The candidate clones generated by these approaches must be tested to confirm unequivocally association with the disease in question. This chapter reviews the techniques currently available to screen and confirm disease genes from a candidate pool of clones. These techniques will include:

1. Heteroduplex mobility in polyacrylamide gels.
2. Single-stranded confirmation analysis (SSCP or SSCA).
3. Chemical cleavage mismatches (CCM).
4. Enzymatic cleavage mismatches (ECM).
5. Denaturing gradient gel electrophoresis (DGGE).
6. Protein truncation test (PTT).
7. Triplet repeat expansions.
8. Automated and DNA chip technology.

General Strategy for Mutation Detection

The region defined as having the gene of interest (delimited by genetic flanking markers), needs to be represented as clones in a test tube before acquisition of ''candidate'' clones can proceed. As detailed in Chapter 21, this typically first results in the isolation of several overlapping ''Yeast Artificial Chromosome'' clones (YACS), cosmids, or other vector constructs containing overlapping cloned human genomic DNA segments. In the case of X-linked rickets a systematic positional cloning approach resulted in the localization of the defective gene (PHEX), to a single YAC *(2,3)*. (For a comprehensive review of the molecular techniques used to localize the defective X-linked rickets gene (PHEX), *see* refs. *4,5,5a*). Cosmids mapping to the YAC and overlapping in a contiguous series were used to screen panels of restriction enzyme digested DNA from normals and patients. In brief, the DNA from 80 patients were digested with seven different restriction enzymes, each of which cleave DNA at sites dependent on specific DNA sequence-motifs recognized by the enzymes. The human DNA fragments generated were then separated by size using agarose gel electrophoresis, and then transferred to nitrocellulose membranes. The cosmids spanning the candidate region were then radiolabeled with P^{32} using standard techniques, and each independently used to hybridize to the immobilized digested blots. Before screening, the cosmids were exhaustively back hybridized with total human DNA to reduce signal to noise from repeat elements present in the cosmids. Using this approach one of the cosmids detected a large 50 kb deletion in one patient. Thus, it was deduced that the gene or part of the gene probably resided on the cosmid. Other patients with deletions were then rapidly found using the same cosmid. Although deletions were found, this was not proof that the gene had been localized. The large deletion may have been associated with genes contiguous with the primary disease gene, and/or independent of the primary disease mutation (benign mutations, or mutations covered by other normal genes fulfilling similar functions). It was therefore essential to characterize single base mutations leading to missense, exon skipping, or premature truncation (stop codons), of coding sequence mapping to the deleted region. The cosmid detecting the mutation (and overlapping cosmids), was therefore used to enrich for cDNA clones from the region using a mixed cDNA library. These clones were then sequenced, overlaps deduced, and sequence compared with the sequenced cosmid(s). Using this data, and a computer-based informatics program (Grail), exon intron boundaries and gene structure were worked out *(6,7)*. This information is essential for the screening and detection of mutations if PCR based techniques are to be used, as discussed below. (For a review of the cloning and function of the rickets gene PHEX, *see* refs. *4,5a*). In other cases (e.g., Alzheimer's disease, Waardenburg syndrome, multiple endocrine neoplasia type 2A), fragments of candidate coding sequence DNA may already be available for mutation testing. With strategies 3 and 4 (CAH and CDS, respectively, *see* Introduction), the entire or substantial part of the candidate gene may be available as a complementary cDNA clone.

Once coding information is available, and/or exon intron structure deduced for candidate clones, the next step is to design primers to amplify portions of coding DNA using PCR from: (1) genomic DNA (if exon/intron boundaries are known); (2) mRNA isolated from patients, using reverse transcriptase-PCR (RT/PCR). The amplified products are then analysed using one of the approaches described below to determine whether any point mutations are likely to be present. This is then confirmed by sequencing the altered amplified products. The mutations are then further analyzed to determine whether they would result in deleterious effects on gene product function or expression.

Interpreting Mutation Data

Rigorous methods must be applied to the interpretation of sequence changes found after screening candidate coding regions. In diseases where most patients have different mutations in the same gene, and where these mutations clearly disrupt function, unequivocal conclusions can be made concerning the genes role in a disease. Diseases falling into this category are generally early onset dominant or recessive X-linked disorders. The PHEX gene, falls into this category, and Fig. 1 shows the range of mutations found after screening 99 patients in a recent study *(7)*. A large number of mutations were identified ranging from deletions, insertions, nonsense mutations, missense mutations, and exon skipping. The interpretation of the mutations was helped considerably by the discovery that the PHEX gene product has high homologies to an M13 family of zinc metallopeptidases (neprilysin, endothelin converting enzyme, kell antigen). The prototypic member of this type II glycoprotein group is neprilysin (MA clan), and much work had already been done using site directed mutagenesis, and other physicochemical techniques on this protein. Consequently, the residues important for structure/function for this family of zinc metallopeptidases were known, and many of the mutations found in PHEX involved these key residues. Also, computer informatics was able to give detailed predictions for functionality, and the nature of the catalytic site

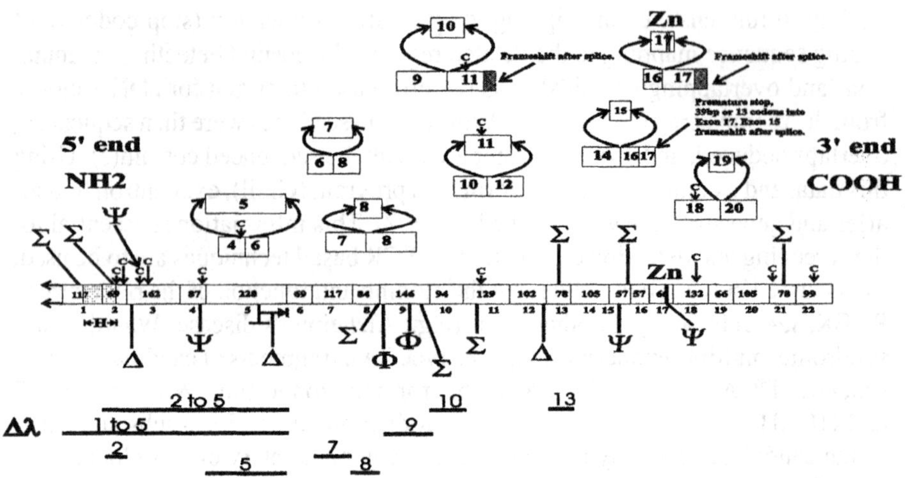

Fig. 1. Linear cDNA sequence structure and primary protein sequence for human PHEX The central bar shows the exon structure of the PHEX gene, with size in base pairs indicated inside each exon compartment. Below each exon and outside the box is the numerical sequence of exons 5' to 3'. Predicted exon skipping mutations (in frame and out of frame), are shown above the central bar representing the PHEX gene/protein. Arrows point to skipped exons, and shaded boxes indicate frameshift. The linear lines below the scheme represent the span of the large deletions found (Δλ), and the numbers above the lines the exons deleted. The following symbols indicate: 1., Δ small deletions < 104 bp); 2., Σ stop mutations; 3., ϕ Insertions; 4.,Ψ missense mutations. The shaded region at the 5' end of the gene partially covering exons 1 and 2 and delimited by the symbol "H", indicates the extent of the hydrophobic 5' region. Also the Zn binding motif in exon 17 (Zn), is marked by a shaded bar. Cysteine residues are represented by the letter C above the central bar, with arrows pointing to their approximate position in the protein.

in PHEX was therefore deduced without purifying the protein. Figure 2 presents a two- dimensional structure prediction profile for PHEX and a mutated form found in a patient with X-linked rickets. The GCG peptide-structure program was used to generate the hydrophobicity/hydrophilicity plot, and clear differences can be seen in the mutant form. Unfortunately, in many cases, the identification of mutations, and their role in disease is much more difficult.

There are four major stumbling blocks or difficulties in interpreting mutation data:

1. Locus heterogeneity: Some disease phenotypes can be caused by mutations in one of a number of different genes. If the candidate gene is derived from one of the rare disease loci then detecting a change in a panel of patients becomes unlikely. To overcome this problem, a large family pedigree with

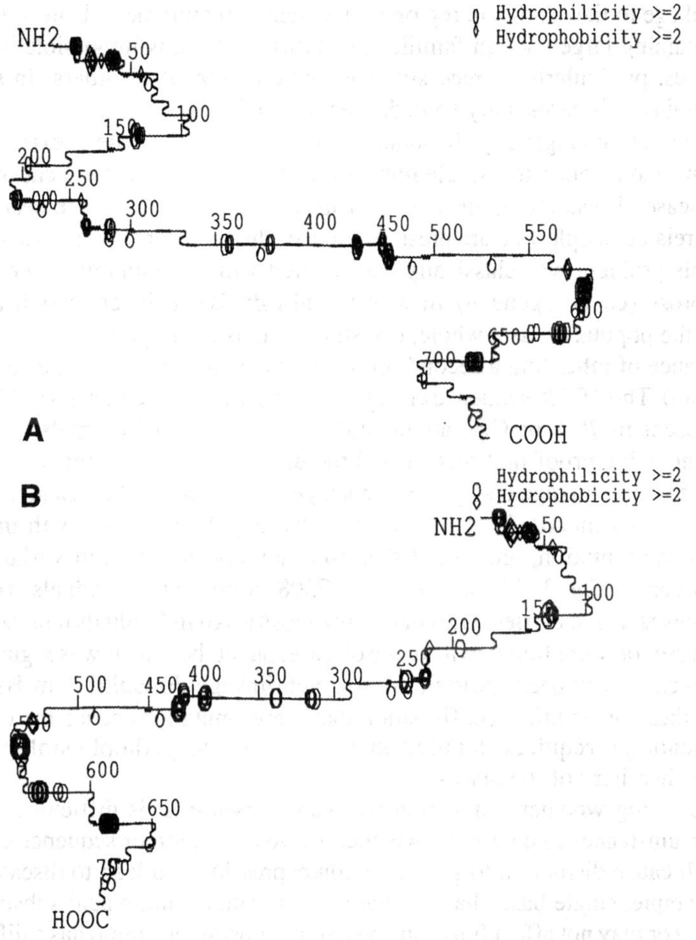

Fig. 2. Secondary structure prediction (GCG/peptidestructure) for PHEX. The profiles were generated from PHEX primary amino acid sequence using the Wisconsin and GCG/EGCG software programs for protein analysis. Surface probability, flexibility, hydrophobicity-hydrophilicity, and antigenicity indices can be generated using this software. In this scheme, Figs. 2A and 2B represent hydrophobicity-hydrophilicity plots and secondary structure predictions. The ellipses drawn over the lines represent regions or nodes of a hydrophilic nature, and the diamonds of a hydrophobic nature. Two distinct regions of high hydrophobic content are present at the N-terminus, and between 550–600 (residues). The N-terminal region is the putative trans-membrane domain, and the region between 550–600 contains the Zn binding motif. The Zn motif region is also delineated by an extended α-helix. In the mutant form (2A), the mutation has resulted in a major change in secondary structure. The predicted profile represents this change as a 180° turn in secondary sequence (compare 2A and 2B). The mutation in this patient was a small deletion of 104 bp involving 54 bp of exon 5 and 50 bp of 3' flanking intron, resulting in a aberrant splicing of exon 6.

linkage to the candidate region is an essential requirement. Unfortunately, obtaining large enough families to confirm linkage is impossible in most cases, particularly in recessive and some dominant disorders. In severe dominant diseases, only sporadic cases are often available.

2. Mutation homogeneity: In some diseases the mutation rate is exceedingly low, and an ancestral single mutation is the predominant form causing the disease. These mutations and associated alleles are present in seemingly unrelated people who are presumed to have had a distant common ancestor. This problem was classically encountered with the cloning of the cystic fibrosis (CFTR), gene *(8)*. In essence, individuals who inherit certain alleles in the population as a whole, can show a statistically greater than random chance of inheriting a second set of associated alleles (linkage disequilibrium). The ΔF508 sequence change (first shown in cystic fibrosis), although present in 70% of CF patients and in only 3–4% of normals, was not conclusive proof that this caused the disease because of this effect *(9)*. The strong linkage disequilibrium suggested that the ΔF508 change might have been inherited by this group of the population along with the real disease mutation, and could therefore have been a benign variation in sequence. The 3–4% presence of ΔF508 in normal individuals we now know is due to carrier status or heterozygosity. All individuals homozygous for ΔF508 were found to have the disease, but at the time it was argued that this could have been due to almost complete linkage-disequilibrium. Because of these difficulties, confirmation that these mutations cause the clinical phenotype requires detailed knowledge of the pathophysiology and biochemistry of the disease.
3. Assessing whether a mutation will cause disease: It is difficult in some circumstances to determine whether a given mutation or sequence change will cause disruption to gene function/expression and lead to disease. For example, single base changes that result in single amino acid substitution may or may not affect function, even if the substituted amino has a different chemistry. Computer software can give good predictions, but without detailed structure function data for the expressed protein, there remains doubt. Adding to the complexity, allelic sequence variation (more than one variant allele at a locus), occurs at a frequency of 1:250 to 1:300 bases in genomic DNA (a mean heterozygosity of 0.0037 across the human genome). This means that a 4000-bp stretch of sequence would have approx 14 potential variations. Although most of these changes will be in noncoding regions since coding sequences are highly conserved due to selection pressure, a few nonpathogenic changes will almost certainly occur. These changes may be present at low frequency in the population, less than 1:5000, for example. Thus >5000 people would need to be screened in order to achieve a reasonable chance of detecting the sequence variant. Thus, functional testing is the only certain way of confirming the role of a sequence variation in disease.
4. Difficulties in finding mutations: Occasionally difficulties are encountered when screening for mutations. Large genes in particular are difficult to

screen. This difficulty may in part be due to the vast area to be covered and the few mutations present.

Mutation Detection Methods

The development of mutation detection methodologies has advanced rapidly in recent years. The core techniques are research laboratory based, and can cope well with a reasonable number of samples. Other approaches have been developed that are suitable for screening much larger number of test DNAs. These highly advanced automated methods are based on ingenious DNA-chip technologies (*see* below). Because of the adaptability of the hardware, and the potential application to other molecular techniques, it is conceivable that the DNA-chip may soon be cost effective for the smaller research laboratories *(10)*.

The main considerations when choosing a mutation detection approach are the end objectives. There are two possible aims: (1) Screening for a single known mutation in a panel of normal and affected individuals (generally diagnostic); (2) The detection of any change in sequence from the standard (screening candidate genes for mutations). This chapter will discuss methods suitable for the second approach.

The main rationale behind mutation screening is a direct comparison of a test sequence with standard sequence. This can be done by sequencing all the test samples directly and comparing them to controls. This method however is laborious, and generates an excessive amount of information (scaling up analysis time). The task is made more difficult by the necessity of sequencing the postulated altered region of at least 100 control samples. This is to ensure that the change is not a benign variation in sequence, but a real mutation. The direct sequencing approach is to a great extent superceded by methods that compare the electrophoretic behavior of mutant and normal single-stranded or duplex DNA molecules. These new elegant techniques can reliably detect single base changes in DNA sequence. One of these approaches directly compares heterozygous-DNA from test and controls using heteroduplex analysis. The heterozygous DNA is melted and allowed to reanneal. Some of the wild-type and mutant alleles form a DNA heteroduplex. Heteroduplex DNA has a different mobility compared to homoduplex strands when separated by electrophoresis through special hydrolink gels (*see* below).

Heteroduplex Mutation Screening

As with most of the techniques used for screening mutations, the first step is amplification of the region of interest using PCR. This is done by designing primers that flank the sequence to be amplified, followed by thermal cycling and amplification using a thermal stable polymerase such as *Taq* DNA polymerase. In most cases the flanking primers are designed from 5' and 3' intronic sequence flanking a specific exon (*see* Fig. 3 for an example

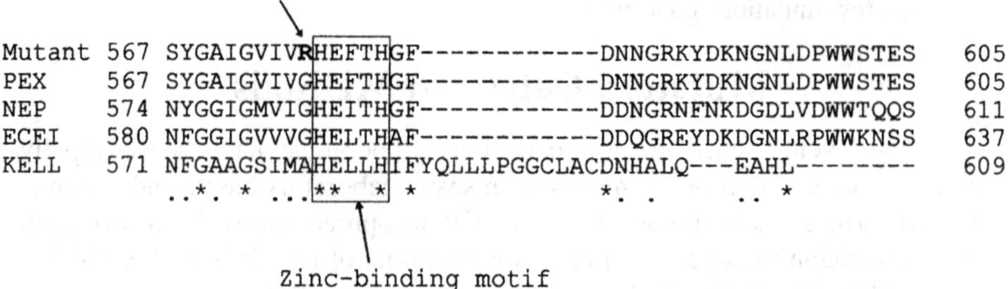

Fig. 3. The scheme shows alignment of exon 17 of the PHEX gene with other members of the M13 Zinc metallopeptidase family (NEP; neprilysin, ECE-1; endothelin converting enzyme, KELL; KELL antigen), and a mutation detected by SSCP in a patient with X-linked rickets (Mutant). The residues are amino acids coding for the exonic sequence, and PCR primers (designed from flanking intron sequence), were used to amplify the complementary DNA coding sequence (not shown). The mutation was detected by SSCP as described in the text (*see* Fig. 4), and involves a substitution of glycine to arginine. A single base change (G to A), in the normal glycine codon GGA converted the glycine to an arginine (AGA), in the patients PHEX protein *(7)*. The change is adjacent to the zinc binding motif (highly conserved in zinc metallopeptidases). A key feature of this region is the clustering of hydrophobic residues, and also some β sheet structure. In this context, replacing glycine that has an uncharged polar R group, with the basic positively charged arginine reduces the hydrophobicity, and also extends predicted b sheet.

from the PHEX gene exon 17). For the heteroduplex method, maximum sensitivity is achieved by designing primers that amplify products smaller than 200 bp. Fragments of this size and smaller will generally detect insertions, deletions, and most single-base substitutions. The amplified DNA from a heterozygous individual is melted and allowed to reanneal as mentioned earlier *(11)*. Heteroduplex DNA has reduced mobility compared to homoduplex DNA in nondenaturing gel electrophoresis experiments. To improve resolution electrophoresis and separation is carried out in specially designed gel matrices such as Hydro-link™, or MDE™ gels. Bands are visualized after ethidium bromide staining. To detect X-linked mutations in hemizygous males, or homozygous mutations in general, the addition of wild-type DNA is necessary prior to the melting and reannealing step. The technique is simple to use, and easy to set up. Disadvantages are short sequence requirements (<200 bp), limited sensitivity, and the technique will not locate the position of the change. Heteroduplex screening is best used in combination with another technique such as SSCP.

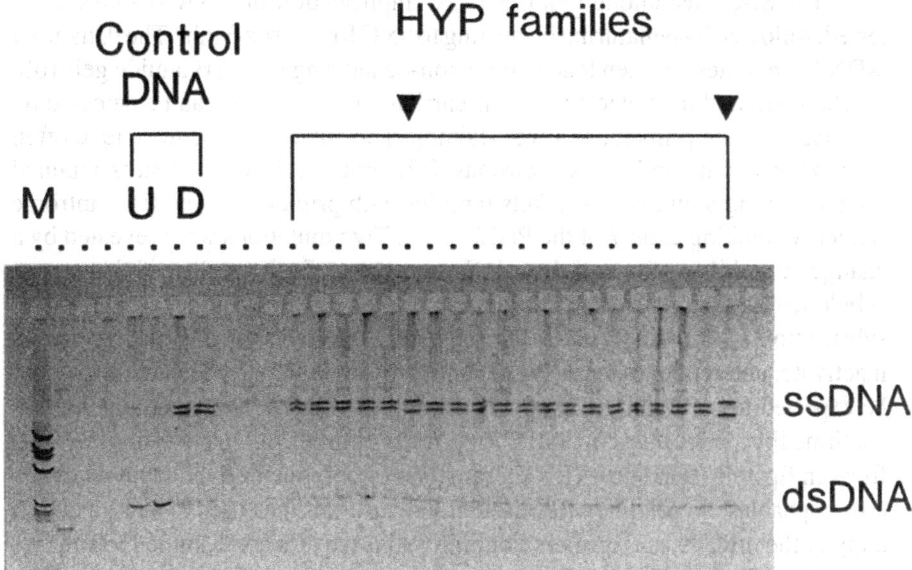

Fig. 4. SSCP analysis of control PCR amplified DNA and test DNA (*see* text). Lane M contains markers (double-stranded). The control lanes (control DNA), contain undenatured double-stranded, PCR amplified DNA (U), and heat denatured single-stranded DNA (normal subjects). The other lanes contained heat denatured amplified DNA from a range of individuals with X-linked hypophosphataemic rickets. All samples (control and rickets), were amplified from genomic DNA (by PCR), using the same set of intronic primers flanking exon 7 (see text). The two lanes marked with triangles contain altered sequence as deduced by the change in mobility of the single-stranded templates compared to controls.

Single-Strand Conformational Polymorphism Analysis (SSCP or SSCA)

As discussed, double-stranded DNA (dsDNA), consists of two strands of complementary DNA forming a heteroduplex. Both strands are held together by hydrogen bonding with purines base pairing with their pyrimidine counterparts. Heating the dsDNA molecule to 95°C in solution melts the heteroduplex into two separate but complementary single-stranded templates (ssDNA). Both ssDNA templates can also form unique complex structures by the formation of weak intramolecular bonds, and base-pairing hydrogen bonds. The resulting conformations adopted by each ssDNA template is dependent on the length of the DNA, and the DNA sequence. Conformation of each ssDNA molecule affects its electrophoretic mobility in a nondenaturing gel. Thus, changes of a single base can easily be detected by comparing the electrophoretic mobility of control- and disease-derived ssDNA templates *(12)*.

The SSCP technique requires PCR amplification of DNA samples to be tested, followed by denaturing by heating to 95°C for approx 5 min. The denatured ssDNA templates are then loaded onto non-denaturing polyacrylamide gels (6% acrylamide), and then electrophoresis carried out. The DNA can be detected by radiolabeling the primers, or silver staining. The silver staining technique often gives better results, and is less hazardous *(2,7)*. Figure 4 shows the results obtained after screening a number of rickets families with primers derived from intronic sequence flanking exon 7 of the PHEX gene. Two mutations were revealed by a change in mobility of one of the ssDNA templates. Both amplified DNAs were subcloned and sequenced, and mutation B was shown to have a single base substitution (C-T). Analysis of the sequence revealed that this change would inactivate, and render defective the flanking exon donor site. This in turn would be expected to cause the skipping of exon 7. The predicted exon 7 skipping was confirmed by reverse transcriptase PCR (RT/PCR). In brief, mRNA, was first extracted from an Epstein-Barr virus (EBV) transformed cell line derived from patient B (B-lymphablastoid cell line). Reverse transcriptase was then used to make a cDNA copy of the mRNA, and primers flanking exons 6 to 7 were designed to amplify control and disease cDNA (primers were complementary to sequence for flanking exons 5 and 8). Electrophoresis of control and patient amplified DNA revealed increased mobility of the patient DNA, indicating a reduced size. Sequencing of the mutant DNA showed conclusively that exon 7 was missing in the patient DNA. As a corollary, many genes are expressed at low (leaky) levels in tissues that are not the primary tissues of expression (ectopic expression). The B-lymphablastoid cell line in this regard is a good model system for generating mRNA from leaky genes like the PHEX gene, and are convenient for RT/PCR analysis/studies. The PHEX gene is thought primarily to be expressed in bone and teeth *(13–15)*.

The main advantages of the SSCP technique are simplicity, versatility, and sensitivity. Disadvantages are short sequence requirement (<200 bp), position of change is not revealed directly, and full range detection may require temperature optimization of electrophoresis runs. In general, approx 80% of mutations are detected using this technique. Differing temperatures during electrophoresis can dramatically affect resolution and detectability of sequence changes. To achieve an 80% detection rate it is necessary to carry out electrophoresis of the PCR products at a range of different temperatures. Some companies (Pharmacia Amersham, Arlington Heights, IL), have developed specialized equipment to do this. The equipment is also designed for high capacity screening of multiple samples, and ready made nondenaturing polyacrylamide gels can also be purchased directly from the manufacturer. An adaptation of the SSCP technique is claimed to give 100% sensitivity *(16)*. In this technique a dideoxy sequencing reaction of amplified sequenced is carried out, and each band in the sequencing ladder is analyzed by SSCP (dideoxy fingerprinting).

Chemical Cleavage of Mismatches (CCM)

This method is one of the most sensitive for the detection of mutations. Large (kilobase size) and small fragments can be analyzed. The position of the mutation is deduced by the size of the cleaved fragments generated by the analysis, and is a major advantage over SSCP and heteroduplex methods. Test DNA is hybridized to a radiolabeled probe derived from wild-type sequence, and a heteroduplex is formed. Mismatches in the heteroduplex (wild-type and test DNA), are detected by the use of specific chemical reactions (hydroxylamine, piperidine, OsO_4), that cleave one of the strands of DNA at the site of the mismatch. The fragments are resolved on a gel, and cleavage (and therefore the site of mismatch and possible mutations), is revealed by the appearance of short labeled fragments. The toxic nature of the chemicals used, and the technical difficulties involved in setting the system up are the main disadvantages.

Enzymatic Cleavage of Mismatches (ECM)

This technique is based on the same principle as the CCM method. The difference is in the use of enzymes instead of chemicals to cleave the mismatches. Bacteriophage resolvases (T4 endonuclease VII, and T7 endonuclease I, for example), have both been used successfully to cleave DNA *(17–19)*, and RNAase A has been used to cleave mismatches in heteroduplexes between the test DNA and an RNA wild-type sequence *(20)*. The utility and power of this technique has been confirmed by a number of papers, particularly when using T4 endonuclease (T4 resolvase). In a recent study a total of 81 of 81 known mutations in the mouse β-globin promotor region were detected using the EMC method and T4 resolvase *(18)*. The method is potentially simple and inexpensive, with the ability to pinpoint mutations on fragments of 1 kilobase or larger.

Denaturing Gradient Gel Electrophoresis (DGGE)

This technique relies on the sequence dependent melting characteristics of DNA duplexes *(21)*. The melting temperature (T_M), or concentration of chemical denaturant required to separate a double-stranded helix is altered dramatically by changes as small as a single base in the DNA sequence. Also, DNA is generally organized into high- and low-melting domains, and the domain with the lower T_M will melt before the high T_M domain in solution. In DGGE, DNA is migrated through an electrophoretic gel in which there is a gradient of increasing amounts of chemical denaturant (urea/formamide), or temperature. The helical double-stranded DNA migrates through the gel until it reaches the concentration of denaturant at which the low temperature domain becomes single-stranded. At this point, the mobility of the partially melted form is reduced greatly compared to the double-stranded molecule. Changes in sequence of a single base is sufficient to cause a change in the melting profile, and thus migration of the DNA template.

Although mutations can only be detected in the low melting domain of the template, mutations in the high melting domain can be resolved by adding on a GC-rich sequence (GC-clamp), to the DNA. The GC sequence becomes the high melting domain, and mutations in the rest of the DNA sequence can then be detected by DGGE.

GC-clamping can be expensive and time consuming, and the choice of primers is critical for good results. As in SSCP, and heteroduplex screening, the position of the mutation is not pinpointed. The sensitivity of this method is very high when optimized.

Protein Truncation Test

The protein truncation test can distinguish between mutations causing disease, and neutral (nonpathogenic), polymorphism variations in sequence *(22)*. This is a major advantage over the other techniques thus far described. The coding sequence from cDNA or large exons from genomic DNA is first amplified by PCR. The PCR forward primer (primer that is contiguous with the translated strand, and complementary to the nontranslated strand), is designed to contain at the 5' end a T7 promotor, and a eukaryotic translation initiator with an ATG start codon. The ATG start codon of the primer is in frame with a gene-specific 3' sequence designed from the test cDNA or genomic exon. The modified forward primer and a gene specific reverse primer are then used to amplify the coding region by PCR, and a coupled transcription-translation system is used to produce a polypeptide from the amplified product. The transcription of the PCR product to produce RNA, is facilitated by the presence of the introduced (nongene specific), T7 promotor (forward primer). The transcribed RNA is then translated into a polypeptide in frame with the ATG (translates to methionine), and initiated by the eukaryotic translation initiation sequence. The translation products (radiolabeled by the introduction of a radiolabeled amino acid), are then size separated by SDS-polyacrylamide gel electrophoresis (PAGE). Mutations resulting in truncations of the polypeptide product will appear as faster running lower molecular weight bands compared to normals. The size of the bands reveal the position of the mutation.

The mutations detected by this method include, frameshifts, splice sites, and nonsense mutations (stop codons), that result in truncation of the protein product. Missense mutations are not detected, as these involve substitution of one amino acid for another and do not alter the size of the product. It is theoretically possible to increase the resolution by incorporating an isoelectro focusing step after SDS-PAGE (SDS-polyacrylamide electrophoresis). The technique is known as two-dimensional isoelectric focusing, and would help to distinguish changes of a single amino acid in potential mutants compared to normals. Unfortunately, the complexity of the second step would be prohibitive when screening a large number of candidate clones.

Missense mutations are relatively rare in some genes (APC, dystrophin, and BRCA1), and PTT is particularly useful for the analysis of mutations in this group of disorders. Mutations involving a single substitution of an amino acid tend to be nonpathogenic in these diseases, and the use of PTT reduces the background by ignoring silent or missense base substitutions.

Triplet Repeat Expansions

A unique class of diseases have been found to be caused by the expansion of highly unstable trinucleotide repeats *(23)*. There are 10 possible permutations of tandem trinucleotide repeats, and most are useful in genetic linkage mapping of diseases because of their polymorphic nature. Repeats below a certain size are stable in meiosis and mitosis, but become unstable when above a certain length resulting in size expansion. Some of the diseases caused by unstable trinucleotide repeats are Huntingtons disease, Spino-cerebellar ataxia, Fragile X, and Myotonic dystrophy. The list is increasing at a fast rate. A key feature of the diseases falling within this mutation class is the phenomenon of "anticipation." Anticipation refers to the early-age presentation of the disease, and the marked increase in severity in successive generations. Disease with this pattern of anticipation are well worth screening for triplet repeat expansions.

The screening for triplet repeat expansions is helped by the fact that there are only 10 possible triplet repeats. Once a sub-chromosomal region has been localized to contain the disease locus, the DNA can be systematically screened with oligonucleotide probes representing the possible repeats. The region flanking a positive hybridization can then be analyzed for evidence of pathological expansion of the triplet repeat. A technique described by Schalling et al., allows the detection but not localization of expanded repeats in genomic DNA extracted from patients *(24)*.

DNA Chip Technology

A new and powerful technology has begun to push forward the frontiers of molecular genetics. This approach has wide application ranging from mutation detection, DNA sequencing, expression analysis, and tagging of genes, and is being pioneered by biotechnology companies, such as Affymetrix (Santa Clara, CA). Central to the methodology is the synthesis and immobilization (as an array) of >500,000 different oligonucleotide probes on a silica support. To achieve this, a combination of photolithography (used in the semiconductor industry), and oligonucleotide synthesis is used *(25,26)*. The silica supports containing the array of oligonucleotides (approx 1.6 cm^2), are then housed in a sealed flow chamber ready for hybridization, and the chips in turn are placed in a specially designed fluidics station. Fluorescently labeled target DNA or RNA is then hybridized to the chips, and washed by a program carried out by the fluidics station. The chips are then transferred to a scanner and the hybridization of target to the oligonucleotide array measured by scanning confocal microscopy.

For sequence analysis or mutation detection the oligonucleotide array has to be designed to interrogate each nucleotide position of a gene. Four oligonucleotides spanning each base in the DNA sequence is synthesized, differing only in the position of the central base. The intensity of the hybridization to each of the four oligonucleotides spanning the sequence position reveals the base at that position. A mutation or change of a single base will result in a different oligonucleotide lighting up. Also, adjacent overlapping oligonucleotides designed to interrogate flanking base sequence will have a reduced hybridization signal, leaving a characteristic gap in the signal emitted (footprint).

Heterozygous mutations can also be screened with a high degree of efficiency using a two-color analysis DNA-chip approach. Mutations in the familial early onset breast cancer gene (BRCA1), have been detected using this method *(27)*. Exon 11 of this gene (3.45 kb), was represented by an array of 96,600 oligonucleotides each 20 nucleotides long. Control DNA, and test samples were labeled with different fluors emitting light at different wavelengths, and co-hybridized to the arrays. The composite image of the hybridized chips highlighted areas of difference between the control and test sequence, and mutations could readily be detected.

This new innovative and powerful technology will play a major role in genetics research in the future. The complete scanner system can now be purchased for the same price as an automated sequencer, and the chips themselves can be bought for approx $56 depending on complexity. This is well within the price range of many research institutions (academic and corporate).

The next few years will see a quantum leap in our knowledge of genetics and the application of that knowledge to medicine. DNA chip technology will play a major role in these advances, in much the same way as the microchip has contributed to advances in computer technology. The rapid progress in molecular genetics and biology, has without doubt laid the foundations for the next phase of biomedical research. This new endeavor will be directed toward the efficient and systematic screening of gene function, and will benefit not only science, but also those afflicted with genetic diseases.

References

1. McKusick, V. A., Francomano, C. A., Antonorakis, S. E. (1992) *Mendelian Inheritance in Man*, The John Hopkins University Press, Baltimore.
2. HYP Consortium, Francis, F., Hennig, S., et al. (1995) A gene (PEX) with homologies to endopeptidases is mutated in patients with X-linked hypophosphatemic rickets. *Nat. Genet.* **11,** 130–136.
3. Rowe, P. S. N., Goulding, J. N., Francis, F., et al. (1996) The gene for X-linked hypophosphataemic rickets maps to a 200–300 kb region in Xp22.1, and is located on a single YAC containing a putative vitamin D response element (VDRE). *Hum. Genet.* **97,** 345–352.
4. Rowe, P. S. (1997) The PEX gene, its role in X-linked rickets, osteomalacia, and bone mineral metabolism. *Exp. Nephrol.* **5,** 355–363.
5. Rowe, P. S. N (1994) Molecular biology of hypophosphataemic rickets and oncogenic osteomalacia. *Hum. Genet.* **94(5),**457–467.

5a. Econs, M. J. and Francis, F. (1997) Positional cloning of the PEX gene, new insights into the pathophysiology of X-linked hypophosphatemic rickets. 1997 *Am. J. Physiol.* **273,** F489–F498.

6. Francis, F., Strom, T. M., Hennig, S., et al. (1997) Genomic organisation of the human PEX gene mutated in X-linked dominant hypophosphataemic rickets. *Genet. Res.* **7(6),** 573–585.
7. Rowe, P. S. N., Oudet, C., Francis, F., et al. (1997) Distribution of mutations in the PEX gene in families with X-linked hypophosphataemic rickets (HYP). *Hum. Mol. Genet.* **6,** 539–549.
8. Anonymous (1994) Population variation of common cystic fibrosis mutations. The Cystic Fibrosis Genetic Analysis Consortium. *Hum. Mutat.* **4,**167–177.
9. Wagner, K., Greil, I., Schneditz, P., et al. (1994) A cystic fibrosis patient with delta F508, G542X and a deletion at the D7S8 locus. *Hum. Mutat.* **3,** 327–329.
10. Anonymous (1996) To affinity ... and beyond! [editorial, comment]. *Nat. Genet.* **14,** 367–370.
11. Keen, J., Lester, D., Inglehearn, C., et al. (1991) Rapid detection of single base mismatches as heteroduplexes on hydrolink gels. *Trends Genet.* **7,** 5.
12. Sheffield, V. C., Beck, J. S., Kwitek, A. S., et al. 1993 The sensitivity of single-strand conformation polymorphism analysis for the detection of single base substitutions. *Genomics* **16,** 325–332.
13. Beck, L., Soumounou, Y., Martel, J., et al. (1997) Pex/PEX tissue distribution and evidence for a deletion in the 3' region of the Pex gene in X–linked hypophosphatemic mice. *J. Clin. Invest.* **99,** 1200–1209.
14. Du, L., Desbarats, M., Viel, J., et al. (1996) cDNA cloning of the murine PEX gene implicated in X-linked hypophosphataemia and evidence for expression in bone. *Genomics* **36,** 22–28.
15. Guo, R. and Quarles, L. D. (1997) Cloning and sequencing of human PEX from a bone cDNA library, evidence for its developmental stage–specific regulation in osteoblasts (In Process Citation). *J. Bone Miner. Res.* **12,** 1009–1017.
16. Sarkar, G., Yoon, H. S., and Sommer, S. S. (1992) Dideoxy fingerprinting (ddE), a rapid and efficient screen for the presence of mutations. *Genomics* **13,** 441–443.
17. Youil, R., Kemper, B. W., and Cotton, R. G. (1995) Screening for mutations by enzyme mismatch cleavage with T4 endonuclease VII. *Proc. Natl. Acad. Sci. USA* **92,** 87–91.
18. Youil, R., Kemper, B., and Cotton, R. G. (1996) Detection of 81 of 81 known mouse beta-globin promoter mutations with T4 endonuclease VII—the EMC method. *Genomics* **32,** 431–435.
19. Babon, J. J., Youil, R., and Cotton, R. G. (1995) Improved strategy for mutation detection—a modification to the enzyme mismatch cleavage method. *Nucleic Acids Res.* **23,** 5082–5084.
20. Myers, R. M., Larin, Z., and Maniatis, T. (1985) Detection of single base substitutions by ribonuclease cleavage at mismatches in RNA,DNA duplexes. *Science* **230,** 1242–1246.
21. Cariello, N. F. and Skopek, T. R. (1993) Mutational analysis using denaturing gradient gel electrophoresis and PCR. *Mutat. Res.* **288,** 103–112.
22. van der Luijt, R., Khan, P. M., Vasen, H., et al. (1994) Rapid detection of translation-terminating mutations at the adenomatous polyposis coli (APC) gene by direct protein truncation test. *Genomics* **20,** 1–4.
23. Fu, Y. H., Kuhl, D. P., Pizzuti, A., et al. (1991) Variation of the CGG repeat at the fragile X site results in genetic instability, resolution of the Sherman paradox. *Cell* **67,** 1047–1058.
24. Schalling, M., Hudson, T. J., Buetow, K. H., et al. (1993) Direct detection of novel expanded trinucleotide repeats in the human genome. *Nat. Genet.* **4,** 135–139.

25. Fodor, S. P., Rava, R. P., Huang, X. C., et al. (1993) Multiplexed biochemical assays with biological chips. *Nature* **364,** 555–556.
26. Lipshutz, R. J., Morris, D., Chee, M., et al. (1995) Using oligonucleotide probe arrays to access genetic diversity. *BioTechniques* **19,** 442–447.
27. Hacia, J. G., Brody, L. C., Chee, M. S., et al. (1996) Detection of heterozygous mutations in BRCA1 using high density oligonucleotide arrays and two–colour fluorescence analysis. *Nat. Genet.* **14,** 441–447.

Index

R

S

9780896037021.